AMERICA'S
TEST KITCHEN

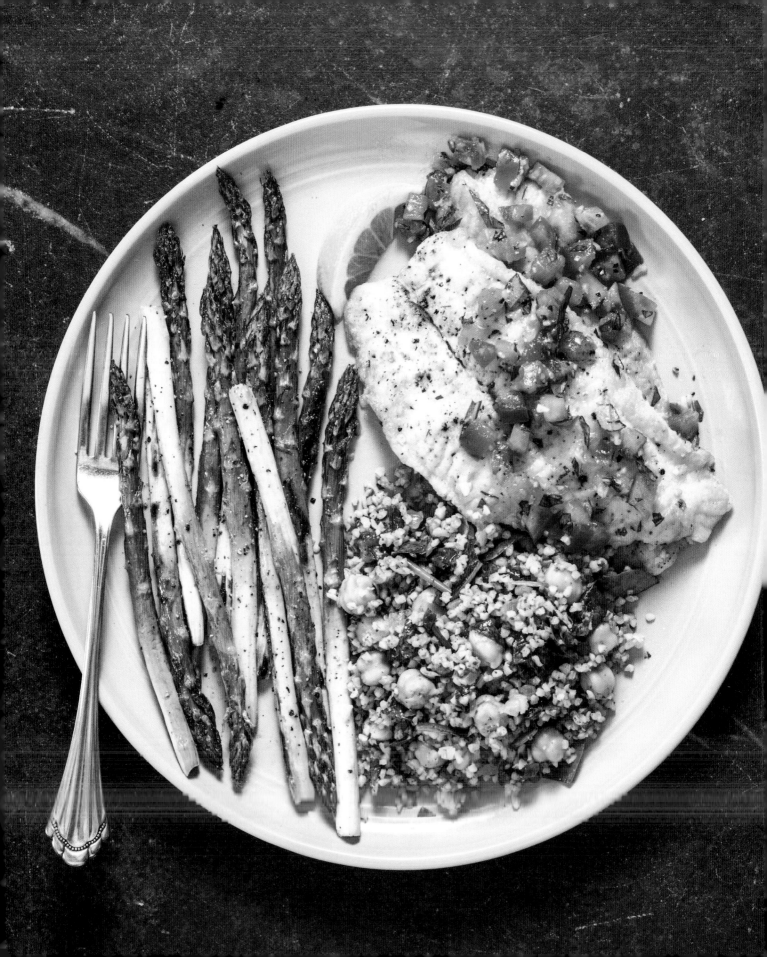

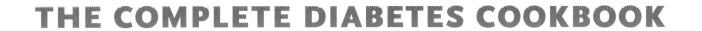

THE COMPLETE DIABETES COOKBOOK

ALSO BY AMERICA'S TEST KITCHEN

The New Essentials Cookbook
Dinner Illustrated
Cook's Illustrated Revolutionary Recipes
Tasting Italy: A Culinary Journey
Cooking at Home with Bridget and Julia
The Complete Slow Cooker
The Complete Make-Ahead Cookbook
The Complete Mediterranean Cookbook
The Complete Vegetarian Cookbook
The Complete Cooking for Two Cookbook
Just Add Sauce
How to Roast Everything
Nutritious Delicious
What Good Cooks Know
Cook's Science
The Science of Good Cooking
The Perfect Cake
The Perfect Cookie
Bread Illustrated
Master of the Grill
Kitchen Smarts
Kitchen Hacks
100 Recipes: The Absolute Best Ways to Make
the True Essentials
The New Family Cookbook
The America's Test Kitchen Cooking School Cookbook
The Cook's Illustrated Meat Book
The Cook's Illustrated Baking Book
The Cook's Illustrated Cookbook
The America's Test Kitchen Family Baking Book
The Best of America's Test Kitchen
(2007–2019 Editions)
The Complete America's Test Kitchen
TV Show Cookbook 2001–2019

Sous Vide for Everybody
Multicooker Perfection
Food Processor Perfection
Pressure Cooker Perfection
Vegan for Everybody
Naturally Sweet
Foolproof Preserving
Paleo Perfected
The How Can It Be Gluten-Free Cookbook: Volume 2
The How Can It Be Gluten-Free Cookbook
The Best Mexican Recipes
Slow Cooker Revolution Volume 2: The Easy-Prep Edition
Slow Cooker Revolution
The Six-Ingredient Solution
The America's Test Kitchen D.I.Y. Cookbook

THE COOK'S ILLUSTRATED ALL-TIME BEST SERIES
All-Time Best Brunch
All-Time Best Dinners for Two
All-Time Best Sunday Suppers
All-Time Best Holiday Entertaining
All-Time Best Appetizers
All-Time Best Soups

COOK'S COUNTRY TITLES
One-Pan Wonders
Cook It in Cast Iron
Cook's Country Eats Local
The Complete Cook's Country TV Show Cookbook

FOR A FULL LISTING OF ALL OUR BOOKS
CooksIllustrated.com
AmericasTestKitchen.com

PRAISE FOR AMERICA'S TEST KITCHEN TITLES

"This is a wonderful, useful guide to healthy eating."
PUBLISHERS WEEKLY ON _NUTRITIOUS DELICIOUS_

"The editors at America's Test Kitchen, known for their meticulous recipe testing and development, are back at it again. This time, they've trained their laser eyed focus on reduced sugar baking Cooks with a powerful sweet tooth should scoop up this well-researched recipe book for healthier takes on classic sweet treats."
BOOKLIST ON _NATURALLY SWEET_

"The sum total of exhaustive experimentation . . . anyone interested in gluten free cookery simply shouldn't be without it."
NIGELLA LAWSON ON _THE HOW CAN IT BE GLUTEN-FREE COOKBOOK_

Selected as an Amazon Best Book of 2015 in the Cookbooks and Food Writing Category
AMAZON ON _THE COMPLETE VEGETARIAN COOKBOOK_

Selected as one of the 10 Best New Cookbooks of 2017
THE LA TIMES ON _THE PERFECT COOKIE_

"Use this charming, focused title to set a showstopping table for special occasions."
LIBRARY JOURNAL ON _ALL-TIME BEST HOLIDAY ENTERTAINING_

Selected as the Cookbook Award Winner of 2017 in the Baking Category
INTERNATIONAL ASSOCIATION OF CULINARY PROFESSIONALS (IACP) ON _BREAD ILLUSTRATED_

"A beautifully illustrated, 318-page culinary compendium showcasing an impressive variety and diversity of authentic Mexican cuisine."
MIDWEST BOOK REVIEW ON _THE BEST MEXICAN RECIPES_

"A one-volume kitchen seminar, addressing in one smart chapter after another the sometimes surprising whys behind a cook's best practices. . . . You get the myth, the theory, the science, and the proof, all rigorously interrogated as only America's Test Kitchen can do."
NPR ON _THE SCIENCE OF GOOD COOKING_

"This comprehensive collection of 800-plus family and global favorites helps put healthy eating In an everyday context, from meatloaf to Indian curry with chicken."
COOKING LIGHT ON _THE AMERICA'S TEST KITCHEN HEALTHY FAMILY COOKBOOK_

"The 21st-century _Fannie Farmer Cookbook_ or _The Joy of Cooking_. If you had to have one cookbook and that's all you could have, this one would do it."
CBS SAN FRANCISCO ON _THE NEW FAMILY COOKBOOK_

"Some 2,500 photos walk readers through 600 painstakingly tested recipes, leaving little room for error."
ASSOCIATED PRESS ON _THE AMERICA'S TEST KITCHEN COOKING SCHOOL COOKBOOK_

"This encyclopedia of meat cookery would feel completely overwhelming if it weren't so meticulously organized and artfully designed. This is Cook's Illustrated at its finest."
THE KITCHN ON _THE COOK'S ILLUSTRATED MEAT BOOK_

"The go-to gift book for newlyweds, small families, or empty nesters."
ORLANDO SENTINEL ON _THE COMPLETE COOKING FOR TWO COOKBOOK_

"This book is a comprehensive, no-nonsense guide . . . a well-thought-out, clearly explained primer for every aspect of home baking."
THE WALL STREET JOURNAL ON _THE COOK'S ILLUSTRATED BAKING BOOK_

"It's all about technique and timing, and the ATK crew delivers their usual clear instructions to ensure success. . . . The thoughtful balance of practicality and imagination will inspire readers of all tastes and skill levels."
PUBLISHERS WEEKLY (STARRED REVIEW) ON _HOW TO ROAST EVERYTHING_

"Further proof that practice makes perfect, if not transcendent. . . . If an intermediate cook follows the directions exactly, the results will be better than takeout or Mom's."
THE NEW YORK TIMES ON _THE NEW BEST RECIPE_

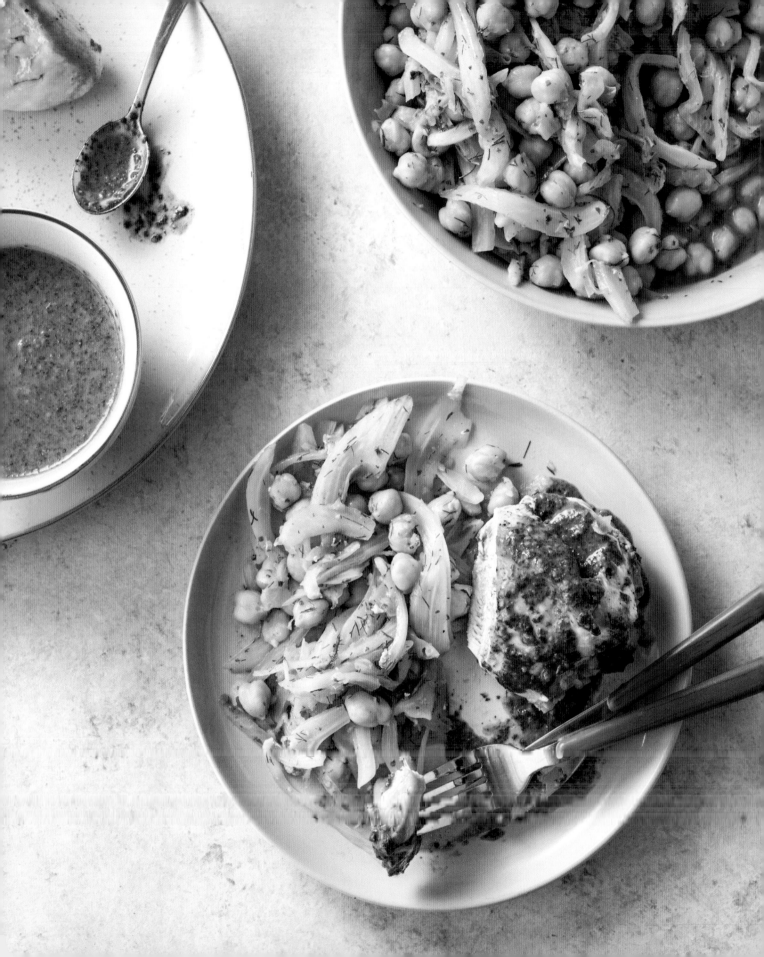

THE COMPLETE DIABETES COOKBOOK

The Healthy Way to Eat the Foods You Love

With a Foreword by Dariush Mozaffarian, MD, DrPH

AMERICA'S TEST KITCHEN

Library of Congress Cataloging-in-Publication Data

Names: America's Test Kitchen (Firm), author.
Title: The complete diabetes cookbook : the healthy way to eat
    the foods you love / America's Test Kitchen ; with a foreword
    by Dariush Mozaffarian, MD, Dr. Ph.
Description: Boston, MA : America's Test Kitchen, 2018. | Includes index.
Identifiers: LCCN 2018022192 | ISBN 9781945256585 (pbk.)
Subjects: LCSH: Diabetes--Diet therapy--Recipes. | LCGFT: Cookbooks.
Classification: LCC RC662 .C626 2018 | DDC 641.5/6314--dc23
LC record available at https://lccn.loc.gov/2018022192

AMERICA'S TEST KITCHEN
21 Drydock Avenue, Boston, MA 02210
Manufactured in Canada
10 9 8 7 6 5 4

Distributed by Penguin Random House Publisher Services
Tel: 800.733.3000

Pictured on front cover (clockwise from top left): Breakfast Tacos (page 21), Roasted Pears with Cider Sauce (page 349), Parmesan-Crusted Chicken Breasts with Warm Bitter Greens and Fennel Salad (page 178), Spiced Basmati Rice with Cauliflower and Pomegranate (page 127), Lemon-Herb Cod Fillets with Garlic Potatoes (page 249), Orange-Sesame Beef and Vegetable Stir-Fry (page 215)

Pictured on back cover: Turkey Burgers (page 200)

Editorial Director, Books ELIZABETH CARDUFF
Executive Food Editors SUZANNAH MCFERRAN AND
  DAN ZUCCARELLO
Deputy Food Editors STEPHANIE PIXLEY AND ANNE WOLF
Senior Editors LEAH COLINS AND SARA MAYER
Senior Managing Editor DEBRA HUDAK
Associate Editors JOSEPH GITTER, LAWMAN JOHNSON, AND
  RUSSELL SELANDER
Test Cooks KATHRYN CALLAHAN AND KATHERINE PERRY
Editorial Assistants KELLY GAUTHIER AND ALYSSA LANGER
Consulting Nutritionist ALICIA ROMANO, MS, RD, LDN
Art Director, Books LINDSEY TIMKO CHANDLER
Deputy Art Director JEN KANAVOS HOFFMAN
Associate Art Director KATIE BARRANGER
Production Designer REINALDO CRUZ
Photography Director JULIE BOZZO COTE
Photography Producers MARY BALL AND MEREDITH MULCAHY
Senior Staff Photographer DANIEL J. VAN ACKERE
Staff Photographers STEVE KLISE AND KEVIN WHITE
Additional Photography KELLER + KELLER AND CARL TREMBLAY
Food Styling CATRINE KELTY, CHANTAL LAMBETH,
  KENDRA MCKNIGHT, ELLE SIMONE SCOTT, AND SALLY STAUB
Photoshoot Kitchen Team
  Manager TIMOTHY MCQUINN
  Lead Test Cook DANIEL CELLUCCI
  Test Cook JESSICA RUDOLPH
  Assistant Test Cooks SARAH EWALD, ERIC HAESSLER,
    MADY NICHAS, AND DEVON SHATKIN
Production Manager CHRISTINE SPANGER
Imaging Manager LAUREN ROBBINS
Production and Imaging Specialists HEATHER DUBE, DENNIS NOBLE,
  AND JESSICA VOAS
Copy Editor DERI REED
Proofreader PAT JALBERT-LEVINE
Indexer ELIZABETH PARSON

Chief Creative Officer JACK BISHOP
Executive Editorial Directors JULIA COLLIN DAVISON AND
  BRIDGET LANCASTER

CONTENTS

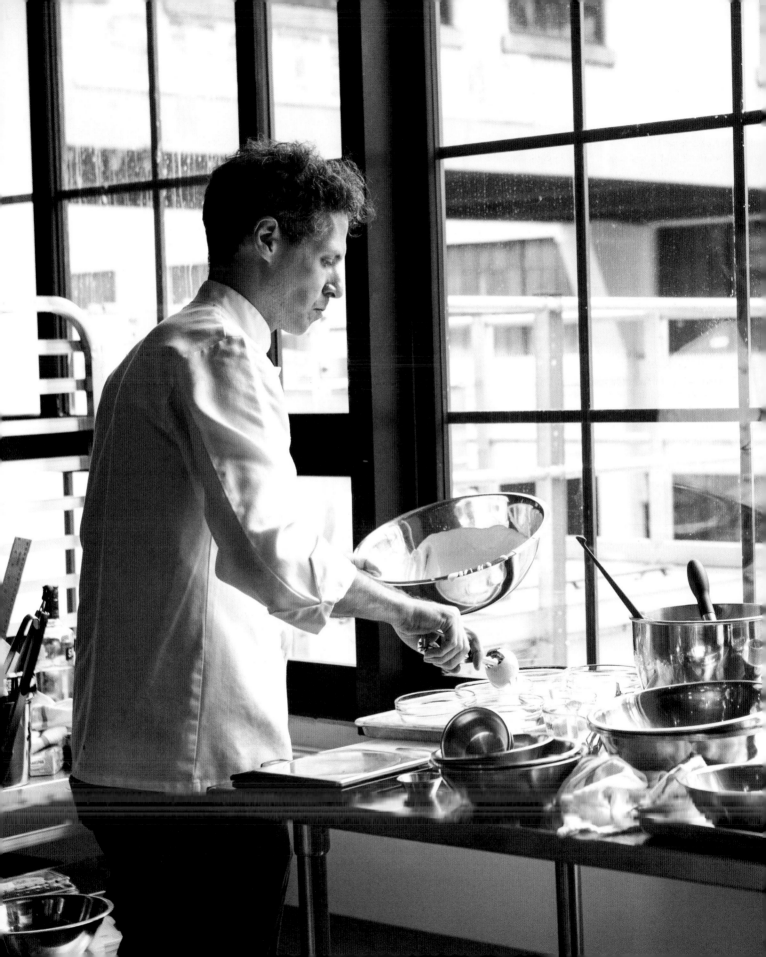

Welcome to America's Test Kitchen

This book has been tested, written, and edited by the folks at America's Test Kitchen, where curious cooks become confident cooks. Located in Boston's Seaport District in the historic Innovation and Design Building, it features 15,000 square feet of kitchen space including multiple photography and video studios. It is the home of *Cook's Illustrated* magazine and *Cook's Country* magazine and is the workday destination for more than 60 test cooks, editors, and cookware specialists. Our mission is to empower and inspire confidence, community, and creativity in the kitchen.

We start the process of testing a recipe with a complete lack of preconceptions, which means that we accept no claim, no technique, and no recipe at face value. We simply assemble as many variations as possible, test a half-dozen of the most promising, and taste the results blind. We then construct our own recipe and continue to test it, varying ingredients, techniques, and cooking times until we reach a consensus. As we like to say in the test kitchen, "We make the mistakes so you don't have to." The result, we hope, is the best version of a particular recipe, but we realize that only you can be the final judge of our success (or failure). We use the same rigorous approach when we test equipment and taste ingredients.

All of this would not be possible without a belief that good cooking, much like good music, is based on a foundation of objective technique. Some people like spicy foods and others don't, but there is a right way to sauté, there is a best way to cook a pot roast, and there are measurable scientific principles involved in producing perfectly beaten, stable egg whites. Our ultimate goal is to investigate the fundamental principles of cooking to give you the techniques, tools, and ingredients you need to become a better cook. It is as simple as that.

To see what goes on behind the scenes at America's Test Kitchen check out our social media channels for kitchen snapshots, exclusive content, video tips, and much more. You can watch us work (in our actual test kitchen) by tuning in to *America's Test Kitchen* or *Cook's Country* on public television or on our websites. Download our award-winning podcast *Proof*, which goes beyond recipes to solve food mysteries (AmericasTestKitchen.com/proof), or listen to test kitchen experts on public radio (SplendidTable.org) to hear insights that illuminate the truth about real home cooking. Want to hone your cooking skills or finally learn how to bake—with an America's Test Kitchen test cook? Enroll in one of our online cooking classes. And you can engage the next generation of home cooks with kid-tested recipes from America's Test Kitchen Kids.

Our community of home recipe testers provides valuable feedback on recipes under development by ensuring that they are foolproof. You can help us investigate the how and why behind successful recipes from your home kitchen. (Sign up at AmericasTestKitchen.com/recipe_testing.)

However you choose to visit us, we welcome you into our kitchen, where you can stand by our side as we test our way to the best recipes in America.

f facebook.com/AmericasTestKitchen
𝕏 twitter.com/TestKitchen
▶ youtube.com/AmericasTestKitchen
⊙ instagram.com/TestKitchen
Ⓟ pinterest.com/TestKitchen

AmericasTestKitchen.com
CooksIllustrated.com
CooksCountry.com
OnlineCookingSchool.com
AmericasTestKitchen.com/kids

Foreword

What we eat is among the most important decisions we make. Food influences nearly every aspect of our well-being: not only our own but that of our families, our communities, and our planet. Food is also intensely personal, connected to our moods, social network, culture, and worldview. For those of us fortunate enough to have some choice in what we eat every day, few things are as profound or important.

In my work as a cardiologist, nutrition scientist, and public health advocate, I've encountered more and more people who recognize the crucial importance of their food choices. Yet, many also feel deeply confused about what actually constitutes a healthier diet. This is especially true for people struggling to control their weight, blood glucose, or other risk factors. An epidemic of obesity and diabetes is sweeping the world. In the United States, one in eight adults has type 2 diabetes or prediabetes (an earlier stage of the disease), and for Americans born after 2000, one in three will develop type 2 diabetes in their lifetime. And this is not unique to the United States. Risk of type 2 diabetes is even higher in Mexico, where it is the leading cause of death. And China faces the world's largest diabetes epidemic: Nearly one in two adults in China has diabetes or prediabetes.

Healthier eating is essential to successfully manage, and even potentially cure, prediabetes and type 2 diabetes. Yet, confusion and uncertainty prevent many people from improving their diets. With all the popular diets that are promoted—low-fat, low-carb, paleo, vegetarian, vegan, gluten-free, organic, non-GMO, local—it's nearly impossible for the average person to sift through the varied and often conflicting recommendations. And things can get even more confusing for individual food choices of grains, fruits, nuts, eggs, meats, cooking oils, and more. In this muddle of uncertainty, the daily crowd of news reports, web blogs, and other voices add to the cacophony of jumbled and often contradictory messages.

Of course, beyond effects on health, a good meal should also nurture the soul. The sights, tastes, aromas, and textures should delight, surprise, and inspire. A good meal can also bring together and bond family and friends, or provide a sanctuary of quiet contemplation when one wishes to dine alone.

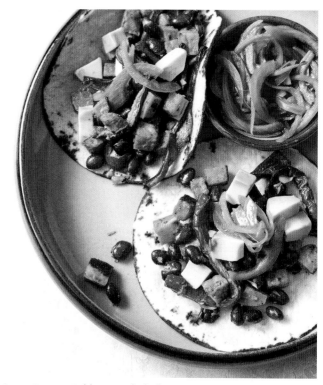

Sweet Potato, Poblano, and Black Bean Tacos

Among ways to achieve healthier, more mindful eating, home cooking is one of the most important. By cooking regularly, a person greatly increases the chances of making better choices while decreasing the burden of excessively processed, packaged, and unhealthy products in their diet. This most human of acts—the bringing together of ingredients, creative preparation, and sharing and enjoying a meal—also engages the mind and the senses in ways that are not otherwise easily achieved.

Yet, while cooking is so important for our health, and so beneficial for our spirit, this seemingly simple and ancient task can intimidate and unnerve even the stoutest foodie. How does one juggle health, taste, cost, and convenience and bring them together to form a meal that is both nurturing and enjoyable? For many, cooking can be a real challenge.

With The Complete Diabetes Cookbook, America's Test Kitchen aims to provide a range of compelling, tasty recipes that are also healthy choices for people with or worried about diabetes. During the creation of this book, America's Test Kitchen asked me and Tufts dietician Alicia Romano to provide input on the core nutrition principles underlying a healthy diabetic diet. Many of these principles can be found across the resulting recipes. They include:

EMPHASIZE THE GOOD Eat more minimally processed foods like beans, nonstarchy vegetables, nuts, seeds, and fruits rich in vitamins, minerals, antioxidants, phenolics, fiber, and other bioactives. And it's worth remembering that many veggies—peppers, zucchini, eggplant, tomatoes, cucumbers, avocados, and so on—are actually fruits, naturally rich in nutrients and phytochemicals in their skin, seeds, and flesh that make them great choices.

EMBRACE HEALTHY FATS Unsaturated fats from plant oils improve glycemic control and other important risk factors, like blood cholesterol levels. Foods like nuts, seeds, avocados, extra-virgin olive oil, canola oil, and seafood should be liberally consumed, especially when in place of starches and sugars.

HIGHLIGHT CARBOHYDRATE AMOUNT *AND* QUALITY While some diabetic diets focus on carb counting, carb quality can be just as important. For example, minimally processed whole grains, beans, and fruits have very different metabolic effects than refined flours, starches, and added sugars. While carb quality is influenced by many factors, a simple rule of thumb is to seek a carbohydrate-to-fiber ratio of 10:1 or lower. In other words: In any food or meal, aim for at least 1 gram of dietary fiber for every 10 grams of total carbohydrate. Most of the recipes in the book achieve this ratio, with plenty of fiber signaling healthful and balancing ingredients. In addition, mixing grains, pasta, rice, and sugars with other healthful ingredients (vegetables, beans, nuts, fruits, plant oils) slows digestion and further reduces spikes in blood sugar.

FOCUS ON FOODS, NOT CALORIES OR SINGLE NUTRIENTS
Advances in science increasingly show that different types of foods have complex effects on long-term weight and metabolic health. Judging a food or meal based on its total calories or a single nutrient greatly oversimplifies these complex influences. Instead, one can focus on eating more of the healthful, minimally processed foods like those described above, and less processed meats and foods rich in refined flours, starches, added sugars, and salt.

Where the science is less certain, this cookbook is more flexible in its recipes. For example, evidence on health effects of different dairy products is rapidly evolving, with emerging findings suggesting that there are metabolic benefits from yogurt (with beneficial probiotics), potential benefits from cheese (possibly due to fermentation), and uncertain health differences between low-fat and whole-fat dairy.

By incorporating these advances in nutrition science with their tested approach to pragmatic cooking, America's Test Kitchen has created engaging, accessible recipes that emphasize not only health but also convenience, taste, color, and creativity. The recipes also recognize that cooking—and eating—should prioritize well-being over weight loss, quality over quantity, and delight over austerity. Read, cook, eat, and enjoy!

Dariush Mozaffarian, MD, DrPH
Friedman School of Nutrition Science and Policy
Tufts University

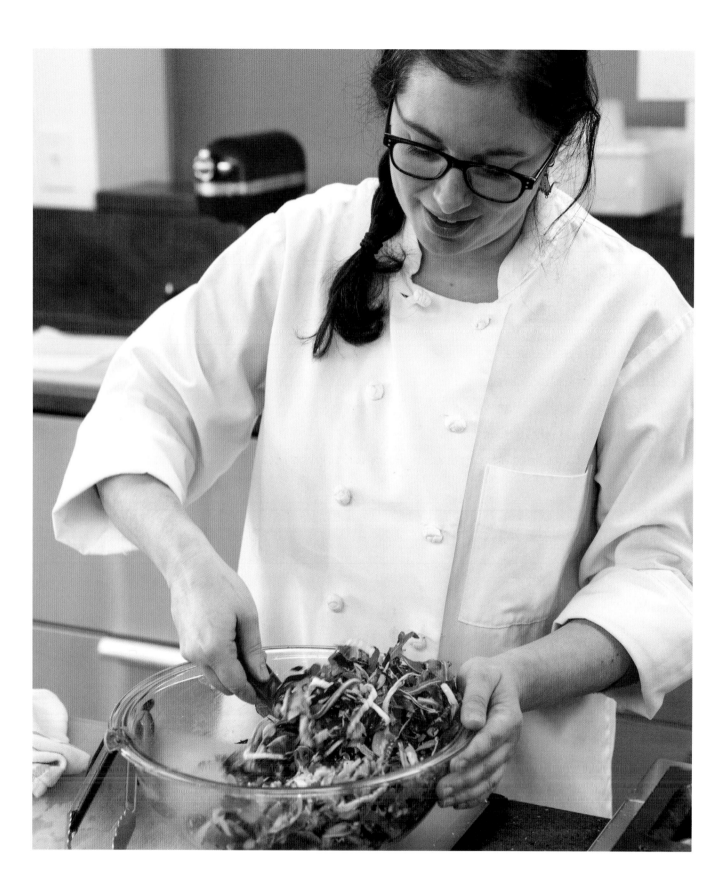

GETTING STARTED

INTRODUCTION

Here at America's Test Kitchen, we develop recipes for books focusing on many dietary needs: gluten-free, paleo, vegetarian, vegan, the Mediterranean diet, and more. Our approach has been to thoroughly research the tenets underlying these diets from a nutritional, scientific, and recipe development perspective. For *The Complete Diabetes Cookbook*, our mission is no different, although perhaps more urgent since more than 30 million Americans suffer with diabetes today. This number continues to climb as the obesity crisis is the prime contributor to the disease. We created this cookbook because we believe that we can make a difference: We believe that a large and varied collection of recipes, all thoughtfully developed and meticulously tested to fit a diabetic diet, will help people forge a path to health, especially if the recipes are accessible and the food tastes great. We also wanted dishes that the entire family, including those without diabetes, would happily eat. We want those who need this book to enjoy their food as much as anyone else, to feel satisfied, and to be able to eat their favorites, including pasta and the occasional dessert.

Since we are cooks first and foremost and not medical professionals, we worked closely with Dr. Dariush Mozaffarian, a world-renowned nutrition scientist, cardiologist, and professor at the Friedman School of Nutrition Science and Policy at Tufts University, and Alicia Romano, a registered dietitian at the Frances Stern Nutrition Center at Tufts Medical Center. The two developed a set of very specific parameters for our test cooks to follow as they developed recipes that limit refined carbohydrates, empty calories, sugar, and unhealthy fat. At the end of every recipe you will find full nutritional information, including the tally of Total Carbohydrate Choices (for those who follow that plan). No diet is one-size-fits-all, which is why anyone using this book will have to mix and match the recipes to fit their very specific needs. We think our great-tasting diabetes-friendly recipes present a healthy way to cook and eat that would truly benefit anyone, whether they have diabetes or not. The recipes are engineered to be controlled in refined carbohydrates (refined starch, added sugar); low in saturated fat and sodium; and high in fiber and heart-healthy whole grains, vegetables, beans, nuts, and fruits. Managing refined carbohydrate intake is obviously an important part of a diabetic diet, so we kept starch and sugars in balance with fiber and healthful ingredients (though it is up to the individual to monitor meals appropriately to avoid unwanted spikes in blood sugar). Want to eat pasta for dinner or possibly indulge in a dessert afterwards? You can easily plan your meals to keep your recommended intake of refined carbs and calories on track and your blood sugar in check.

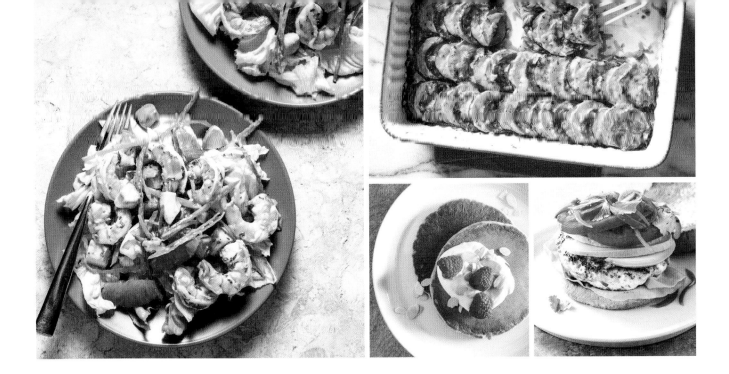

DIABETES: AN OVERVIEW

When you have diabetes, the food you eat cannot be used normally for energy because your body is not making enough insulin, or because the insulin you make is not used properly by your body. Insulin is the hormone made in the pancreas that responds to rising levels of blood glucose—a key component of starch and sugar. When starch and sugar are eaten, they are broken down into their components, in particular glucose, a main source of the body's energy. Within minutes of eating refined carbohydrates, glucose enters the bloodstream. In people with diabetes, lack of available insulin or inadequately functioning insulin does not allow the glucose to enter the cells. The result: Glucose is trapped in the bloodstream, leading to abnormally high levels. High glucose levels are just the tip of the iceberg; the most common form of diabetes is also linked to high blood pressure, harmful blood cholesterol levels, chronic inflammation, and more—all risk factors for poor health. And all of these risk factors can be improved by healthier eating.

TYPE 1 VERSUS TYPE 2

There are two different forms of diabetes. Type 1 diabetes, most often diagnosed in childhood, occurs in 5 to 10 percent of people with diabetes and is characterized by the body making little or no insulin on its own. People with type 1 diabetes rely on insulin injections for management and often are not overweight. Type 1 diabetes is caused by the body's own immune system attacking the pancreas (the home of insulin production). The causes of this auto-immunity are not clearly defined, and appear to be influenced by both genetics and environmental factors.

Type 2 diabetes is much more common, affecting 90 to 95 percent of all people with diabetes; it is characterized by insulin that does not function properly in the body. There is a strong link between excess body fat and the risk of developing type 2 diabetes, as excess fat, especially in the abdominal area, is associated with insulin resistance. In fact, three out of every four individuals with diabetes are at least overweight and nearly half of them are obese. An important part of the diabetic diet focuses on healthier eating and reducing refined carbohydrates and empty calories to promote weight management.

EATING WELL IS KEY

A cornerstone to managing type 2 diabetes is eating a healthy diet. Learning how to eat well is essential and includes an understanding of the foods that help with weight management, affect blood sugar level and/or keep blood sugars at a steady level, and improve other diabetes-related health problems with an emphasis on heart-healthy eating. There is no one-size-fits all eating pattern for people with diabetes, therefore individualized nutritional education and counseling with a registered dietitian or certified diabetes educator is recommended. A personalized plan should promote and support healthful eating patterns and emphasize a wide variety of nutrient-dense foods in appropriate portion sizes, while maintaining the pleasure of eating. Our serving sizes are carefully calculated to be sensible portions that emphasize quality over quantity.

THE ROLE OF CARBOHYDRATES

Refined carbohydrates are the body's quickest form of energy and have the most immediate effect on glucose levels in people with diabetes. Monitoring total carbohydrate intake (quantity) in addition to type of carbohydrate intake (quality) have both been recommended as key strategies for glycemic control. In our recipes we chose carbohydrates from minimally processed, higher-fiber, nutrient-rich food sources such as whole grains, beans, seeds, and fruits and also dairy, rather than those from more highly processed sources containing excess refined starch, added sugar, and additives such as salt.

Because both quality and quantity of carbohydrates appear to be important, the ideal amount of carbohydrates you eat each day and at each meal can be established with the help of your dietitian or certified diabetes educator. Let's refer to this amount of carbohydrates as your "carbohydrate bank." One aim could be to budget your carbohydrate bank evenly throughout the day between meals and snacks. To help you budget your carbohydrate bank using the recipes in this book, we include grams of Total Carbs as well as Total Carbohydrate Choices for each recipe. These conversions were used to establish carbohydrate choices:

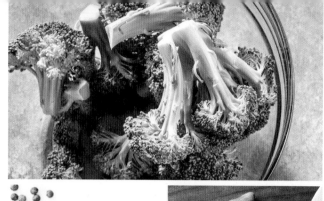

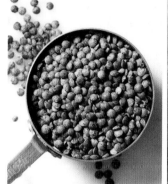

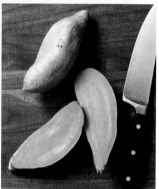

CARBOHYDRATE CHOICES	CARBOHYDRATE GRAMS
<0.5	<5g
0.5	6–10g
1	11–20g
1.5	21–25g
2	26–35g
2.5	36–40g
3	41–50g

Note: 1 Carbohydrate Choice or serving = 15g carbohydrates

CARBOHYDRATE QUALITY: FIBER IS USEFUL

Carbohydrate quality can be influenced by several different factors, making it difficult to define simply. Such factors include, for example, the extent of processing, the fiber content, the amount of starch and sugar, the rapidity of digestion (glycemic response), the whole grain content, and the form (solid or liquid). In developing our recipes we focused on two reasonable rules of thumb: to emphasize minimally processed, fiber-rich, nutrient-rich foods; and to balance the overall content of carbohydrate versus fiber (i.e., refined starch and sugar versus more healthful components).

Fiber is an important part of the diabetic diet. It is an indigestible carbohydrate that improves satiety, slows down digestion, and nurtures healthy gut bacteria, which together can help lower blood sugar, improve bowel function, and lower blood pressure and blood cholesterol. People with diabetes are encouraged to consume at least the amount of fiber recommended to the general public, between 25 to 38 grams per day. High-fiber foods included in this book's recipes are nuts and seeds, berries, whole grains such as brown rice and wheat berries, dried beans and lentils, and vegetables such as artichokes, cauliflower, onions, and sweet potatoes. We made sure that there was meaningful fiber in our recipes, even in the dessert treats.

As a basic rule, look for at least a 10:1 carb to fiber ratio when you are evaluating a food, whether through nutrition labels at the grocery store or the nutrition information given in a recipe. Using the 10:1 carbohydrate to fiber rule is a useful and relatively simple tool for quickly identifying whether a packaged food or a given recipe is delivering on the nutritional front. This ratio simply means that for every 10 grams of carbohydrate there should be at least 1 gram of fiber; the tighter this ratio (i.e., 5:1) the better. This tool can also be used throughout the book when choosing to incorporate some of the carb-based side dishes into a meal. So if a recipe or product is falling short on the fiber scale, it's important to add a source of fiber, such as fresh fruit or non starchy vegetables (such as broccoli, spinach, or tomatoes), to aid in delayed digestion and improved glycemic control.

LIMITING REFINED STARCH AND SUGAR

When digested, all starches and sugars are broken down into simpler forms, such as glucose and fructose. Foods that contain carbohydrates contain these compounds in different forms whether they are naturally occurring, such as sugar found in milk products (lactose) and fruits (fructose), or added to the food. Refined starches and added sugars are the most problematic for diabetics. Refined starches can include white bread, white rice, crackers, most breakfast cereals, and foods made with cornstarch and potato starch. Added sugars can include anything from cane sugar, beet sugar, and brown sugar to honey, agave, maple syrup, and corn syrup. Generally speaking, when refined starch and sugar are added to foods and drinks, they add rapidly digested calories without adding nutrition, which may contribute to weight gain, high cholesterol, and other risk factors for developing heart disease. Additionally, refined starches and added simple sugars tend to be digested quickly and impact blood glucose levels more abruptly. Added sugar should be limited to less than 10 percent of total calories daily (that's around 200 calories on a 2000-calorie diet). Because there is no accepted limit on refined starches, we aimed to use as little as possible; thus, throughout this book, we limit refined starch and added sugars. In recipes where their use is inevitable, such as desserts or baked goods, the amounts are vastly reduced, and also balanced whenever possible with healthful ingredients.

If incorporating a sweet treat in your diet, account for it in your daily carb bank and combine it with foods from other food groups to aid in delaying digestion and the glycemic response. For example, if you have a total of 60 grams of carbohydrates (4 Total Carb Choices) budgeted for your dinner meal, and you want a dessert with 30 grams of carbohydrates (2 Carb Choices), you can account for it by removing 30 grams of carbohydrates (2 Carb Choices) from the starches in your dinner meal. You should then aim to fill your plate with protein and non-starchy vegetables (higher in fiber and nutrients) plus the remaining 30 grams of carbohydrates (2 Carb Choices) from high-fiber sources. Dessert should be eaten as part of your meal (instead of on its own) to aid in delayed digestion and

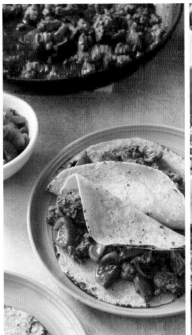
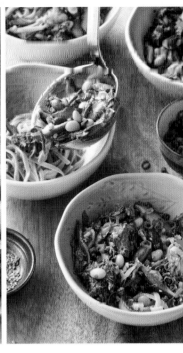

improved glucose tolerance at that meal. Remember, sweets are labeled as "treats" for a reason and should be reserved for a special occasion and not as part of a regular diabetic diet.

THE BENEFITS OF BALANCE

The most optimal glycemic control is achieved when smaller amounts of less-processed, fiber-rich carbohydrates are eaten in combination with lean protein and healthy fats. That is why throughout the book you will find many complete meals or dishes re-engineered to include the right balance of fiber, protein, and healthy fats. The recipes in the pasta chapter are a good example of how we achieve this balance: We use only fiber-rich 100 percent whole-wheat pasta, limit the amount of pasta per serving, and incorporate an abundance of non-starchy vegetables, beans, lean proteins, and/or healthy fats into all our pasta recipes.

THE ROLE OF PROTEIN

Protein plays an important role in the diabetic diet by improving satiety and slowing down digestion, which can help lower blood sugars after a meal. There is no "ideal" amount of protein for optimal glycemic control; however, we aimed to include healthier, protein-rich foods in our recipes. These include skinless poultry, fish, leaner red meat, eggs, nuts, and tofu.

Lean protein promotes a lower saturated fat intake and leaner calorie intake, while fatty fish such as salmon improve intake of omega-3 fatty acids. Some foods are considered proteins, such as milk, plain yogurt, and beans, as they contain both protein and about 1 Carb Choice (15g) per serving.

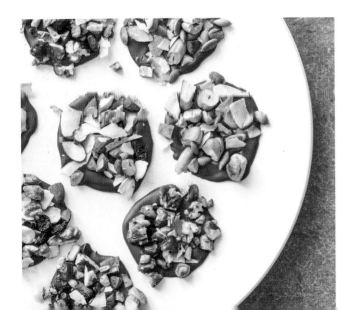

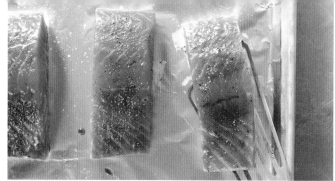

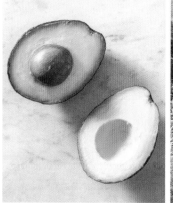

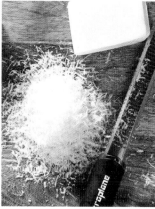

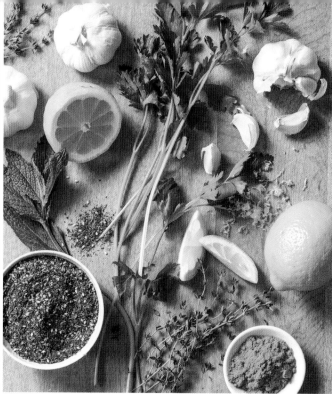

FAT IS NO LONGER THE ENEMY, JUST CHOOSE WISELY

Recent research indicates that a low-fat diet is not necessary for people with diabetes or anyone else—as long as the right type of fat is consumed. This means that fats in a diabetic diet should come from healthy foods rich in unsaturated fats, with an emphasis on monounsaturated fats, polyunsaturated fats, and omega-3 fatty acids, as these may benefit glycemic control and limit cardiovascular risk factors.

There should be much more unsaturated fat than saturated fat in a food or meal, so people with diabetes should actively seek out foods rich in healthy unsaturated fats. And dairy is not as bad as people think since it contains both protein and carbs and may also benefit diabetic control in other ways due to probiotics (yogurt) and fermentation (cheese).

Foods rich in unsaturated fats should replace foods high in saturated fats and refined carbohydrates, which are known to have negative effects on cholesterol levels and weight. Throughout the recipes in the book, we restrict the use of foods such as butter, processed meats, and high-fat cuts of red meat. Priority is placed on the liberal use of unsaturated fats from a number of sources, including nuts and seeds, avocados, extra-virgin olive oil, canola oil, and fatty fish like salmon.

GETTING SODIUM UNDER CONTROL

Given the high risk of hypertension and cardiovascular disease associated with type 2 diabetes, we were very mindful of the sodium content in our recipes, especially for well-known sodium offenders like soups and grains. The average American takes in over 3400mg of sodium per day, far exceeding the 2300mg per day recommended for the general public. (Note: 2300mg of sodium is the equivalent to about 1 teaspoon of salt.)

In order to meet the sodium guidelines for the recipes across the book, we employed a few tactics when developing the recipes. First, we didn't season meat or fish before cooking. We also used the smallest amount of salt we deemed necessary to add flavor during the cooking process and did not season to taste at the end. And since salt acts as a flavor enhancer, we found other ways to make up for not using it. These included boosting flavor with aromatics (like garlic and herbs), Dijon mustard, high-quality olive oil with more robust flavor, and bold seasonings like za'atar, curry, and turmeric; adding lemon or orange zest or citrus juice or other acid at the end to brighten the dish; and relying on techniques like deeply browning vegetables, tomato paste, and meat to add layers of flavor. We also call for no-salt-added store-bought products like broth, beans, and canned tomatoes (see the Kitchen section on pages 10–11).

PUTTING THE GUIDELINES INTO PRACTICE: BUILDING A COMPLETE MEAL

THE PLATE METHOD

With all the information about what you can eat, how do you put it all together into a healthy and great-tasting diabetic meal? The Plate Method is a valuable tool for proper meal planning. It encourages a large serving (half the plate) of fiber-rich healthy foods—like non-starchy vegetables, beans, nuts and seeds, and fruits—in combination with healthy, protein-rich foods (one quarter of the plate) and higher-fiber starches or grains (one quarter of the plate), as well as heart-healthy unsaturated fats. Milk, yogurt, and cheese can also make their way onto the plate based on your individualized meal plan. As you work through the recipes, you will notice that not all recipes will fill all sections of the plate; the Plate Method is a great tool to use to help fill in and balance out a complete meal.

THE BREAKFAST EQUATION

Breakfast can be approached in a similar way when it comes to meal balance, often with different choices of specific foods than at other meals. For a more traditional American breakfast, the breakfast equation should include healthy protein-rich foods paired with portion-controlled high-fiber starches/grains and a serving of fruit and/or nuts. This model can also be used to balance out recipes in the book that lack all parts of the equation. For example, for a carb-only breakfast recipe, adding a high-protein food such as Scrambled Eggs (page 14) or Homemade Turkey Breakfast Sausage (page 23) or 6 ounces plain Greek-style yogurt and one serving of fruit can help you balance this meal to aid in glycemic control and general health.

THE PLATE METHOD

1/2 PLATE OF NON-STARCHY VEGETABLES, BEANS, NUTS AND SEEDS, AND FRUITS

Fill half of your plate with a liberal amount of minimally processed, higher-fiber, nutrient-rich foods like non-starchy vegetables (such as broccoli, spinach, tomatoes, and salad greens); nuts and seeds; and berries and other fruits.

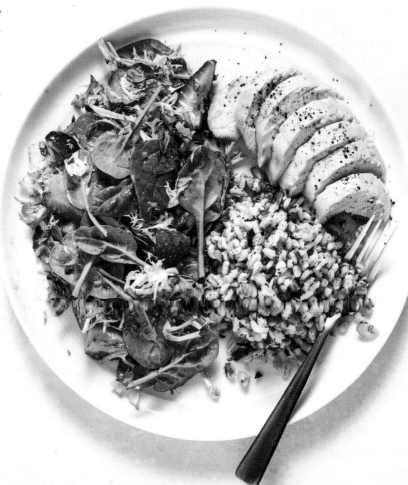

1/4 PLATE OF PROTEIN

Fill one quarter of your plate with heart-healthy protein such as skinless chicken breast, ground turkey, or salmon. Flank steak is also reasonable a few times per week. Our portion sizes are 6 ounces for fish and shellfish, 3–6 ounces for poultry, and 4 ounces for meat.

1/4 PLATE OF STARCH

Fill about one quarter of your plate with whole grains like barley or starchier vegetables such as potatoes or corn. This portion may vary according to your individual meal plan.

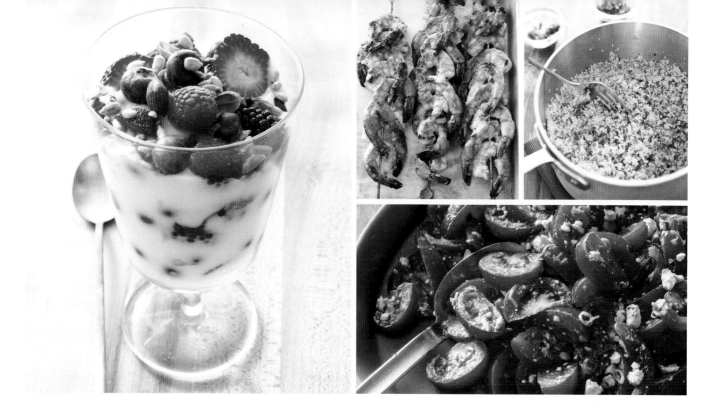

MEAL PLANNING

When using this book, people with diabetes may find it useful to keep their whole day in mind. These sample menus show how to compose a meal, with choices for breakfast, lunch, and dinner, indicating how such foods might fit into the total quality diet over a whole day.

BREAKFAST	
MENUS	**TOTALS PER MEAL**
• Homemade Turkey Breakfast Sausages (per 2 sausages) (page 23) • Blueberry Oat Pancakes (per pancake with about 1 tablespoon Orange-Honey Yogurt) (page 26)	**Cal** 230 • **Total Fat** 7g • **Sat Fat** 2g • **Chol** 45mg **Sodium** 480mg • **Total Carbs** 21g • **Fiber** 2g • **Total Sugar** 9g **Added Sugar** 5g • **Protein** 20g • **Total Carbohydrate Choices** 1.5
• Spinach and Feta Omelet (page 18) • Green Smoothie (page 33)	**Cal** 490 • **Total Fat** 26g • **Sat Fat** 7g • **Chol** 390mg **Sodium** 450mg • **Total Carbs** 45g • **Fiber** 7g • **Total Sugar** 25g **Added Sugar** 0g • **Protein** 24g • **Total Carbohydrate Choices** 3
• Scrambled Eggs with Goat Cheese, Sun-Dried Tomatoes, and Oregano (page 14) • Cheesy Baked Grits (page 23)	**Cal** 410 • **Total Fat** 24g • **Sat Fat** 10g • **Chol** 470mg **Sodium** 580mg • **Total Carbs** 25g • **Fiber** 3g • **Total Sugar** 3g **Added Sugar** 0g • **Protein** 23g • **Total Carbohydrate Choices** 1.5
• Yogurt Parfait (page 28)	**Cal** 480 • **Total Fat** 29g • **Sat Fat** 4g • **Chol** 10mg **Sodium** 130mg • **Total Carbs** 39g • **Fiber** 11g • **Total Sugar** 24g **Added Sugar** 0g • **Protein** 22g • **Total Carbohydrate Choices** 2.5

LUNCH

MENUS	TOTALS PER MEAL
• Classic Chicken Salad (page 119) • Creamy Carrot-Ginger Soup (page 59)	Cal 400 • **Total Fat** 20g • **Sat Fat** 3g • **Chol** 90mg **Sodium** 580mg • **Total Carbs** 22g • **Fiber** 6g • **Total Sugar** 12g **Added Sugar** 0g • **Protein** 32g • **Total Carbohydrate Choices** 1.5
• Southwestern Brown Rice and Pinto Bean Bowl (page 275)	Cal 410 • **Total Fat** 20g • **Sat Fat** 2.5g • **Chol** 5mg **Sodium** 460mg • **Total Carbs** 53g • **Fiber** 13g • **Total Sugar** 8g **Added Sugar** 0g • **Protein** 12g • **Total Carbohydrate Choices** 3.5
• Mediterranean Tuna Salad (page 119) • Farro Salad with Asparagus, Snap Peas, and Tomatoes (page 134)	Cal 420 • **Total Fat** 22g • **Sat Fat** 4g • **Chol** 30mg **Sodium** 420mg • **Total Carbs** 34g • **Fiber** 5g • **Total Sugar** 5g **Added Sugar** 0g • **Protein** 22g • **Total Carbohydrate Choices** 2

WEEKNIGHT DINNERS

MENUS	TOTALS PER MEAL
• Spinach Lasagna (page 167) • Arugula Salad with Fennel and Shaved Parmesan (page 89)	Cal 490 • **Total Fat** 27g • **Sat Fat** 10g • **Chol** 60mg **Sodium** 740mg • **Total Carbs** 41g • **Fiber** 7g • **Total Sugar** 11g **Added Sugar** 0g • **Protein** 26g • **Total Carbohydrate Choices** 3
• Weeknight Skillet Roast Chicken (page 192) • Spinach Salad with Frisée and Strawberries (page 92) • Barley with Lemon and Herbs (page 128)	Cal 580 • **Total Fat** 22g • **Sat Fat** 3.5g • **Chol** 160mg **Sodium** 530mg • **Total Carbs** 47g • **Fiber** 11g • **Total Sugar** 3g **Added Sugar** 0g • **Protein** 49g • **Total Carbohydrate Choices** 3
• Pan-Seared Sirloin Steak (page 208) • Sautéed Snow Peas with Lemon and Parsley (page 310) • Bibb Lettuce Salad with Endive and Cucumber (page 89) • Oatmeal Cookie with Chocolate and Goji Berries (page 355)	Cal 530 • **Total Fat** 27g • **Sat Fat** 5g • **Chol** 90mg **Sodium** 600mg • **Total Carbs** 39g • **Fiber** 7g • **Total Sugar** 19g **Added Sugar** 8g • **Protein** 35g • **Total Carbohydrate Choices** 2.5
• Meatloaf with Mushroom Gravy (page 218) • Pan-Roasted Broccoli (page 293) • Roasted Pears with Cider Sauce (page 349)	Cal 510 • **Total Fat** 27g • **Sat Fat** 7g • **Chol** 115mg **Sodium** 600mg • **Total Carbs** 39g • **Fiber** 7g • **Total Sugar** 20g **Added Sugar** 0g • **Protein** 33g • **Total Carbohydrate Choices** 2.5
• Garlic Pork Roast (page 225) • Warm Wheat Berries with Zucchini, Red Bell Pepper, and Oregano (page 141)	Cal 420 • **Total Fat** 14g • **Sat Fat** 3.5g • **Chol** 75mg **Sodium** 420mg • **Total Carbs** 41g • **Fiber** 7g • **Total Sugar** 2g **Added Sugar** 0g • **Protein** 33g • **Total Carbohydrate Choices** 3
• Sautéed Sole (page 247) Bulgur with Chickpeas, Spinach, and Za'atar (page 132) • Roasted Asparagus (page 290)	Cal 450 • **Total Fat** 28g • **Sat Fat** 4g • **Chol** 50mg **Sodium** 610mg • **Total Carbs** 28g • **Fiber** 6g • **Total Sugar** 3g **Added Sugar** 0g • **Protein** 22g • **Total Carbohydrate Choices** 2
• Grilled Marinated Shrimp Skewers (page 263) • Tomato Salad with Feta and Cumin-Yogurt Dressing (page 106) • Quinoa Pilaf with Lemon and Thyme (page 139)	Cal 470 • **Total Fat** 25g • **Sat Fat** 5g • **Chol** 115mg **Sodium** 600mg • **Total Carbs** 40g • **Fiber** 6g • **Total Sugar** 8g **Added Sugar** 0g • **Protein** 22g • **Total Carbohydrate Choices** 2.5

STOCKING A DIABETES-FRIENDLY KITCHEN

We use a lot of familiar ingredients in our recipes, but reach for their lower salt and sometimes lower-fat versions in order to meet our nutritional guidelines. That means using no-salt-added or unsalted store-bought products like broth, beans, and tomatoes and some low-fat dairy products (milk, yogurt, and sour cream). To increase the amount of protein and fiber while keeping empty calories in check, we call for 100 percent whole-wheat bread and pasta, more white than red meats, and more whole grains and non-starchy vegetables.

NO-SALT-ADDED PRODUCTS

The convenience of buying commercial items at the supermarket can't be beat; but that convenience can come with a high-sodium price tag. That's why we call for no-salt-added canned ingredients in the recipes in this book.

UNSALTED CHICKEN BROTH Unsalted means that no salt was added during processing. Even so, unsalted broth still contains sodium. Our winning unsalted broth is **Swanson Unsalted Chicken Stock,** which has subtle but distinct chicken flavor.

UNSALTED VEGETABLE BROTH Double-check the nutrition label since unsalted vegetable broths still have quite a bit of naturally occurring sodium. Look for a broth that lists vegetable content first on the ingredient list. We used Edward & Sons Low Sodium Not-Chick'n Bouillon Cubes when testing our recipes.

NO-SALT-ADDED CANNED BEANS (chickpeas, black beans, cannellini beans, pinto beans, etc.) Beans are a great source of fiber. Canned beans are made by pressure-cooking dried beans directly in the can with water, salt, and preservatives. That is why it's important to use canned beans that were processed without any added salt. We had good luck using canned beans from Eden Organics.

NO-SALT-ADDED CANNED TOMATOES Canned tomatoes are processed at the height of freshness so they deliver better flavor than off-season fresh tomatoes. We call for no-salt-added diced, crushed, and whole peeled tomatoes as well as tomato paste. We used Hunt's brand no-salt-added tomato products when testing the recipes.

NATURAL PEANUT BUTTER Peanut butter (and other nut butters) is a convenient source of both protein and healthy fats. Be sure to look for nut butters with no salt or sugar added. We used Teddie Smooth Unsalted All Natural Peanut Butter to develop the recipes for this book.

FLAVOR BOOSTERS

We aimed to limit our use of salt in the recipes in the book. Since salt is a flavor enhancer, we found creative ways to replace it. In addition to creating flavor with aromatics like garlic, ginger, and fresh herbs and acidic ingredients like citrus and vinegar, we employed bolder-flavored spices and seasonings.

BOLD SPICES We reach into the spice rack for high-performance spices like bay leaves, cumin, curry, cayenne, smoked paprika, and za'atar.

SUPER-FLAVORFUL SEASONINGS We use very small amounts of high-test ingredients like these to help build great flavor: Dijon mustard, capers, low-sodium soy sauce, and sun-dried tomatoes.

HEART-HEALTHY OILS

Plant-based oils are rich in either mono- or polyunsaturated fats (or both) and are a good choice for a diabetic diet. Cold-pressed or expeller-pressed oils are more nutritious because they retain more of their antioxidants but they spoil more quickly and have lower smoking points.

EXTRA VIRGIN OLIVE OIL Extra-virgin olive oil is high in healthy fats (monounsaturated fatty acids) as well as antioxidants. Studies have shown that people who regularly include olive oil in their diet have reduced rates of diabetes. Our winning supermarket EVOO is **California Olive Ranch Everyday Extra Virgin Olive Oil.**

CANOLA OIL This vegetable oil has become a kitchen standard. It comes from rapeseed plants that have been bred to have a neutral taste and are a good source of plant omega-3s.

MAYONNAISE Full-fat mayo is actually loaded with healthy fats; it has the same ratio of unsaturated to saturated fats as avocado. Our winner is **Blue Plate Mayonnaise.**

LIGHT COCONUT MILK We use light coconut milk when developing our recipes because it has less saturated fat than full-fat coconut milk. The light version still adds plenty of rich flavor and body. We like using Thai Kitchen Lite Coconut Milk in the test kitchen.

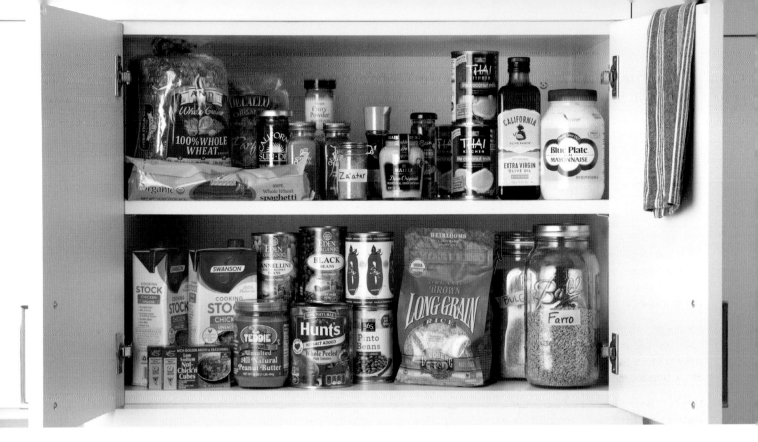

WHOLE GRAINS

Whole grains are often less processed and contain both bran and germ. This means that they contain more fiber and nutrients and so are a healthier choice than their white counterparts (for more information, see page 126).

BROWN RICE Brown rice is whole-grain, gluten-free, and inexpensive. It is less processed than white rice so it has more fiber, although it still can be digested rapidly and should be eaten in moderation. We only use brown rice in the book. Our winning brand is **Lundberg Organic Brown Long Grain Rice.**

BULGUR Bulgur is a highly nutritious grain made from partially cooked wheat berries that are dried and only partially stripped of their outer bran layer.

FARRO Farro is hulled whole-wheat kernels.

WHEAT BERRIES Wheat berries are whole, unprocessed kernels of wheat. They are an excellent source of nutrition because none of the grain has been removed.

100 PERCENT WHOLE-WHEAT BREAD AND PASTA

Because it includes the bran and germ, whole-wheat flour contains proteins, fats, fiber, vitamins, and minerals that refined white flour lacks.

100 PERCENT WHOLE-WHEAT BREAD Whole-wheat bread has a flavor and nutrient profile more complex than that of white bread. Our winner is **Arnold Whole Grains 100% Whole Wheat Bread.**

100 PERCENT WHOLE-WHEAT PASTA Made from 100-percent whole durum wheat, whole-wheat pasta has more protein and fiber than the best white pastas. Our winner is **Bionaturae Organic 100% Whole Wheat Spaghetti.**

DAIRY PRODUCTS

Dairy products are a great way to get high-quality protein into a recipe.

LOW-FAT MILK, YOGURT, AND SOUR CREAM We use low-fat versions of these to help us keep within our nutritional guidelines for saturated fat.

FULL-FAT CHEESES, COTTAGE CHEESE, CREAM CHEESE, AND RICOTTA CHEESE We use the full-fat versions of these because we like their flavor better. Most hard cheeses are also fermented, and cheeses and other fermented foods are also increasingly linked to lower risk of diabetes.

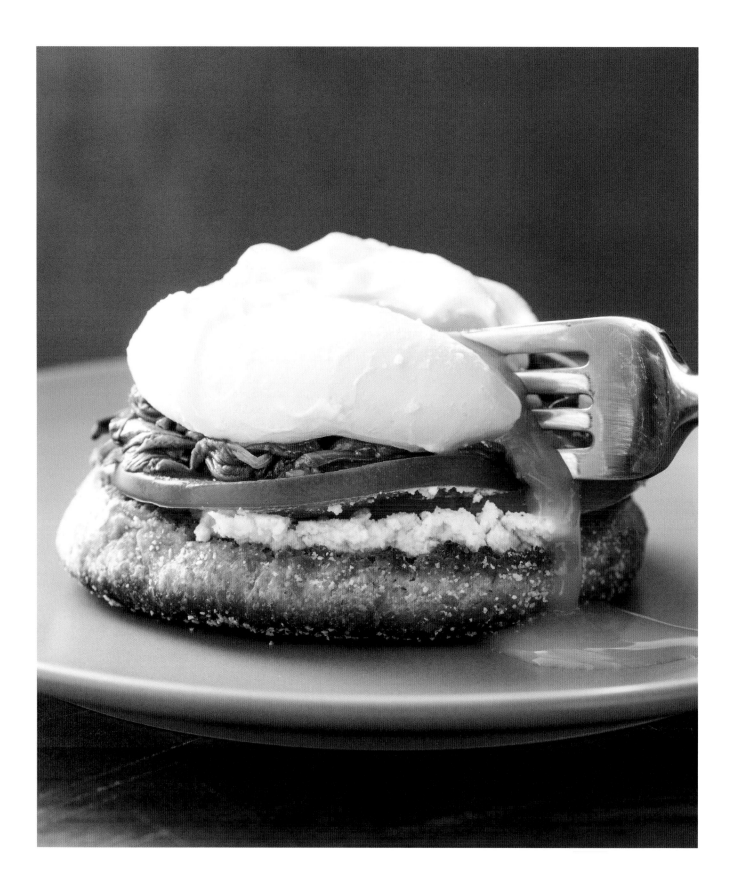

BREAKFAST

Photo: Open-Faced Poached Egg Sandwich

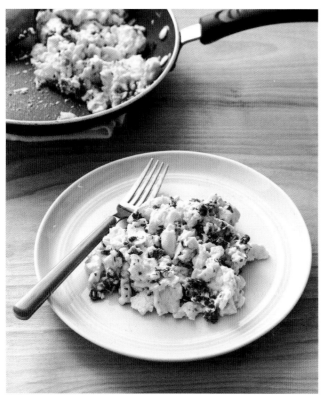

Cooking our scrambled eggs in extra-virgin olive oil gives them rich flavor and also helps to keep them tender.

Scrambled Eggs with Herbs
SERVES 2

WHY THIS RECIPE WORKS Fluffy and creamy scrambled eggs are the perfect foundation for a good breakfast whether you have diabetes or not. We found that the best way to reduce calories and the saturated fat in our traditional scrambled eggs, without ruining their flavor or texture, was to not include any extra yolks. We replaced the half-and-half we would usually use with low-fat milk and used healthier extra-virgin olive oil instead of butter when cooking. (These slight changes also freed up space nutritionally to add flavor-packed ingredients when it came to creating variations.) Cooking our eggs in olive oil gave them rich flavor and ensured that they remained tender throughout cooking. We don't recommend substituting skim milk in this recipe. Be sure to remove the eggs from the skillet as soon as they are done to prevent overcooking. We like a combination of fresh herbs in these eggs, but you can use only one if you prefer.

4 large eggs
2 teaspoons 1 percent low-fat milk
Pinch salt
Pinch pepper
1 teaspoon extra-virgin oil
2 tablespoons minced fresh chives, basil, and tarragon

1. Beat eggs, milk, salt, and pepper with fork in bowl until eggs are thoroughly combined and color is pure yellow; do not overbeat.

2. Heat oil in 10-inch nonstick skillet over medium-high heat until shimmering, swirling to coat pan. Add egg mixture and, using rubber spatula, constantly and firmly scrape along bottom and sides of skillet until eggs begin to clump and spatula just leaves trail on bottom of pan, 45 to 75 seconds. Reduce heat to low and gently but constantly fold eggs until clumped and just slightly wet, 30 to 60 seconds. Quickly fold in herbs, then immediately transfer eggs to individual warmed plates. Serve immediately.

PER SERVING

Cal 170 • **Total Fat** 12g • **Sat Fat** 3.5g • **Chol** 370mg **Sodium** 220mg • **Total Carbs** 1g • **Fiber** 0g • **Total Sugar** 1g **Added Sugar** 0g • **Protein** 13g • **Total Carbohydrate Choices** 0

VARIATIONS
Scrambled Eggs with Feta, Shallot, and Basil
Omit salt and herbs. Before adding egg mixture to oil in skillet, cook 1 minced shallot until softened, about 2 minutes. Before removing cooked eggs from skillet, quickly fold in 2 tablespoons crumbled feta cheese and 2 tablespoons chopped fresh basil.

PER SERVING

Cal 200 • **Total Fat** 13g • **Sat Fat** 4.5g • **Chol** 380mg **Sodium** 210mg • **Total Carbs** 4g • **Fiber** 1g • **Total Sugar** 2g **Added Sugar** 0g • **Protein** 14g • **Total Carbohydrate Choices** 0

Scrambled Eggs with Goat Cheese, Sun-Dried Tomatoes, and Oregano
Omit salt and herbs. Before removing eggs from skillet, quickly fold in ¼ cup crumbled goat cheese, 2 tablespoons minced oil-packed sun-dried tomatoes, and 2 teaspoons minced fresh oregano.

PER SERVING

Cal 220 • **Total Fat** 16g • **Sat Fat** 6g • **Chol** 380mg **Sodium** 230mg • **Total Carbs** 3g • **Fiber** 0g • **Total Sugar** 1g **Added Sugar** 0g • **Protein** 16g • **Total Carbohydrate Choices** 0

Scrambled Eggs with Parmesan and Asparagus

Omit salt and herbs. Microwave 4 ounces asparagus, sliced thin on bias, with ½ cup water in small covered bowl until bright green and tender, 1 to 3 minutes; drain, pat dry, and set aside while cooking eggs. Before removing eggs from skillet, quickly fold in asparagus and 2 tablespoons grated Parmesan cheese.

PER SERVING

Cal 210 • **Total Fat** 14g • **Sat Fat** 4.5g • **Chol** 375mg
Sodium 270mg • **Total Carbs** 3g • **Fiber** 1g • **Total Sugar** 2g
Added Sugar 0g • **Protein** 17g • **Total Carbohydrate Choices** 0

SCRAMBLING EGGS

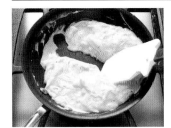

When your spatula just leaves a trail through the eggs, that's your cue in our dual-heat method to turn the dial from medium-high to low.

Tofu Scramble with Bell Pepper, Shallot, and Herbs

SERVES 4

WHY THIS RECIPE WORKS A great tofu scramble will satisfy your craving for scrambled eggs but with very little fat and plenty of plant-based protein. But while recipes for tofu scrambles are numerous, some seem like bland or boring imitations of their eggy counterparts. We wanted a recipe that offered a creamy, egg-like texture and a subtle but satisfying flavor, made more interesting with the addition of some fresh vegetables. We tried silken, soft, medium, and firm tofu, and the soft tofu proved to have a texture closest to eggs, yielding pieces that, when crumbled, were smooth and creamy. (Silken tofu produced a looser scramble, and firmer tofu varieties developed into hard curds.) A small amount of curry powder was key, contributing depth of flavor and a nice touch of color without overwhelming the dish with actual curry flavor. We also found that the tofu could be crumbled into smaller or larger pieces to resemble egg curds of different sizes. If you cannot find soft tofu, you can use silken tofu but your scramble will be significantly wetter. Do not use firm tofu in this recipe.

All About Eggs

When eggs are the focal point of a dish, their quality makes a big difference. Here's what we've learned in the test kitchen about buying eggs.

Color
The shell's hue depends on the breed of the chicken. The run-of-the-mill leghorn chicken produces the typical white egg. Brown-feathered birds, such as Rhode Island Reds, produce ecru- to coffee-colored eggs. Despite marketing hype extolling the virtues of nonwhite eggs, our tests proved that shell color has no effect on flavor.

Farm-Fresh and Organic
In our taste tests, farm-fresh eggs were standouts. The large yolks were bright orange and sat very high above the comparatively small whites, and the flavor was exceptionally rich and complex. Organic eggs followed in second place, with eggs from hens raised on a vegetarian diet in third, and the standard supermarket eggs last. Differences were easily detected in egg-based dishes like a scramble or a frittata, but not in baked goods.

Eggs and Omega-3s
Several companies are marketing eggs with a high level of omega-3 fatty acids, the healthful unsaturated fats also found in some fish. In our taste test, we found that more omega-3s translated into a richer egg flavor. Why? Commercially raised chickens usually peck on corn and soy, but chickens on an omega-3-enriched diet have supplements of greens, flaxseeds, and algae, which also add flavor, complexity, and color to their eggs. Read labels carefully and look for brands that guarantee at least 200 milligrams of omega-3s per egg.

How Old Are My Eggs?
Egg cartons are marked with both a sell-by date and a pack date. The pack date is the day the eggs were packed, which is generally within a week of when they were laid but may be as much as 30 days later. The sell-by date is within 30 days of the pack date, which is the legal limit set by the U.S. Department of Agriculture (USDA). In short, a carton of eggs may be up to two months old by the end of the sell-by date. But according to the USDA, eggs are still fit for consumption for an additional three to five weeks past the sell-by date.

14 ounces soft tofu, drained and patted dry
1½ teaspoons canola oil
  1 small red bell pepper, stemmed, seeded, and chopped fine
  1 shallot, minced
  ½ teaspoon salt
  ¼ teaspoon ground curry powder
  ⅛ teaspoon pepper
  2 tablespoons minced fresh basil, parsley, tarragon, or marjoram

1. Crumble tofu into ¼- to ½-inch pieces. Spread tofu on paper towel–lined baking sheet and let drain for 20 minutes, then gently press dry with additional paper towels. Heat oil in 10-inch nonstick skillet over medium heat until shimmering. Add bell pepper and shallot and cook until softened, about 5 minutes.

2. Stir in tofu, salt, curry powder, and pepper and cook until tofu is heated through, about 2 minutes. Off heat, stir in basil. Serve.

PER SERVING
Cal 100 • **Total Fat** 6g • **Sat Fat** 0g • **Chol** 0mg
Sodium 290mg • **Total Carbs** 4g • **Fiber** 1g • **Total Sugar** 1g
Added Sugar 0g • **Protein** 8g • **Total Carbohydrate Choices** 0

VARIATION
Tofu Scramble with Tomato and Scallions
Omit bell pepper and basil. Add 1 seeded and finely chopped tomato and 1 minced garlic clove to skillet with shallot and cook until tomato is no longer wet, 3 to 5 minutes. Add 2 tablespoons minced scallions to skillet with tofu.

PER SERVING
Cal 100 • **Total Fat** 6g • **Sat Fat** 0g • **Chol** 0mg
Sodium 290mg • **Total Carbs** 4g • **Fiber** 1g • **Total Sugar** 1g
Added Sugar 0g • **Protein** 8g • **Total Carbohydrate Choices** 0

Fried Eggs with Garlicky Swiss Chard and Bell Pepper
SERVES 4

WHY THIS RECIPE WORKS Greens for breakfast? When considering options for weekday mornings, Swiss chard doesn't immediately come to mind. However, the hearty leaves made an ideal partner (instead of toast) for a fried egg, especially when the rich, drippy yolk broke and mingled with the earthy greens. To keep our breakfast quick, we simply bloomed minced garlic in olive oil, then wilted handfuls of chard before adding red bell pepper for sweetness and a pinch of red pepper flakes to perk everything up. The greens became tender and vibrant in 5 minutes. We then drained our vegetables to banish excess liquid before portioning them out, and used the same skillet to quickly fry 4 eggs before sliding them atop our greens. A complementary spritz from a lemon wedge added pleasant brightness. You will need a 12-inch nonstick skillet with a tight-fitting lid for this recipe.

  2 tablespoons extra-virgin olive oil
  5 garlic cloves, minced
  2 pounds Swiss chard, stemmed, 1 cup stems chopped fine, leaves sliced into ½-inch-wide strips
  1 small red bell pepper, stemmed, seeded, and cut into ¼-inch pieces
    Pinch salt
  ⅛ teaspoon red pepper flakes
  4 large eggs
    Lemon wedges

1. Heat 1 tablespoon oil and garlic in 12-inch nonstick skillet over medium-low heat, stirring occasionally, until garlic is light golden, 3 to 5 minutes. Increase heat to high, add chard stems, then chard leaves, 1 handful at a time, and cook until wilted, about 2 minutes. Stir in bell pepper, salt, and pepper flakes and cook, stirring often, until chard is tender and peppers are softened, about 3 minutes. Transfer to colander set in bowl and let drain while preparing eggs; discard liquid. Wipe skillet clean with paper towels.

2. Crack 2 eggs into small bowl. Repeat with remaining 2 eggs in second bowl. Heat remaining 1 tablespoon oil in now-empty skillet over medium-high heat until shimmering; quickly swirl to coat skillet. Working quickly, pour one bowl of eggs in one side of skillet and second bowl of eggs in other side. Cover and cook for 1 minute.

3. Remove skillet from heat and let sit, covered, 15 to 45 seconds for runny yolks (white around edge of yolk will be barely opaque), 45 to 60 seconds for soft but set yolks, and about 2 minutes for medium-set yolks.

4. Divide chard mixture between individual plates and top with eggs. Serve immediately with lemon wedges.

PER SERVING
Cal 190 • **Total Fat** 12g • **Sat Fat** 2.5g • **Chol** 185mg
Sodium 550mg • **Total Carbs** 11g • **Fiber** 4g • **Total Sugar** 3g
Added Sugar 0g • **Protein** 10g • **Total Carbohydrate Choices** 1

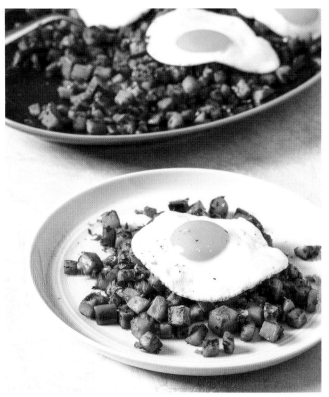

Using sweet potatoes instead of white in this hash provides it with an earthy, natural sweetness and adds extra nutrients.

Fried Eggs with Sweet Potatoes and Turkey Sausage
SERVES 6

WHY THIS RECIPE WORKS Given that traditional hash is comprised of white potatoes and fatty meat and is loaded with salt, it wouldn't be amiss to assume that it's not a great choice for a diabetic diet; but we wanted to make sure that wasn't the case for our recipe. We started by replacing regular white potatoes with diced sweet potatoes, which are significantly lower in carbohydrates. We paired the sweet potatoes with fresh Italian turkey sausage; the leaner turkey sausage added richness and flavor to our hash without overdoing it on sodium or fat. For extra flavor we sautéed onion, garlic, thyme, sage, lemon zest, and a pinch of red pepper flakes to add to our potato base. We fried eggs in just a teaspoon of olive oil and served them atop our finished hash for extra protein. You will need a 12-inch nonstick skillet with a tight-fitting lid for this recipe.

1½ pounds sweet potatoes, peeled and cut into ¼-inch pieces
2 tablespoons extra-virgin olive oil
¼ teaspoon pepper
8 ounces sweet Italian turkey sausage, casings removed
1 onion, chopped fine
2 garlic cloves, minced
1 teaspoon minced fresh thyme
1 teaspoon minced fresh sage
¼ teaspoon grated lemon zest, plus lemon wedges for serving
Pinch red pepper flakes
6 large eggs
2 tablespoons minced fresh parsley

1. Microwave potatoes, 1 teaspoon oil, and pepper in covered bowl, stirring occasionally, until potatoes begin to soften, 6 to 8 minutes. Drain potatoes well and return to bowl.

2. Heat 1 teaspoon oil in 12-inch nonstick skillet over medium-high heat until shimmering. Add sausage and onion and cook, breaking up sausage with wooden spoon, until sausage is lightly browned and onion is softened, 5 to 7 minutes. Stir in garlic, thyme, sage, lemon zest, and pepper flakes and cook until fragrant, about 30 seconds. Transfer sausage mixture to separate bowl.

3. Wipe skillet clean with paper towel. Heat 1 tablespoon oil in now-empty skillet over medium heat until shimmering. Add potatoes and cook, stirring occasionally, until tender and well browned, about 4 minutes. Stir in sausage mixture and cook until heated through, about 2 minutes. Transfer to serving platter and tent with aluminum foil.

4. Wipe skillet clean with paper towel. Crack 3 eggs into bowl. Crack remaining 3 eggs into second bowl. Heat remaining 1 teaspoon oil in now-empty skillet and heat over medium-low heat until shimmering. Working quickly, pour 1 bowl of eggs into one side of pan and second bowl of eggs into other side of pan. Cover and cook for 1 minute. Remove skillet from heat and let sit, covered, 15 to 45 seconds for runny yolks (white around edge of yolk will be barely opaque), 45 to 60 seconds for soft but set yolks, and about 2 minutes for medium-set yolks. Using rubber spatula, gently transfer eggs on top of hash. Sprinkle with parsley and serve.

PER SERVING
Cal 270 • **Total Fat** 14g • **Sat Fat** 2g • **Chol** 210mg
Sodium 380mg • **Total Carbs** 23g • **Fiber** 4g • **Total Sugar** 7g
Added Sugar 0g • **Protein** 15g • **Total Carbohydrate Choices** 1.5

Spinach and Feta Omelets

SERVES 2

WHY THIS RECIPE WORKS A classic filled omelet uses multiple whole eggs, butter (used to cook with as well as brush on the omelet before serving), and a generous amount of cheese. We wanted a nutritionally streamlined version with a foolproof cooking method. Starting with the eggs, we first considered everyone's leaner go-to, the all-egg-white omelet, but lackluster flavor and leathery texture quickly put an end to that. Instead, we borrowed from our scrambled eggs recipe that had won over tasters. In keeping our omelet diabetes-friendly, we decided to do away with butter altogether, opting to cook with a little canola oil. Ditching the milk (found in our scrambled eggs recipe) meant more structure and a better foil for our delicious vegetable fillings. As for a foolproof cooking method, we found that a good-quality nonstick skillet was essential and a heatproof rubber spatula kept the eggs from tearing as we shaped the omelet with the sides of the pan. To ensure the cheese melted before the eggs overcooked, we crumbled the cheese into small pieces for quick melting and removed the pan from the heat after adding the cheese. The residual heat was enough to melt the cheese without overcooking the eggs. This technique gave us the omelets we had been looking for: moist and creamy with just enough perfectly melted cheese to satisfy any omelet lover.

4 large eggs
1 tablespoon canola oil
1 shallot, minced
4 ounces (4 cups) baby spinach
1 ounce feta cheese, crumbled (¼ cup)

1. Beat 2 eggs with fork in bowl until eggs are thoroughly combined and color is pure yellow; do not overbeat. Repeat with remaining 2 eggs in second bowl.

2. Heat 1 teaspoon oil in 10-inch nonstick skillet over medium heat until shimmering. Add shallot and cook until softened, about 2 minutes. Stir in spinach and cook until wilted, about 1 minute. Using tongs, squeeze out any excess moisture from spinach mixture, then transfer to bowl and cover to keep warm. Wipe skillet clean with paper towels and let cool slightly.

3. Heat 1 teaspoon oil in now-empty skillet over medium heat until shimmering. Add 1 bowl of eggs and cook until edges begin to set, 2 to 3 seconds. Using rubber spatula, stir eggs in circular motion until slightly thickened, about 10 seconds. Use spatula to pull cooked edges of eggs in toward center, then tilt skillet to 1 side so that uncooked eggs run to edge of skillet. Repeat until omelet is just set but still moist on surface, 20 to 25 seconds. Sprinkle 2 tablespoons feta and half of spinach mixture across center of omelet.

4. Off heat, use spatula to fold lower third (portion nearest you) of omelet over filling; press gently with spatula to secure seam, maintaining fold. Run spatula between outer edge of omelet and skillet to loosen. Pull skillet sharply toward you few times to slide

SHAPING A FILLED OMELET

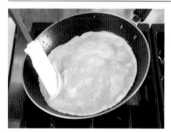

1. Pull cooked eggs from edges of skillet toward center, tilting skillet so any uncooked eggs run to skillet's edges.

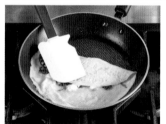

2. Sprinkle cheese and filling across center of omelet. Off heat, fold lower third of omelet over filling, then press seam to secure.

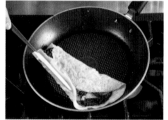

3. Pull skillet sharply toward you so that unfolded edge of omelet slides up far side of skillet.

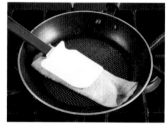

4. Fold far edge of omelet toward center and press to secure seam. Invert omelet onto plate.

unfolded edge of omelet up far side of skillet. Jerk skillet again so that unfolded edge folds over itself, or use spatula to fold edge over. Invert omelet onto plate. Tidy edges with spatula and serve immediately.

5. Wipe skillet clean with paper towels and repeat with remaining 1 teaspoon oil, remaining eggs, remaining 2 tablespoons feta, and remaining filling.

PER SERVING

Cal 270 • **Total Fat** 20g • **Sat Fat** 6g • **Chol** 385mg
Sodium 320mg • **Total Carbs** 6g • **Fiber** 2g • **Total Sugar** 2g
Added Sugar 0g • **Protein** 16g • **Total Carbohydrate Choices** 0

VARIATION
Mushroom and Gruyère Omelets

Substitute 4 ounces white mushrooms, trimmed and sliced thin, for spinach; cook until lightly browned and dry, 5 to 7 minutes. Stir ¼ teaspoon minced fresh thyme into mushroom mixture and cook until fragrant, about 30 seconds. Transfer filling to bowl and proceed with recipe as directed, substituting ¼ cup shredded Gruyère cheese for feta.

PER SERVING

Cal 270 • **Total Fat** 19g • **Sat Fat** 6g • **Chol** 390mg
Sodium 250mg • **Total Carbs** 5g • **Fiber** 1g • **Total Sugar** 3g
Added Sugar 0g • **Protein** 18g • **Total Carbohydrate Choices** 0

Frittata with Spinach, Bell Pepper, and Basil
SERVES 4

WHY THIS RECIPE WORKS Loaded with eggs and cheese, the classic frittata is not the healthiest breakfast option. To transform this dish we looked to reduce the amount of saturated fat and also pack it with vegetables for extra fiber and nutrition. Whole eggs plus small amounts of Parmesan cheese and low-fat milk helped keep our frittata creamy without adding too much fat. We found that starting the frittata on the stovetop and finishing it in the oven set it evenly so it didn't burn or dry out. Conventional skillets required so much oil to prevent sticking that frittatas cooked in them were likely to be greasy, so we used a nonstick skillet to ensure a clean release. Do not substitute skim milk here. You will need a 10-inch ovensafe nonstick skillet for this recipe.

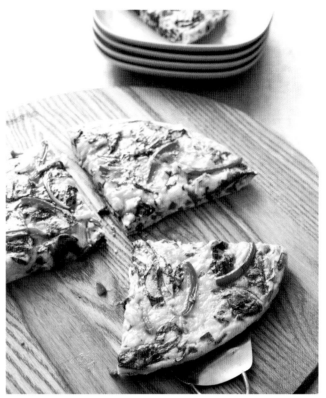

To ensure our frittata doesn't dry out or burn, we move it from the stovetop to the oven to set and finish cooking.

8 large eggs
1 ounce Parmesan cheese, grated (½ cup)
3 tablespoons 1 percent low-fat milk
2 tablespoons chopped fresh basil
⅛ teaspoon salt
¼ teaspoon pepper
2 teaspoons extra-virgin olive oil
1 small onion, chopped fine
1 red bell pepper, stemmed, seeded, and cut into 2-inch matchsticks
1 garlic clove, minced
3 ounces (3 cups) baby spinach

1. Adjust oven rack to middle position and heat oven to 350 degrees. Beat eggs, Parmesan, milk, basil, salt, and pepper with fork in bowl until eggs are thoroughly combined and color is pure yellow; do not overbeat.

2. Heat oil in 10-inch ovensafe nonstick skillet over medium heat until shimmering. Add onion and bell pepper and cook until softened, about 5 minutes. Stir in garlic and cook until fragrant, about 30 seconds. Stir in spinach and cook until wilted, about 1 minute.

3. Add egg mixture and, using rubber spatula, constantly and firmly scrape along bottom and sides of skillet until eggs begin to clump and spatula just leaves trail on bottom of pan but eggs are still very wet, about 30 seconds. Smooth curds into even layer and cook, without stirring, for 30 seconds.

4. Transfer skillet to oven and bake until frittata is slightly puffy and surface is dry and bounces back when lightly pressed, 6 to 9 minutes. Run spatula around edge of skillet to loosen frittata, then carefully slide it out onto serving plate. Let sit for 5 minutes before slicing and serving.

PER SERVING

Cal 230 • **Total Fat** 14g • **Sat Fat** 4.5g • **Chol** 380mg
Sodium 370mg • **Total Carbs** 7g • **Fiber** 2g • **Total Sugar** 3g
Added Sugar 0g • **Protein** 17g • **Total Carbohydrate Choices** 0.5

VARIATION
Frittata with Asparagus, Mushrooms, and Goat Cheese

Omit bell pepper and spinach and substitute ½ cup crumbled goat cheese for Parmesan. Add 4 ounces mushrooms, trimmed and sliced thin, and 4 ounces asparagus, trimmed and cut on bias into ¼-inch pieces, to skillet with onion; increase vegetable cooking time to 6 to 8 minutes.

PER SERVING

Cal 230 • **Total Fat** 15g • **Sat Fat** 6g • **Chol** 380mg
Sodium 290mg • **Total Carbs** 6g • **Fiber** 1g • **Total Sugar** 3g
Added Sugar 0g • **Protein** 17g • **Total Carbohydrate Choices** 0.5

Open-Faced Poached Egg Sandwiches
SERVES 4

WHY THIS RECIPE WORKS An open-faced egg sandwich is a good choice for the diabetic diet and here a whole-wheat English muffin spread with goat cheese makes a great base for a poached egg. To make it hearty and add a nutritional punch, we added sliced tomato and a generous helping of sautéed spinach. The vinegar in the egg poaching water adds more than just flavor—it lowers the pH in the water, ensuring that the egg whites stay intact during cooking. You will need a 12-inch nonstick skillet with a tight-fitting lid for this recipe.

  2 ounces goat cheese, crumbled and softened (½ cup)
½ teaspoon lemon juice
⅛ teaspoon pepper

  2 whole-wheat English muffins, split in half, toasted, and still warm
  1 small tomato, cored, seeded, and sliced thin (about 8 slices)
  2 teaspoons extra-virgin olive oil
  1 shallot, minced
  1 garlic clove, minced
  4 ounces (4 cups) baby spinach
⅛ teaspoon salt
  2 tablespoons distilled vinegar
  4 large eggs

1. Adjust oven rack to middle position and heat oven to 300 degrees. Stir goat cheese, lemon juice, and pepper together in bowl until smooth. Spread goat cheese mixture evenly over warm English muffin halves and top with tomato slices. Arrange English muffins on rimmed baking sheet and keep warm in oven while preparing spinach and eggs.

2. Heat oil in 12-inch nonstick skillet over medium heat until shimmering. Add shallot and cook until softened, about 2 minutes. Stir in garlic and cook until fragrant, about 30 seconds. Stir in spinach and salt and cook until wilted, about 1 minute. Using tongs, squeeze out any excess moisture from spinach, then divide evenly among English muffins.

3. Wipe skillet clean with paper towels, then fill it nearly to rim with water. Add vinegar and bring to boil over high heat. Meanwhile, crack eggs into two teacups (2 eggs in each). Reduce water to simmer. Gently tip cups so eggs slide into skillet simultaneously. Remove skillet from heat, cover, and poach eggs for 4 minutes (add 30 seconds for firm yolks).

4. Using slotted spoon, gently lift eggs from water and let drain before laying them on top of spinach. Serve immediately.

PER SANDWICH

Cal 210 • **Total Fat** 11g • **Sat Fat** 4g • **Chol** 195mg
Sodium 350mg • **Total Carbs** 17g • **Fiber** 3g • **Total Sugar** 4g
Added Sugar 0g • **Protein** 13g • **Total Carbohydrate Choices** 1

POACHING EGGS

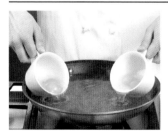

Crack two eggs into each teacup and tip cups simultaneously into simmering water.

Breakfast Tacos
SERVES 2

WHY THIS RECIPE WORKS We love tacos for lunch and dinner. So why not for the most important meal of the day? Inherent to all tacos is the tortilla, specifically a flour tortilla. It should be tender and chewy yet sturdy enough to hold the substantial fillings with a clean, non-distracting flavor. Unfortunately, most store-bought flour tortillas tip the scales in calories, fat, sodium, and carbohydrates. Homemade tortillas would be better nutritionally but didn't seem practical for only two people, beside the best-tasting versions still contained shortening. Store-bought corn tortillas, which are whole grain, made a great and easy substitute for flour ones. With the tortillas squared away, we focused on arguably the second most important part of a taco—the filling. We wanted to keep the filling pretty simple; it's breakfast, after all. Most breakfast tacos feature scrambled eggs with a few add-ins. Four eggs and two tablespoons of low-fat milk made up the egg-based portion of our tacos. The addition of cheese folded into the eggs helped boost flavor and avoided the need to fuss with cheese later when building the tacos. As for the rest of the filling, we ditched the typical greasy processed breakfast meats (bacon and sausage) in favor of something lighter-tasting. Refreshing pico de gallo (fresh tomato, shallot, cilantro leaves, jalapeño, lime juice, and a pinch of salt) and avocado slices made up the rest of our delicious and healthy dish. A few more bright cilantro leaves on top completed these perfect breakfast tacos for two. Do not substitute skim milk here. Be sure to remove the eggs from the skillet as soon as they are done to prevent them from overcooking.

- 1 plum tomato, cored and chopped fine
- 1 shallot, minced
- ¼ cup fresh cilantro leaves
- 1 tablespoon minced jalapeño chile
- 1 tablespoon lime juice
- Salt
- 4 large eggs
- 2 tablespoons 1 percent low-fat milk
- 1 teaspoon canola oil
- 1 ounce cheddar cheese, shredded (¼ cup)
- 4 (6-inch) corn tortillas, warmed
- ½ avocado, sliced ¼ inch thick

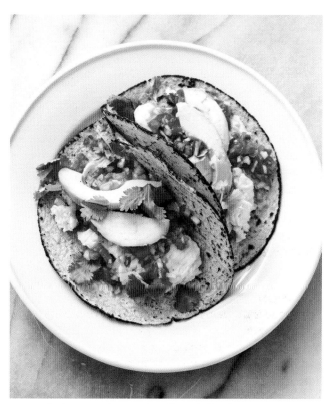

We opt for homemade pico de gallo and sliced avocado to keep our taco filling fresh.

1. Combine tomato, shallot, 2 tablespoons cilantro, jalapeño, lime juice, and pinch salt in bowl; set pico de gallo aside for serving.

2. Beat eggs, milk, and pinch salt with fork in bowl until eggs are thoroughly combined and color is pure yellow; do not overbeat.

3. Heat oil in 10-inch nonstick skillet over medium-high heat until shimmering, swirling to coat pan. Add egg mixture and, using rubber spatula, constantly and firmly scrape along bottom and sides of skillet until eggs begin to clump and spatula just leaves trail on bottom of pan, 45 to 75 seconds. Reduce heat to low and gently but constantly fold eggs until clumped and just slightly wet, 30 to 60 seconds. Quickly fold in cheddar, then immediately transfer eggs to medium bowl.

4. Divide egg mixture between tortillas and top with pico de gallo, avocado, and remaining 2 tablespoons cilantro leaves. Serve immediately.

PER SERVING (2 TACOS)
Cal 440 • **Total Fat** 26g • **Sat Fat** 7g • **Chol** 390mg
Sodium 430mg • **Total Carbs** 33g • **Fiber** 6g • **Total Sugar** 4g
Added Sugar 0g • **Protein** 20g • **Total Carbohydrate Choices** 2

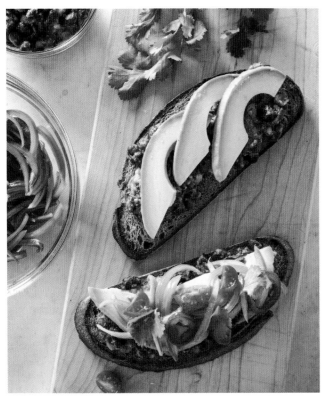

Mashed black beans are the perfect protein- and fiber-rich base for sliced avocado, marinated red onion, and tomatoes.

Avocado and Bean Toast
SERVES 4

WHY THIS RECIPE WORKS Avocado toast is one of our favorite healthy snacks, but we wanted a topped toast that was a bit more substantial and could stand alone as breakfast. We chose a bold Southwestern flavor profile to liven up our morning: Mashed black beans on toast elevated with a bit of spice, fresh tomato, and a squeeze of lime is hard to argue with. By simply mashing our beans with hot water, oil, and lime zest and juice, we were able to get a flavorsome, well-textured base. We really liked the addition of spicy quick-pickled onions, but didn't appreciate the added sugar and salt they supply. By marinating some red onion in vinegar and red pepper, we were able to add pops of brightness, color, and spice without the extra carbs or sodium.

1 small red onion, halved and sliced thin
½ cup red wine vinegar
½ teaspoon red pepper flakes
4 ounces grape or cherry tomatoes, quartered
4 teaspoons extra-virgin olive oil

Salt and pepper
1 (15-ounce) can no-salt-added black beans, rinsed
¼ cup boiling water
½ teaspoon grated lime zest plus 1 tablespoon juice
4 (2-ounce) slices rustic 100 percent whole-grain bread, toasted
1 ripe avocado, halved, pitted, and sliced thin
¼ cup fresh cilantro leaves

1. Combine onion, vinegar, and pepper flakes in small bowl and let sit at room temperature for at least 20 minutes. (Onions can be refrigerated for up to 3 days.)

2. Combine tomatoes, 1 teaspoon oil, pinch salt, and pinch pepper in second bowl. Using potato masher in third bowl, mash beans, boiling water, lime zest and juice, ½ teaspoon salt, pinch pepper, and remaining 1 tablespoon oil to coarse paste, leaving some whole beans intact.

3. Spread mashed bean mixture evenly on toast and shingle avocado on top. Drain onions, then arrange on top of avocado along with tomatoes and cilantro. Serve.

PER SERVING
Cal 350 • **Total Fat** 15g • **Sat Fat** 2g • **Chol** 0mg
Sodium 560mg • **Total Carbs** 42g • **Fiber** 12g • **Total Sugar** 6g
Added Sugar 0g • **Protein** 13g • **Total Carbohydrate Choices** 3

NOTES FROM THE TEST KITCHEN

Getting to Know Avocados

Although avocados are high in fat, it is largely the monounsaturated kind important in heart-healthy diets. They also are high in fiber and a source of lutein, a natural antioxidant known to be beneficial to healthy eyes and skin. We favor small, rough-skinned California Hass avocados over the larger, smooth-skinned Florida avocados, which taste watery and bland. Avocados are typically sold relatively hard and unripe and require at least a day or two in a dark, warm spot to soften and develop their characteristically creamy texture and flavor. When ripe, the skins of Hass avocados turn from green to dark purplish-black and the fruit will yield slightly to a gentle squeeze when held in the palm of your hand. Another way to identify ripeness involves the small stem on the small end of the avocado. If you can easily flick it off with your finger, and you can see green underneath it, the avocado is ripe. If the stem is not easily removed, save the avocado for another day.

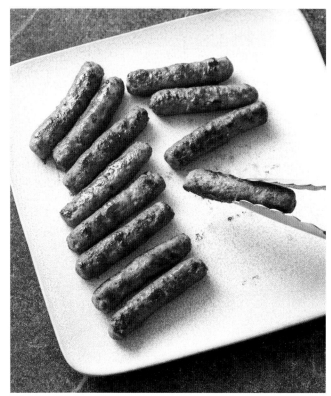
Our lean turkey breakfast sausages are a great add-on to many of the carb-only recipes in this chapter.

Homemade Turkey Breakfast Sausage
MAKES 16 LINKS

WHY THIS RECIPE WORKS These homemade turkey sausages are infused with the flavor of sage and maple, are easy to make, and have just 3 grams of fat for a serving of two sausages. They beat out any store-bought variety hands-down in terms of flavor and fit easily into the diabetic diet. To keep the fat on the low side we turned to 93 percent lean ground turkey, sautéing a quarter of it first with a little canola oil then adding flavorful minced fresh sage. The precooked bits of meat provided both chewy texture and rich flavor throughout the sausage. To bind our sausages together, a mixture of buttermilk and whole-wheat bread mashed to a paste worked perfectly (the buttermilk added welcome tang). Be sure to use ground turkey, not ground turkey breast (also labeled 99 percent fat-free), in this recipe.

1 tablespoon canola oil
1 pound ground turkey
2 teaspoons minced fresh sage or ½ teaspoon dried

1½ (1-ounce) slices hearty whole-wheat sandwich bread, crusts removed, torn into small pieces
¼ cup buttermilk
1 tablespoon maple syrup
1 garlic clove, minced
1 teaspoon salt
½ teaspoon pepper
1 teaspoon minced fresh thyme or ¼ teaspoon dried
Pinch cayenne pepper
Pinch ground nutmeg

1. Heat 1 teaspoon oil in 12-inch nonstick skillet over medium heat until shimmering. Add 4 ounces ground turkey and cook, breaking up meat with wooden spoon, until well browned, 6 to 8 minutes. Stir in sage and cook until fragrant, about 30 seconds; transfer to bowl and let cool slightly. Wipe skillet clean with paper towels.

2. Using fork, mash bread and buttermilk into paste in large bowl. Stir in cooked turkey, maple syrup, garlic, salt, pepper, thyme, cayenne, and nutmeg. Add remaining uncooked turkey and knead with hands until thoroughly combined. Working with 1 heaping tablespoon of mixture at a time, use wet hands to shape mixture into sixteen 4-inch-long links. (Sausages can be wrapped tightly in plastic wrap and aluminum foil and frozen for up to 1 month; thaw before cooking.)

3. Heat remaining 2 teaspoons oil in skillet over medium heat until shimmering. Add sausages and cook until well browned on all sides, about 10 minutes. Transfer sausages to paper towel–lined plate and let drain briefly before serving.

PER SERVING (2 LINKS)
Cal 100 • **Total Fat** 2.5g • **Sat Fat** 1g • **Chol** 25mg
Sodium 350mg • **Total Carbs** 3g • **Fiber** 0g • **Total Sugar** 2g
Added Sugar 2g • **Protein** 15g • **Total Carbohydrate Choices** 0

Cheesy Baked Grits
SERVES 10

WHY THIS RECIPE WORKS Rich and cheesy, baked grits would generally be off limits for anyone aiming to eat healthfully as they are usually packed with shredded cheese, not to mention cream. And while this version is still a treat, we were able to keep butter and cheese to a minimum and swap in low-fat milk for cream. To start, we built a flavorful base in which to cook the grits. A little finely chopped onion sautéed in a just a tablespoon of butter was first.

To that, we added water, the milk, and some hot sauce, bringing it all to a boil before adding old-fashioned grits. Once the grits were thick and creamy and had absorbed all the liquid, we added half the cheese and the eggs and poured it all into a baking dish. A topping of an additional ½ cup shredded cheese turned appealingly golden in the oven and ensured cheesy flavor in every bite. Smoked cheddar or Gouda both work nicely here in place of the cheddar.

    1 tablespoon unsalted butter
    1 onion, chopped fine
    1 teaspoon salt
4½ cups water
1½ cups 1 percent low-fat milk
 ¾ teaspoon hot sauce
1½ cups old-fashioned grits
    4 ounces extra-sharp cheddar cheese, shredded (1 cup)
    4 large eggs, lightly beaten
 ¼ teaspoon pepper

1. Adjust oven rack to lower-middle position and heat oven to 350 degrees. Lightly spray 13 by 9-inch baking dish with canola oil spray. Melt butter in large saucepan over medium heat. Add onion and salt and cook until softened, about 5 minutes. Stir in water, milk, and hot sauce and bring to boil.

2. Pour grits into boiling liquid in very slow stream while whisking constantly in circular motion to prevent clumping. Reduce heat to low, cover, and cook, stirring often and vigorously (make sure to scrape corners of pot), until grits are thick and creamy, 10 to 15 minutes.

3. Off heat, whisk in ½ cup cheddar, eggs, and pepper. Pour mixture into prepared dish, smooth top, and sprinkle with remaining ½ cup cheddar. Bake until top is browned and grits are hot, 35 to 45 minutes. Let cool for 10 minutes before serving.

PER SERVING
Cal 190 • **Total Fat** 8g • **Sat Fat** 4g • **Chol** 90mg
Sodium 360mg • **Total Carbs** 22g • **Fiber** 2g • **Total Sugar** 3g
Added Sugar 0g • **Protein** 7g • **Total Carbohydrate Choices** 1

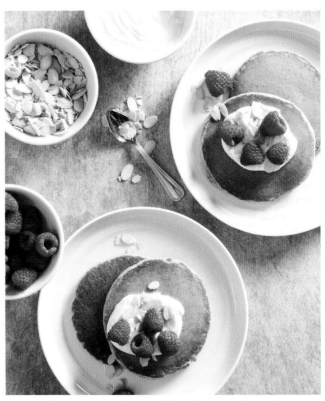

Instead of covering our hearty whole-wheat pancakes with sugary syrup, we top them with flavored yogurt, berries, and almonds.

100 Percent Whole-Wheat Pancakes
MAKES 15 PANCAKES

WHY THIS RECIPE WORKS Pancakes seemed like the perfect opportunity to showcase whole-wheat flour for a healthier breakfast with more nutrients and fiber than its all-purpose flour counterpart. While most whole-wheat pancake recipes shy away from using only whole-wheat flour, we prepared a batch of 100 percent whole-wheat pancakes. Rather than being leaden, they turned out light and fluffy, thanks to the bran present in the whole-wheat flour that cuts through any gluten strands that form, preventing the batter from becoming tough. The robust flavor of our pancakes paired perfectly with our fragrant Orange-Honey Yogurt, which added sweetness without all the sugar of syrup. Adding a sprinkle of fresh berries and nuts improved the nutritional content of the dish. An electric griddle set at 350 degrees can be used in place of a skillet.

    2 cups (11 ounces) whole-wheat flour
    2 tablespoons sugar
1½ teaspoons baking powder
 ½ teaspoon baking soda
 ¼ teaspoon salt

2¼ cups buttermilk
5 tablespoons plus 2 teaspoons canola oil
2 large eggs
1 recipe Orange-Honey Yogurt (recipe follows)
5 ounces (1 cup) raspberries
1 cup sliced almonds, toasted

1. Adjust oven rack to middle position and heat oven to 200 degrees. Set wire rack in rimmed baking sheet.

2. Whisk flour, sugar, baking powder, baking soda, and salt together in large bowl. In separate bowl, whisk buttermilk, 5 tablespoons oil, and eggs together until combined. Whisk buttermilk mixture into flour mixture until smooth. Make well in center of dry ingredients, add all of wet ingredients to well, and gently stir until just combined. Mixture will be thick; do not add more buttermilk.

3. Heat 1 teaspoon oil in 12-inch nonstick skillet over medium heat until shimmering, 3 to 5 minutes. Using paper towels, wipe out oil, leaving thin film in skillet. Using ¼-cup measure, portion batter into skillet, spreading each into 4-inch round using back of spoon. Cook until edges are set, first side is golden, and bubbles on surface are just beginning to break, 2 to 3 minutes.

4. Flip pancakes and cook until second side is golden, 1 to 3 minutes. Transfer to prepared rack and keep warm in oven. Repeat with remaining batter, adding remaining oil to skillet as needed. Serve, dolloping each pancake with 1 rounded tablespoon of orange-honey yogurt and sprinkling with raspberries and almonds.

PER PANCAKE WITH ABOUT 1 TABLESPOON
ORANGE-HONEY YOGURT

Cal 200 • **Total Fat** 10g • **Sat Fat** 1.5g • **Chol** 30mg
Sodium 180mg • **Total Carbs** 24g • **Fiber** 4g • **Total Sugar** 7g
Added Sugar 4g • **Protein** 8g • **Total Carbohydrate Choices** 1.5

Orange-Honey Yogurt
MAKES ABOUT 1¼ CUPS
Do not substitute 0 percent Greek yogurt.

1 cup 2 percent Greek yogurt
2 tablespoons honey
¼ teaspoon grated orange zest plus 2 tablespoons juice

Whisk ingredients together in bowl. (Yogurt can be refrigerated for up to 3 days.) Serve.

PER TABLESPOON

Cal 15 • **Total Fat** 0 g • **Sat Fat** 0g • **Chol** 0mg
Sodium 0mg • **Total Carbs** 2g • **Fiber** 0g • **Total Sugar** 2g
Added Sugar 2g • **Protein** 1g • **Total Carbohydrate Choices** 0

NOTES FROM THE TEST KITCHEN

Making Better Pancakes

Here are our tips for getting perfectly fluffy, golden-brown pancakes every time.

Make a Well When Mixing Make a well in the center of the dry ingredients, pour the liquid ingredients into the well, and gently whisk together until just incorporated. We like this method when making liquidy batters, because it helps incorporate the wet ingredients into the dry without overmixing.

Leave Some Lumps When stirring the batter, be careful not to overmix it—the batter should actually have a few lumps. Overmixed batter makes for dense pancakes.

Get the Skillet Hot But Not Scorching Heat the oil in a 12 inch nonstick skillet over medium heat for 3 to 5 minutes. If the skillet is not hot enough, the pancakes will be pale and dense. Knowing when the skillet is hot enough can take some practice; if you're not sure if the skillet is ready, try cooking just one small pancake to check.

Wipe Out Excess Oil Before adding the batter, use a wad of paper towels to carefully wipe out the excess oil, leaving a thin film of oil in the pan. If you use too much oil, the delicate cakes will taste greasy and dense.

Use a ¼-Cup Measure Add the batter to the skillet in ¼-cup increments (two or three pancakes will fit at a time). Using a measuring cup ensures that the pancakes are the same size and that they cook at the same rate. Don't crowd the pan or the pancakes will run together and be difficult to flip.

Flip When You See Bubbles Cook the pancakes on the first side until bubbles on the surface just begin to break, about 2 minutes. The bubbles indicate that the pancakes are ready to be flipped. If the pancakes are not browned when flipped, the skillet needs to be hotter; if the pancakes are too brown, turn down the heat.

Blueberry Oat Pancakes
MAKES 18 PANCAKES

WHY THIS RECIPE WORKS A classic pancake makes for a delicious component in a breakfast but doesn't offer much in the way of nutrition. To give this breakfast a boost, we turned to whole grains and zeroed in on oats for their nutty flavor, hearty texture, and high fiber content. We were able to create a smooth base for our batter using three-quarters oat flour, with ½ cup all-purpose flour providing structure and lift. We stirred whole rolled oats into our batter as well. Pre-soaked until just softened, they gave our pancakes a satisfying, nubby texture. Fresh blueberries, cinnamon, and nutmeg paired nicely with the toasty oats. Lastly, switching from whole milk to low-fat buttermilk kept our pancakes light and fluffy. We prefer using store-bought oat flour, as it has a very fine grind and creates the most fluffy pancakes, but you can make your own in a pinch: Grind 1½ cups (4½ ounces) old-fashioned rolled oats in a food processor to a fine meal, about 2 minutes; note pancakes will be denser if using ground oats. Do not use toasted oat flour, or quick, instant, or thick-cut oats in this recipe. An electric griddle set at 350 degrees can be used in place of a skillet.

    2 cups buttermilk, plus extra as needed
    1 cup (3 ounces) old-fashioned rolled oats
1½ cups (4½ ounces) oat flour
    ½ cup (2½ ounces) all-purpose flour
2½ teaspoons baking powder
    1 teaspoon ground cinnamon
    ¼ teaspoon salt
    ⅛ teaspoon ground nutmeg
    2 large eggs
    3 tablespoons plus 2 teaspoons canola oil
    3 tablespoons sugar
    2 teaspoons vanilla extract
7½ ounces (1½ cups) blueberries
    1 recipe Orange-Honey Yogurt (page 25)

1. Adjust oven rack to middle position and heat oven to 200 degrees. Set wire rack in rimmed baking sheet. Combine 1 cup buttermilk and oats in bowl and let sit at room temperature until softened, about 15 minutes.

2. Whisk oat flour, all-purpose flour, baking powder, cinnamon, salt, and nutmeg together in large bowl. In separate bowl, whisk remaining 1 cup buttermilk, eggs, 3 tablespoons oil, sugar, and vanilla together until frothy, about 1 minute. Make well in center of dry ingredients, add all of egg mixture to well, and gently stir until just combined. Using rubber spatula, fold in oat-buttermilk mixture until just combined.

3. Heat 1 teaspoon oil in 12-inch nonstick skillet over medium heat until shimmering, 3 to 5 minutes. Using paper towels, wipe out oil, leaving thin film in skillet. Using ¼-cup measure, portion batter into skillet, spreading each into 4-inch round using back of spoon. Sprinkle each pancake with 1 rounded tablespoon blueberries. Cook until edges are set, first side is golden, and bubbles on surface are just beginning to break, 2 to 3 minutes.

4. Flip pancakes and cook until second side is golden, 1 to 3 minutes. Transfer to prepared rack and keep warm in oven. Repeat with remaining batter, whisking additional buttermilk into batter as needed to loosen, and adding remaining oil to pan as necessary. Serve, dolloping each pancake with 1 tablespoon of orange-honey yogurt.

PER PANCAKE WITH ABOUT 1 TABLESPOON
ORANGE-HONEY YOGURT
Cal 130 • **Total Fat** 4.5g • **Sat Fat** 1g • **Chol** 25mg
Sodium 135mg • **Total Carbs** 19g • **Fiber** 2g • **Total Sugar** 7g
Added Sugar 4g • **Protein** 5g • **Total Carbohydrate Choices** 1

Steel-Cut Oatmeal with Blueberries and Almonds
SERVES 4

WHY THIS RECIPE WORKS Steel-cut oats, which are dried oat kernels cut crosswise into coarse bits, create an oatmeal that is full of texture while still being luscious and creamy, and have the added benefit of being a whole grain. Normally steel-cut oats require a long cooking time, so we sped up the process by soaking them overnight and then heating them through in the morning. We replaced whole milk with lighter 1 percent, which was amply rich and creamy. We cut down significantly on both salt and sugar, finding a mere ¼ teaspoon of salt was plenty and 1 tablespoon of brown sugar (which packs more of a flavorful punch than white sugar) was more than enough to sweeten our oatmeal. Cinnamon and nutmeg provided the classic, warm spice flavor we were searching for. We topped our finished oatmeal with blueberries and chopped, lightly toasted almonds. Do not substitute rolled oats for steel-cut oats. This oatmeal reheats well, so you can quickly serve it up again later in the week.

    3 cups water
    1 cup steel-cut oats
    ¼ teaspoon salt
    ½ cup 1 percent low-fat milk
    1 tablespoon packed brown sugar

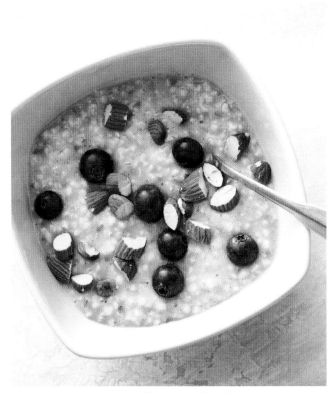

For a quick nutritious breakfast, we soak steel-cut oats overnight then cook them the next morning.

¼ teaspoon ground cinnamon
  Pinch ground nutmeg
2½ ounces (½ cup) blueberries
⅓ cup whole almonds, toasted and chopped coarse

1. Bring water to boil in large saucepan over high heat. Off heat, stir in oats and salt, cover, and let sit for at least 12 hours or up to 24 hours.

2. Stir milk, sugar, cinnamon, and nutmeg into oats and bring to boil over medium-high heat. Reduce heat to medium and cook, stirring occasionally, until oats are softened but still retain some chew and mixture thickens and resembles warm pudding, 4 to 6 minutes.

3. Remove saucepan from heat and let sit for 5 minutes. Stir to recombine and serve, sprinkling individual portions with blueberries and almonds.

PER SERVING (½ CUP)
Cal 270 • **Total Fat** 8g • **Sat Fat** 1g • **Chol** 0mg
Sodium 170mg • **Total Carbs** 42g • **Fiber** 6g • **Total Sugar** 8g
Added Sugar 3g • **Protein** 9g • **Total Carbohydrate Choices** 3

VARIATION
Steel-Cut Oatmeal with Raspberries, Orange, and Pistachios

Substitute 1 teaspoon grated orange zest for cinnamon and nutmeg, ½ cup raspberries for blueberries, and ⅓ cup shelled pistachios, toasted and chopped, for almonds.

PER SERVING (½ CUP)
Cal 260 • **Total Fat** 7g • **Sat Fat** 1g • **Chol** 0mg
Sodium 170mg • **Total Carbs** 41g • **Fiber** 7g • **Total Sugar** 7g
Added Sugar 3g • **Protein** 9g • **Total Carbohydrate Choices** 3

NOTES FROM THE TEST KITCHEN

Understanding Oats

We found only one type of oat that was just right for our ideal bowl of oatmeal. Also called Scottish or Irish oats, steel-cut oats are simply whole oats that have been cut into smaller pieces. They take longer to cook than regular rolled oats, but the outcome is worth the wait—and with our easy recipe, most of the time is hands-off. The hot cereal made with steel-cut oats had a faint nutty flavor, and while its consistency was surprisingly creamy, it also had a pleasing chewy quality. Rolled oats, on the other hand, resulted in bland, gummy oatmeal.

	UNCOOKED	**COOKED**
Oat Groats	Whole oats hulled and cleaned	These have a flavor reminiscent of brown rice and a very coarse texture.
Steel-Cut Oats	Groats cut crosswise into a few pieces	These make a creamy yet chewy hot cereal with a nutty flavor.
Rolled Oats	Groats steamed and pressed into flat flakes; also known as old-fashioned or regular	These American-style oats make a drab, gummy bowl of oatmeal.
Quick Oats	Groats rolled extra-thin	Cooked, these are flavorless and quick to cool into a flabby, pastelike consistency.
Instant Oats	Precooked rolled oats	These make a gummy, gelatinous cereal.

Yogurt Parfaits
SERVES 4

WHY THIS RECIPE WORKS Creamy yogurt, fresh fruit, and crunchy, toasted nuts make an easy and healthy start to the day—and layering them in a tall glass makes a simple breakfast feel like a special occasion. The bright flavor of lower-carb and fiber-rich fresh berries perfectly complemented the plain yogurt. We also added low-calorie, high-protein almonds and sunflower seeds, which we toasted to bring out their flavor and crunch. Almost any combination of fruits, nuts, and seeds will work well here. Do not substitute frozen fruit. Serve the parfaits within 15 minutes of assembling or the nuts and seeds will begin to turn soggy.

    1 cup whole almonds, toasted and chopped
    ½ cup raw sunflower seeds, toasted
    3 cups low-fat plain yogurt
    20 ounces (4 cups) blackberries, blueberries, raspberries,
       and/or sliced strawberries

Combine almonds and sunflower seeds in bowl. Using four 16-ounce glasses, spoon ¼ cup yogurt into each glass, then top with ⅓ cup berries, followed by 2 tablespoons nut mixture. Repeat layering process 2 more times with remaining yogurt, berries, and nut mixture. Serve.

PER SERVING

Cal 480 • **Total Fat** 29g • **Sat Fat** 4g • **Chol** 10mg
Sodium 130mg • **Total Carbs** 39g • **Fiber** 11g • **Total Sugar** 24g
Added Sugar 0g • **Protein** 22g • **Total Carbohydrate Choices** 2.5

NOTES FROM THE TEST KITCHEN

Chia Seeds

Chia seeds, from the flowering chia plant, look unassuming, like gray poppy seeds. But when they meet liquid, they swell into tapioca-like beads. Why do you want to eat them? They're full of protein, omega-3 fatty acids, and fiber, along with other nutrients. Almost all of the carbs in chia seeds is fiber, which means that almost none of those carbs are sugar or starch. This is great for people on a diabetes-friendly diet.

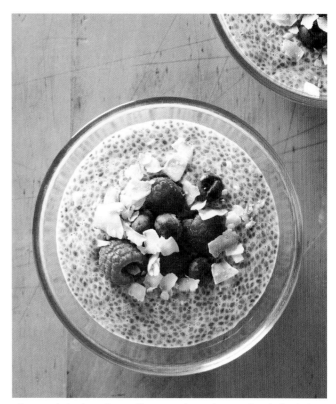

Chia seeds hydrated in milk overnight and topped with fresh fruit and toasted coconut make an easy, hands-off breakfast.

Chia Pudding with Fresh Fruit and Coconut
SERVES 4

WHY THIS RECIPE WORKS Chia pudding comes together by what seems like Jack and the Beanstalk–level magic. When chia seeds are combined with liquid and left to soak overnight they create a gel, which thickens and produces a no-cook tapioca-like pudding—a spectacular base for a simple, healthy breakfast. Pudding alchemy aside, chia is great because it's a nutritional powerhouse, packed with fiber, protein, and omega-3 fatty acids; plus, it has a neutral flavor that's the perfect canvas for fruity toppings. This recipe took little effort, just time. We tried to cut back on that by scalding the milk to speed up the thickening process. And indeed we could: After just 15 minutes the pudding had thickened as much as it had after a cold overnight soak. But that speed came with downsides: a decidedly grassier, "seedier" flavor and the loss of the fresh, milky notes we enjoyed in the soaked pudding. So we stuck with the hands-off overnight method. Before we put it to bed for the night, we gave the pudding a quick second whisk 15 minutes after its initial mixing to make sure all the chia hydrated and to prevent clumping. To flavor the pudding, we kept things simple with vanilla extract and maple syrup, which pair nicely with almost any toppings you have at your breakfast table. You have to soak the chia seeds for at least 8 hours or up to 1 week.

- 2 cups 1 percent low-fat milk, plus extra for serving
- ½ cup chia seeds
- 2 tablespoons maple syrup
- 1½ teaspoons vanilla extract
- ¼ teaspoon salt
- 2 cups (10 ounces) blueberries, raspberries, blackberries, sliced strawberries, and/or sliced bananas
- ¼ cup unsweetened flaked coconut, toasted

1. Whisk milk, chia seeds, maple syrup, vanilla, and salt together in bowl. Let mixture sit for 15 minutes, then whisk again to break up any clumps. Cover and refrigerate for at least 8 hours or up to 1 week.

2. Stir pudding to recombine and adjust consistency with extra milk as needed. Top individual portions with fruit and coconut before serving.

PER SERVING (½ CUP)
Cal 250 • Total Fat 11g • Sat Fat 4.5g • Chol 5mg
Sodium 210mg • Total Carbs 30g • Fiber 11g • Total Sugar 16g
Added Sugar 6g • Protein 9g • Total Carbohydrate Choices 2

NOTES FROM THE TEST KITCHEN

Flaxseeds

Flaxseeds are one of the highest sources known for the omega-3 fatty acid called alpha-linolenic acid (ALA), which is found only in certain plant foods and oils, and must be supplied by our diet for good health. (The other two omega-3 fatty acids are found in fish.) Similar in size to sesame seeds, they have a sweet, wheaty flavor and are sold both whole and ground. Whole seeds have a longer shelf life, but grinding the seeds will improve the release of the omega-3s and other nutrients once consumed. You can grind the whole seeds in a spice grinder or food processor. We store flaxseeds, like other nuts and seeds, in the freezer.

Omega-3 Granola
MAKES ABOUT 6 CUPS; SERVES 12

WHY THIS RECIPE WORKS Store-bought granola is often packed with sugar in various forms, so we wanted to make our own granola at home, with crunchy clusters that wouldn't end up being a starch bomb. To bulk up our oats, we used a healthy amount of nutritionally rich almonds, walnuts, sunflower seeds, and sesame seeds, all full of good unsaturated fats. We also appreciated that the protein in the nuts would keep us fuller, longer. Flaxseeds provided an additional punch of omega-3s, and also helped bind the granola. Using canola oil and honey also helped bind our oats together. We were able to avoid the often sandy texture of oats by cooling our granola en masse and breaking it apart once cooled. Do not substitute quick oats, instant oats, or steel-cut oats in this recipe.

- ⅓ cup slivered almonds
- ⅓ cup walnuts, chopped
- 3 cups (9 ounces) old-fashioned rolled oats
- 3 tablespoons canola oil
- ¼ cup raw sunflower seeds
- 2 tablespoons sesame seeds
- ½ cup honey
- 2 tablespoons ground flaxseeds
- ¼ teaspoon salt
- ½ cup raisins

1. Adjust oven rack to middle position and heat oven to 325 degrees. Line rimmed baking sheet with parchment paper and lightly spray with canola oil spray. Toast almonds and walnuts in 12-inch skillet over medium heat, stirring often, until fragrant and beginning to darken, about 3 minutes. Stir in oats and oil and continue to toast until oats begin to turn golden, about 2 minutes. Stir in sunflower seeds and sesame seeds and continue to toast until mixture turns golden, about 2 minutes.

2. Off heat, stir in honey, flaxseeds, and salt until well coated. Spread granola evenly over prepared sheet. Bake, stirring every few minutes, until granola is light golden brown, about 15 minutes.

3. Stir in raisins. With lightly greased stiff metal spatula, push granola onto one-half of baking sheet and press gently into ½-inch-thick slab. Let granola cool to room temperature, about

30 minutes. Loosen dried granola with spatula, break into small clusters, and serve. (Granola can be stored at room temperature in airtight container for up to 2 weeks.)

PER ½-CUP SERVING
Cal 240 • **Total Fat** 11g • **Sat Fat** 1g • **Chol** 0mg
Sodium 55mg • **Total Carbs** 32g • **Fiber** 4g • **Total Sugar** 16g
Added Sugar 11g • **Protein** 5g • **Total Carbohydrate Choices** 2

VARIATIONS
Omega-3 Granola with Cherries
Substitute 1 cup unsweetened dried cherries for raisins.

PER ½-CUP SERVING
Cal 250 • **Total Fat** 11g • **Sat Fat** 1g • **Chol** 0mg
Sodium 55mg • **Total Carbs** 34g • **Fiber** 4g • **Total Sugar** 16g
Added Sugar 11g • **Protein** 5g • **Total Carbohydrate Choices** 2

Omega-3 Granola with Peanut Butter
Substitute ⅔ cup peanuts, chopped, for almonds and walnuts. Reduce amount of oil to 2 tablespoons and stir ¼ cup natural unsweetened creamy peanut butter into oat mixture with honey and flaxseed.

PER ½-CUP SERVING
Cal 270 • **Total Fat** 13g • **Sat Fat** 1.5g • **Chol** 0mg
Sodium 80mg • **Total Carbs** 34g • **Fiber** 4g • **Total Sugar** 17g
Added Sugar 11g • **Protein** 7g • **Total Carbohydrate Choices** 2

Quinoa Granola
MAKES ABOUT 9 CUPS; SERVES 18

WHY THIS RECIPE WORKS For a new take on granola we decided to turn to quinoa, a seed known to be a protein powerhouse. We loved the crunch toasted quinoa added, and balanced it with quinoa flakes, which mimicked the texture of rolled oats and added a more delicate crunch, which we found appealing. Almonds and sunflower seeds were mild enough to pair well with the quinoa, while unsweetened flaked coconut contributed flavor without making our granola too sweet. Maple syrup and a hefty amount

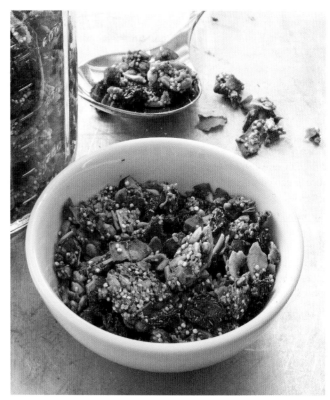

For a new spin on granola, we use protein-packed quinoa flakes instead of traditional rolled oats.

of vanilla rounded things out. Stirring in unsweetened dried tart cherries gave the finished quinoa granola pleasant fruitiness. If you buy unwashed quinoa (or if you are unsure whether it has been washed), be sure to rinse it before cooking to remove its bitter protective coating (called saponin).

½ cup maple syrup
4 teaspoons vanilla extract
½ teaspoon salt
¼ cup extra-virgin olive oil
2 cups whole almonds, chopped
2 cups unsweetened flaked coconut
1 cup quinoa flakes
1 cup prewashed white quinoa, rinsed
1 cup raw sunflower seeds
2 cups unsweetened dried tart cherries, chopped

1. Adjust oven rack to upper-middle position and heat oven to 325 degrees. Line rimmed baking sheet with parchment paper and lightly spray with canola oil spray.

2. Whisk maple syrup, vanilla, and salt together in large bowl. Whisk in oil. Fold in almonds, coconut, quinoa flakes, quinoa, and sunflower seeds until thoroughly coated.

3. Transfer mixture to prepared sheet and spread into thin, even layer. Using lightly greased stiff metal spatula, press on quinoa mixture until very compact. Bake until deep golden, 45 to 55 minutes.

4. Remove granola from oven and let cool on wire rack for 1 hour. Break cooled granola into pieces of desired size and stir in dried cherries. Serve. (Granola can be stored at room temperature in airtight container for up to 2 weeks.)

PER ½ CUP SERVING

Cal 350 • **Total Fat** 22g • **Sat Fat** 7g • **Chol** 0mg
Sodium 70mg • **Total Carbs** 34g • **Fiber** 6g • **Total Sugar** 13g
Added Sugar 5g • **Protein** 8g • **Total Carbohydrate Choices** 2

Granola Bars
MAKES 16 BARS

WHY THIS RECIPE WORKS It can be hard to find granola bars that aren't packed with sugar, and even homemade ones tend to be overzealous with honey and dried fruit. For a lower-sugar version, honey seemed like a good option, but its relatively high sugar content meant we couldn't use nearly enough to hold the bars together. We ultimately settled on just ⅓ cup of brown sugar, which gave our bars a hint of molasses flavor. To keep the bars cohesive, we turned to egg whites, which contain both water and protein. The egg whites coated the nuts and seeds, and when the water baked off, the protein that was left formed a crisp binding layer. To prevent our bars from drying out, we ground some of the oats into an oat flour, which helped hold on to some of the moisture. For our nuts and seeds, we chose a combination of pecans, pepitas, sunflower seeds, and unsweetened flaked coconut. Do not substitute quick oats, instant oats, or steel-cut oats in this recipe.

2 cups (6 ounces) old-fashioned rolled oats
⅓ cup packed (2¼ ounces) brown sugar
3 large egg whites
⅓ cup canola oil
1 tablespoon vanilla extract
¼ teaspoon salt
¼ teaspoon ground cinnamon
   Pinch ground nutmeg
½ cup pecans, chopped fine
½ cup raw pepitas
½ cup raw sunflower seeds
½ cup (1 ounce) unsweetened flaked coconut

1. Adjust oven rack to middle position and heat oven to 300 degrees. Make foil sling for 13 by 9-inch baking pan by folding 2 long sheets of aluminum foil; first sheet should be 13 inches wide and second sheet should be 9 inches wide. Lay sheets of foil in pan perpendicular to each other, with extra foil hanging over edges of pan. Push foil into corners and up sides of pan, smoothing foil flush to pan. Lightly spray foil with canola oil spray.

2. Process ½ cup oats in food processor until finely ground, about 30 seconds. Whisk sugar, egg whites, oil, vanilla, salt, cinnamon, and nutmeg together in large bowl. Stir in processed oats, remaining 1½ cups whole oats, pecans, pepitas, sunflower seeds, and coconut until thoroughly coated.

3. Transfer mixture to prepared pan and spread into even layer. Using lightly greased stiff metal spatula, press firmly on mixture until very compact. Bake granola bars until light golden brown and fragrant, about 40 minutes, rotating pan halfway through baking.

4. Remove bars from oven and let cool in pan for 15 minutes; do not turn oven off. Using foil overhang, lift bars from pan and transfer to cutting board. Cut into 16 bars. Space bars evenly on parchment paper–lined baking sheet and continue to bake until deep golden brown, 15 to 20 minutes, rotating sheet halfway through baking.

5. Transfer bars to wire rack and let cool completely, about 1 hour. Serve. (Bars can be stored at room temperature in airtight container for up to 1 week.)

PER BAR

Cal 180 • **Total Fat** 13g • **Sat Fat** 2.5g • **Chol** 0mg
Sodium 50mg • **Total Carbs** 13g • **Fiber** 2g • **Total Sugar** 5g
Added Sugar 4g • **Protein** 4g • **Total Carbohydrate Choices** 1

Muesli
SERVES 4

WHY THIS RECIPE WORKS Today's mueslis include all manner of ingredients (we counted as many as 20 in some recipes), but we saw no reason to get fussy. An oat-forward mixture of 3 parts oats to 2 parts add-ins—a nut, a seed, and two dried fruits—offered an ideal balance of flavor and texture. While traditional methods leave everything raw, we found that toasting the nuts and seeds brought greater depth and complexity to this simple dish. For our nut, sliced almonds required almost no prep work. Picking a seed proved trickier. Soaked flaxseed and chia seeds had overpowering flavor. Pepitas were ideal; we loved the big flavor they took on from toasting. To round out our muesli, we added raisins and antioxidant-packed goji berries, which benefit from the soaking, as it softens their chewy texture. Muesli can also be served like cereal (no soaking overnight). You can find goji berries in the natural foods section of most well-stocked supermarkets. This recipe can easily be doubled. To make a single serving, combine ½ cup muesli with ⅓ cup milk in bowl, cover, and refrigerate overnight.

1½ cups (4½ ounces) old-fashioned rolled oats
¼ cup raisins
¼ cup goji berries
¼ cup sliced almonds, toasted and chopped
¼ cup roasted pepitas
1⅔ cups 1 percent low-fat milk
5 ounces (1 cup) blueberries, raspberries, and/or blackberries

1. Combine oats, raisins, goji berries, almonds, and pepitas in bowl. (Muesli can be stored at room temperature for up to 2 weeks.)

2. Stir milk into muesli until combined. Cover and refrigerate for at least 12 hours or up to 24 hours.

3. Top individual portions with berries before serving.

PER 1-CUP SERVING
Cal 310 • **Total Fat** 10g • **Sat Fat** 2g • **Chol** 5mg
Sodium 65mg • **Total Carbs** 46g • **Fiber** 6g • **Total Sugar** 20g
Added Sugar 0g • **Protein** 12g • **Total Carbohydrate Choices** 3

VARIATION
Sunflower Seed, Hazelnut, and Cherry Muesli
Substitute unsweetened dried tart cherries for goji berries; toasted, skinned, and chopped hazelnuts for almonds; and roasted sunflower seeds for pepitas.

PER 1-CUP SERVING
Cal 330 • **Total Fat** 12g • **Sat Fat** 2g • **Chol** 5mg
Sodium 50mg • **Total Carbs** 48g • **Fiber** 7g • **Total Sugar** 20g
Added Sugar 0g • **Protein** 11g • **Total Carbohydrate Choices** 3

NOTES FROM THE TEST KITCHEN

Goji Berries

Native to China, once-exotic goji berries are now more widely available. Though fresh and frozen berries do exist in the U.S., they're difficult to find; the berries are most often available dried. Studies have explored their possible connection to preventing vision degeneration, defeating cancer cells, and even combating the flu. Whether or not they are more powerful than other nutrient-dense foods, the sweet-tart berries are rich sources of vitamins, minerals, fiber, and phytonutrients.

Berry Smoothies
SERVES 2

WHY THIS RECIPE WORKS Making a smoothie is easy, but we didn't want our berry smoothie to just taste great—it had to be filling enough to call it breakfast too. Low-fat yogurt was an easy addition; not only did it provide some protein and lean fat, it also created a smooth, creamy texture. For an additional protein boost (without adding distracting flavors or textures) we looked to hemp seed hearts, the hulled center of the hemp seed. On their own these taste subtly nutty, but blended into a smoothie they're hardly perceptible and 2 tablespoons was enough to contribute an additional 6 grams of protein. For a flavor combination that everyone could get behind, we liked a mix of blackberries, blueberries, raspberries, and a whole banana. We like the neutral flavor and color of hemp seed hearts, but you can use 2 tablespoons almond butter or ¼ cup wheat germ in their place.

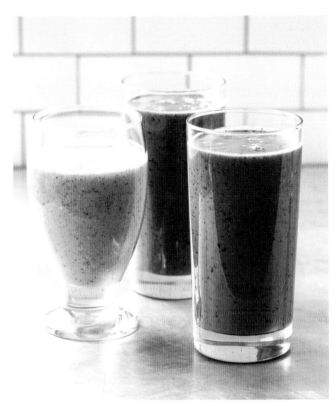

Smoothies full of fruit, leafy greens, low-fat yogurt, and hemp seed hearts start your day with plenty of fiber and protein.

3⅓ ounces (⅔ cup) frozen blackberries
3⅓ ounces (⅔ cup) frozen blueberries
3⅓ ounces (⅔ cup) frozen raspberries
 1 cup plain low-fat yogurt
 1 cup water
 1 ripe banana, peeled and halved lengthwise
 2 tablespoons hemp seed hearts
 ⅛ teaspoon salt

Process all ingredients in blender on low speed until mixture is combined but still coarse in texture, about 10 seconds. Increase speed to high and process until completely smooth, about 1 minute. Serve.

PER SERVING

Cal 270 • Total Fat 7g • Sat Fat 1.5g • Chol 5mg
Sodium 240mg • Total Carbs 44g • Fiber 9g • Total Sugar 27g
Added Sugar 0g • Protein 11g • Total Carbohydrate Choices 3

Green Smoothies
SERVES 2

WHY THIS RECIPE WORKS Green smoothies usually get their bright hue from green vegetables like spinach or kale, and while they may look healthy, they're often loaded with sweeteners to mask their grassy, bitter flavor. For our own green smoothie, we turned to convenient baby kale. Not only does it require little to no prep (no chef's knife needed for stemming), we found it was also less chewy and broke down easily in our smoothie, all while retaining the healthful qualities of the curly adult variety. As for the rest of the smoothie, a small amount of yogurt added body and creaminess, while a combination of apple, banana, and frozen pineapple provided just enough sweetness and additional fiber to balance the kale. Hemp seeds hearts again proved to be an easy stir in for a protein boost. We like the neutral flavor and color of hemp seed hearts, but you can use 2 tablespoons almond butter or ¼ cup wheat germ in their place.

1½ cups (1½ ounces) baby kale
 ½ cup plain low-fat yogurt
 ½ cup frozen pineapple
 1 Fuji, Gala, or Golden Delicious apple, peeled, cored, and quartered
 1 ripe banana, peeled and halved lengthwise
 ¼ cup water
 2 tablespoons hemp seed hearts
 Pinch salt

Process all ingredients in blender on low speed until mixture is combined but still coarse in texture, about 10 seconds. Increase speed to high and process until completely smooth, about 1 minute. Serve.

PER SERVING

Cal 230 • Total Fat 6g • Sat Fat 1g • Chol 5mg
Sodium 130mg • Total Carbs 39g • Fiber 6g • Total Sugar 22g
Added Sugar 0g • Protein 8g • Total Carbohydrate Choices 2.5

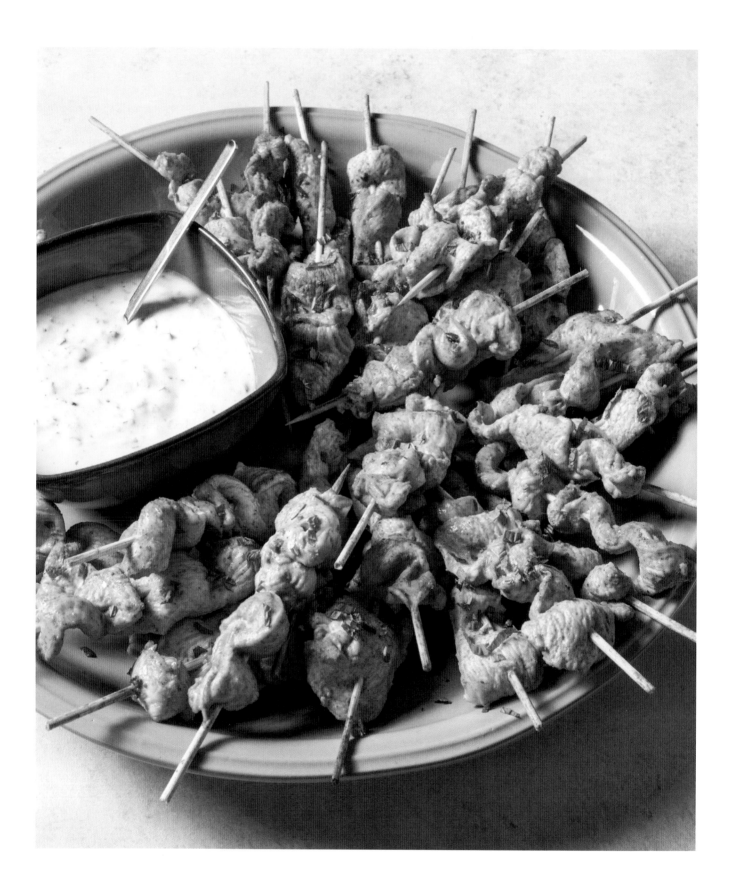

APPETIZERS AND SNACKS

Photo: Curried Chicken Skewers with Yogurt Dipping Sauce

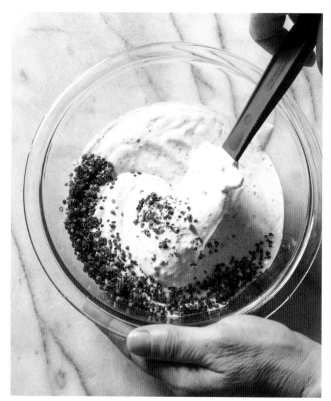

Cottage cheese, quickly processed with boiling water to smooth out its curds, is the key to a rich but light dip.

Green Goddess Dip

MAKES ABOUT 2½ CUPS

WHY THIS RECIPE WORKS Most creamy dips rely on sour cream, mayonnaise, or both for their rich flavor and smooth texture, which means that a traditional creamy dip can contain a whopping amount of calories. Substituting nonfat sour cream and mayonnaise seemed logical but this produced dips that were gluey and bland. After trying a mix of low-fat and nonfat dairy, we found that a blend of full-fat cottage cheese, processed with boiling water to eliminate its curds, and low-fat sour cream, to help keep the dip's nutritional numbers on target, produced a velvety base. Fresh herbs gave our quick and easy dip its fresh flavor and distinctive color; do not substitute dried herbs. For an accurate measurement of boiling water, bring a full kettle of water to a boil, then measure out the desired amount. Serve with Crudités (page 43) or 1 ounce of whole-grain tortilla chips or whole-wheat pita chips per serving of dip.

1 cup cottage cheese
¼ cup boiling water
1 cup low-fat sour cream

2 tablespoons extra-virgin olive oil
1 tablespoon lemon juice, plus extra for seasoning
¼ cup fresh parsley leaves
1 tablespoon fresh tarragon leaves
1 garlic clove, minced
¼ teaspoon salt
⅛ teaspoon pepper
¼ cup minced fresh chives

Process cottage cheese and boiling water in food processor until smooth, about 30 seconds, scraping down sides of bowl as needed. Add sour cream, oil, lemon juice, parsley, tarragon, garlic, salt, and pepper and process until well combined, about 30 seconds. Transfer dip to serving bowl and stir in chives. Cover and refrigerate until flavors meld, at least 1 hour or up to 24 hours. Season with extra lemon juice to taste before serving.

PER ¼-CUP SERVING DIP
Cal 70 • **Total Fat** 5g • **Sat Fat** 2g • **Chol** 5mg
Sodium 160mg • **Total Carbs** 3g • **Fiber** 0g • **Total Sugar** 2g
Added Sugar 0g • **Protein** 4g • **Total Carbohydrate Choices** <0.5

Artichoke and White Bean Dip

MAKES ABOUT 2½ CUPS

WHY THIS RECIPE WORKS Bean dips are usually the healthy alternative at a party, but they tend to disappoint unless they are loaded with cheese. We wanted a bean-based dip that was healthy but had our company coming back for more. Here we paired canned cannellini beans with artichokes, one of the highest-fiber vegetables. We processed the beans with just enough extra-virgin olive oil for richness and binding, along with a shallot, lemon juice, and water. The chopped artichokes gave our dip a nice, chunky texture and lemon zest and parsley completed our zesty dip. Do not substitute canned or jarred artichokes for the frozen artichokes. Be sure to puree the beans to a smooth texture before stirring in the artichokes. Serve with Crudités (page 43) or 1 ounce of whole-grain tortilla chips or whole-wheat pita chips per serving of dip.

1 (15-ounce) can no-salt-added cannellini beans, rinsed
3 tablespoons extra-virgin olive oil
1 shallot, minced
1 tablespoon water
1½ teaspoons grated lemon zest plus 1½ tablespoons juice, plus extra juice for seasoning
1 garlic clove, minced
½ teaspoon salt

⅛ teaspoon pepper
  Cayenne pepper
9 ounces frozen artichoke hearts, thawed, patted dry, and chopped fine
1 tablespoon minced fresh parsley or mint

Process beans, oil, shallot, water, lemon zest and juice, garlic, salt, pepper, and pinch cayenne in food processor until smooth, about 30 seconds, scraping down sides of bowl as needed. Transfer dip to medium serving bowl and stir in artichokes and parsley. Cover and refrigerate until flavors meld, at least 1 hour or up to 2 days. Season with extra lemon juice and cayenne to taste before serving.

PER ¼-CUP SERVING DIP

Cal 80 • **Total Fat** 4.5g • **Sat Fat** 0.5g • **Chol** 0mg
Sodium 150mg • **Total Carbs** 7g • **Fiber** 3g • **Total Sugar** 1g
Added Sugar 0g • **Protein** 2g • **Total Carbohydrate Choices** <0.5

Spicy Whipped Feta with Roasted Red Peppers

MAKES ABOUT 2 CUPS

WHY THIS RECIPE WORKS Salty, tangy feta cheese packs a punch so a little goes a long way. This classic meze is appealingly simple: Feta is processed to a smooth consistency along with roasted red peppers to make a rich yet light dip. Jarred roasted red peppers offered big flavor with minimal effort. To keep the flavor profile streamlined, we kept the additional flavors simple and straightforward. A hefty dose of cayenne pepper gave the dip a well-rounded heat while olive oil imparted fruity notes and some richness and bright lemon juice balanced the saltiness of the cheese. This dip is fairly spicy; to make it less so, reduce the amount of cayenne to ¼ teaspoon. Serve with Crudités (page 43) or 1 ounce of whole-grain tortilla chips or whole-wheat pita chips per serving of dip.

8 ounces feta cheese, crumbled (2 cups)
1 cup jarred roasted red peppers, rinsed, patted dry, and chopped
⅓ cup extra-virgin olive oil
1 tablespoon lemon juice
½ teaspoon cayenne pepper
¼ teaspoon pepper

Process feta, red peppers, oil, lemon juice, cayenne, and pepper in food processor until smooth, about 30 seconds, scraping down

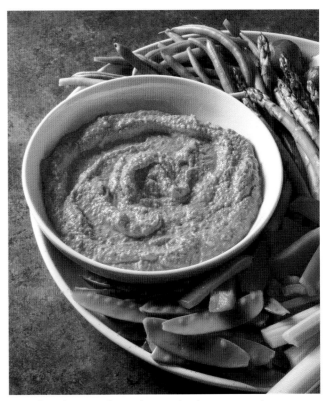

Briny feta cheese and jarred roasted red peppers make a supereasy and flavorful, light and tangy dip.

sides of bowl as needed. Transfer mixture to serving bowl and serve. (Dip can be refrigerated for up to 2 days; bring to room temperature before serving.)

PER 2-TABLESPOON SERVING DIP

Cal 80 • **Total Fat** 8g • **Sat Fat** 3g • **Chol** 15mg
Sodium 170mg • **Total Carbs** 1g • **Fiber** 0g • **Total Sugar** 1g
Added Sugar 0g • **Protein** 2g • **Total Carbohydrate Choices** <0.5

NOTES FROM THE TEST KITCHEN

Buying Feta

In Greece, feta must be made from at least 70 percent sheep's milk. This rule doesn't apply stateside, so imitators abound; but none of them beat the real deal. Our favorite, **Mt Vikos Traditional Feta**, is from Greece and boasts plenty of tang with just enough salt.

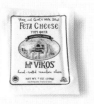

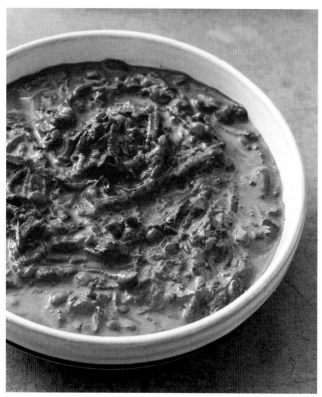

Raw, grated beets add fiber, vitamins, and vibrant color to traditional tzatziki.

Tzatziki
MAKES ABOUT 2 CUPS

WHY THIS RECIPE WORKS Tzatziki is a traditional Greek sauce made from strained yogurt and cucumber, as delicious eaten as a dip for raw vegetables as it is dolloped over grilled chicken or lamb. To make our own classic version, we started by shredding a cucumber on a coarse grater, salting it, and letting it drain to keep any excess liquid from watering down the dip. Greek yogurt gives tzatziki its pleasant tang and richness, but before stirring in our drained cucumber, we enhanced its flavor with minced fresh herbs and garlic. Using Greek yogurt here is key; do not substitute regular plain yogurt or the sauce will be very watery. Serve with Crudités (page 43) or 1 ounce of whole-grain tortilla chips or whole-wheat pita chips per serving of tzatziki.

1 (12-ounce) cucumber, peeled, halved lengthwise, seeded, and shredded
¼ teaspoon salt
1 cup 2 percent Greek yogurt
2 tablespoons extra-virgin olive oil
2 tablespoons minced fresh mint or dill
1 small garlic clove, minced
⅛ teaspoon pepper

1. Toss cucumber with salt in colander and let drain for 15 minutes.

2. Whisk yogurt, oil, mint, and garlic together in medium serving bowl, then stir in cucumber. Cover and refrigerate until chilled, at least 1 hour or up to 2 days. Stir in pepper before serving.

PER ¼-CUP SERVING TZATZIKI
Cal 60 • **Total Fat** 4g • **Sat Fat** 1g • **Chol** 0mg
Sodium 85mg • **Total Carbs** 2g • **Fiber** 0g • **Total Sugar** 2g
Added Sugar 0g • **Protein** 3g • **Total Carbohydrate Choices** <0.5

VARIATION
Beet Tzatziki
Reduce amount of cucumber to 6 ounces and add 6 ounces raw beets, peeled and grated, to cucumber and salt in step 1.

PER ¼-CUP SERVING TZATZIKI
Cal 60 • **Total Fat** 4g • **Sat Fat** 1g • **Chol** 0mg
Sodium 95mg • **Total Carbs** 3g • **Fiber** 1g • **Total Sugar** 2g
Added Sugar 0g • **Protein** 3g • **Total Carbohydrate Choices** <0.5

SEEDING CUCUMBERS

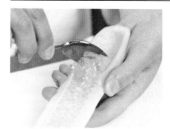

Peel and halve cucumber lengthwise. Run small spoon inside each cucumber half to scoop out seeds and any surrounding excess liquid.

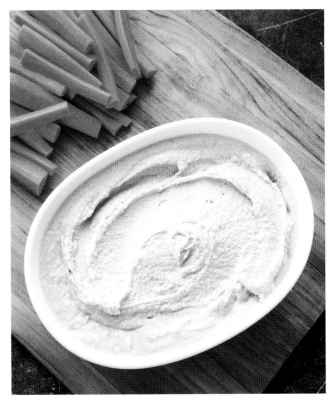

It's easy to turn convenient canned chickpeas into a protein- and fiber-filled hummus.

Classic Hummus
MAKES ABOUT 2 CUPS

WHY THIS RECIPE WORKS With protein and fiber from the chickpeas, hummus makes a healthy snack especially if paired with vegetables or whole-grain crackers. Classic hummus is composed of only a few simple ingredients: chickpeas, tahini, olive oil, garlic, and lemon juice. But many traditional recipes are surprisingly complex: The chickpeas must be soaked overnight and then skinned. We wanted a simple, streamlined recipe for hummus with a light, silky-smooth texture and balanced flavor profile. We employed convenient canned chickpeas and got out the food processor to make quick work of turning them into a smooth puree. But when we pureed the chickpeas alone, the hummus turned out grainy. The key to the best texture was to create an emulsion. We started by grinding the chickpeas, then slowly added a mixture of water and lemon juice. We whisked the olive oil and a generous amount of tahini together and drizzled the mixture into the chickpeas while processing; this created a lush, light, and flavorful puree.

Earthy cumin, garlic, and a pinch of cayenne kept the flavors balanced. If desired, garnish the hummus with 1 tablespoon of minced fresh cilantro or parsley and/or 2 tablespoons of reserved whole chickpeas. Serve with Crudités (page 43) or 1 ounce of whole-wheat pita chips per serving of hummus.

¼ cup water, plus extra as needed
3 tablespoons lemon juice
6 tablespoons tahini
2 tablespoons extra-virgin olive oil
1 (15-ounce) can no-salt-added chickpeas, rinsed
1 small garlic clove, minced
½ teaspoon salt
¼ teaspoon ground cumin
Pinch cayenne pepper

1. Combine water and lemon juice in small bowl. In separate bowl, whisk tahini and oil together.

2. Process chickpeas, garlic, salt, cumin, and cayenne in food processor until almost fully ground, about 15 seconds. Scrape down sides of bowl with rubber spatula. With machine running, add lemon juice mixture in steady stream. Scrape down sides of bowl and continue to process for 1 minute. With machine running, add tahini mixture in steady stream and process until hummus is smooth and creamy, about 15 seconds, scraping down sides of bowl as needed.

3. Transfer hummus to serving bowl, cover with plastic wrap, and let sit at room temperature until flavors meld, about 30 minutes. (Hummus can be refrigerated for up to 5 days; adjust consistency with up to 1 tablespoon warm water as needed.) Serve.

PER ¼-CUP SERVING HUMMUS
Cal 140 • **Total Fat** 10g • **Sat Fat** 1.5g • **Chol** 0mg
Sodium 160mg • **Total Carbs** 9g • **Fiber** 2g • **Total Sugar** 0g
Added Sugar 0g • **Protein** 4g • **Total Carbohydrate Choices** 0.5

VARIATIONS
Roasted Red Pepper Hummus
Omit water and cumin. Add ¼ cup jarred roasted red peppers, rinsed and patted dry, to food processor with chickpeas. Garnish hummus with 2 tablespoons toasted sliced almonds and 2 teaspoons minced fresh parsley.

PER ¼-CUP SERVING HUMMUS
Cal 150 • **Total Fat** 10g • **Sat Fat** 1.5g • **Chol** 0mg
Sodium 180mg • **Total Carbs** 9g • **Fiber** 2g • **Total Sugar** 1g
Added Sugar 0g • **Protein** 4g • **Total Carbohydrate Choices** 0.5

Artichoke-Lemon Hummus

Omit cumin and increase lemon juice to ¼ cup (2 lemons). Add ¾ cup frozen artichoke hearts, thawed and patted dry, and ¼ teaspoon grated lemon zest to food processor with chickpeas. Garnish hummus with additional ¼ cup thawed frozen artichoke hearts, patted dry and chopped, and 2 teaspoons minced fresh parsley or mint.

PER ¼-CUP SERVING HUMMUS

Cal 150 • **Total Fat** 10g • **Sat Fat** 1.5g • **Chol** 0mg
Sodium 180mg • **Total Carbs** 11g • **Fiber** 3g • **Total Sugar** 1g
Added Sugar 0g • **Protein** 4g • **Total Carbohydrate Choices** 1

Roasted Garlic Hummus

Remove outer papery skins from 2 heads garlic; cut top quarters off heads and discard. Wrap garlic in aluminum foil and roast in 350-degree oven until browned and very tender, about 1 hour; let cool, then squeeze out cloves from skins (you should have about ¼ cup). Meanwhile, heat 2 tablespoons extra-virgin olive oil and 2 thinly sliced garlic cloves in 8-inch skillet over medium-low heat. Cook, stirring occasionally, until garlic is golden brown, about 15 minutes; transfer garlic slices to paper towel–lined plate and reserve oil. Substitute garlic cooking oil for olive oil in step 1. Add roasted garlic to food processor with chickpeas. Garnish hummus with toasted garlic slices and 2 teaspoons minced fresh parsley.

PER ¼-CUP SERVING HUMMUS

Cal 140 • **Total Fat** 10g • **Sat Fat** 1.5g • **Chol** 0mg
Sodium 230mg • **Total Carbs** 11g • **Fiber** 2g • **Total Sugar** 1g
Added Sugar 0g • **Protein** 4g • **Total Carbohydrate Choices** 0.5

ROASTING GARLIC

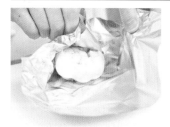 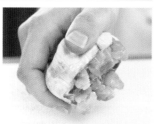

1. Cut off top of head so cloves are exposed. Place head, cut side up, in center of square of aluminum foil and seal.

2. Once heads have roasted and cooled, squeeze cloves from skins, starting from root and working up.

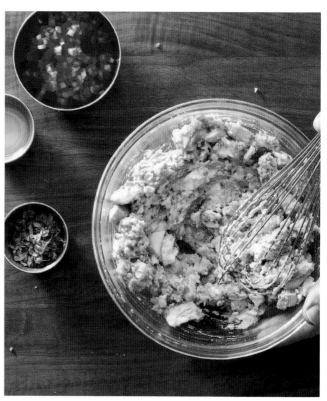

Rich in heart-healthy fats, avocados don't require much to become a crowd-pleasing dip.

Guacamole
MAKES ABOUT 2 CUPS

WHY THIS RECIPE WORKS Although avocados are high in fat, there is no reason to shy away from them as their fat is the good kind: They are packed with heart-healthy monounsaturated fats as well as a variety of vitamins and other nutrients. For the ultimate creamy, big-flavor guacamole, we looked at the traditional methods that typically make a smooth guacamole using the coarse surface of a *molcajete*, a three-legged Mexican mortar made of volcanic rock. Hoping to make ours without any special equipment, we minced the onion and chile by hand with kosher salt; the coarse crystals broke down the aromatics, releasing their juices and flavors and transforming them into a paste that was easy to combine with the avocado and other ingredients. (The salt will also help the aromatics break down if you use a regular mortar and pestle.) A bit of lime zest added further brightness without acidity. We used a whisk to mix and mash the avocado into the paste, creating a creamy but still chunky dip. Chopped tomato and cilantro added fruity flavor and freshness. For a spicier version, mince and add the serrano ribs and seeds to the onion mixture. A mortar and pestle can be used to process the onion mixture. Be sure to use Hass avocados here; Florida, or "skinny," avocados are too watery for dips. Serve with 1 ounce of whole-grain tortilla chips or whole-wheat pita chips per serving of guacamole.

2 tablespoons finely chopped onion
1 serrano chile, stemmed, seeded, and minced
1 teaspoon kosher salt
¼ teaspoon grated lime zest plus 1½–2 tablespoons juice
3 ripe avocados, halved, pitted, and cut into ½-inch pieces
1 plum tomato, cored, seeded, and minced
2 tablespoons chopped fresh cilantro

Place onion, serrano, salt, and lime zest on cutting board and chop until very finely minced. Transfer onion mixture to medium serving bowl and stir in 1½ tablespoons lime juice. Add avocados and, using sturdy whisk, mash and stir mixture until well combined with some ¼- to ½-inch chunks of avocado remaining. Stir in tomato and cilantro. (Guacamole can be refrigerated for up to 1 day by pressing plastic wrap directly against its surface.) Season with up to additional 1½ teaspoons lime juice to taste before serving.

PER ¼-CUP SERVING GUACAMOLE
Cal 120 • Total Fat 11g • Sat Fat 1.5g • Chol 0mg
Sodium 160mg • Total Carbs 7g • Fiber 5g • Total Sugar 1g
Added Sugar 0g • Protein 2g • Total Carbohydrate Choices <0.5

Fresh Tomato Salsa
MAKES ABOUT 2 CUPS

WHY THIS RECIPE WORKS Salsa is already a great option for the appetizer table; it's low carb, easy to make, and, if made well, packed with flavor. But salsa can go wrong in a number of ways: too watery, bland, spicy, or generally out of balance. We set out to solve the problem of watery salsa, trying numerous techniques before stumbling upon one that worked—draining diced tomatoes (skin, seeds, and all) in a colander. Doing so rid them of excess liquid, giving us a thicker, more substantial salsa. Next, we turned the spotlight on the supporting ingredients in a typical salsa recipe, choosing red onions over white, yellow, and sweet onions for their bright color and stronger flavor; jalapeño chiles over serrano, habanero, and poblano chiles because of their wide availability, slight vegetal flavor, and moderate heat; and lime juice over red wine vinegar, rice vinegar, or lemon juice for its authentic flavor that complements the rest of the ingredients. To make this salsa spicier, add the seeds from the chile. Serve with 1 ounce of whole-grain tortilla chips or whole-wheat pita chips per serving of salsa.

1 pound ripe tomatoes, cored and cut into ½-inch pieces
1 jalapeño chile, stemmed, seeded, and minced
⅓ cup finely chopped red onion
1 small garlic clove, minced
3 tablespoons minced fresh cilantro
1 tablespoon lime juice, plus extra for seasoning
¼ teaspoon salt

PREPARING AVOCADOS

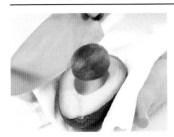 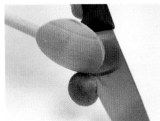 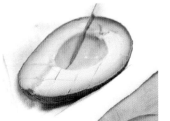 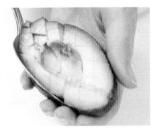

1. After slicing avocado in half around pit, lodge edge of knife blade into pit and twist to remove.

2. Don't pull pit off with your hands. Instead, use large wooden spoon to pry pit safely off knife.

3. Use dish towel to hold avocado steady. Make ½-inch crosshatch incisions in flesh of each avocado half with knife, cutting down to but not through skin.

4. Separate diced flesh from skin with large spoon inserted between skin and flesh, gently scooping out avocado cubes.

Place tomatoes in large colander and let drain for 30 minutes. As tomatoes drain, layer jalapeño, onion, garlic, and cilantro on top. Shake colander to drain off excess juice, then transfer to serving bowl. Stir in lime juice and salt. (Salsa can be refrigerated for up to 3 days.) Season with extra lime juice to taste before serving.

PER ¼-CUP SERVING SALSA

Cal 15 • **Total Fat** 0g • **Sat Fat** 0g • **Chol** 0mg
Sodium 75mg • **Total Carbs** 3g • **Fiber** 1g • **Total Sugar** 2g
Added Sugar 0g • **Protein** 1g • **Total Carbohydrate Choices** <0.5

Toasted Corn Salsa
MAKES ABOUT 2 CUPS

WHY THIS RECIPE WORKS Very low in carbs and calories, this salsa is a great option when trying to eat more healthfully. The combo of fresh toasted corn kernels and chopped red bell pepper gives the salsa its hearty texture, while jalapeño, shallot, and garlic ensure it is anything but dull. In keeping with the Mexican theme, we rounded it out with lime juice, cilantro, and cumin. Do not substitute frozen corn for the fresh corn here. Be sure to use a nonstick skillet when toasting the corn. To make this salsa spicier, add the seeds from the chile. Serve with 1 ounce of whole-grain tortilla chips or whole-wheat pita chips per serving of salsa.

4½ teaspoons extra-virgin olive oil
  2 ears corn, kernels cut from cobs
  1 red bell pepper, stemmed, seeded, and chopped fine
½ jalapeño chile, stemmed, seeded, and minced
  1 scallion, sliced thin
  2 garlic cloves, minced
  2 tablespoons lime juice, plus extra for seasoning
  2 tablespoons minced fresh cilantro
½ teaspoon ground cumin
¼ teaspoon salt
⅛ teaspoon pepper

1. Heat 1½ teaspoons oil in 12-inch nonstick skillet over medium-high heat until shimmering. Add corn and cook, stirring occasionally, until golden brown, 6 to 8 minutes.

2. Transfer corn to medium serving bowl and stir in remaining 1 tablespoon oil, bell pepper, jalapeño, scallion, garlic, lime juice, cilantro, cumin, salt, and pepper. Cover and refrigerate until flavors meld, at least 1 hour or up to 2 days. Season with extra lime juice to taste before serving.

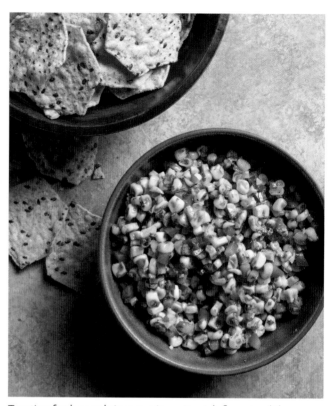

Toasting fresh corn brings out its nutty, rich flavor, and the kernels give this lively salsa its hearty texture.

PER ¼-CUP SERVING SALSA

Cal 50 • **Total Fat** 3.5g • **Sat Fat** 0g • **Chol** 0mg
Sodium 75mg • **Total Carbs** 6g • **Fiber** 1g • **Total Sugar** 2g
Added Sugar 0g • **Protein** 1g • **Total Carbohydrate Choices** <0.5

VARIATION
Toasted Corn and Black Bean Salsa
Reduce amount of corn to 1 ear; use 10-inch skillet when cooking corn in step 1 and reduce cooking time to 4 minutes. Add ¾ cup canned no-salt-added black beans, rinsed, to corn with remaining ingredients.

PER ¼-CUP SERVING SALSA

Cal 60 • **Total Fat** 3g • **Sat Fat** 0g • **Chol** 0mg
Sodium 75mg • **Total Carbs** 7g • **Fiber** 2g • **Total Sugar** 1g
Added Sugar 0g • **Protein** 2g • **Total Carbohydrate Choices** <0.5

Crudités

When done right, a platter of crudités can give you a lot of nutritional bang for your buck and be beautiful, if not downright irresistible. There are just three basic rules to keep in mind when preparing crudités. First and foremost, do not buy one of those prepackaged vegetable "rings" at the supermarket. They look bad, the vegetables taste old, and they are simply a waste of money because they rarely are eaten. The other two rules are equally simple: Prep fresh vegetables properly and arrange them so that the platter looks attractive and everything is within reach.

Preparing Vegetables for Crudités

In order to make appealing (and edible) crudités, some vegetables must first be blanched, then shocked in ice water. Prepping your vegetables properly is half the battle when it comes to crudités. Below are some specific instructions for particular vegetables.

TO BLANCH Bring 6 quarts water and 2 tablespoons salt to boil in large pot. Cook vegetables, one variety at a time, until slightly softened but still crunchy at core, following times given below. Transfer blanched vegetables immediately to bowl of ice water until completely cool, then drain and pat dry.

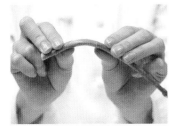

Asparagus To remove tough, fibrous ends of asparagus, bend thick end of each stalk until it snaps off. Blanch asparagus for 30 to 60 seconds.

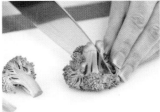

Broccoli and Cauliflower Cut broccoli and cauliflower florets into bite-size pieces by slicing down through stem. Blanch broccoli and cauliflower (separately) for 1 to 1½ minutes.

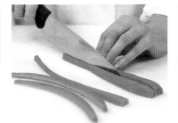

Carrots and Celery Slice both celery and peeled carrots lengthwise into long, elegant lengths rather than short, stumpy pieces.

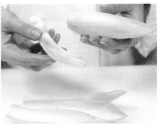

Endive Gently pull off leaves one at a time, trimming root end as you work your way toward heart of endive.

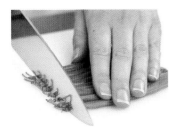

Green Beans Line beans up in a row and trim off inedible stem ends with just one cut. Blanch beans for 1 minute.

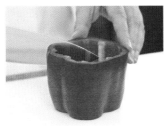

Peppers Slice off top and bottom of pepper and remove seeds and stem. Slice down through side of pepper, unroll it so that it lies flat, then slice into ½-inch-wide strips.

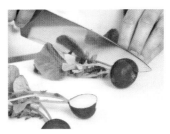

Radishes Choose radishes with green tops still attached so that each half has a leafy handle for grasping and dipping. Slice each radish in half through stem.

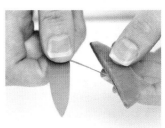

Snow and Snap Peas Remove tough, fibrous string that runs along straight side of snow and snap peas. Blanch snow or snap peas for 15 seconds.

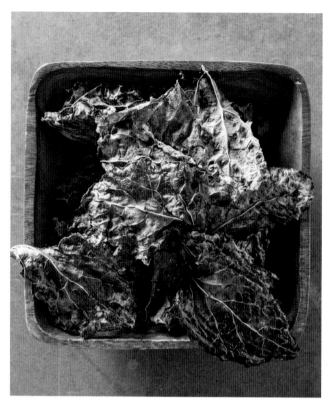

Baking kale chips on a wire rack distributes air flow above and beneath the leaves and makes them ultra-crisp.

were a super-satisfying snack. We prefer to use Lacinato (Tuscan) kale in this recipe, but curly-leaf kale can be substituted; chips made with curly-leaf kale will taste a bit chewy at the edges and won't keep as well. We prefer the larger crystal size of kosher salt here; if using table salt, reduce the amount by half.

12 ounces Lacinato kale, stemmed and torn into 3-inch pieces
1 tablespoon extra-virgin olive oil
½ teaspoon kosher salt

1. Adjust oven racks to upper-middle and lower-middle positions and heat oven to 200 degrees. Set wire racks in 2 rimmed baking sheets. Dry kale thoroughly between dish towels, transfer to large bowl, and toss with oil and salt.

2. Arrange kale on prepared racks, making sure leaves overlap as little as possible. Bake kale until very crisp, 45 to 60 minutes, switching and rotating sheets halfway through baking. Let kale chips cool completely before serving. (Kale chips can be stored in paper towel–lined airtight container for up to 1 day.)

PER 2-CUP SERVING
Cal 60 • **Total Fat** 4g • **Sat Fat** 0.5g • **Chol** 0mg
Sodium 160mg • **Total Carbs** 5g • **Fiber** 2g • **Total Sugar** 1g
Added Sugar 0g • **Protein** 3g • **Total Carbohydrate Choices** <0.5

Kale Chips
MAKES 8 CUPS

WHY THIS RECIPE WORKS A nutritious alternative to potato chips, kale chips have become all the rage. But store-bought versions are often deep fried and loaded with salt, and homemade ones never turn out crispy enough. We wanted a light-as-air, earthy kale chip that remained crispy. We discovered three keys to getting kale chips to the perfect texture. First, we lengthened the cooking time and lowered the oven temperature to mimic the effects of a dehydrator. Next, we baked the kale on wire racks to allow the oven air to circulate above and beneath the leaves. Finally, we started with completely dry leaves—we blotted them between two dish towels to make sure no water was left clinging. Tossed with olive oil and seasoned lightly with crunchy kosher salt, these ultracrisp kale chips

Popcorn with Olive Oil
MAKES ABOUT 14 CUPS

WHY THIS RECIPE WORKS Popcorn can be a naturally healthy snack. But add some oil to the pot when cooking, sprinkle a hearty dash of salt, and drizzle a little melted butter over the top before serving and suddenly you've turned this healthy food into a high fat, high sodium no-no. Looking for the healthiest way to make popcorn, we discovered an interesting trick: You can actually cook popcorn on the stovetop without any oil at all. Just adding a small amount of water to the pot along with the kernels was enough to do the trick. And for a classic popcorn profile, we found that a modest amount of olive oil and salt tossed before serving gave us just the flavor we craved. When cooking the popcorn, be sure to keep the lid on tight and shake the pot vigorously to prevent scorching.

1 tablespoon water
½ cup popcorn kernels
2 tablespoons extra-virgin olive oil
½ teaspoon salt
½ teaspoon pepper

Heat Dutch oven over medium-high heat for 2 minutes. Add water and popcorn, cover, and cook, shaking frequently, until first few kernels begin to pop. Continue to cook, shaking vigorously, until popping slows to about 2 seconds between pops. Transfer popcorn to large serving bowl and toss with oil, salt, and pepper. Serve.

PER 2-CUP SERVING
Cal 90 • **Total Fat** 4.5g • **Sat Fat** 0.5g • **Chol** 0mg
Sodium 170mg • **Total Carbs** 10g • **Fiber** 2g • **Total Sugar** 0g
Added Sugar 0g • **Protein** 1g • **Total Carbohydrate Choices** 0.5

VARIATIONS
Popcorn with Warm Spices and Garlic
Heat oil, 2 teaspoons garlic powder, ½ teaspoon ground coriander, and ½ teaspoon ground cumin in small skillet over medium-low heat until fragrant, about 1 minute; toss spiced oil with popcorn, salt, and pepper.

PER 2-CUP SERVING
Cal 90 • **Total Fat** 4.5g • **Sat Fat** 0.5g • **Chol** 0mg
Sodium 170mg • **Total Carbs** 10g • **Fiber** 2g • **Total Sugar** 0g
Added Sugar 0g • **Protein** 2g • **Total Carbohydrate Choices** 0.5

Popcorn with Parmesan and Black Pepper
We like to use a rasp-style grater for the Parmesan here because it makes small, delicate shreds of cheese that stick nicely to the warm popcorn.

Heat oil and pepper in small skillet over medium-low heat until fragrant, about 1 minute. Toss popcorn with pepper oil, salt, and ½ cup finely grated Parmesan cheese.

PER 2-CUP SERVING
Cal 100 • **Total Fat** 6g • **Sat Fat** 1g • **Chol** 5mg
Sodium 220mg • **Total Carbs** 10g • **Fiber** 2g • **Total Sugar** 0g
Added Sugar 0g • **Protein** 3g • **Total Carbohydrate Choices** 0.5

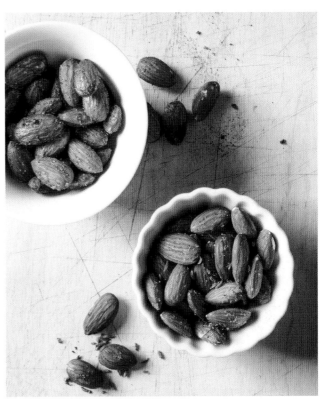

We dress up protein-packed almonds with orange zest and fennel seeds for a simple and superflavorful snack.

Orange-Fennel Spiced Almonds
MAKES ABOUT 2 CUPS

WHY THIS RECIPE WORKS Making your own spiced nuts is a great way to enjoy them without all the added sugar and salt that usually comes along with the store-bought varieties. You can almost eat them with abandon but, beware, nuts *are* calorie-dense. But they are also filling, high in protein, low in carbs, and just a handful can be satisfying. Watch the nuts carefully during toasting as they go from golden and fragrant to burnt very quickly.

1 tablespoon extra-virgin olive oil
1 teaspoon grated orange zest
1 teaspoon fennel seeds
1 teaspoon salt
¼ teaspoon pepper
2 cups raw whole almonds

Adjust oven rack to middle position and heat oven to 350 degrees. Combine oil, orange zest, fennel seeds, salt, and pepper in bowl. Toss almonds with oil mixture until well coated, then spread into single layer on rimmed baking sheet. Bake, stirring often, until fragrant and lightly browned, about 10 minutes. Transfer almonds to serving bowl and let cool completely before serving. (Almonds can be stored in airtight container for up to 1 week.)

PER ¼-CUP SERVING

Cal 220 • Total Fat 20g • Sat Fat 1.5g • Chol 0mg
Sodium 290mg • Total Carbs 8g • Fiber 5g • Total Sugar 2g
Added Sugar 0g • Protein 8g • Total Carbohydrate Choices 0.5

VARIATION
Spicy Chipotle Almonds

Substitute 1 teaspoon ground cumin, ¾ teaspoon chipotle chile powder, and ½ teaspoon garlic powder for orange zest and fennel seeds.

PER ¼-CUP SERVING

Cal 230 • Total Fat 20g • Sat Fat 1.5g • Chol 0mg
Sodium 290mg • Total Carbs 8g • Fiber 5g • Total Sugar 2g
Added Sugar 0g • Protein 8g • Total Carbohydrate Choices 0.5

Cherry, Chocolate, and Orange Trail Mix
MAKES ABOUT 3 CUPS

WHY THIS RECIPE WORKS Trail mix is often a fat, sugar, and calorie bomb unless you make it yourself—which is surprisingly simple. Here we start with raw pepitas, almonds, and walnuts, which we toast until fragrant and golden brown. To keep the sugar under control, we used unsweetened dried cherries and just a little chopped semisweet chocolate. To pull all the flavors together, a hefty dose of orange zest added brightness that complemented the nuts and the chocolate while just a tiny amount of salt and cinnamon completed our mix. Watch the nuts carefully during toasting as they go from golden and fragrant to burnt very quickly.

½ cup raw pepitas
2 tablespoons grated orange zest
¼ teaspoon ground cinnamon
⅛ teaspoon salt
¾ cup raw whole almonds
¾ cup raw walnuts, broken into large pieces
½ cup unsweetened dried cherries
1 ounce semisweet chocolate, chopped

1. Adjust oven rack to middle position and heat oven to 350 degrees. Line rimmed baking sheet with parchment paper. Combine pepitas, orange zest, cinnamon, and salt in bowl.

2. Spread almonds and walnuts into single layer on rimmed baking sheet and bake, stirring often, until beginning to turn fragrant, about 6 minutes. Stir in pepita mixture and continue to bake until nuts are fragrant and lightly browned, 3 to 4 minutes. Transfer nut mixture to large bowl and let cool completely, about 20 minutes.

3. Add dried cherries and chocolate to nut mixture and toss to combine. (Trail mix can be stored in airtight container for up to 1 week). Serve.

PER ¼-CUP SERVING

Cal 150 • Total Fat 12g • Sat Fat 1.5g • Chol 0mg
Sodium 30mg • Total Carbs 9g • Fiber 2g • Total Sugar 4g
Added Sugar 1g • Protein 5g • Total Carbohydrate Choices 0.5

VARIATION
Cherry, Coconut, Chili, and Lime Trail Mix

Omit chocolate. Substitute lime zest for orange zest and cayenne pepper for cinnamon. Add ⅓ cup unsweetened flaked coconut to pepita mixture in step 1.

PER ¼-CUP SERVING

Cal 150 • Total Fat 12g • Sat Fat 2.5g • Chol 0mg
Sodium 30mg • Total Carbs 7g • Fiber 2g • Total Sugar 3g
Added Sugar 0g • Protein 5g • Total Carbohydrate Choices <0.5

Stuffed Mushrooms
SERVES 6

WHY THIS RECIPE WORKS Forget about leathery, dried-out stuffed mushrooms with a bland, watery filling; we were able to create meaty bites full of savory flavor without a lot of sodium or bad fat. To rid the mushrooms of excess moisture, we tossed them in a bit of salt, which seasoned them and drew out their moisture. Then we roasted the mushrooms gill side up until their juice was released; we then flipped them gill side down to let the liquid evaporate. For the filling, we chopped the mushroom stems (a low-carb alternative to bread crumbs) in the food processor and sautéed them with garlic and wine. Cheese bound the filling together while a hit of acid brightened it. We topped the mushrooms with a pinch more cheese, cooked them until browned for more umami flavor, and sprinkled them with parsley for an attractive, fresh finish.

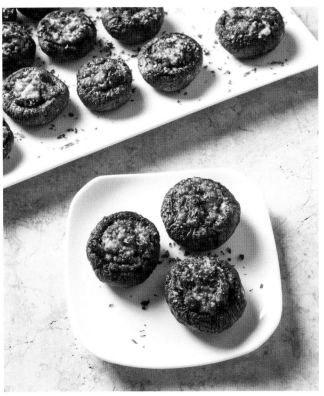

For a lower-carb and more flavorful filling, we use chopped mushroom stems in place of traditional bread crumbs.

24 large white mushrooms (1¾ to 2 inches in diameter), stems removed and reserved
2 tablespoons extra-virgin olive oil
¼ teaspoon salt
¼ teaspoon pepper
1 small shallot, minced
2 garlic cloves, minced
¼ cup dry white wine
1 ounce Parmesan cheese, grated (½ cup)
1 teaspoon minced fresh thyme
1 teaspoon lemon juice
1 tablespoon minced fresh parsley

1. Adjust oven rack to middle position and heat oven to 425 degrees. Line rimmed baking sheet with aluminum foil. Toss mushroom caps with 1 tablespoon oil, salt, and ⅛ teaspoon pepper and arrange gill side up on prepared sheet. Bake until mushrooms release their moisture and shrink in size, about 15 minutes. Flip caps and continue to bake until well browned, about 5 minutes; set aside.

All About Mushrooms

With their substantial, meaty texture, great flavor, and wide variety of vitamins and minerals, mushrooms add complex meatiness to soups, sauces, and stuffings. They are also enjoyed simply sautéed, stuffed, marinated, or grilled on their own. Here's everything you need to know about buying, storing, and cleaning mushrooms.

Buying Mushrooms

There are many varieties of fresh mushrooms available at the supermarket now: the humble white button mushroom, as well as cremini, shiitake, oyster, and portobello mushrooms, for starters. We find cremini mushrooms to be firmer and more flavorful than less expensive white button mushrooms, but the two are interchangeable in any recipe. If possible, always buy mushrooms loose so that you can inspect their quality. When buying button or cremini mushrooms, look for mushrooms with whole, intact caps; avoid those with discoloration or dry, shriveled patches. Pick mushrooms with large caps and minimal stems.

Storing Mushrooms

Because of their high moisture content, mushrooms are very perishable; most mushrooms can be kept fresh for only a few days. To extend their shelf life as long as possible, store loose mushrooms in the crisper drawer in a partially open zipper-lock bag. Store packaged mushrooms in their original containers, as these are designed to "breathe," maximizing the life of the mushrooms. Once the package has been opened, simply rewrap it with plastic wrap.

Cleaning Mushrooms

When it comes to cleaning, you can ignore the advice against washing mushrooms, which exaggerates their ability to absorb water. As long as they are washed before they are cut, we found that 6 ounces of mushrooms gain only about a quarter-ounce of water. However, rinsing can cause discoloration, so don't wash mushrooms that will be eaten raw; simply brush dirt away with a soft pastry brush or cloth. If you are cooking the mushrooms, rinse away dirt and grit with cold water just before using, then spin dry in a salad spinner.

2. Meanwhile, pulse reserved mushroom stems, shallot, garlic, and ⅛ teaspoon pepper in food processor until finely chopped, 10 to 14 pulses. Heat remaining 1 tablespoon oil in 8-inch nonstick skillet over medium heat until shimmering. Add stem mixture and cook until dry and golden brown, about 5 minutes. Stir in wine and cook until evaporated and mixture thickens, about 2 minutes. Transfer to bowl and let cool slightly. Stir in 6 tablespoons Parmesan, thyme, and lemon juice.

3. Flip caps gill side up. Divide stuffing evenly among caps and top with remaining 2 tablespoons Parmesan. Bake until stuffing is heated through and Parmesan is golden brown, about 15 minutes. Transfer to serving platter and sprinkle with parsley. Serve.

PER 4-PIECE SERVING
Cal 90 • **Total Fat** 6g • **Sat Fat** 1.5g • **Chol** 5mg
Sodium 190mg • **Total Carbs** 3g • **Fiber** 0g • **Total Sugar** 2g
Added Sugar 0g • **Protein** 3g • **Total Carbohydrate Choices** <0.5

Crispy Polenta Squares with Olives and Sun-Dried Tomatoes
MAKES 24 SQUARES

WHY THIS RECIPE WORKS With their crispy crust and creamy interior, bite-size polenta squares serve as a perfect base for a hearty appetizer that goes beyond the usual things-on-bread recipes. We poured the polenta into a loaf pan and let it firm up in the refrigerator. Once firm, it was easy to slice into bite-size squares. Broiling the polenta on a preheated baking sheet proved to be the best (and most hands-off) method for achieving a nicely browned exterior. We topped the crispy squares with a quick tapenade of sun-dried tomatoes and kalamata olives, brightened with a dash of red wine vinegar. A sprinkle of basil added the perfect herbal and aesthetic finishing touch. Be sure to use instant or quick-cooking polenta; traditional polenta will not work in this recipe.

  2 tablespoons plus 1 teaspoon extra-virgin olive oil
  4 garlic cloves, minced
 ½ teaspoon minced fresh rosemary
  2 cups water
 ½ teaspoon salt
 ½ cup instant polenta
 ¼ teaspoon pepper
 ⅓ cup pitted kalamata olives, chopped fine
 ⅓ cup oil-packed sun-dried tomatoes, patted dry
    and chopped fine
 ½ teaspoon red wine vinegar
  1 tablespoon minced fresh basil

1. Line 8½ by 4½-inch loaf pan with parchment paper and lightly coat with canola oil spray. Cook 4 teaspoons oil and three-quarters of garlic in 8-inch nonstick skillet over low heat, stirring often, until garlic is golden and fragrant, about 10 minutes. Off heat, stir in rosemary; set aside.

2. Bring water to boil in large saucepan. Reduce heat to low and stir in salt. Slowly add polenta while whisking constantly in circular motion to prevent clumping. Continue to cook, stirring often, until polenta is soft and smooth, 3 to 5 minutes. Off heat, stir in oil-garlic mixture and ⅛ teaspoon pepper.

3. Pour polenta into prepared pan, smooth top, and let cool to room temperature, about 2 hours. Wrap pan tightly in plastic wrap and refrigerate until polenta is very firm, at least 2 hours or up to 24 hours.

4. Combine olives, tomatoes, vinegar, remaining 1 tablespoon oil, remaining garlic, and remaining ⅛ teaspoon pepper in bowl; set aside.

5. Run small knife around edge of polenta, then flip onto cutting board; discard parchment. Trim polenta loaf as needed to create uniform edges. Cut loaf in half lengthwise, then cut each strip crosswise into 6 pieces. Slice polenta pieces in half to form ¼-inch-thick squares. (You should have 24 squares.)

6. Adjust oven rack 3 inches from broiler element. (If necessary, set overturned rimmed baking sheet on oven rack to get closer to broiler element.) Place rimmed baking sheet on rack and heat broiler for 10 minutes. Carefully remove sheet from oven. Spray canola oil evenly on hot sheet and arrange squares in single layer. Broil polenta until spotty brown and crisp, 8 to 10 minutes. Transfer polenta to serving platter, top each square with olive mixture, sprinkle with basil, and serve.

PER 3-PIECE SERVING
Cal 90 • **Total Fat** 5g • **Sat Fat** 0.5g • **Chol** 0mg
Sodium 180mg • **Total Carbs** 10g • **Fiber** 1g • **Total Sugar** 0g
Added Sugar 0g • **Protein** 1g • **Total Carbohydrate Choices** 0.5

MAKING POLENTA SQUARES

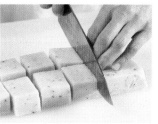 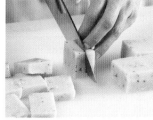

1. Cut trimmed loaf in half lengthwise, then cut each strip crosswise into 6 pieces.

2. Slice polenta pieces in half to form ¼-inch-thick squares.

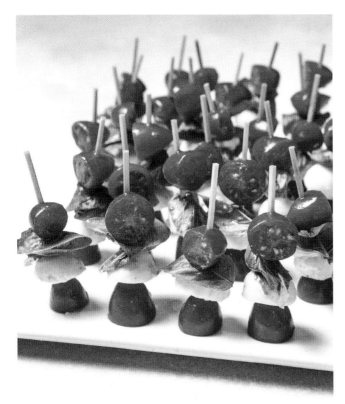

Fresh tomatoes, mozzarella balls, and basil threaded on toothpicks make perfect bite-size appetizers.

Caprese Skewers
SERVES 10

WHY THIS RECIPE WORKS For a tasty and lighter alternative to many skewered appetizers we turned to baby fresh mozzarella balls and bright grape tomatoes. This appetizer take on the caprese salad uses toothpicks to stand bite-size portions upright on a halved grape tomato pedestal. We found that a quick garlic-infused oil, which we made by mincing garlic into a paste and stirring it into fruity extra-virgin olive oil, boosted the flavor of the mozzarella and tomatoes, as did a bit of salt and pepper. Basil leaves, skewered onto our toothpicks whole, completed the caprese flavor profile and added a fresh touch. You will need about 40 sturdy wooden toothpicks for this recipe; avoid using very thin, flimsy toothpicks. Placing a halved grape tomato, with its flat side facing down, on the bottom of the toothpick makes it easy to stand the skewers upright on a serving platter. You can use larger fresh mozzarella balls, but they should be cut into ¾- to 1-inch pieces.

¼ cup extra-virgin olive oil
1 garlic clove, minced
¼ teaspoon salt
⅛ teaspoon pepper
10 ounces grape or cherry tomatoes, halved
8 ounces baby mozzarella balls, halved
1 cup fresh basil leaves

1. Combine oil, garlic, salt, and pepper in small bowl. Toss tomatoes and mozzarella with 2 tablespoons of garlic oil in separate bowl.

2. Skewer tomatoes, mozzarella, and basil leaves on sturdy wooden toothpicks in following order from top to bottom: tomato half, basil leaf (folded if large), mozzarella half, and tomato half with flat side facing down. (You should have about 40 skewers.) Stand skewers upright on serving platter. Drizzle remaining garlic oil over skewers just before serving.

PER 4-SKEWER SERVING
Cal 120 • **Total Fat** 11g • **Sat Fat** 4g • **Chol** 15mg
Sodium 70mg • **Total Carbs** 1g • **Fiber** 0g • **Total Sugar** 1g
Added Sugar 0g • **Protein** 4g • **Total Carbohydrate Choices** <0.5

ASSEMBLING CAPRESE SKEWERS

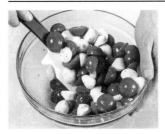

1. After mincing garlic to paste and combining it with olive oil, toss halved tomatoes and mozzarella balls in garlic oil to infuse them with flavor.

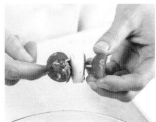

2. Skewer a tomato half, basil leaf (folded if large), mozzarella ball half, and second tomato half, with flat side facing out, onto toothpick. Stand skewers on platter and drizzle with remaining garlic oil.

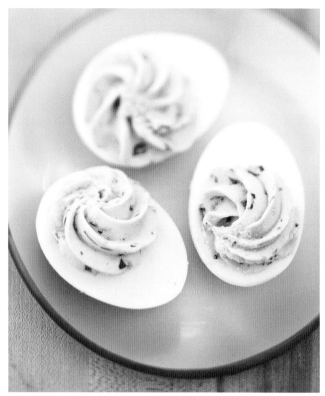

Replacing some of the egg yolks with cottage cheese makes the filling in our deviled eggs smooth and creamy.

Herbed Deviled Eggs
SERVES 6

WHY THIS RECIPE WORKS An essential part of any picnic or cookout, deviled eggs are easy to make, requiring just a handful of ingredients: eggs, mayonnaise, mustard, and a few flavorings. We kept the good fat of regular mayonnaise but took out some of the egg yolks and replaced them with cottage cheese. Pressing the cottage cheese and yolks through a fine-mesh strainer ensured our filling stayed smooth and creamy. A pinch of turmeric reinforced the golden hue of the yolks, and chopped herbs added fresh flavor. For a traditional look, dust the filled eggs with paprika. For filling the eggs, a spoon works fine, but for eggs that look their Sunday best, we prefer to use a pastry bag fitted with a large open-star tip, or make our own pastry bag by pressing the filling into the corner of a zipper-lock bag and snipping off the corner with scissors.

6 large eggs
¼ cup cottage cheese
2 tablespoons mayonnaise
1 tablespoon minced fresh parsley, chives, or cilantro
½ teaspoon white wine vinegar
½ teaspoon Dijon mustard
⅛ teaspoon ground turmeric
⅛ teaspoon ground coriander
⅛ teaspoon salt
⅛ teaspoon pepper

1. Bring 1 inch water to rolling boil in medium saucepan over high heat. Place eggs in steamer basket. Transfer basket to saucepan. Cover, reduce heat to medium-low, and cook eggs for 13 minutes.

2. When eggs are almost finished cooking, combine 2 cups ice cubes and 2 cups cold water in medium bowl. Using tongs or spoon, transfer eggs to ice bath. Let sit for 15 minutes, then peel.

3. Halve eggs lengthwise. Transfer 3 yolks to fine-mesh strainer set over medium bowl (reserve remaining yolks for another use or discard). Arrange whites on large serving platter. Using spatula, press yolks and cottage cheese through fine-mesh strainer into bowl. Stir in mayonnaise, parsley, 1 tablespoon warm water, vinegar, mustard, turmeric, coriander, salt, and pepper until well combined and smooth. (Egg whites and yolk filling can be refrigerated, separately, for up to 2 days.)

4. Fit pastry bag with large open-star tip. Fill bag with yolk mixture, twisting top of pastry bag to help push mixture toward tip of bag. Pipe yolk mixture into egg white halves, mounding filling about ½ inch above flat surface of whites. Serve at room temperature.

PER 2-PIECE SERVING
Cal 110 • **Total Fat** 8g • **Sat Fat** 2.5g • **Chol** 190mg
Sodium 190mg • **Total Carbs** 1g • **Fiber** 0g • **Total Sugar** 1g
Added Sugar 0g • **Protein** 7g • **Total Carbohydrate Choices** <0.5

PIPING DEVILED EGGS FILLING

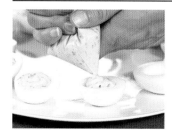

A piping bag can make quick work of filling deviled eggs. But if you don't have one, substitute a zipper-lock bag. Spoon filling into bag and push into one corner. Use scissors to snip off corner of bag, then squeeze filling into each egg.

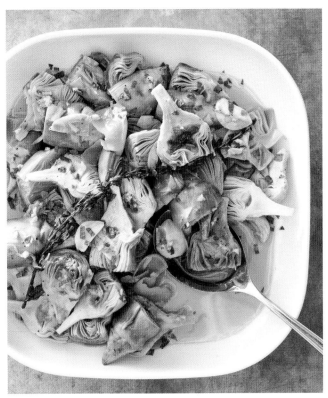

We like to marinate fiber-rich artichokes in olive oil infused with aromatic lemon zest, garlic, red pepper flakes, and thyme.

Marinated Artichokes
SERVES 8

WHY THIS RECIPE WORKS Marinated artichokes have so many uses that they should be considered a pantry staple; they're perfect for everything from throwing on pizzas, to tossing into a salad or pasta, to eating on an antipasto platter. But store-bought versions tend to be mushy and bland—and expensive. We set out to make our own recipe for easy, inexpensive, and boldly flavorful marinated artichokes. To get the best tender-yet-meaty texture and sweet, nutty artichoke flavor, we started with fresh baby artichokes. We simmered them gently in olive oil with strips of lemon zest, garlic, red pepper flakes, and thyme, then let them sit off the heat until they were perfectly fork-tender and infused with the aromatic flavors. Then we stirred in fresh lemon juice and more zest, minced garlic, and mint before transferring the artichokes to a bowl and topping them with some of the infused oil for serving and storage.

PREPARING ARTICHOKES

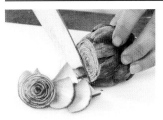

1. Using chef's knife, cut off top quarter of each artichoke.

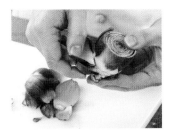

2. Snap off tough outer leaves; trim any remaining dark parts using paring knife.

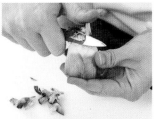

3. Using paring knife, peel stem and trim end.

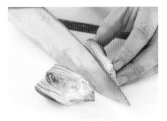

4. Once trimmed, cut artichoke in half.

NOTES FROM THE TEST KITCHEN

Assessing Artichokes

When selecting fresh artichokes at the market, examine the leaves for some clues that will help you pick the best specimens. The leaves should look tight, compact, and bright green; they should not appear dried out or feathery at the edges. If you give an artichoke a squeeze, its leaves should squeak as they rub together (evidence that the artichoke still possesses much of its moisture). The leaves should also snap off cleanly; if they bend, the artichoke is old.

2 lemons

2½ cups extra-virgin olive oil

3 pounds baby artichokes (3 ounces each)

8 garlic cloves (6 peeled and smashed, 2 minced)

¼ teaspoon red pepper flakes

2 sprigs fresh thyme

½ teaspoon salt

¼ teaspoon pepper

2 tablespoons minced fresh mint

1. Using vegetable peeler, remove three 2-inch strips zest from 1 lemon. Grate ½ teaspoon zest from second lemon and set aside. Halve and juice lemons to yield ¼ cup juice, reserving spent lemon halves.

2. Combine oil and lemon zest strips in large saucepan. Working with 1 artichoke at a time, cut top quarter off each, snap off outer leaves, and trim away dark parts. Peel and trim stem, then cut artichoke in half lengthwise (quarter artichoke if large). Rub each artichoke half with spent lemon half and place in saucepan.

3. Add smashed garlic, pepper flakes, thyme sprigs, salt, and pepper to oil in saucepan and bring to rapid simmer over high heat. Reduce heat to medium-low and simmer, stirring occasionally to submerge all artichokes, until artichokes can be pierced with fork but are still firm, about 5 minutes. Remove from heat, cover, and let sit until artichokes are fork-tender and fully cooked, about 20 minutes.

4. Transfer artichokes and ¼ cup oil to serving bowl and gently stir in ½ teaspoon reserved grated lemon zest, ¼ cup reserved lemon juice, and minced garlic. Discard remaining oil or reserve for another use. Let artichokes cool to room temperature. Sprinkle with mint and serve. (Artichokes and reserved oil can be refrigerated separately for up to 4 days.)

PER ¼-CUP SERVING

Cal 100 • **Total Fat** 7g • **Sat Fat** 1g • **Chol** 0mg
Sodium 135mg • **Total Carbs** 8g • **Fiber** 4g • **Total Sugar** 1g
Added Sugar 0g • **Protein** 2g • **Total Carbohydrate Choices** 0.5

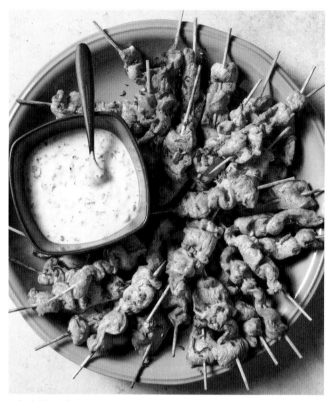

A little bit of plain yogurt tenderizes lean chicken breast and helps to protect it from the high heat of the broiler.

Curried Chicken Skewers with Yogurt Dipping Sauce
MAKES 30

WHY THIS RECIPE WORKS Chicken skewers are often coated in a salty-sugary glaze. Our Indian-inspired rub uses curry powder, paprika, red pepper flakes, garlic powder, and just enough salt. Mixing in a little yogurt coated the chicken to protect it from the heat of the broiler and its acidity tenderized the chicken. The result was moist chicken bursting with flavor. Slicing the chicken thin is essential. A combination of sour cream and yogurt created a tangy base for a sauce, while garlic, fresh mint, and scallions added complementary flavors. The cooking time will depend on the strength and type of your broiler. Under-the-oven drawer broilers tend to take a few minutes longer than in-oven broilers. To make slicing the chicken easier, freeze it first for 30 minutes.

DIPING SAUCE

¾ cup low-fat plain yogurt

¼ cup low-fat sour cream

2 small garlic cloves, minced

3 tablespoons minced fresh mint

2 scallions, sliced thin

¼ teaspoon salt

⅛ teaspoon pepper

CHICKEN

3 tablespoons low-fat plain yogurt

1 tablespoon curry powder

½ teaspoon salt

½ teaspoon paprika

¼ teaspoon red pepper flakes

¼ teaspoon garlic powder

2 pounds boneless, skinless chicken breasts, trimmed

30 (6-inch) wooden skewers

1 tablespoon minced fresh mint

1. FOR THE DIPPING SAUCE Whisk all ingredients together in bowl until smooth. Cover and refrigerate until flavors meld, at least 30 minutes or up to 2 days.

2. FOR THE CHICKEN Combine yogurt, curry powder, salt, paprika, pepper flakes, and garlic powder in a large bowl. Slice chicken diagonally into ¼-inch-thick strips. Add chicken to yogurt mixture and toss to coat. Cover and refrigerate for at least 1 hour or up to 24 hours.

3. Position oven rack 6 inches from broiler element and heat broiler. Set wire rack in aluminum foil–lined rimmed baking sheet and lightly spray with canola oil spray. Weave chicken onto skewers. Lay skewers on prepared rack and cover skewer ends with foil. Broil until chicken is fully cooked, 6 to 8 minutes, flipping skewers halfway through broiling. Transfer skewers to serving platter and sprinkle with mint. Serve with sauce.

PER 3-SKEWER SERVING

Cal 140 • **Total Fat** 3.5g • **Sat Fat** 1g • **Chol** 70mg
Sodium 240mg • **Total Carbs** 3g • **Fiber** 1g • **Total Sugar** 2g
Added Sugar 0g • **Protein** 22g • **Total Carbohydrate Choices** <0.5

ASSEMBLING CHICKEN SKEWERS

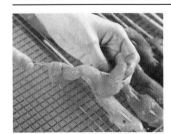

Weave chicken onto skewers, leaving portion of blunt end exposed.

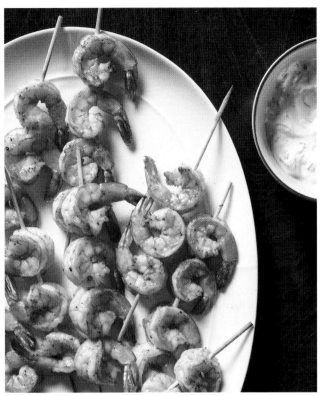

For easy shrimp cocktail that's perfect for entertaining, we skip the usual fussy poaching and let the broiler do the work instead.

Coriander Shrimp Skewers with Lemon-Tarragon Dipping Sauce
MAKES 8

WHY THIS RECIPE WORKS A classic, splurge-worthy crowd-pleasing appetizer, shrimp are a great source of lean, flavorful protein, but are known for being high in sodium. We found through testing that we could develop a shrimp appetizer with big flavor without loading in additional sodium. For the easiest-ever version of a diabetes-friendly shrimp cocktail, we bypassed the traditional method of poaching the shrimp in a work-intensive and salty broth known as a court bouillon, and instead put the high heat of the broiler to work. A simple rub of pepper, coriander, and cayenne infused the shrimp with big flavor without the need for additional salt. Threading 3 or 4 shrimp onto each skewer made for a fun party presentation and helped to ensure proper portions. Instead

Shrimp Basics

Buying Shrimp

Virtually all of the shrimp sold in supermarkets today have been previously frozen, either in large blocks of ice or by a method called "individually quick-frozen," or IQF for short. Supermarkets simply defrost the shrimp before displaying them on ice at the fish counter. We highly recommend purchasing bags of still-frozen shrimp and defrosting them as needed at home, since there is no telling how long "fresh" shrimp may have been kept on ice at the market. IQF shrimp have a better flavor and texture than shrimp frozen in blocks, and they are convenient because it's easy to defrost just the amount you need. Shrimp are sold both with and without their shells, but we find shell-on shrimp to be firmer and sweeter. Also, shrimp should be the only ingredient listed on the bag or box. Some packagers add preservatives, but we find treated shrimp to have an unpleasant texture and sometimes a chemical taste.

Sorting Out Shrimp Sizes

Shrimp are sold both by size (small, medium, etc.) and by the number needed to make 1 pound, usually given in a range. Choosing shrimp by the numerical rating is more accurate, because the size labels vary from store to store. Here's how the two sizing systems generally compare:

SMALL	51 to 60 per pound
MEDIUM	41 to 50 per pound
MEDIUM-LARGE	31 to 40 per pound
LARGE	26 to 30 per pound
EXTRA-LARGE	21 to 25 per pound
JUMBO	16 to 20 per pound

Defrosting Shrimp

You can thaw frozen shrimp overnight in the refrigerator in a covered bowl. For a quicker thaw, place them in a colander under cold running water; they will be ready in a few minutes. Thoroughly dry the shrimp before cooking.

of a traditional cocktail sauce, a creamy herb and lemon dipping sauce was the perfect balance to the broiled shrimp. It's important to dry the shrimp thoroughly before broiling. Covering the exposed ends of the skewers with aluminum foil protects them from burning.

DIPPING SAUCE

- ⅓ cup 2 percent Greek yogurt
- 2 tablespoons mayonnaise
- 1 tablespoon minced fresh tarragon, dill, or basil
- ½ teaspoon grated lemon zest plus 1 teaspoon juice
- 1 garlic clove, minced
  Pepper

SHRIMP

- 1 pound large shrimp (26 to 30 per pound), peeled and deveined
- 2 tablespoons extra-virgin olive oil
- ¾ teaspoon ground coriander
- ¼ teaspoon pepper
  Pinch cayenne pepper
- 8 wooden skewers

1. FOR THE DIPPING SAUCE Whisk all ingredients together in bowl until smooth and season with pepper to taste. Cover and refrigerate until flavors meld, at least 30 minutes or up to 2 days.

2. FOR THE SHRIMP Adjust oven rack 3 inches from broiler element and heat broiler. (If necessary, set overturned rimmed baking sheet on oven rack to get closer to broiler element.) Pat shrimp dry with paper towels, then toss with oil, coriander, pepper, and cayenne in bowl. Thread 3 or 4 shrimp onto each skewer.

3. Set wire rack in aluminum foil–lined rimmed baking sheet and lightly spray with canola oil spray. Lay skewers on prepared rack and cover skewer ends with foil. Broil until shrimp are opaque throughout, 3 to 5 minutes. Transfer skewers to serving platter and serve with sauce.

PER 1-SKEWER SERVING

Cal 90 • **Total Fat** 7g • **Sat Fat** 1g • **Chol** 55mg
Sodium 90mg • **Total Carbs** 1g • **Fiber** 0g • **Total Sugar** 0g
Added Sugar 0g • **Protein** 7g • **Total Carbohydrate Choices** <0.5

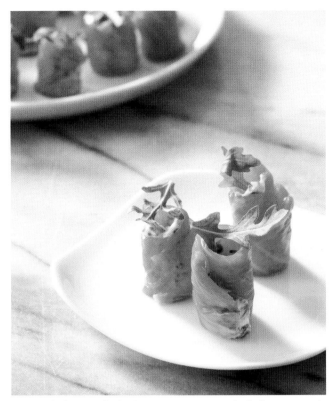

For a carb-free smoked salmon appetizer, we ditch the toast and focus on filling the fish with flavor-packed cream cheese.

Smoked Salmon Rolls
MAKES ABOUT 18

WHY THIS RECIPE WORKS Who doesn't love toast points smeared with cream cheese or crème fraîche and topped with a pile of salty smoked salmon? But that can really tip the scales. This clever little recipe allows you to get your smoked salmon fix without all the unwanted carbs and calories. We flavored cream cheese with lemon juice and pepper, and stirred in minced shallot, capers, and chives so their flavors would be evenly distributed. It's easy then to spread this savory mixture across slices of salmon and simply roll them up for an irresistible appetizer. Be sure to use good-quality, fresh smoked salmon for this recipe; it should glisten and have a bright, rosy color.

- 1 tablespoon cream cheese, softened
- 1 tablespoon low-fat sour cream
- ½ teaspoon lemon juice
    Pinch pepper
- 1 teaspoon minced shallot
- 1 teaspoon capers, rinsed and minced
- 1 teaspoon minced fresh chives or dill
- 9 slices smoked salmon (about 8 ounces)
- 18 small sprigs baby arugula

1. Stir cream cheese, sour cream, lemon juice, and pepper in bowl until smooth, then stir in shallot, capers, and chives.

2. Spread about 1 teaspoon cream cheese mixture evenly over each slice of salmon. Roll salmon around cream cheese mixture. (Salmon rolls can be covered tightly with plastic wrap and refrigerated for up to 4 hours.)

3. Slice each salmon roll in half with sharp knife. Stand each roll on its cut end, garnish with arugula sprig, and serve.

PER 3-PIECE SERVING
Cal 60 • **Total Fat** 2.5g • **Sat Fat** 1g • **Chol** 10mg
Sodium 280mg • **Total Carbs** 1g • **Fiber** 0g • **Total Sugar** 0g
Added Sugar 0g • **Protein** 7g • **Total Carbohydrate Choices** <0.5

MAKING SALMON ROLLS

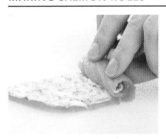

1. Roll the salmon up around the filling.

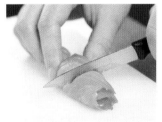

2. Using a sharp knife, slice the salmon roll in half.

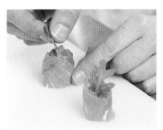

3. Stand up each roll up on its cut end and garnish with a small sprig of arugula.

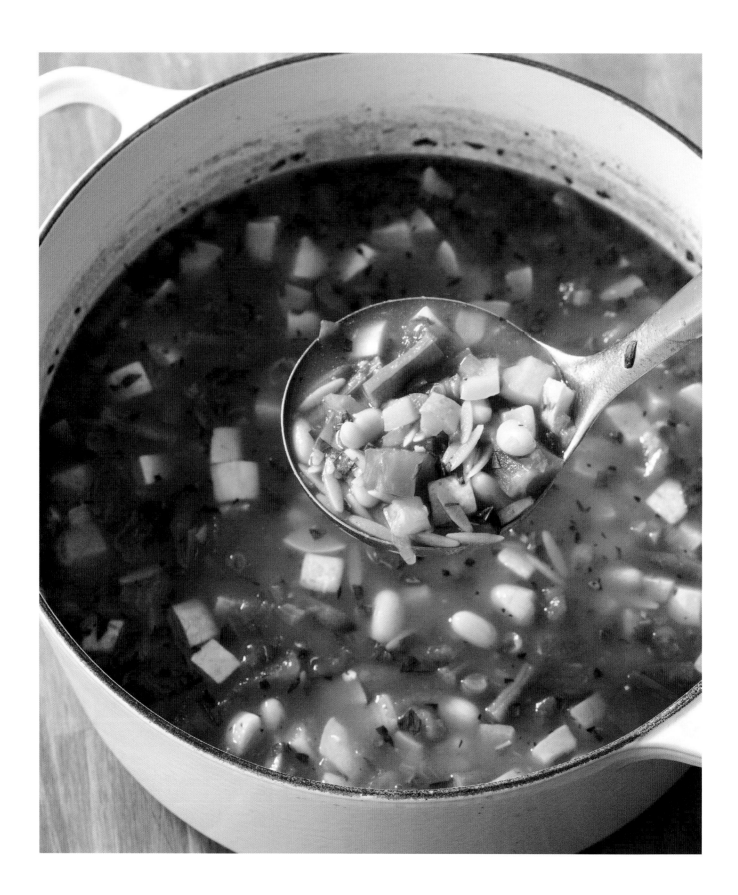

Photo: Garden Minestrone

Creamy Asparagus and Pea Soup
SERVES 6

WHY THIS RECIPE WORKS Creamy vegetable soups don't need to be fancy or laden with cream to be delicious and on target nutritionally. For a creamy asparagus soup, we wanted the sweet, nutty flavor of the asparagus to be the star. We found that sautéing the asparagus spears on medium-low heat coaxed out their flavor. But there was a fine line between perfect and overcooked; for its fresh flavor to translate to the soup, the asparagus needed to be just tender enough to puree, but no more. For the soup's base, we quickly discovered that water was bland (no surprise). A homemade asparagus stock wasn't worth the extra effort, and additions of wine or vermouth turned a delicate soup grassy and acidic. Ultimately, our tasters liked store-bought chicken broth the best. We tested a number of "cream" components, from yogurt to sour cream, crème fraîche, and rice milk, but they were all too heavy, too tangy, or too weird. In the end, just 2 tablespoons of heavy cream tasted just right. To give our pureed soup velvety body and a sweet undertone, we switched from a base of onions to leeks. When pureed they made the soup creamier and added heft. Adding a handful of frozen peas to the asparagus before pureeing improved both the soup's color and body. A small amount of Parmesan echoed the nuttiness of the asparagus, while lemon juice added brightness. Peel the asparagus spears with a vegetable peeler if they are thicker than ½ inch.

- 2 pounds asparagus, trimmed
- 2 tablespoons extra-virgin olive oil
- 12 ounces leeks, white and light green parts only, halved lengthwise and sliced thin
  Salt and pepper
- 3½ cups unsalted chicken broth
- ½ cup frozen peas
- 2 tablespoons grated Parmesan cheese
- 2 tablespoons heavy cream
- 1 teaspoon lemon juice

1. Cut tips off asparagus and chop spears into ½-inch pieces. Heat 1 tablespoon oil in Dutch oven over medium-high heat until shimmering. Add asparagus tips and cook, stirring occasionally, until just tender, about 2 minutes. Transfer tips to bowl and set aside.

2. Add remaining 1 tablespoon oil, asparagus spears, leeks, ¼ teaspoon salt, and ⅛ teaspoon pepper to now-empty pot and cook over medium-low heat, stirring occasionally, until vegetables are softened, about 10 minutes.

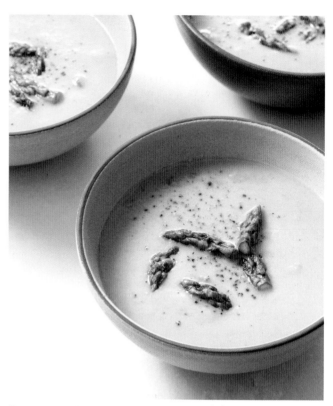

Frozen peas give our asparagus soup a subtle sweetness and a boost of green.

3. Add broth to pot and bring to boil over medium-high heat. Reduce heat to medium-low and simmer until vegetables are tender, about 5 minutes. Stir in peas and Parmesan. Working in batches, process soup in blender until smooth, 1 to 2 minutes. Return soup to clean pot. Stir in cream, lemon juice, asparagus tips, and ⅛ teaspoon salt and cook until warmed through, about 2 minutes. Season with pepper to taste and serve. (Soup can be refrigerated in airtight container for 2 days.)

PER 1-CUP SERVING
Cal 130 • **Total Fat** 7g • **Sat Fat** 2g • **Chol** 5mg
Sodium 270mg • **Total Carbs** 10g • **Fiber** 4g • **Total Sugar** 4g
Added Sugar 0g • **Protein** 7g • **Total Carbohydrate Choices** 0.5

Creamy Carrot-Ginger Soup

SERVES 4

WHY THIS RECIPE WORKS Sometimes the simplest recipes become overcomplicated as more and more versions appear. Case in point: carrot-ginger soup, whose flavors often get pushed aside with the addition of other vegetables and fruits, plus a generous amount of heavy cream. For a fresh, clean-tasting soup, we decided to focus on the basics. A combination of cooked carrots and onion provided depth of flavor and a fresh, pleasantly sweet soup base. Grated ginger contributed brightness and a moderate kick of heat that nicely complemented the carrots' sweetness. A mere 2 tablespoons of orange juice provided brightness and acidity that tasters felt was lacking in previous versions. We kept the fat in check by adding some low-fat milk, which gave our soup the perfect creamy feel and allowed all the flavors to meld. For a little texture and freshness, we finished with a simple garnish of minced chives. Do not substitute ground ginger for the fresh ginger here.

2 tablespoons canola oil
1½ pounds carrots, peeled and chopped
1 onion, chopped fine
   Salt and pepper
1½ tablespoons grated fresh ginger
3 cups unsalted chicken broth
½ cup 1 percent low-fat milk
2 tablespoons orange juice
1 tablespoon minced fresh chives

1. Heat oil in Dutch oven over medium heat until shimmering. Add carrots, onion, and ⅛ teaspoon salt and cook until softened, 8 to 10 minutes.

2. Stir in ginger and cook until fragrant, about 30 seconds. Stir in broth and bring to simmer. Reduce heat to medium-low, cover, and cook until carrots are very tender, about 16 minutes.

3. Working in batches, process soup in blender until smooth, about 1 minute. Return soup to clean pot, stir in milk and orange juice, and bring to brief simmer over medium-low heat. Season with pepper to taste. Sprinkle individual portions with chives before serving.

PER 1½-CUP SERVING
Cal 170 • **Total Fat** 8g • **Sat Fat** 1g • **Chol** 0mg
Sodium 280mg • **Total Carbs** 20g • **Fiber** 5g • **Total Sugar** 11g
Added Sugar 0g • **Protein** 6g • **Total Carbohydrate Choices** 1

Store-Bought Broths

Soup can be a nutritious option, but only if its sodium is in check. The biggest culprit, of course, is the broth. A typical store-bought broth can have 500 milligrams or more of sodium per cup. Because minimizing salt intake is an important part of the diabetes diet, we call for unsalted and low-sodium broths in our recipes. Amping up a soup's flavor in other creative ways means we don't miss the salt. (Note that a label boasting "no salt added" or "unsalted" means that no salt was added during processing; some of these products can still contain quite a bit of naturally occurring sodium, so double-check the label.)

Chicken Broth

We prefer chicken broth to vegetable broth and beef broth for its stronger, cleaner flavor and look for broth with a short ingredient list. Our winning unsalted chicken broth, **Swanson Unsalted Chicken Stock,** contains 130 milligrams of sodium per cup. (The U.S. Department of Agriculture's ceiling for low-sodium foods is 140 milligrams.)

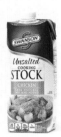

Vegetable Broth

Though most vegetable broths on the market contain excessive amounts of salt, our winning commercial low-sodium vegetable broth, **Edward & Sons Low Sodium Not-Chick'n Natural Bouillon Cubes,** contains 130 milligrams of sodium per cup. This broth contains yeast extract, which is full of glutamates and nucleotides that boost savory umami flavor. It is an important ingredient for manufacturers of low-sodium products, as it enhances the perception of saltiness without any increase in salt.

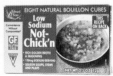

Beef Broth

We have found that the best beef broths have flavor-enhancing ingredients such as tomato paste and yeast extract near the top of their ingredient list and include concentrated beef stock. We had good luck using **Better Than Bouillon Reduced Sodium Beef Base,** which contains 510 milligrams of sodium per serving (their traditional Beef Base contains 680 milligrams).

Creamy Butternut Squash Soup
SERVES 8

WHY THIS RECIPE WORKS Butternut squash soup should be a simple soup—little more than squash, cooking liquid, and a few aromatic ingredients—that comes together easily, yet is creamy and deeply flavorful. But many squash soups fail to live up to their potential, often ending up too sweet or with too little squash flavor. We got the most flavor out of our squash by first roasting it along with onion; the natural sugars caramelized (no need for added sugar) and the flavor intensified. Sautéing the roasted vegetables in oil rather than butter helped to keep the saturated fat minimal. We further enhanced the squash's flavor by adding garlic and deglazing the pot with a splash of wine. A quick spin in the blender transformed the squash into a smooth puree, and a bit of half-and-half added richness. We finished the soup with a drizzle of balsamic vinegar, which balanced the squash's earthy flavor with a punch of brightness and tang. For a variation with a more savory flavor profile that didn't stray too far from its origin, we reduced the amount of squash in favor of fennel.

    3 pounds butternut squash, peeled, seeded,
      and cut into ½-inch pieces (8 cups)
    1 onion, halved and sliced ½ inch thick
    4 teaspoons canola oil
    ¼ teaspoon salt
    3 garlic cloves, minced
    ¼ cup dry white wine
 7½ cups low-sodium vegetable broth
    1 bay leaf
    ½ cup half-and-half
    4 teaspoons balsamic vinegar

1. Adjust oven racks to upper-middle and lower-middle positions and heat oven to 450 degrees. Toss squash and onion with 1 tablespoon oil and salt and spread into even layer on two rimmed baking sheets. Roast, stirring occasionally, until vegetables are softened and lightly browned, 30 to 40 minutes.

2. Heat remaining 1 teaspoon oil in Dutch over medium heat until shimmering. Add squash and onion and cook, stirring often, until squash begins to break down, 3 to 5 minutes. Stir in garlic and cook until fragrant, about 30 seconds.

3. Stir in wine, scraping up any browned bits, and cook until nearly evaporated, about 1 minute. Stir in broth and bay leaf and bring to simmer. Reduce heat to medium-low, cover, and cook until flavors meld, about 5 minutes.

4. Discard bay leaf. Working in batches, process soup in blender until smooth, about 1 minute. Return soup to clean pot, stir in half-and-half, and bring to brief simmer over medium-low heat. Drizzle individual portions with vinegar before serving.

PER 1-CUP SERVING

Cal 120 • **Total Fat** 5g • **Sat Fat** 1.5g • **Chol** 5mg
Sodium 210mg • **Total Carbs** 18g • **Fiber** 3g • **Total Sugar** 4g
Added Sugar 0g • **Protein** 2g • **Total Carbohydrate Choices** 1

VARIATION
Creamy Butternut Squash Soup with Fennel
Reduce squash to 2 pounds (5 cups). Toss squash and onion mixture with 2 fennel bulbs, stalks discarded, bulbs halved, cored, and chopped, and 1 teaspoon fennel seeds before roasting.

PER 1-CUP SERVING

Cal 130 • **Total Fat** 5g • **Sat Fat** 1.5g • **Chol** 5mg
Sodium 240mg • **Total Carbs** 18g • **Fiber** 4g • **Total Sugar** 6g
Added Sugar 0g • **Protein** 2g • **Total Carbohydrate Choices** 1

CUTTING UP BUTTERNUT SQUASH

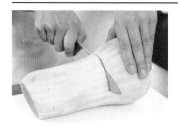 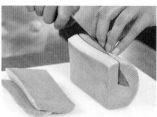 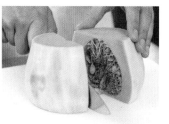 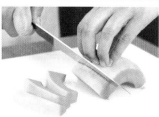

1. After peeling squash, trim off top and bottom and cut squash in two between narrow neck and wide curved bottom.

2. Cut squash neck into evenly sized planks, then cut planks into evenly sized pieces, according to recipe.

3. Cut squash base in half lengthwise, then scoop out and discard seeds and fibers.

4. Slice each base half into evenly sized lengths. Cut lengths into evenly sized pieces, according to recipe.

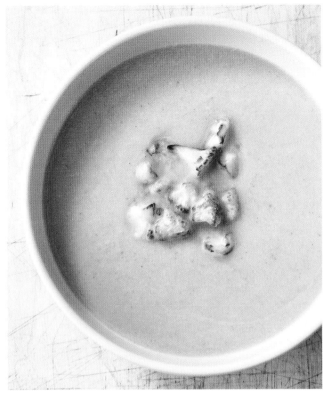

Because cauliflower is low in insoluble fiber, when it is cooked and pureed it is creamy and silky without any cream.

Creamy Curried Cauliflower Soup
SERVES 8

WHY THIS RECIPE WORKS Cauliflower soups are often loaded with cream and thickened with flour, making them neither healthy nor appealing. We wanted a nourishing soup with a creamy texture that wouldn't weigh us down. Though cauliflower is high in soluble fiber, it's lower in insoluble fiber, which helps the vegetable easily blend into a velvety puree, so no cream was needed. We added the cauliflower to simmering water in two stages to bring out the grassy flavor of just-cooked cauliflower and the sweeter, nuttier flavor of longer-cooked cauliflower. Curry powder and ginger bloomed in olive oil gave our soup a unique flavor profile. Light coconut milk and lime juice complemented the spices and rounded out the soup. For an attractive, nutritious garnish, we sautéed some reserved florets until perfectly caramelized. Be sure to thoroughly trim the cauliflower's core of green leaves and leaf stems, which can be fibrous and contribute to a grainy texture in the soup.

1 head cauliflower (2 pounds)
¼ cup extra-virgin olive oil
1 tablespoon grated fresh ginger
1 tablespoon curry powder
1 leek, white and light green parts only, halved lengthwise, sliced thin, and washed thoroughly
1 small onion, halved and sliced thin
Salt and pepper
4½ cups water
½ cup canned light coconut milk
1 teaspoon lime juice

1. Pull off outer leaves of cauliflower and trim stem. Using paring knife, cut around core to remove; slice core thin and reserve. Cut heaping 1 cup of ½-inch florets from head of cauliflower; set aside. Cut remaining cauliflower crosswise into ½-inch-thick slices.

2. Heat 3 tablespoons oil in large saucepan over medium heat until shimmering. Add ginger and curry powder and cook until fragrant, about 1 minute. Add leek, onion, and ¼ teaspoon salt and cook, stirring often, until softened but not browned, about 7 minutes. Stir in water, sliced core, and half of sliced cauliflower. Bring to simmer and cook for 15 minutes. Stir in remaining sliced cauliflower and simmer until cauliflower is tender and crumbles easily, 15 to 20 minutes.

3. Meanwhile, heat remaining 1 tablespoon oil in 8-inch skillet over medium heat until shimmering. Add reserved florets and cook, stirring often, until golden brown, 6 to 8 minutes; transfer to bowl and season with pepper to taste.

4. Working in batches, process soup in blender until smooth, about 1 minute. Return soup to clean saucepan and bring to brief simmer over medium-low heat. Off heat, stir in coconut milk, lime juice, and ½ teaspoon salt. Top individual portions with florets before serving.

PER 1-CUP SERVING
Cal 130 • **Total Fat** 9g • **Sat Fat** 2g • **Chol** 0mg
Sodium 270mg • **Total Carbs** 11g • **Fiber** 3g • **Total Sugar** 4g
Added Sugar 0g • **Protein** 3g • **Total Carbohydrate Choices** 1

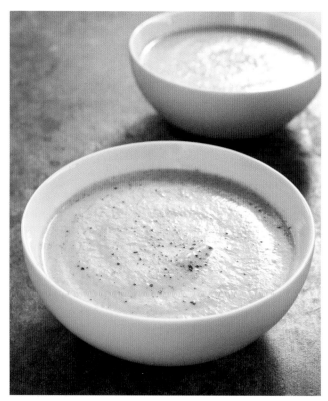

Swapping out regular cheddar for extra-sharp allows us to use less cheese without compromising the soup's cheesy flavor.

Creamy Broccoli-Cheddar Soup
SERVES 8

WHY THIS RECIPE WORKS Though broccoli is one of the most nutritious foods out there, broccoli-cheddar soup can clock in at over 600 calories thanks to an abundance of cheese and heavy cream. We wanted to transform this classic into a lighter dish more reminiscent of its healthy roots. To get the same velvety texture without cream, we'd have to find a substitute. Simply replacing the cream with milk or half-and-half resulted in thin, watery soup. Fat-free evaporated milk, on the other hand, worked like a charm. As for the cheddar, some recipes call for as much as a pound. But we found that switching to a bolder cheese—extra-sharp cheddar— infused our soup with so much flavor that we were able to cut back to just 3 ounces. For more broccoli flavor, we made use of the often-discarded stalks and added them to the pot. Once pureed, our broccoli-cheddar soup offered the rich texture, subtle broccoli flavor, and bold cheddar taste that we were craving.

1 tablespoon extra-virgin olive oil
1½ pounds broccoli, florets cut into 1-inch pieces, stalks peeled and sliced ¼ inch thick
1 pound leeks, white and light green parts only, halved lengthwise, sliced thin, and washed thoroughly
2 garlic cloves, minced
3 cups unsalted chicken broth
1 cup water
¾ cup fat-free evaporated milk
3 ounces extra-sharp cheddar cheese, shredded (¾ cup)
1 tablespoon Dijon mustard
Salt and pepper

1. Heat oil in Dutch oven over medium heat until shimmering. Add broccoli stalks and leeks and cook until softened, 8 to 10 minutes. Stir in garlic and cook until fragrant, about 30 seconds.

2. Stir in broth and water and bring to simmer. Reduce heat to medium-low, cover, and cook until broccoli stalks are softened, about 8 minutes. Stir in broccoli florets, cover, and cook until tender, about 5 minutes.

PREPARING BROCCOLI

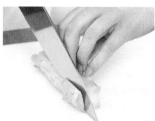

1. Place broccoli head upside down on cutting board and, with large knife, trim off florets very close to their heads. Cut florets into 1-inch pieces.

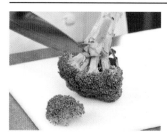

2. Trim four sides of stalk, removing tough outer layer.

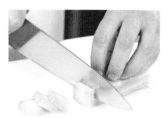

3. Continue to cut squared stalk into pieces as directed.

3. Working in batches, process soup in blender with milk, cheddar, mustard, and ¼ teaspoon salt until cheese is melted and soup is smooth, about 1 minute. Return soup to clean pot and bring to gentle simmer over medium-low heat. Season with pepper to taste. Serve.

PER 1-CUP SERVING

Cal 130 • **Total Fat** 6g • **Sat Fat** 2.5g • **Chol** 10mg
Sodium 300mg • **Total Carbs** 13g • **Fiber** 3g • **Total Sugar** 6g
Added Sugar 0g • **Protein** 8g • **Total Carbohydrate Choices** 1

Creamy Mushroom Soup
SERVES 6

WHY THIS RECIPE WORKS For a lighter creamy mushroom soup that boasted the deep, woodsy flavor and luxurious, velvety texture of the full-fat favorite, we started with a substantial amount of nutrient-dense mushrooms. We cooked them, covered, in a bit of olive oil, then removed the lid so the moisture could evaporate and the mushrooms could brown. Thinly sliced leeks added a delicate sweetness to the soup. For the liquid, beef broth and Madeira proved to be the perfect combination—the beef broth accentuated the mushrooms' meaty, savory notes, while the Madeira complemented their earthiness. After trying many types of dairy options to thin out the soup, we settled on half-and-half, which gave the soup the right richness and silky texture without overwhelming the mushroom flavor. A squeeze of lemon juice cut through the richness. For some textural interest, we crisped some finely chopped mushrooms and sprinkled them on before serving. You can use brandy or dry sherry in place of the Madeira.

    4 teaspoons extra-virgin olive oil
    2 pounds white mushrooms, trimmed and quartered
    1 pound leeks, white and light green parts only, halved
      lengthwise, sliced thin, and washed thoroughly
      Pepper
    4 garlic cloves, minced
    2 teaspoons minced fresh thyme or ½ teaspoon dried
    3 cups low-sodium beef broth
    2 cups water
    ½ cup Madeira
    ½ cup half-and-half
    2 teaspoons lemon juice
    2 tablespoons minced fresh chives

1. Heat 1 tablespoon oil in Dutch oven over medium heat until shimmering. Add mushrooms, leeks, and ¼ teaspoon pepper, cover, and cook until mushrooms have released their liquid, 8 to 10 minutes. Uncover, increase heat to medium-high, and continue to cook, stirring occasionally, until mushrooms are dry and browned, 8 to 12 minutes. Transfer ⅔ cup of mushroom mixture to cutting board and chop fine; set aside.

2. Stir garlic and thyme into pot and cook until fragrant, about 30 seconds. Stir in broth, water, and Madeira and bring to simmer. Reduce heat to low, cover, and cook until mushrooms and leeks are completely tender, 20 to 25 minutes.

3. Working in batches, process soup in blender until smooth, about 1 minute. Return soup to clean pot, stir in half-and-half and lemon juice, and bring to brief simmer over medium-low heat. Season with pepper to taste.

4. Meanwhile, heat remaining 1 teaspoon oil in 8-inch nonstick skillet over medium-high heat until shimmering. Add reserved mushroom mixture and cook, stirring often, until dried and well browned, 5 to 7 minutes. Sprinkle individual portions with mushroom mixture and chives before serving.

PER 1¼-CUP SERVING

Cal 130 • **Total Fat** 6g • **Sat Fat** 2g • **Chol** 5mg
Sodium 290mg • **Total Carbs** 12g • **Fiber** 1g • **Total Sugar** 6g
Added Sugar 0g • **Protein** 4g • **Total Carbohydrate Choices** 1

NOTES FROM THE TEST KITCHEN

Pureeing Soup

Because pureeing hot soup can be dangerous, follow our safety tips.

Blender Is Best
The blade on the blender does the best job with soups because it pulls ingredients down from the top of the container. No stray bits go untouched by the blade. And as long as plenty of headroom is left at the top of the blender, there is no leakage. Immersion blenders and food processors can leave unblended bits of food behind (though this may be intentional for some recipes).

Wait Before Blending, and Blend in Batches
When blending hot soup, wait 5 minutes for moderate cooling, and fill the blender only two-thirds full; otherwise, the soup can explode out the top. Hold the lid securely with a dish towel to keep it in place and to protect your hand from steam. Pulse a few times before blending continuously.

Successful Soup Making

Making a great pot of soup, stew, or chili requires attention to detail, the right ingredients, well-made equipment, and a good recipe.

Sauté Aromatics

The first step in making many soups is sautéing aromatics such as onion and garlic. Sautéing softens their texture so that there is no unwelcome crunch in the soup, and it tames harsh flavors and develops complex flavors in the process.

Start with Good Broth

Store-bought broth is a convenient option, and many brands now offer low-sodium options. To learn more and for our recommended brands, see page 59.

Cut Vegetables to the Right Size

Haphazardly cut vegetables will cook unevenly; larger pieces will be underdone and crunchy, while smaller ones will be mushy. Cutting vegetables evenly to the size specified in the recipe ensures that they will be perfectly cooked.

Stagger the Addition of Vegetables

When a soup contains a variety of vegetables, they are often added in stages to account for their varied cooking times. Hardy vegetables like potatoes and winter squash need much more cooking than delicate asparagus and spinach.

Simmer, Don't Boil

The fine line between simmering and boiling can make a big difference in your soups. A simmer is a restrained version of a boil; fewer bubbles break the surface. Simmering heats food through more gently and more evenly; boiling can cause vegetables such as potatoes to break apart.

Season Just Before Serving

For the recipes in this book we kept a close eye on sodium and developed our recipes with flavor boosters that would keep them tasting bright and well seasoned without a heavy hand with salt. But we still like to give finished dishes a flavor boost at the end since pepper and delicate herbs and lemon juice can have their maximum impact just before serving. For our simple vegetable soups, particularly pureed soups, we also like to include easy garnishes like chopped chives, caramelized vegetables, or a splash of vinegar.

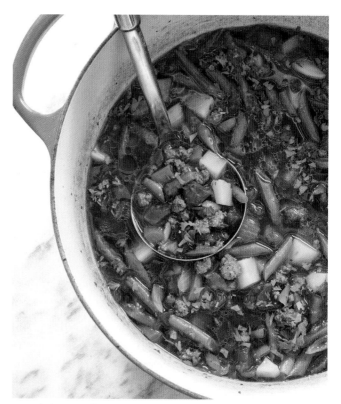

For a lighter beef soup, we turn to quick-cooking lean ground beef simmered with plenty of veggies and flavorful aromatics.

Quick Beef and Vegetable Soup
SERVES 6

WHY THIS RECIPE WORKS Beef-based soups and stews tend to be heavy, but we wanted a hearty beef soup that was full of vegetables and didn't weigh us down. We opted for quick-cooking ground beef, a great alternative to beef cubes that still offered plenty of meatiness. Cutting the vegetables into small pieces sped up their cooking time and cooking the beef, carrots, and aromatics simultaneously over medium-high heat meant this family-pleasing soup could come together quickly. Canned tomatoes and tomato paste provided a flavorful backbone. Once the potatoes cooked through in the simmering broth, we stirred in the green beans, which didn't need quite as much time to cook through as the potatoes. A final sprinkle of parsley added freshness, and our soup was ready in only half an hour.

1 pound 93 percent lean ground beef
2 carrots, peeled and cut into ½-inch pieces
1 onion, chopped

2 garlic cloves, minced

1 tablespoon no-salt-added tomato paste

2 teaspoons minced fresh thyme or ½ teaspoon dried
  Salt and pepper

4 cups low-sodium beef broth

2 cups water

1 (14.5-ounce) can no-salt-added diced tomatoes

8 ounces Yukon Gold potatoes, peeled and cut into
  ½-inch pieces

6 ounces green beans, trimmed and cut into 1-inch lengths

2 tablespoons chopped fresh parsley

1. Cook beef, carrots, onion, garlic, tomato paste, thyme, ⅛ teaspoon salt, and ¼ teaspoon pepper in Dutch oven over medium-high heat, breaking up beef with wooden spoon, until beef is no longer pink, about 6 minutes. Stir in broth, water, tomatoes and their juice, and potatoes. Bring to simmer, then reduce heat to low, cover, and cook until potatoes are almost tender, about 10 minutes.

2. Stir in green beans and cook, uncovered, until vegetables are tender and soup has thickened slightly, 10 to 12 minutes. Stir in parsley and season with pepper to taste. Serve.

PER 2-CUP SERVING

Cal 200 • **Total Fat** 5g • **Sat Fat** 2g • **Chol** 50mg
Sodium 470mg • **Total Carbs** 18g • **Fiber** 4g • **Total Sugar** 5g
Added Sugar 0g • **Protein** 19g • **Total Carbohydrate Choices** 1

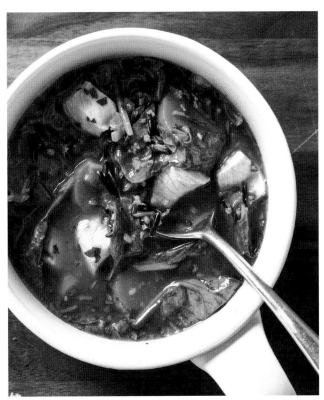

Nutrient-dense wild rice takes the place of white pasta or rice in this comforting garlicky chicken soup.

Garlic-Chicken and Wild Rice Soup
SERVES 6

WHY THIS RECIPE WORKS There's nothing like a bowl of steaming chicken soup when you're feeling under the weather, or even simply when fall turns to winter. But we wanted to transform this soup, often made with white rice or pasta and lacking in veggies, into a comforting, nutrient-dense meal. We started by infusing our chicken broth with a megadose of garlic, before adding tender morsels of chicken. We tested our way through increasing amounts of garlic, starting with what we thought was a hefty amount—2 tablespoons. Much to our surprise and satisfaction, tasters rallied behind a whopping half cup of minced garlic, praising its bright yet balanced presence in our full-flavored soup. Mincing and blooming the garlic before adding liquid gave it a toasty sweetness without having to roast it. To build flavor, we added aromatic vegetables, thyme, bay leaves, and tomato paste along with our chicken broth. To incorporate a whole grain, we opted for toothsome wild rice, cooking it directly in the soup to infuse it with garlicky flavor. To keep our chicken tender, we simmered it during the last few minutes of cooking. Baby spinach and a generous amount of chopped parsley gave the soup a vegetal boost that complemented the deep garlic notes.

3 tablespoons extra-virgin olive oil

½ cup minced garlic (about 25 cloves)

2 carrots, peeled and sliced ¼ inch thick

1 onion, chopped fine

1 celery rib, minced
  Salt and pepper

2 teaspoons minced fresh thyme or ½ teaspoon dried

1 teaspoon no-salt-added tomato paste

6 cups unsalted chicken broth

2 bay leaves

⅔ cup wild rice, rinsed

8 ounces boneless, skinless chicken breasts, trimmed of
  all visible fat and cut into ¾-inch pieces

3 ounces (3 cups) baby spinach

¼ cup chopped fresh parsley

1. Heat oil and garlic in Dutch oven over medium-low heat, stirring occasionally, until garlic is light golden and fragrant, 3 to 5 minutes. Increase heat to medium and add carrots, onion, celery, and ¼ teaspoon salt. Cook, stirring occasionally, until vegetables are softened and lightly browned, 10 to 12 minutes.

2. Stir in thyme and tomato paste and cook until fragrant, about 30 seconds. Stir in broth and bay leaves, scraping up any browned bits. Stir in rice and bring to simmer. Reduce heat to medium-low, cover, and cook until rice is tender, 40 to 50 minutes.

3. Discard bay leaves. Reduce heat to low and stir in chicken and spinach. Cook, stirring occasionally, until chicken is cooked through and spinach is wilted, 3 to 5 minutes. Off heat, stir in parsley and season with pepper to taste. Serve.

PER 1½-CUP SERVING

Cal 240 • **Total Fat** 9g • **Sat Fat** 1g • **Chol** 30mg
Sodium 280mg **Total Carbs** 25g • **Fiber** 4g • **Total Sugar** 3g
Added Sugar 0g • **Protein** 17g • **Total Carbohydrate Choices** 1.5

Chicken Tortilla Soup with Greens
SERVES 8

WHY THIS RECIPE WORKS With its brothy base, bold flavors, and lean protein, chicken tortilla soup has the potential to be a great diabetes-friendly dinner choice. To keep the salt in check, we used unsalted chicken broth and no-salt-added canned diced tomatoes as the soup's base. We also lightly seasoned our tortilla strips with just a quarter teaspoon of salt. For the meat, we used bone-in, skin-on chicken breasts, which we browned first, then poached in the broth after removing the skin. Once cooked and cooled, we shredded the meat and added it back into the soup. Chipotle chiles added a subtle punch of heat. For a deeper vegetal flavor and heartier texture, we sautéed chard stems with onion and garlic, then stirred the chard leaves into the soup at the end of cooking. Different brands of corn tortillas come in varying thicknesses; the cooking time for the tortilla strips may vary based on how thick yours are. For a spicier soup, use the larger amount of chipotle.

  8 (6-inch) corn tortillas, cut into ½-inch strips
  2 tablespoons canola oil
    Salt
1½ pounds bone-in split chicken breasts, trimmed
 12 ounces Swiss chard, stems chopped, leaves cut into 1-inch pieces
  1 onion, chopped fine
  1 tablespoon no-salt-added tomato paste

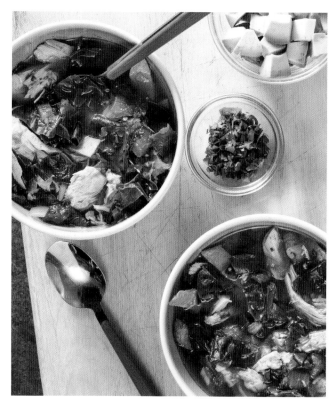

For a heartier chicken tortilla soup, we incorporate Swiss chard, using both the stems and leaves.

1–3 tablespoons minced canned chipotle chile in adobo sauce
  1 (14.5-ounce) can no-salt-added diced tomatoes, drained
  2 garlic cloves, minced
  8 cups unsalted chicken broth
  1 avocado, halved, pitted, and cut into ½-inch pieces
  1 cup fresh cilantro leaves

1. Adjust oven rack to middle position and heat oven to 425 degrees. Toss tortilla strips with 1 tablespoon oil and spread evenly onto rimmed baking sheet. Bake, stirring occasionally, until strips are deep golden brown and crisp, 8 to 12 minutes. Sprinkle tortillas with ¼ teaspoon salt and transfer to paper towel–lined plate.

2. Pat chicken dry with paper towels. Heat remaining 1 tablespoon oil in Dutch oven over medium-high heat until just smoking. Brown chicken, 3 to 5 minutes per side; transfer to plate and discard skin.

3. Add chard stems, onion, and ½ teaspoon salt to fat left in pot and cook until softened, about 5 minutes. Stir in tomato paste, chipotle plus sauce, and tomatoes and cook until mixture is dry and slightly darkened, 5 to 7 minutes. Stir in garlic and cook until fragrant, about 30 seconds.

4. Stir in broth, scraping up any browned bits. Nestle chicken into pot along with any accumulated juices and bring to simmer. Reduce heat to medium-low, cover, and cook until chicken registers 160 degrees, 16 to 18 minutes. Transfer chicken to plate, let cool slightly, then shred into bite-size pieces using 2 forks.

5. Return soup to simmer, stir in chard leaves, and cook until mostly tender, about 5 minutes. Off heat, stir in chicken and let sit until heated through, about 5 minutes. Divide tortilla strips among individual serving bowls and ladle soup over top. Top with avocado and cilantro before serving.

PER 1½-CUP SERVING

Cal 270 • **Total Fat** 10g • **Sat Fat** 1.5g • **Chol** 60mg
Sodium 500mg • **Total Carbs** 19g • **Fiber** 5g • **Total Sugar** 3g
Added Sugars 0g • **Protein** 26g • **Total Carbohydrate Choices** 1

Italian Vegetable Soup
SERVES 6

WHY THIS RECIPE WORKS A rich-tasting Italian soup complete with pasta and vegetables usually requires lots of time for all the prep. For a streamlined version, we started with store-bought chicken broth and looked for ways to enhance its flavor. Upping our aromatics to 6 cloves of garlic and 3 bay leaves gave the soup backbone, but we found that reserving some of the garlic and stirring it in raw at the end of cooking is what really punched up the flavor profile. A healthy combination of zucchini, curly-leaf spinach, peas, and fresh basil added substance and allowed us to rely less on carb-heavy pasta. We prefer the flavor and texture of whole-wheat pasta shells in this soup.

- 2 **tablespoons extra-virgin olive oil**
- 1 **onion, chopped fine**
- ¼ **teaspoon salt**
- 1 **teaspoon minced fresh thyme or ¼ teaspoon dried**
- 6 **garlic cloves, minced**
- 8 **cups unsalted chicken broth**
- 3 **bay leaves**
- 8 **ounces (3¼ cups) medium whole-wheat shells**
- 1 **zucchini, halved lengthwise, seeded, and cut into ½-inch pieces**
- 12 **ounces curly-leaf spinach, stemmed and chopped coarse**
- 2 **cups frozen peas**
- ¼ **cup chopped fresh basil**
- ¼ **teaspoon grated lemon zest**
- 6 **tablespoons grated Parmesan cheese**

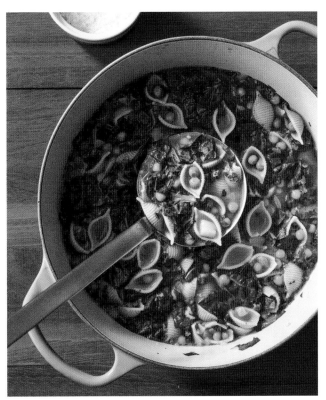

We take the time to remove the seeds from the zucchini so it will have a more appealing texture in the soup.

1. Heat 1 tablespoon oil in Dutch oven over medium heat until simmering. Add onion and salt and cook until softened, about 5 minutes. Stir in thyme and two-thirds of garlic and cook until fragrant, about 30 seconds. Stir in broth and bay leaves, scraping up any browned bits, and bring to simmer.

2. Stir in pasta and cook for 8 minutes. Stir in zucchini and cook until pasta and zucchini are just tender, 3 to 5 minutes. Stir in spinach and peas and cook until spinach is wilted, about 3 minutes.

3. Discard bay leaves. Stir in basil, lemon zest, remaining 1 tablespoon oil, and remaining garlic. Sprinkle individual portions with Parmesan before serving.

PER 1½-CUP SERVING

Cal 280 • **Total Fat** 8g • **Sat Fat** 1.5g • **Chol** 5mg
Sodium 440mg • **Total Carbs** 36g • **Fiber** 9g • **Total Sugar** 6g
Added Sugar 0g • **Protein** 18g • **Total Carbohydrate Choices** 2.5

Hearty Cabbage Soup
SERVES 8

WHY THIS RECIPE WORKS Often a dieter's frenemy, cabbage has the bad reputation of being overbearing in taste, limp in texture, and smelly when cooked. But this humble vegetable has loads of potential for a healthy and satisfying soup. Too often, though, cabbage soup tastes weak and one-dimensional, consisting of little besides cabbage and broth. For a satisfying version, we started with ground chicken, a great lean source of protein with much less sodium than sausage (a common pairing with cabbage). Sweating the aromatics helped to amp up the flavor of the soup. Caraway seeds were a perfect pairing with the cabbage while hot smoked paprika provided depth of flavor. Cooking the cabbage for about 30 minutes rendered it tender but still holding its texture. The addition of potatoes helped turn this soup into a hearty meal. Before serving we add ½ cup low-fat sour cream for richness and tang. If added directly to the soup, the sour cream may curdle and create unattractive lumps; adding a little hot broth to the sour cream (a technique known as tempering) raises its temperature and helps stabilize it so it can be slowly stirred into the soup without fear of curdling. Avoid red cabbage; it will discolor the soup.

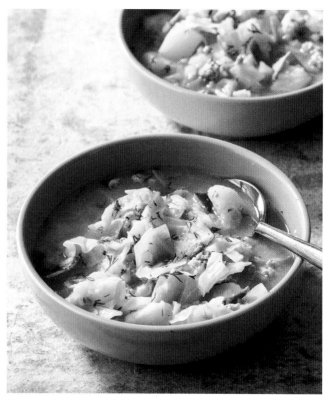

Ground chicken contributes good lean protein and heartiness to our cabbage soup.

3 tablespoons canola oil
1 pound ground chicken
1 onion, chopped fine
2 teaspoons caraway seeds, toasted
  Salt and pepper
5 garlic cloves, minced
1 teaspoon minced fresh thyme or ¼ teaspoon dried
½ teaspoon hot smoked paprika
¼ cup dry white wine
1 head green cabbage (2 pounds), cored and cut into ¾-inch pieces
8 cups unsalted chicken broth
1 bay leaf
12 ounces red potatoes, unpeeled, cut into ¾-inch pieces
½ cup low-fat sour cream
1 tablespoons minced fresh dill

1. Heat oil in Dutch oven over medium heat until shimmering. Add chicken, onion, caraway seeds, and ¼ teaspoon salt and cook, breaking up chicken with wooden spoon, until chicken is no longer pink and onion is softened, 7 to 9 minutes.

2. Stir in garlic, thyme, and paprika and cook until fragrant, about 30 seconds. Stir in wine, scraping up any browned bits, and cook until nearly evaporated. Stir in cabbage, broth, and bay leaf and bring to simmer. Reduce heat to medium-low, cover, and cook for 15 minutes. Stir in potatoes and continue to cook until vegetables are tender, 15 to 20 minutes.

3. Discard bay leaf. Stir a few tablespoons of hot broth into sour cream to temper, then stir sour cream mixture and ½ teaspoon salt into pot. Stir in dill and season with pepper to taste. Serve.

PER 1½-CUP SERVING
Cal 240 • **Total Fat** 11g • **Sat Fat** 2g • **Chol** 40mg
Sodium 430mg • **Total Carbs** 18g • **Fiber** 5g • **Total Sugar** 7g
Added Sugar 0 • **Protein** 17g • **Total Carbohydrate Choices** 1

Mushroom and Wheat Berry Soup
SERVES 8

WHY THIS RECIPE WORKS This hearty soup features a combination of mushrooms and wheat berries that makes it taste satisfying and substantial but not heavy. Wheat berries, whole unprocessed kernels of wheat, are an excellent source of nutrients. To bring out their nutty flavor, we toasted them in a dry Dutch oven. Next we slowly cooked our cremini mushrooms in the covered pot to concentrate their flavors and extract the juices. To amplify the earthiness of the wheat berries and creminis, we built a flavorful base from ground dried shiitake mushrooms, tomato paste, soy sauce, dry sherry, and plenty of garlic. Grinding the shiitakes ensured that their flavor permeated the broth. After simmering the wheat berries, we finished the soup with fiber-rich mustard greens and some lemon zest and juice for freshness. White mushrooms can be substituted for the cremini. We used a spice grinder to process the dried shiitake mushrooms, but a blender also works.

1 cup wheat berries, rinsed
3 tablespoons extra-virgin olive oil
1½ pounds cremini mushrooms, trimmed and sliced thin
¼ teaspoon salt
1 onion, chopped fine
6 garlic cloves, minced
2 teaspoons no-salt-added tomato paste
1 cup dry sherry
8 cups unsalted chicken broth
1 tablespoon low-sodium soy sauce
1 sprig fresh thyme
1 bay leaf
½ ounce dried shiitake mushrooms, finely ground using spice grinder
4 ounces mustard greens, stemmed and chopped
¼ teaspoon grated lemon zest plus 2 teaspoons juice

1. Toast wheat berries in Dutch oven over medium heat, stirring often, until fragrant and beginning to darken, about 5 minutes; transfer to bowl.

2. Heat 2 tablespoons oil in now-empty pot over medium heat until shimmering. Add cremini mushrooms and salt, cover, and cook until mushrooms have released their liquid, about 3 minutes. Uncover, increase heat to medium-high, and continue to cook, stirring occasionally, until mushrooms are dry and begin to brown, 5 to 7 minutes; transfer to plate.

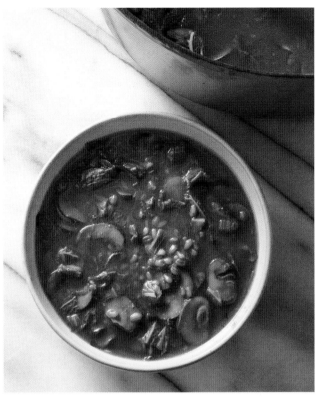

We briefly toast fiber-rich wheat berries to bring out their nutty flavor before cooking them in the soup.

3. Heat remaining 1 tablespoon oil in now-empty pot over medium heat until shimmering. Add onion and cook until softened, about 5 minutes. Stir in garlic and tomato paste and cook until slightly darkened, about 2 minutes.

4. Stir in sherry, scraping up any browned bits, and cook until nearly evaporated, about 2 minutes. Stir in wheat berries, broth, soy sauce, thyme sprig, bay leaf, and shiitakes and bring to simmer. Reduce heat to low, cover, and cook until wheat berries are tender but still chewy, 45 minutes to 1 hour.

5. Discard thyme sprig and bay leaf. Off heat, stir in cremini mushrooms and any accumulated juices, mustard greens, and lemon zest. Cover and let sit until greens are wilted, about 5 minutes. Stir in lemon juice. Serve.

PER 1¼-CUP SERVING
Cal 210 • **Total Fat** 6g • **Sat Fat** 1g • **Chol** 0mg
Sodium 280mg • **Total Carbs** 26g • **Fiber** 5g • **Total Sugar** 4g
Added Sugar 0g • **Protein** 10g • **Total Carbohydrate Choices** 2

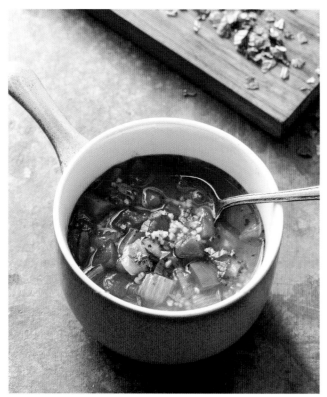

Nutritious whole-grain bulgur enriches our tomato soup and its starch provides a creamy texture.

Turkish Tomato, Bulgur, and Red Pepper Soup
SERVES 8

WHY THIS RECIPE WORKS This simple tomato and red pepper soup, inspired by Turkish flavors, relies on herbs, spices, and grains to yield an irresistible flavor. We started by softening onion and red bell peppers before creating a solid flavor backbone with garlic, tomato paste, white wine, dried mint, smoked paprika, and red pepper flakes. To impart additional smokiness, canned fire-roasted tomatoes did the trick. Wanting to incorporate a quick-cooking whole grain, we turned to fiber-rich bulgur. When stirred into the soup, this quick-cooking grain absorbs the surrounding flavors and gives off starch that creates a silky texture—no cream needed. We added the bulgur toward the end, giving it just enough time to become tender. A sprinkle of fresh mint gave the soup a final punch of flavor. When shopping, don't confuse bulgur with cracked wheat, which has a much longer cooking time and will not work in this recipe.

2 tablespoons extra-virgin olive oil
2 red bell peppers, stemmed, seeded, and chopped
1 onion, chopped
　Salt and pepper
3 garlic cloves, minced
1 tablespoon no-salt-added tomato paste
1 teaspoon dried mint, crumbled
½ teaspoon smoked paprika
⅛ teaspoon red pepper flakes
½ cup dry white wine
1 (28-ounce) can no-salt-added diced fire-roasted tomatoes
4 cups unsalted chicken broth
2 cups water
¾ cup medium-grind bulgur, rinsed
⅓ cup chopped fresh mint

1. Heat oil in Dutch oven over medium heat until shimmering. Add bell peppers, onion, ¾ teaspoon salt, and ¼ teaspoon pepper and cook until softened and lightly browned, 6 to 8 minutes. Stir in garlic, tomato paste, dried mint, smoked paprika, and pepper flakes and cook until fragrant, about 1 minute.

2. Stir in wine, scraping up any browned bits, and cook until reduced by half, about 1 minute. Add tomatoes and their juice and cook, stirring occasionally, until tomatoes soften and begin to break apart, about 10 minutes.

3. Stir in broth, water, and bulgur and bring to simmer. Reduce heat to low, cover, and cook until bulgur is tender, about 20 minutes. Season with pepper to taste. Sprinkle individual portions with fresh mint before serving.

PER 1¼-CUP SERVING
Cal 140 • **Total Fat** 4g • **Sat Fat** 0.5g • **Chol** 0mg
Sodium 300mg • **Total Carbs** 20g • **Fiber** 5g • **Total Sugar** 5g
Added Sugar 0g • **Protein** 5g • **Total Carbohydrate Choices** 1

Classic Lentil Soup
SERVES 6

WHY THIS RECIPE WORKS Lentils boast plenty of nutritional benefits, are quite filling, and pair well with many vegetables. We wanted to keep the flavors of our soup classic, so we used just two strips of bacon to create a meaty base, then layered in aromatic onions, garlic, thyme, and a bay leaf. White wine and no-salt-added canned tomatoes added a bit of acidity to complement the earthy lentils. We cooked the lentils in a combination of broth and water to maximize flavor without overdoing it on salt. And we finished the

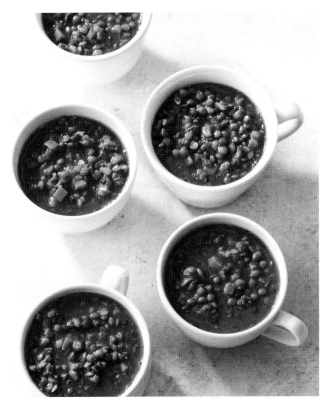

We use no-salt-added canned tomatoes and unsalted chicken broth to moderate the amount of sodium in our lentil soup.

soup with a bit of balsamic vinegar, which brightened the final dish and added just a bit of sweetness. We prefer the flavor and texture of French green lentils (*lentilles du Puy*) in this soup, but brown lentils can be used.

- 1 tablespoon canola oil
- 2 slices bacon, chopped fine
- 3 garlic cloves, minced
- 1 teaspoon minced fresh thyme or ¼ teaspoon dried
- 1¼ cups French green lentils, picked over and rinsed
- 1 (14.5 ounce) can no-salt-added diced tomatoes, drained
- 1 onion, chopped fine
- 1 carrot, peeled and cut into ¼-inch pieces
- ¼ teaspoon salt
- ¼ teaspoon pepper
- 1 bay leaf
- ¾ cup dry white wine
- 4 cups unsalted chicken broth
- 1½ cups water
- Balsamic vinegar

1. Heat oil in Dutch oven over medium heat until shimmering. Add bacon and cook until rendered and crisp, about 3 minutes. Stir in garlic and thyme and cook until fragrant, about 30 seconds.

2. Stir in lentils, tomatoes, onion, carrot, salt, pepper, and bay leaf and cook until vegetables are softened and lentils are darkened in color, 8 to 10 minutes.

3. Stir in wine, scraping up any browned bits, and cook until nearly evaporated, about 3 minutes. Stir in broth and water and bring to simmer. Reduce heat to medium-low, partially cover, and cook until lentils are tender but still hold their shape, 30 to 45 minutes.

4. Discard bay leaf. Stir in up to 1 tablespoon vinegar to taste. Serve.

PER 1-CUP SERVING

Cal 250 • **Total Fat** 7g • **Sat Fat** • 1.5g • **Chol** 5mg
Sodium 270mg • **Total Carbs** 30g • **Fiber** 8g • **Total Sugar** 4g
Added Sugar 0g • **Protein** 13g • **Total Carbohydrate Choices** 2

NOTES FROM THE TEST KITCHEN

Storing and Reheating Soups, Stews, and Chilis

Soups, stews, and chilis yield a generous number of servings, making it convenient to stock your freezer with last night's leftovers so you can reheat them whenever you like. First you'll need to cool the pot. As tempting as it might seem, don't transfer hot contents straight to the refrigerator. This can increase the fridge's internal temperature to unsafe levels. Letting the pot cool on the countertop for an hour helps the temperature drop to about 75 degrees, at which point you can transfer it safely to the fridge. If you don't have an hour to cool the whole pot, you can divide the contents into several storage containers so the heat dissipates more quickly, or you can cool it rapidly by using a frozen bottle of water to stir the contents of the pot.

To reheat, we prefer to simmer gently on the stovetop in a sturdy, heavy-bottomed pot, but a spin in the microwave works too. Be sure to cover the dish to prevent a mess. While most soups, stews, and chilis store just fine, those that contain dairy or pasta do not—the dairy curdles as it freezes, and the pasta turns mushy. Instead, make and freeze the dish without the dairy or pasta component. After you have thawed the dish and it has been heated through, you can stir in the uncooked pasta and simmer until just tender, or stir in the dairy and continue to heat gently until hot (do not boil).

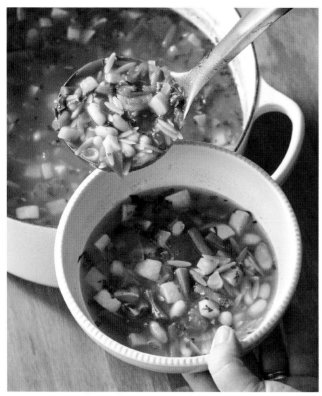

We choose protein-rich cannellini beans and whole-wheat orzo to round out our vegetable-filled minestrone soup.

Garden Minestrone
SERVES 8

WHY THIS RECIPE WORKS Good minestrone recipes capture the fleeting flavors of summer vegetables in a bowl. So we were after a soup that hewed closely to this principle and was packed with plenty of fresh, healthy vegetables. Yellow squash was a given, so to preserve its delicate texture while maximizing its subtle sweetness, we browned the seeded squash and removed it from the pot—we'd add it back later. To keep the soup from becoming thin and watery, we next built a backbone of tomato flavor: tomato paste cooked with the aromatics, and then fresh tomatoes simmered gently with green beans and cannellini beans. To add a punch of savoriness to the broth instead of adding salt, we tossed in a rind of Parmesan, a classic trick. And finally, a whole cup of chopped basil, along with the reserved squash, ensured our minestrone had a bright herbal flavor through and through.

3 tablespoons extra-virgin olive oil
1½ pounds yellow summer squash, halved lengthwise, seeded, and cut into ½-inch pieces
Salt and pepper
1 large onion, chopped fine
6 garlic cloves, minced
2 tablespoons no-salt-added tomato paste
2 teaspoons minced fresh thyme or ½ teaspoon dried
½ cup dry white wine
8 cups unsalted chicken broth
1½ pounds tomatoes, cored, seeded, and chopped coarse
2 (15-ounce) cans no-salt-added cannellini beans, rinsed
8 ounces green beans, trimmed and cut into 1-inch lengths
1 Parmesan cheese rind (optional), plus 1 ounce Parmesan, grated (½ cup)
1⅓ cups whole-wheat orzo
1 cup coarsely chopped fresh basil

1. Heat 1 tablespoon oil in Dutch oven over medium heat until shimmering. Add squash and ¼ teaspoon salt, cover, and cook until squash has released its liquid, about 3 minutes. Uncover, increase heat to medium-high, and continue to cook, stirring occasionally, until squash is dry and lightly browned, about 3 minutes. Transfer squash to plate and wipe pot clean with paper towels.

2. Heat 1 tablespoon oil in now-empty pot over medium heat until shimmering. Add onion and ¼ teaspoon salt and cook until softened and lightly browned, 5 to 7 minutes. Stir in two-thirds of garlic, tomato paste, thyme, and ½ teaspoon pepper and cook until fragrant, about 1 minute. Stir in wine, scraping up any browned bits.

3. Stir in broth, tomatoes, cannellini beans, green beans, and Parmesan rind, if using. Bring to simmer and cook for 4 minutes. Stir in orzo, reduce heat to low, cover, and cook until green beans are just tender, 8 to 10 minutes.

4. Discard Parmesan rind, if using. Stir in squash and let sit until heated through, about 1 minute. Stir in basil, ⅛ teaspoon salt, remaining garlic, and remaining 1 tablespoon oil and season with pepper to taste. Sprinkle individual portions with grated Parmesan before serving.

PER 2-CUP SERVING
Cal 300 • **Total Fat** 8g • **Sat Fat** 1.5g • **Chol** 5mg
Sodium 410mg • **Total Carbs** 42g • **Fiber** 10g • **Total Sugar** 9g
Added Sugar 0g • **Protein** 15g • **Total Carbohydrate Choices** 3

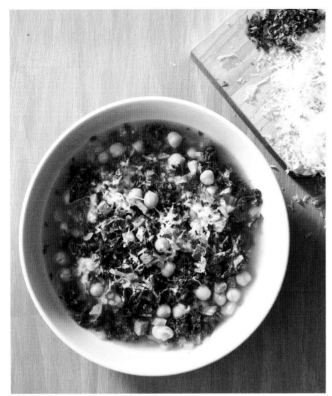

We incorporate a hefty amount of nutrient-dense kale into our soup; a quick simmer perfectly tenderizes the leaves.

Chickpea and Kale Soup
SERVES 8

WHY THIS RECIPE WORKS When considering kale, a salad often comes to mind before a hearty soup. But a soup featuring beans and hearty greens is a winning and nutritious combo. We set out to pair nutty chickpeas and earthy kale along with some chorizo in a soup that would make for a great, satisfying meal. First, we built a flavorful foundation of onions and fennel, which we lightly browned for a deeper flavor. We added our aromatics—garlic and red pepper flakes—and then our broth, before our canned chickpeas (for extra heft and to keep things streamlined) and handfuls of kale. A quick simmer turned the kale tender and melded all the flavors. We were happy with the soup's depth of flavor, but wanted a little more savoriness. A sprinkle of Pecorino at the end did the trick, adding a pleasant hint of salt.

¼ cup extra-virgin olive oil

2 onions, chopped

2 fennel bulbs, stalks discarded, bulbs halved, cored, and chopped

4 ounces Spanish-style chorizo sausage, cut into ¼-inch pieces
Salt and pepper

6 garlic cloves, minced

¼ teaspoon red pepper flakes

8 cups unsalted chicken broth

2 (15-ounce) cans no-salt-added chickpeas, rinsed

12 ounces kale, stemmed and chopped

1 teaspoon sherry vinegar, plus extra for seasoning

1 ounce Pecorino Romano cheese, grated (½ cup)

¼ cup chopped fresh parsley

1. Heat oil in Dutch oven over medium heat until shimmering. Add onions, fennel, chorizo, ¼ teaspoon salt, and 1 teaspoon pepper and cook until vegetables are softened and lightly browned, 8 to 10 minutes. Stir in garlic and pepper flakes and cook until fragrant, about 30 seconds.

2. Stir in broth, chickpeas, and kale and bring to simmer. Reduce heat to medium-low, cover, and cook until kale is tender, about 15 minutes. Stir in vinegar and season with extra vinegar and pepper to taste. Sprinkle individual portions with Pecorino and parsley before serving.

PER 1½-CUP SERVING
Cal 280 • **Total Fat** 14g • **Sat Fat** 3.5g • **Chol** 15mg
Sodium 500mg • **Total Carbs** 24g • **Fiber** 7g • **Total Sugar** 6g
Added Sugar 0g • **Protein** 15g • **Total Carbohydrate Choices** 1.5

Moroccan Chickpea Soup
SERVES 6

WHY THIS RECIPE WORKS This healthy, weeknight-friendly soup is easy to assemble and packed with bold flavor. We wanted to build a soup around hearty canned chickpeas because we love their convenience, buttery taste, and the fact that they easily take on the flavors of a broth without breaking down or getting mushy. For a bold broth, we decided to give it a Moroccan spin, blooming a handful of spices—hot paprika, saffron, ginger, and cumin. With so many fragrant spices, we were able to limit the amount of added salt. As for the vegetables, canned diced tomatoes, plus potatoes and zucchini, rounded out the mix and paired well with the chickpeas. To thicken our soup, we simply smashed some of the potatoes in the pot with a potato masher. If you don't have hot paprika, substitute ½ teaspoon sweet paprika and a pinch of cayenne pepper.

1 tablespoon canola oil
1 onion, chopped fine
  Salt and pepper
4 garlic cloves, minced
½ teaspoon hot paprika
¼ teaspoon saffron threads, crumbled
¼ teaspoon ground ginger
¼ teaspoon ground cumin
4 cups unsalted chicken broth
1 pound red potatoes, unpeeled, cut into ½-inch pieces
2 (15-ounce) cans no-salt-added chickpeas, rinsed
1 (14.5-ounce) can no-salt-added diced tomatoes
1 zucchini, halved lengthwise, seeded, and cut into
  ½-inch pieces
¼ cup minced fresh parsley or mint
  Lemon wedges

1. Heat oil in Dutch oven over medium heat until shimmering. Add onion and ½ teaspoon salt and cook until softened, about 5 minutes. Stir in garlic, paprika, saffron, ginger, and cumin and cook until fragrant, about 30 seconds.

2. Stir in broth, potatoes, chickpeas, and tomatoes and their juice and bring to simmer. Reduce heat to medium-low, partially cover, and cook until potatoes are tender, about 25 minutes. Stir in zucchini, partially cover, and cook until tender, 5 to 10 minutes.

3. Using potato masher, mash some of potatoes to thicken soup to desired consistency. Stir in parsley and season with pepper to taste. Serve with lemon wedges.

PER 1½-CUP SERVING
Cal 220 • **Total Fat** 3.5g • **Sat Fat** 0g • **Chol** 0mg
Sodium 330 • **Total Carbs** 35g • **Fiber** 8g • **Total Sugar** 6g
Added Sugar 0g • **Protein** 11g • **Total Carbohydrate Choices** 2

SEEDING A ZUCCHINI

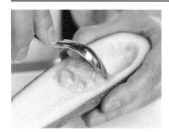

Halve zucchini lengthwise. Run small spoon inside each half to scoop out seeds.

Butternut Squash and White Bean Soup with Sage Pesto
SERVES 8

WHY THIS RECIPE WORKS While a smooth and creamy butternut squash soup (page 60) is a fantastic, elegant starter, we wanted a heartier soup featuring the squash as well. We paired our squash with creamy cannellini beans, which added a smooth, delicate texture to the soup; using no-salt-added beans helped the sodium stay within a healthy range. For an even heartier texture, we cubed the neck of the squash (which ensured even cooking) and added it to our soup with the beans. We simmered the bulb section of our squash in broth until very soft and then mashed it by hand and stirred it into the broth for body. For an extra boost of flavor, we topped the soup with a simple pesto made of sage, parsley, and walnuts, punched up with garlic and Parmesan cheese. Just 1 teaspoon of white wine vinegar at the end of cooking rounded out all the flavors and beautifully complemented the rich pesto.

PESTO
⅓ cup walnuts, toasted
2 garlic cloves, minced
¾ cup fresh parsley leaves
⅓ cup fresh sage leaves
⅓ cup extra-virgin olive oil
1 ounce Parmesan cheese, grated (½ cup)

SOUP
1 (2- to 2½-pound) butternut squash
4 cups unsalted chicken broth
3 cups water
1 tablespoon extra-virgin olive oil
1 pound leeks, white and light green parts only, halved
  lengthwise, sliced thin, and washed thoroughly
1 tablespoon no-salt-added tomato paste
2 garlic cloves, minced
  Salt and pepper
2 (15-ounce) cans no-salt-added cannellini beans
1 teaspoon white wine vinegar

1. FOR THE PESTO Pulse walnuts and garlic in food processor until coarsely chopped, about 5 pulses. Add parsley and sage. With processor running, slowly add oil and process until smooth, about 1 minute, scraping down sides of bowl as needed. Transfer pesto to bowl and stir in Parmesan; set aside. (Pesto can be refrigerated for up to 3 days. To prevent browning, press plastic wrap flush to surface or top with thin layer of olive oil. Bring to room temperature before using.)

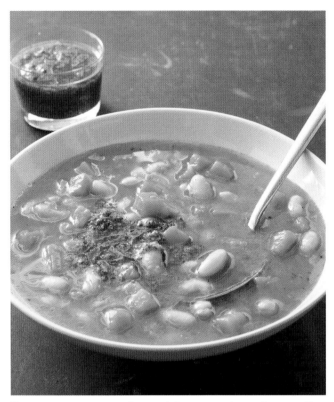

For great texture, we cook squash two ways, simmering a portion in broth until soft and cubing and sautéing the remainder.

2. FOR THE SOUP Using sharp vegetable peeler or chef's knife, remove skin and fibrous threads just below skin from squash (peel until squash is completely orange with no white flesh remaining, roughly ⅛ inch deep). Cut round bulb section off squash and cut in half lengthwise. Scoop out and discard seeds; cut each half into 4 wedges.

3. Bring broth, water, and squash wedges to boil in medium saucepan over high heat. Reduce heat to medium, partially cover, and simmer vigorously until squash is very tender and starting to fall apart, about 20 minutes. Using potato masher, mash squash, still in broth, until completely broken down. Cover to keep warm; set aside.

4. Meanwhile, cut neck of squash into ⅓-inch cubes. Heat oil in Dutch oven over medium heat until shimmering. Add leeks and tomato paste and cook, stirring occasionally, until leeks are softened and tomato paste is darkened, about 5 minutes. Stir in garlic and cook until fragrant, about 30 seconds. Add squash pieces, ¼ teaspoon salt, and ¼ teaspoon pepper and cook, stirring occasionally, for 5 minutes. Add squash broth and bring to simmer. Partially cover and cook for 10 minutes.

5. Stir in beans and their liquid, partially cover, and cook, stirring occasionally, until squash is just tender, 15 to 20 minutes. Stir in vinegar. Top each individual portion with 1 tablespoon pesto before serving.

PER 1½-CUP SERVING
Cal 270 • **Total Fat** 16g • **Sat Fat** 2.5g • **Chol** 5mg
Sodium 240mg • **Total Carbs** 26g • **Fiber** 6g • **Total Sugar** 5g
Added Sugars 0g • **Protein** 9g • **Total Carbohydrate Choices** 2

Hearty Chicken Stew with Leeks, Fennel, and Saffron
SERVES 6

WHY THIS RECIPE WORKS A chicken stew should include tender chunks of meat accompanied by a few bright, savory elements and enveloped in a glossy, flavorful sauce. We opted for bone-in breasts as they offered more flavor than the boneless variety. Browning them with skin allowed fond to form at the bottom of the pan, while protecting the delicate white meat from overcooking. We then discarded the skin so little fat actually made it into the stew. Leeks made for a neutral base, while chopped fennel introduced some anise sweetness. For a Spanish profile, sherry, saffron, and smoked paprika added intense savoriness. Just a few potatoes and a little flour helped add body. Parsley, minced fennel fronds, and a splash of sherry vinegar at the end brightened this homey dish.

- 3 **pounds bone-in split chicken breasts, trimmed**
- 2 **teaspoons canola oil**
- 1 **pound leeks, white and light green parts only, halved lengthwise, sliced thin, and washed thoroughly**
- 1 **fennel bulb, 1 tablespoon fronds minced, stalks discarded, bulb halved, cored, and cut into ½-inch pieces**
- 1 **teaspoon salt**
- ¼ **teaspoon pepper**
- 3 **tablespoons all-purpose flour**
- 1 **tablespoon no-salt-added tomato paste**
- 4 **garlic cloves, minced**
- 2 **teaspoons smoked paprika**
  Pinch saffron threads, crumbled
- ½ **cup dry sherry**
- 4 **cups unsalted chicken broth**
- 1 **pound red potatoes, unpeeled, cut into 1-inch pieces**
- 2 **bay leaves**
- 2 **tablespoons minced fresh parsley**
- 2 **teaspoons sherry vinegar**

1. Pat chicken dry with paper towels. Heat oil in Dutch oven over medium-high heat until just smoking. Brown chicken, 3 to 5 minutes per side; transfer to plate and discard skin.

2. Add leeks, fennel, salt, and pepper to fat left in pot. Reduce heat to medium and cook until vegetables are softened, 7 to 9 minutes. Stir in flour, tomato paste, three-quarters of garlic, paprika, and saffron and cook until fragrant, about 1 minute. Slowly whisk in sherry, scraping up any browned bits and smoothing out any lumps.

3. Stir in broth, potatoes, and bay leaves. Nestle chicken into pot along with any accumulated juices and bring to simmer. Cover, reduce heat to medium-low, and cook until chicken registers 160 degrees, 20 to 25 minutes.

4. Discard bay leaves. Transfer chicken to cutting board, let cool slightly, then shred into bite-size pieces using 2 forks; discard bones. Off heat, stir chicken into stew and let sit until heated through, about 5 minutes. Stir in fennel fronds, remaining garlic, parsley, and vinegar. Serve.

PER 1½-CUP SERVING

Cal 330 • **Total Fat** 6g • **Sat Fat** 1g • **Chol** 110mg
Sodium 600mg • **Total Carbs** 26g • **Fiber** 5g • **Total Sugar** 6g
Added Sugar 0g • **Protein** 39g • **Total Carbohydrate Choices** 2

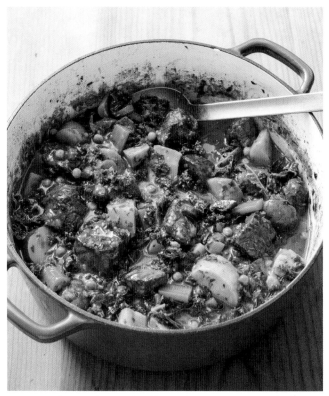

Umami-rich ingredients plus fiber-rich kale and peas let us use less meat in our stew, minimizing the saturated fat.

Beef and Vegetable Stew
SERVES 6

WHY THIS RECIPE WORKS Beef and vegetable stew, at its heart, is simple but rich and satisfying, thanks to tender chunks of meat surrounded by a rich, deeply flavorful, and slightly thickened broth. Chuck roast is our preferred cut—it is flavorful, tender, juicy, and more consistent than precut stew meat. Browning the meat was the first step in creating complex flavor in the stew. Then, searing umami-rich mushrooms and tomato paste allowed us to cut back on the quantity of meat without sacrificing meatiness. Some reduced red wine emphasized the stew's bright, rich flavors. A combination of parsnips, carrots, and potatoes provided sweetness and heft to the stew while some hearty braised kale and sweet peas, stirred in at the end, bolstered the fiber content.

2 pounds boneless beef chuck-eye roast, trimmed of all visible fat and cut into 1½-inch pieces
  Salt and pepper
5 teaspoons canola oil
1 portobello mushroom cap, cut into ½-inch pieces
2 onions, chopped fine

3 tablespoons all-purpose flour
3 garlic cloves, minced
1 tablespoon no-salt-added tomato paste
1 tablespoon minced fresh thyme or 1 teaspoon dried
1½ cups dry red wine
4 cups unsalted chicken broth
2 bay leaves
4 carrots, peeled and cut into 1-inch pieces
12 ounces red potatoes, unpeeled, cut into 1-inch pieces
12 ounces parsnips, peeled and cut into 1-inch pieces
1 pound kale, stemmed and cut into ½-inch pieces
½ cup frozen peas
¼ cup minced fresh parsley

1. Adjust oven rack to lower-middle position and heat oven to 300 degrees. Pat beef dry with paper towels and sprinkle with ½ teaspoon salt and ¼ teaspoon pepper. Heat 1 teaspoon oil in Dutch oven over medium-high heat until just smoking. Brown half of beef on all sides, 5 to 7 minutes; transfer to bowl. Repeat with 1 teaspoon oil and remaining beef; transfer to bowl.

2. Add mushroom and ¼ teaspoon salt to fat left in pot, cover, and cook until mushroom has released its liquid, about 3 minutes. Uncover, increase heat to medium-high, and continue to cook, stirring occasionally, until mushroom is dry and well browned, about 10 minutes.

3. Stir in onions and remaining 1 tablespoon oil and cook until softened, about 5 minutes. Stir in flour, garlic, tomato paste, and thyme and cook until fragrant, about 1 minute. Slowly whisk in wine, scraping up any browned bits and smoothing out any lumps. Stir in broth, bay leaves, and beef and any accumulated juices and bring to simmer. Cover, transfer pot to oven, and cook for 1½ hours.

4. Stir in carrots, potatoes, and parsnips, cover, and cook until meat and vegetables are tender, about 1 hour.

5. Stir in kale, cover, and cook until tender, about 10 minutes. Remove pot from oven and discard bay leaves. Stir in peas and let sit until heated through, about 5 minutes. Stir in parsley and serve.

PER 1½-CUP SERVING

Cal 480 • **Total Fat** 12g • **Sat Fat** 3.5g • **Chol** 100mg
Sodium 570mg • **Total Carbs** 39g • **Fiber** 9g • **Total Sugar** 10g
Added Sugar 0g • **Protein** 42g • **Total Carbohydrate Choices** 2.5

CUTTING STEW MEAT

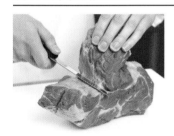

1. Pull apart roast at its major seams (delineated by lines of fat and silver skin). Use knife as necessary.

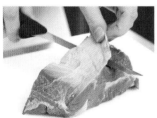

2. With sharp knife, trim off excess fat and silver skin.

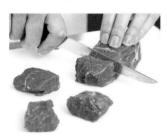

3. Cut meat into 1½-inch pieces.

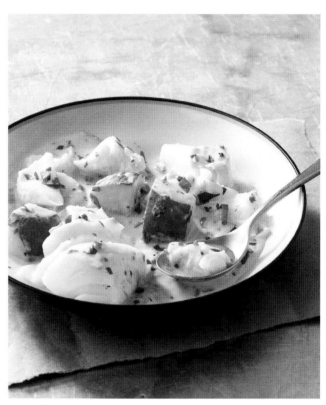

A bit of half-and-half replaces the usual heavy cream to provide body and richness to this fish stew.

New England Fish Stew
SERVES 4

WHY THIS RECIPE WORKS In New England, fish stew is similar to clam chowder. Chunks of white fish take the place of the clams, but otherwise the two are fairly similar—onions, potatoes, and bacon or salt pork are added with fish to a briny, creamy broth. We set out to lighten up this main course stew without sacrificing flavor. First, for the flavor base, one slice of bacon, chopped fine, was enough to infuse our soup. In addition, cooking the bacon first allowed us to use the rendered fat to cook the onion, giving the stew a smoky flavor that oil alone could not match. Next we added a mix of clam juice, water, and wine, let it simmer, then added the potatoes and herbs, and finally the fish once the potatoes were just tender. For richness and body, we swapped out the usual heavy cream for a splash of half-and-half, which we added at the end of cooking. Our finished stew was healthy and quick, while maintaining its restrained and dignified New England pedigree. Halibut and haddock are good substitutes for cod.

1 teaspoon canola oil

1 slice bacon, chopped fine

1 onion, chopped

Salt and pepper

4½ teaspoons all-purpose flour

½ teaspoon minced fresh thyme or ⅛ teaspoon dried

2 (8-ounce) bottles clam juice

½ cup water

¼ cup dry white wine

8 ounces red potatoes, unpeeled, cut into 1-inch pieces

1 bay leaf

1½ pounds skinless cod fillets, ¾ to 1 inch thick, cut into 1½-inch pieces

⅓ cup half-and-half

2 tablespoons chopped fresh parsley

1. Heat oil in Dutch oven over medium heat until shimmering. Add bacon and cook until rendered and crisp, 5 to 7 minutes. Stir in onion and ⅛ teaspoon salt and cook until softened, about 5 minutes. Stir in flour and thyme and cook until fragrant, about 1 minute. Slowly whisk in clam juice, water, and wine, scraping up any browned bits and smoothing out any lumps.

2. Stir in potatoes and bay leaf and bring to simmer. Cover, reduce heat to medium-low, and cook until potatoes are almost tender, about 15 minutes.

3. Nestle cod pieces into stew, cover, and cook until fish flakes apart when gently prodded with paring knife and registers 140 degrees, 8 to 10 minutes.

4. Discard bay leaf. Off heat, stir in half-and-half and parsley and season with pepper to taste. Serve.

PER 1½-CUP SERVING

Cal 280 • **Total Fat** 7g • **Sat Fat** 2.5g • **Chol** 90mg
Sodium 480mg • **Total Carbs** 15g • **Fiber** 2g • **Total Sugar** 3g
Added Sugar 0g • **Protein** 34g • **Total Carbohydrate Choices** 1

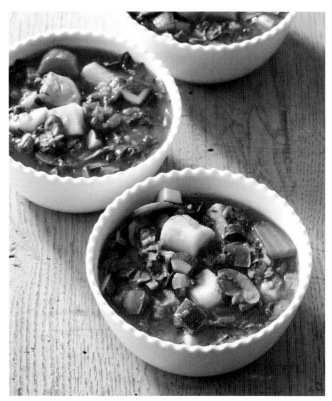

A variety of perfectly cooked vegetables gives this meatless stew complex flavor and a hearty texture.

Hearty Ten Vegetable Stew
SERVES 8

WHY THIS RECIPE WORKS Great vegetable stews marry hearty vegetables with a richly flavored broth and herbs that complement the vegetables. But all too often, they are little more than a jumble of soggy vegetables devoid of color and flavor. We wanted a healthy vegetable stew that could be as soul-satisfying in the dead of winter as a beef stew. When making a vegetable stew, you can't simply throw a handful of vegetables into a pot and simmer them until tender; the resulting flavor would be muted and muddy. We found the key to a really good vegetable stew is to use a wide variety of vegetables and to add them to the pot based on their relative cooking times. This way, each vegetable retains its distinct flavor and shape. To start, we worked on developing a great base of flavor. We selected a number of aromatics—onion, celery, and bell pepper—and sautéed them until brown to coax out their natural sweetness. Garlic, thyme, and tomato paste contributed further depth. At this point, a little bit of flavorful fond had built up, so we deglazed the pot with wine, which picked up the browned bits and added complexity.

Unsalted vegetable broth with a splash of low-sodium soy sauce added more savory flavor, while an abundance of hearty root vegetables simmered until perfectly tender and the flavors of the stew were fully developed. We then added delicate zucchini and earthy Swiss chard, utilizing both the stems and leaves. We sautéed the stems with the aromatics and added the leaves toward the end of the cooking to ensure they didn't disintegrate.

2 tablespoons canola oil
1 pound white mushrooms, trimmed and sliced thin
  Salt and pepper
8 ounces Swiss chard, stems chopped fine, leaves cut into ½-inch pieces
2 onions, chopped fine
1 celery rib, cut into ½-inch pieces
1 carrot, peeled, halved lengthwise, and sliced 1 inch thick
1 red bell pepper, stemmed, seeded, and cut into ½-inch pieces
6 garlic cloves, minced
2 tablespoons all-purpose flour
1 tablespoon no-salt added tomato paste
2 teaspoons minced fresh thyme or ½ teaspoon dried
½ cup dry white wine
6 cups low-sodium vegetable broth
1 tablespoon low-sodium soy sauce
8 ounces red potatoes, unpeeled, cut into 1-inch pieces
8 ounces celery root, peeled and cut into 1-inch pieces
2 parsnips, peeled and cut into 1-inch pieces
2 bay leaves
1 zucchini, halved lengthwise, seeded, and cut into ½-inch pieces
1 tablespoon lemon juice

1. Heat oil in Dutch oven over medium heat until shimmering. Add mushrooms and ¼ teaspoon salt, cover, and cook until mushrooms have released their liquid, about 3 minutes. Uncover, increase heat to medium-high, and continue to cook, stirring occasionally, until mushrooms are dry and well browned, 8 to 12 minutes.

2. Stir in chard stems, onions, celery, carrot, bell pepper, and ⅛ teaspoon salt and cook until vegetables are softened and well browned, 7 to 10 minutes. Stir in garlic, flour, tomato paste, and thyme and cook until fragrant, about 1 minute. Slowly whisk in wine, scraping up any browned bits and smoothing out any lumps, and cook until nearly evaporated, about 2 minutes.

3. Stir in broth, soy sauce, potatoes, celery root, parsnips, and bay leaves and bring to simmer. Reduce heat to medium-low, partially cover, and cook until stew is thickened and vegetables are tender, about 45 minutes.

4. Stir in chard leaves and zucchini, cover, and cook until tender, 5 to 10 minutes. Discard bay leaves. Stir in lemon juice and ¼ teaspoon salt and season with pepper to taste. Serve.

PER 1½-CUP SERVING

Cal 160 • **Total Fat** 5g • **Sat Fat** 0.5g • **Chol** 0mg
Sodium 460mg • **Total Carbs** 23g • **Fiber** 4g • **Total Sugar** 6g
Added Sugar 0g • **Protein** 4g • **Total Carbohydrate Choices** 1.5

Ultimate Beef Chili
SERVES 6

WHY THIS RECIPE WORKS Full of tender chunks of meat and creamy beans coated with a rich, heady, spice-laden sauce, chili is the epitome of comfort food. In lieu of store-bought chili powder, which can give chili a gritty, dusty texture and a subpar flavor, we found we were far better off making our own chili powder. Of the dried chiles available in most supermarkets, we chose anchos for their earthiness and arbols for their smooth heat. Toasting the anchos brought out their deep, fruity flavors, and adding hefty doses of cumin and oregano, along with a little cocoa, enhanced their complexity. A little cornmeal added subtle corn flavor plus some thickening power. We blitzed jalapeños, onion, and mushrooms in the food processor to give the chili a meaty backbone. Dried pinto beans, brined overnight, lent superior texture and creaminess without overcooking. Light lager complemented the flavor profile well while a final splash of fresh lime juice brightened up the dish. For a spicier chili, use the larger amount of arbols.

Salt and pepper
8 ounces (1¼ cups) dried pinto beans, picked over and rinsed
6 dried ancho chiles, stemmed, seeded, and torn into ½-inch pieces (1½ cups)
1–4 dried arbol chiles, stemmed and seeded
3 tablespoons cornmeal
2 teaspoons dried oregano
2 teaspoons ground cumin
2 teaspoons unsweetened cocoa powder
4 cups unsalted chicken broth
2 onions, chopped coarse
12 ounces cremini mushrooms, trimmed and chopped coarse
1–3 small jalapeño chiles, stemmed, seeded, and chopped
4 teaspoons canola oil

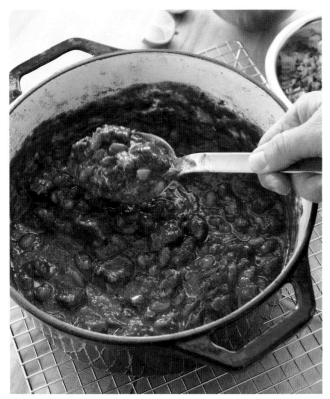

For the best flavor, we make our own chili powder and brine the beans in our ultimate beef chili.

4. Heat 2 teaspoons oil in Dutch oven over medium heat until shimmering. Add onion mixture, cover, and cook until vegetables have released their liquid, about 5 minutes. Uncover, increase heat to medium-high, and continue to cook, stirring occasionally, until vegetables are dry and beginning to brown, 7 to 9 minutes. Stir in garlic and cook until fragrant, about 30 seconds. Stir in chili paste and tomatoes and their juice until thoroughly combined. Stir in beans and remaining 3½ cups broth and bring to simmer.

5. Meanwhile, pat beef dry with paper towels and sprinkle with ½ teaspoon salt and ⅛ teaspoon pepper. Heat 1 teaspoon oil in now-empty skillet over medium-high heat until just smoking. Brown half of beef on all sides, 4 to 7 minutes; transfer to pot. Repeat with remaining 1 teaspoon oil and remaining beef; transfer to pot. Add lager to again-empty skillet, scraping up any browned bits, and bring to simmer; transfer to pot.

6. Cover pot and transfer to oven. Cook until meat and beans are fully tender, 1½ to 2 hours. Remove pot from oven and let chili sit, uncovered, for 10 minutes. Stir in lime juice and serve.

PER 1½-CUP SERVING

Cal 520 • **Total Fat** 13g • **Sat Fat** 3.5g • **Chol** 100mg
Sodium 440mg • **Total Carbs** 48g • **Fiber** 16g • **Total Sugar** 7g
Added Sugar 0g • **Protein** 49g • **Total Carbohydrate Choices** 3

- 4 **garlic cloves, minced**
- 1 **(14.5-ounce) can no-salt-added diced tomatoes**
- 2 **pounds boneless beef chuck-eye roast, trimmed of all visible fat and cut into ¾-inch pieces**
- 1 **(12-ounce) bottle mild lager, such as Budweiser**
- 2 **teaspoons lime juice**

1. Dissolve 1½ tablespoons salt in 2 quarts cold water in large bowl or container. Add beans and soak at room temperature for at least 8 hours or up to 24 hours. Drain and rinse well.

2. Adjust oven rack to lower-middle position and heat oven to 300 degrees. Toast anchos in 12-inch skillet over medium-high heat, stirring frequently, until fragrant, 2 to 6 minutes; transfer to bowl and let cool slightly. Do not wash skillet.

3. Process anchos, arbols, cornmeal, oregano, cumin, and cocoa in food processor until finely ground, about 2 minutes. With processor running, slowly add ½ cup broth until smooth paste forms, about 45 seconds, scraping down sides of bowl as needed; transfer to bowl. Pulse onions, mushrooms, and jalapeños in now-empty processor until chopped, 9 to 12 pulses.

White Chicken Chili
SERVES 8

WHY THIS RECIPE WORKS White chicken chili is a fresher, lighter cousin of the thick red chili most of us know and love. Its appeal is not surprising because it is a healthier alternative and, when made well, packed with vibrant flavors and spiciness. All too often, however, this chili is lackluster. We found not one but three solutions to bland chicken chili recipes. To fix what is often a watery sauce, we pureed some of our sautéed chile-onion mixture and beans with the broth to thicken the base. To avoid floating bits of rubbery chicken, we browned, poached, and shredded bone-in, skin-on chicken breasts, which gave the chicken a hearty texture and full flavor. And to solve the problem of insufficient chile flavor, we used a trio of fresh chiles: jalapeño, poblano, and Anaheim. For a spicier chile, add the jalapeño seeds. If you can't find Anaheim chiles, add an additional poblano and jalapeño to the chili.

- 2 **onions, chopped**
- 3 **Anaheim chiles, stemmed, seeded, and chopped**
- 3 **poblano chiles, stemmed, seeded, and chopped**

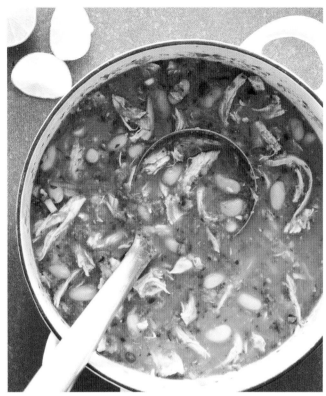

Pureeing a portion of the cooked vegetables, beans, and broth adds body to this chicken chili.

3 jalapeño chiles, stemmed, seeded, and minced
3 pounds bone-in split chicken breasts, trimmed
2 tablespoons canola oil
6 garlic cloves, minced
1 tablespoon ground cumin
1½ teaspoons ground coriander
  Salt and pepper
2 (15-ounce) cans no-salt-added cannellini beans, rinsed
4 cups unsalted chicken broth
¼ cup minced fresh cilantro
4 scallions, sliced thin
2 tablespoons lime juice, plus lime wedges
  for serving
1 tablespoon minced fresh oregano

1. Toss onions, Anaheims, poblanos, and two-thirds of jalapeños together in bowl. Working in two batches, pulse vegetables in food processor to consistency of chunky salsa, about 12 pulses; set aside.

2. Pat chicken dry with paper towels. Heat oil in Dutch oven over medium-high heat until just smoking. Brown chicken, 3 to 5 minutes per side; transfer to plate and discard skin.

3. Add processed vegetable mixture, garlic, cumin, coriander, ¾ teaspoon salt, and ¼ teaspoon pepper to fat left in pot and cook over medium heat, stirring often, until vegetables are softened, about 10 minutes. Remove pot from heat.

4. Process 1 cup cooked vegetable mixture, 1 cup beans, and 1 cup broth in food processor until smooth, about 20 seconds, scraping down sides of bowl as needed. Return pureed mixture to pot and stir in remaining 3 cups broth, scraping up any browned bits. Nestle chicken into pot along with any accumulated juices and bring to simmer. Reduce heat to medium-low, cover, and cook until chicken registers 160 degrees, 10 to 15 minutes.

5. Transfer chicken to carving board, let cool slightly, then shred into bite-size pieces using 2 forks; discard bones.

6. Stir remaining beans into chili, bring to simmer over medium heat, and cook, uncovered, until chili has thickened slightly, about 10 minutes. Off heat, stir in chicken and let sit until heated through, about 5 minutes. Stir in cilantro, scallions, lime juice, oregano, and remaining jalapeño and season with pepper to taste. Serve with lime wedges.

PER 1½-CUP SERVING
Cal 260 • **Total Fat** 7g • **Sat Fat** 1g • **Chol** 80mg
Sodium 460mg • **Total Carbs** 16g • **Fiber** 5g • **Total Sugar** 4g
Added Sugar 0g • **Protein** 31g • **Total Carbohydrate Choices** 1

Pumpkin Turkey Chili
SERVES 8

WHY THIS RECIPE WORKS Beef chili can turn out heavy and greasy, but lighter turkey chilis often lack depth and richness. We wanted a satisfying turkey chili that wouldn't leave us missing the beef. To safeguard against rubbery turkey, we treated the meat with a bit of salt and baking soda, which helped it hold onto moisture. Then, to give our dish a smoky, aromatic backbone, we made our own chili powder by grinding toasted ancho chiles, cumin, coriander, paprika, and oregano. We loaded the chili with red bell peppers and black beans for extra fiber and protein. Still, our chili needed more richness. We found the answer in a unique ingredient— convenient canned pumpkin puree. Folding the puree into the chili gave it a rich, silky texture and subtle squash-y flavor, along with a dose of vitamins. Be sure to use ground turkey, not ground turkey breast (also labeled 99 percent fat-free) in this recipe.

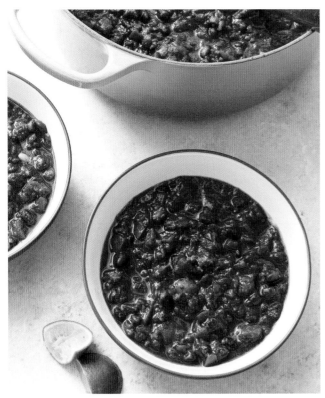

An unexpected ingredient—canned pumpkin—contributes depth of flavor, nutrients, and heartiness to turkey chili.

1. Toss turkey, 1 tablespoon water, ¼ teaspoon salt, and baking soda in bowl until thoroughly combined. Set aside for 20 minutes.

2. Toast anchos in Dutch oven over medium-high heat, stirring frequently, until fragrant, 4 to 6 minutes; transfer to food processor and let cool slightly. Add cumin, coriander, oregano, paprika, and 1 teaspoon pepper and process until finely ground, about 2 minutes; transfer to bowl. Process tomatoes and their juice in now-empty food processor until smooth, about 30 seconds.

3. Heat oil in now-empty pot over medium heat until shimmering. Add onions, bell peppers, and ¾ teaspoon salt and cook until softened, 8 to 10 minutes. Increase heat to medium-high, add turkey, and cook, breaking up meat with wooden spoon, until no longer pink, 4 to 6 minutes. Stir in spice mixture and garlic and cook until fragrant, about 30 seconds. Stir in tomatoes, pumpkin, and remaining 2 cups water and bring to simmer. Reduce heat to low, cover, and cook, stirring occasionally, for 1 hour.

4. Stir in beans, cover, and cook until slightly thickened, about 45 minutes. (If chili begins to stick to bottom of pot or looks too thick, stir in extra water as needed.) Season with pepper to taste. Sprinkle individual portions with cilantro and serve with lime wedges.

PER 1½-CUP SERVING

Cal 240 • **Total Fat** 6g • **Sat Fat** 1.5g • **Chol** 20mg
Sodium 460mg • **Total Carbs** 26g • **Fiber** 9g • **Total Sugar** 6g
Added Sugar 0g • **Protein** 22g • **Total Carbohydrate Choices** 2

1	pound ground turkey
1	tablespoon plus 2 cups water, plus extra as needed
	Salt and pepper
¼	teaspoon baking soda
4	dried ancho chiles, stemmed, seeded, and torn into ½-inch pieces (1 cup)
1½	tablespoons ground cumin
1½	teaspoons ground coriander
1½	teaspoons dried oregano
1½	teaspoons paprika
1	(28-ounce) can no-salt-added whole peeled tomatoes
2	tablespoons extra-virgin olive oil
2	onions, chopped fine
2	red bell peppers, stemmed, seeded, and cut into ½-inch pieces
6	garlic cloves, minced
1	cup canned unsweetened pumpkin puree
2	(15-ounce) cans no-salt-added black beans, rinsed
¼	cup chopped fresh cilantro
	Lime wedges

Tasting Chili Powder

Chili powder is a seasoning blend made from ground dried chiles and an assortment of other ingredients such as cumin, garlic, and oregano. Considering that most chili recipes rely so heavily on it, we thought it was necessary to gather up as many brands as possible to find our favorite. To assess each sample uncooked, we sprinkled them over potatoes; and then we cooked each one in beef-and-bean chili. **Morton & Bassett Chili Powder** was the clear winner, with deep, complex flavor, subtle sweetness, and just the right amount of heat. This "smoky, sizzling, full-flavored" chili powder was "much more dimensional than others."

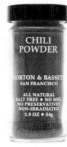

Vegetarian Chili
SERVES 6

WHY THIS RECIPE WORKS There are countless ways to make a meatless chili, and for a diabetic-friendly version we turned to tempeh as our starting point. Tempeh, which is made from cooked and fermented soybeans, is high in protein, vitamins, and minerals, but low in sodium and carbs. We treated it like ground meat, crumbling it and cooking it in a little oil until browned, then building a flavorful base for our chili. A hefty tablespoon of cumin seeds added a bold flavor backbone while traditional aromatics rounded out the classic chili flavor profile. A chopped bell pepper and a couple of cut-up carrots added texture and a subtle sweetness that paired well with the tempeh. To give our chili a burst of freshness and color, we added zucchini and frozen corn at the end along with the cooked tempeh. We prefer 5-grain tempeh in this chili, but any type of tempeh will work well.

4 teaspoons canola oil
1 (8-ounce) package 5-grain tempeh, crumbled into ¼-inch pieces
1 tablespoon cumin seeds
2 carrots, peeled and cut into ½-inch pieces
1 onion, chopped fine
1 red bell pepper, stemmed, seeded, and cut into ½-inch pieces
9 garlic cloves, minced
2 tablespoons chili powder
1 teaspoon minced canned chipotle chile in adobo sauce
   Salt and pepper
3 cups water
1 (28-ounce) can no-salt-added crushed tomatoes
1 (15-ounce) can no-salt-added kidney beans, rinsed
1 teaspoon dried oregano
1 cup frozen corn
1 zucchini, halved lengthwise, seeded, and cut into ½-inch pieces
½ cup minced fresh cilantro
   Lime wedges

1. Heat 1 teaspoon oil in Dutch oven over medium-high heat until shimmering. Add tempeh and cook until browned, about 5 minutes; transfer to plate and set aside.

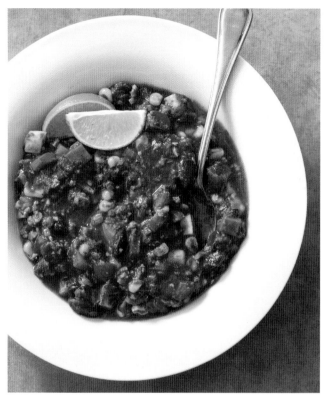

To make a killer vegetarian chili, we use crumbled tempeh, a great source of plant-based protein.

2. Add cumin seeds to now-empty pot and cook over medium heat, stirring often, until fragrant, about 1 minute. Stir in remaining 1 tablespoon oil, carrots, onion, bell pepper, garlic, chili powder, chipotle, and ¼ teaspoon salt and cook until vegetables are softened, 8 to 10 minutes.

3. Stir in water, tomatoes, beans, and oregano, scraping up any browned bits. Bring to simmer and cook until chili is slightly thickened, about 45 minutes.

4. Stir in corn, zucchini, and tempeh and cook until zucchini is tender, 5 to 10 minutes. Stir in cilantro and season with pepper to taste. Serve with lime wedges.

PER 1½-CUP SERVING

Cal 240 • **Total Fat** 6g • **Sat Fat** 0.5g • **Chol** 0mg
Sodium 220mg • **Total Carbs** 35g • **Fiber** 10g • **Total Sugar** 9g
Added Sugar 0g • **Protein** 13g • **Total Carbohydrate Choices** 2

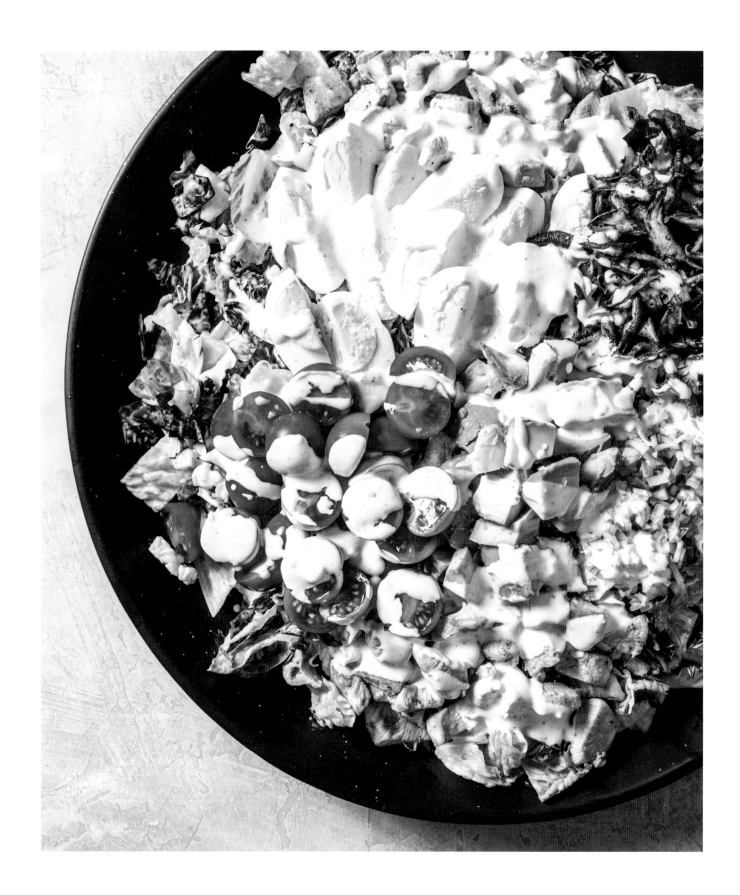

SALADS

Photo: Cobb Salad

A good vinaigrette makes all the difference between a salad that is just OK and one you really enjoy. And when you are trying to eat more healthfully, it's best to make your own salad dressing; store-bought versions are often packed with chemicals and emulsifiers and loaded with added sugar and sodium. For a well-balanced vinaigrette that doesn't separate, we whisk the oil and vinegar together with a little mayonnaise. You can use red wine vinegar, white wine vinegar, or champagne vinegar here; however, it is important to use high-quality ingredients. Each vinaigrette or dressing makes enough to dress 8 to 10 cups of greens; you will need about 2 tablespoons of Parmesan-Peppercorn Dressing for every 2 cups of greens.

Classic Vinaigrette

MAKES ¼ CUP

This vinaigrette works well with all types of greens. To make an herb vinaigrette, whisk in 1 tablespoon minced fresh parsley or chives and ½ teaspoon minced fresh thyme, tarragon, marjoram, or oregano before serving.

1	tablespoon wine vinegar
1½	teaspoons minced shallot
½	teaspoon mayonnaise
½	teaspoon Dijon mustard
⅛	teaspoon salt
	Pinch pepper
3	tablespoons extra-virgin olive oil

Whisk vinegar, shallot, mayonnaise, mustard, salt, and pepper together in bowl. While whisking constantly, drizzle in oil until completely emulsified. (Vinaigrette can be refrigerated for up to 1 week; whisk to recombine.)

PER 1-TABLESPOON SERVING

Cal 100 • **Total Fat** 11g • **Sat Fat** 1.5g • **Chol** 0mg
Sodium 90mg • **Total Carbs** 0g • **Fiber** 0g • **Total Sugar** 0g
Added Sugar 0g • **Protein** 0g • **Total Carbohydrate Choices** 0

Lemon Vinaigrette

MAKES ¼ CUP

This vinaigrette is best for dressing mild greens.

¼	teaspoon grated lemon zest plus 1 tablespoon juice
½	teaspoon mayonnaise
½	teaspoon Dijon mustard
⅛	teaspoon salt
	Pinch pepper
3	tablespoons extra-virgin olive oil

Whisk lemon zest and juice, mayonnaise, mustard, salt, and pepper together in bowl. While whisking constantly, drizzle in oil until completely emulsified. (Vinaigrette can be refrigerated for up to 1 week; whisk to recombine.)

PER 1-TABLESPOON SERVING

Cal 100 • **Total Fat** 11g • **Sat Fat** 1.5g • **Chol** 0mg
Sodium 90mg • **Total Carbs** 0g • **Fiber** 0g • **Total Sugar** 0g
Added Sugar 0g • **Protein** 0g • **Total Carbohydrate Choices** 0

Balsamic-Mustard Vinaigrette

MAKES ¼ CUP

This vinaigrette is best for dressing assertive greens.

1	tablespoon balsamic vinegar
2	teaspoons Dijon mustard
1½	teaspoons minced shallot
½	teaspoon mayonnaise
½	teaspoon minced fresh thyme
⅛	teaspoon salt
	Pinch pepper
3	tablespoons extra-virgin olive oil

Whisk vinegar, mustard, shallot, mayonnaise, thyme, salt, and pepper together in bowl. While whisking constantly, drizzle in oil until completely emulsified. (Vinaigrette can be refrigerated for up to 1 week; whisk to recombine.)

PER 1-TABLESPOON SERVING

Cal 110 • **Total Fat** 11g • **Sat Fat** 1.5g • **Chol** 0mg
Sodium 140mg • **Total Carbs** 1g • **Fiber** 0g • **Total Sugar** 1g
Added Sugar 0g • **Protein** 0g • **Total Carbohydrate Choices** 0

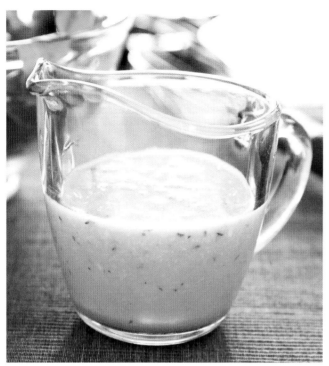

Our easy-to-make salad dressings are very flavorful and use a minimum of salt.

Walnut Vinaigrette

MAKES ¼ CUP

This vinaigrette is best for dressing mild greens.

1 tablespoon white wine vinegar
1½ teaspoons minced shallot
½ teaspoon mayonnaise
½ teaspoon Dijon mustard
⅛ teaspoon salt
Pinch pepper
1½ tablespoons roasted walnut oil
1½ tablespoons extra-virgin olive oil

Whisk vinegar, shallot, mayonnaise, mustard, salt, and pepper together in bowl. While whisking constantly, drizzle in oils until completely emulsified. (Vinaigrette can be refrigerated for up to 1 week; whisk to recombine.)

PER 1-TABLESPOON SERVING

Cal 100 • **Total Fat** 11g • **Sat Fat** 1g • **Chol** 0g
Sodium 90mg • **Total Carbs** 0g • **Fiber** 0g • **Total Sugar** 0g
Added Sugar 0g • **Protein** 0g • **Total Carbohydrate Choices** 0

Tahini-Lemon Dressing

MAKES ½ CUP

This dressing is best for dressing mild greens.

2½ tablespoons lemon juice
2 tablespoons tahini
1 tablespoon water
1 garlic clove, minced
½ teaspoon salt
⅛ teaspoon pepper
¼ cup extra-virgin olive oil

Whisk lemon juice, tahini, water, garlic, salt, and pepper together in bowl. While whisking constantly, drizzle in oil until completely emulsified. (Dressing can be refrigerated for up to 1 week; whisk to recombine.)

PER 1-TABLESPOON SERVING

Cal 90 • **Total Fat** 9g • **Sat Fat** 1.5g • **Chol** 0mg
Sodium 150mg • **Total Carbs** 1g • **Fiber** 0g • **Total Sugar** 0g
Added Sugar 0g • **Protein** 1g • **Total Carbohydrate Choices** 0

Parmesan-Peppercorn Dressing

MAKES ½ CUP

This dressing works well with all types of greens.

2 tablespoons buttermilk
2 tablespoons mayonnaise
2 tablespoons low-fat sour cream
2 tablespoons grated Parmesan cheese
1 tablespoon water
1½ teaspoons lemon juice
½ teaspoon Dijon mustard
½ teaspoon minced shallot
¼ teaspoon pepper
¼ teaspoon garlic powder

Whisk all ingredients in bowl until smooth. (Dressing can be refrigerated for up to 1 week; whisk to recombine.)

PER 2-TABLESPOON SERVING

Cal 70 • **Total Fat** 6g • **Sat Fat** 1.5g • **Chol** 5mg
Sodium 135mg • **Total Carbs** 1g • **Fiber** 0g • **Total Sugar** 1g
Added Sugar 0g • **Protein** 2g • **Total Carbohydrate Choices** 0

Basic Green Salad
SERVES 4

WHY THIS RECIPE WORKS A simple formula for making a perfect leafy green salad is a vital recipe to have in your arsenal. We wanted to develop a recipe for a basic salad—a mix of well-chosen greens tossed with a light vinaigrette that was neither harsh nor oily. Leafy green salad sounds simple, but in reality, the dressing often soaks the greens, resulting in a muddy salad that's too acidic from the vinegar. We went back to the basics and revisited standard vinaigrette proportions. In most cases, 4 parts oil to 1 part vinegar produces the best balance of flavors in a vinaigrette. To keep our salad bold in flavor, we used a ratio of 3 parts oil to 2 parts vinegar. We also rubbed the bowl with cut garlic to impart just a hint of flavor. It is important to use high-quality ingredients as there are no bells or whistles to camouflage old lettuce, flavorless oil, or harsh vinegar. You can also use interesting leafy greens, such as mesclun, arugula, or Bibb lettuce, but avoid those with a more neutral flavor, such as iceberg lettuce.

½ garlic clove, peeled
3 tablespoons extra-virgin olive oil
2 tablespoons vinegar
¼ teaspoon salt
⅛ teaspoon pepper
8 ounces (8 cups) green leaf lettuce, torn into bite-size pieces if necessary

Rub inside of salad bowl with garlic. Whisk oil, vinegar, salt, and pepper in bowl until combined. Add lettuce and gently toss to coat. Serve.

PER SERVING
Cal 100 • Total Fat 11g • Sat Fat 1.5g • Chol 0mg
Sodium 150mg • Total Carbs 1g • Fiber 1g • Total Sugar 1g
Added Sugar 0g • Protein 1g • Total Carbohydrate Choices 0

Mesclun Salad with Goat Cheese and Almonds
SERVES 4

WHY THIS RECIPE WORKS Mesclun greens feature a mix of nutritious leafy greens and are best served with a vinaigrette that lets their delicate flavors shine through. The greens are tossed with the

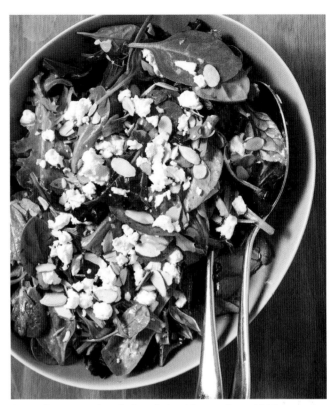

A simple green side salad, with or without a few add-ins, rounds out any meal.

vinaigrette and toasted sliced almonds, which add flavor, crunch, and protein. The salad is then topped with pungent goat cheese, which is more flavorful than many other cheeses.

5 ounces (5 cups) mesclun
3 tablespoons toasted sliced almonds
1 recipe Classic Vinaigrette (page 86)
2 ounces goat cheese, crumbled (½ cup)

Gently toss mesclun with almonds and vinaigrette in bowl until well coated. Sprinkle with goat cheese. Serve.

PER SERVING
Cal 170 • Total Fat 16g • Sat Fat 4g • Chol 5mg
Sodium 160mg • Total Carbs 1g • Fiber 1g • Total Sugar 0g
Added Sugar 0g • Protein 4g • Total Carbohydrate Choices 0

Romaine Salad with Chickpeas and Feta
SERVES 4

WHY THIS RECIPE WORKS This nutritious salad features hearty romaine lettuce and protein-rich canned chickpeas. Just a little feta cheese goes a long way and makes the salad feel indulgent.

- 3 romaine lettuce hearts (18 ounces), torn into bite-size pieces
- 1 cup canned no-salt-added chickpeas, rinsed
- 1 recipe Balsamic-Mustard Vinaigrette (page 86)
- 2 ounces feta cheese, crumbled (½ cup)

Gently toss lettuce and chickpeas with vinaigrette in bowl until well coated. Sprinkle with feta. Serve.

PER SERVING
Cal 230 • Total Fat 14g • Sat Fat 3.5g • Chol 15mg
Sodium 290mg • Total Carbs 17g • Fiber 3g • Total Sugar 5g
Added Sugar 0g • Protein 7g • Total Carbohydrate Choices 1

Bibb Lettuce Salad with Endive and Cucumber
SERVES 4

WHY THIS RECIPE WORKS Bibb lettuce is a nice alternative to romaine and makes for an elegant side salad. Here we pair it with pieces of crunchy endive and sliced cucumber as well as halved cherry tomatoes. Our Parmesan-Peppercorn Dressing makes it taste rich without breaking the bank on fat and calories.

- 12 ounces cherry tomatoes, halved
- 1 head Bibb lettuce (8 ounces), leaves separated and torn into bite-size pieces
- 1 head Belgian endive (4 ounces), cut into ½-inch pieces
- 1 cucumber, peeled, halved lengthwise, seeded, and sliced ¼ inch thick
- 1 recipe Parmesan-Peppercorn Dressing (page 87)

Gently toss cherry tomatoes, lettuce, endive, and cucumber with dressing until well coated. Serve.

PER SERVING
Cal 110 • Total Fat 7g • Sat Fat 1.5g • Chol 5mg
Sodium 140mg • Total Carbs 8g • Fiber 3g • Total Sugar 4g
Added Sugar 0g • Protein 4g • Total Carbohydrate Choices 1

Arugula Salad with Fennel and Shaved Parmesan
SERVES 6

WHY THIS RECIPE WORKS This simple salad features assertive arugula with crisp sliced fennel. To flatter the bright flavor of the arugula, we made a vinaigrette using tart lemon juice, shallot, a little chopped thyme, and a touch of Dijon to help emulsify everything. A bit of shaved Parmesan was the perfect finishing touch.

- 1½ tablespoons lemon juice
- 1 small shallot, minced
- 1 teaspoon Dijon mustard
- 1 teaspoon minced fresh thyme
- 1 small garlic clove, minced
  Salt and pepper
- ¼ cup extra-virgin olive oil
- 6 ounces (6 cups) baby arugula
- 1 large fennel bulb, stalks discarded, bulb halved, cored, and sliced thin
- 1 ounce Parmesan cheese, shaved

Whisk lemon juice, shallot, mustard, thyme, garlic, ⅛ teaspoon salt, and pinch pepper together in large bowl. While whisking constantly, drizzle in oil until completely emulsified. Add arugula and fennel and gently toss to coat. Season with pepper to taste. Sprinkle with Parmesan. Serve.

PER SERVING
Cal 130 • Total Fat 11g • Sat Fat 2g • Chol 5mg
Sodium 190mg • Total Carbs 6g • Fiber 2g • Total Sugar 3g
Added Sugar 0g • Protein 4g • Total Carbohydrate Choices <0.5

All About Salad Greens

With such a wide array of greens to choose from, it's good to know how to mix and match them to build interesting salads. Many are great on their own, but others are generally best used to add texture or color to other salads. Below are some of the most common salad greens you'll find at the market. No matter what type of greens you buy, make sure to select the freshest ones possible and avoid any that are wilted, bruised, or discolored.

Arugula (also called Rocket and Roquette)
Delicate dark green leaves with a peppery bite. Sold in bunches, usually with roots attached, or prewashed in cellophane bags. Bruises easily and can be very sandy, so wash thoroughly in several changes of water before using.

Bibb Lettuce
Small, compact heads of pale- to medium-green leaves and soft, buttery outer leaves. Inner leaves have a surprising crunch and a sweet, mild flavor.

Iceberg
A large, round, tightly packed head of pale green leaves; very crisp and crunchy, with minimal flavor.

Loose-Leaf Lettuces (specifically Red Leaf and Green Leaf)
Ruffled dark red or green leaves that grow in big, loose heads; versatile, with a soft yet crunchy texture. Green leaf is crisp and mild; red leaf is earthier.

Mesclun (also called Mesclune, Spring Mix, Field Greens)
A mix of up to 14 different baby greens, including spinach, red leaf, oak leaf, frisée, radicchio, green leaf. Delicate leaves; flavors range from mild to slightly bitter.

Romaine
Long, full heads with stiff, deep green leaves that are crisp and crunchy with a mild, earthy flavor. Also sold in bags of three romaine hearts. Tough outer leaves should be discarded from full heads.

Spinach (Flat-Leaf, Curly-Leaf, and Baby)
All varieties are vibrant green with an earthy flavor. Choose tender flat-leaf or baby spinach for raw salads; tough curly-leaf spinach is better steamed and sautéed. Rinse loose spinach well to remove dirt. Varieties available prewashed in bags.

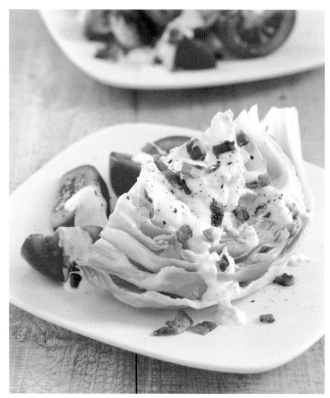

To cut down on the amount of cheese in our dressing, we replace mild blue cheese with more flavorful Roquefort.

Classic Wedge Salad
SERVES 6

WHY THIS RECIPE WORKS The pairing of crisp iceberg lettuce and creamy, tangy, blue cheese dressing is what makes this steakhouse staple so popular. But that thick, rich dressing usually makes this salad off limits for those watching their diet. Typically made with mayonnaise, sour cream, and blue cheese, we wanted to make this salad more accessible. We liked the unsaturated fat in the mayo but needed to replace full-fat sour cream with its lighter counterpart to help us trim calories. Since we couldn't find a good low-fat substitute for blue cheese, we reduced the amount of cheese and traded the mild blue cheese usually called for in wedge salad with more pungent Roquefort or Stilton. Now our dressing offered big, bold, blue cheese flavor.

3 slices uncured bacon, cut into ¼-inch pieces
⅓ cup buttermilk
1 ounce strong blue cheese, such as Roquefort or Stilton, crumbled (¼ cup)
⅓ cup mayonnaise
⅓ cup low-fat sour cream
3 tablespoons water
1 tablespoon white wine vinegar
¼ teaspoon garlic powder
¼ teaspoon pepper
1 head iceberg lettuce (2 pounds), cored and cut into 6 wedges
3 tomatoes, cored and cut into ½-inch-thick wedges
2 tablespoons minced fresh chives

1. Cook bacon in 12-inch nonstick skillet over medium-high heat until rendered and crisp, about 5 minutes. Using slotted spoon, transfer bacon to paper towel–lined plate.

2. Mash buttermilk and blue cheese together with fork in small bowl until mixture resembles cottage cheese with small curds. Stir in mayonnaise, sour cream, water, vinegar, garlic powder, and pepper until combined.

3. Divide lettuce and tomatoes among individual plates. Spoon dressing over top, then sprinkle with bacon and chives. Serve.

PER SERVING

Cal 170 • **Total Fat** 13g • **Sat Fat** 3g • **Chol** 15mg
Sodium 270mg • **Total Carbs** 7g • **Fiber** 2g • **Total Sugar** 5g
Added Sugar 0g • **Protein** 6g • **Total Carbohydrate Choices** 0.5

Spinach Salad with Carrots, Oranges, and Sesame
SERVES 6

WHY THIS RECIPE WORKS Spinach salad can go in many directions: from a simple classic salad with red onion and a bright vinaigrette, to a warm salad enhanced with bacon, to an Asian-inspired salad such as this one. Since spinach and oranges make a great pairing, we decided to add orange juice to our vinaigrette and segments to the salad itself. For a bold Asian dressing, we combined the orange juice with rice vinegar and toasted sesame oil, with neutral tasting canola oil as its base. Shaved carrot blended easily into the spinach, adding flavor and nutrients. A sprinkling of toasted sesame seeds added a healthy bit of crunch.

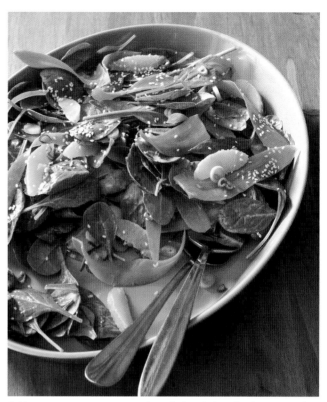

Adding orange segments to the salad and their fresh juice to the dressing brings bright citrus flavor to spinach salad.

2 oranges
2 carrots, peeled
2 tablespoons rice vinegar
1 small shallot, minced
1 teaspoon Dijon mustard
¾ teaspoon mayonnaise
⅛ teaspoon salt
2½ tablespoons canola oil
¾ teaspoon toasted sesame oil
6 ounces (6 cups) baby spinach
2 scallions, sliced thin
1½ teaspoons toasted sesame seeds

1. Grate ½ teaspoon zest from 1 orange; set zest aside. Cut away peel and pith from oranges. Holding fruit over fine-mesh strainer set in bowl, use paring knife to slice between membranes to release segments. Measure out and reserve 2 tablespoons juice; discard remaining juice. Using vegetable peeler, shave carrots lengthwise into ribbons.

2. Whisk orange zest and reserved juice, vinegar, shallot, mustard, mayonnaise, and salt together in large bowl. While whisking constantly, drizzle in oils until completely emulsified. Add orange segments, carrots, spinach, and scallions and gently toss to coat. Sprinkle with sesame seeds. Serve.

PER SERVING

Cal 110 • **Total Fat** 7g • **Sat Fat** 0.5g • **Chol** 0mg
Sodium 110mg • **Total Carbs** 10g • **Fiber** 3g • **Total Sugar** 5g
Added Sugar 0g • **Protein** 2g • **Total Carbohydrate Choices** 1

SEGMENTING CITRUS

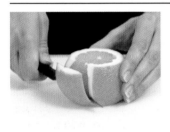 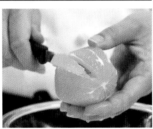

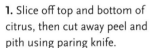

1. Slice off top and bottom of citrus, then cut away peel and pith using paring knife.

2. Holding fruit over bowl, slice between membranes to release individual segments.

VARIATION
Spinach Salad with Frisée and Strawberries
SERVES 6

WHY THIS RECIPE WORKS For a healthy spinach salad with a touch of sweetness, we paired the baby spinach with cut-up strawberries and chopped fresh basil. We chose to make a balsamic vinaigrette rather than the traditional creamy poppyseed dressing often served with this type of salad. To round out the dish, we chopped up a head of frisée, which bulked it up and gave the salad a nice texture overall.

    2 tablespoons chopped fresh basil
    5 teaspoons balsamic vinegar
    1 small shallot, minced
    1 teaspoon Dijon mustard
    ¾ teaspoon mayonnaise
    ½ teaspoon grated orange zest plus 2 tablespoons juice
    ½ teaspoon pepper
    ⅛ teaspoon salt
    3 tablespoons extra-virgin olive oil
    6 ounces (6 cups) baby spinach
    1 head frisée (6 ounces), chopped
    5 ounces strawberries, hulled and quartered (1 cup)

Whisk basil, vinegar, shallot, mustard, mayonnaise, orange zest and juice, pepper, and salt together in large bowl. While whisking constantly, drizzle in oil until completely emulsified. Add spinach, frisée, and strawberries and gently toss to coat. Serve.

PER SERVING

Cal 100 • **Total Fat** 8g • **Sat Fat** 1g • **Chol** 0mg
Sodium 95mg • **Total Carbs** 6g • **Fiber** 2g • **Total Sugar** 2g
Added Sugar 0g • **Protein** 1g • **Total Carbohydrate Choices** 0.5

Warm Spinach Salad with Feta and Pistachios
SERVES 6

WHY THIS RECIPE WORKS Served wilted in a salad, spinach takes on a milder flavor, perfect for pairing with bold mix-ins—so long as the leaves don't reduce to mush. We experimented with various types of spinach and found that flat-leaf and baby spinach became overly soft, but heartier curly-leaf spinach could withstand the heat. To make the dressing, we began by heating 3 tablespoons of fruity extra-virgin olive oil in a Dutch oven along with some minced shallot. For a burst of bright citrus, we also simmered a strip of lemon zest in the oil, then we added fresh lemon juice before tossing in the spinach off the heat. The residual heat in the pot steamed the spinach until it was warm and just wilted. Peppery sliced radishes, crumbled feta, and toasted pistachios rounded out our salad. We freeze the feta so it doesn't get too warm from the spinach. Do not substitute flat-leaf or baby spinach here. Be sure to cook the spinach just until it begins to wilt; any longer and the leaves will overcook and clump.

    1½ ounces feta cheese, crumbled (⅓ cup)
     3 tablespoons extra-virgin olive oil
     1 (3-inch) strip lemon zest plus 1½ tablespoons juice
     1 shallot, minced
    10 ounces curly-leaf spinach, stemmed and torn into bite-size pieces
     6 radishes, trimmed and sliced thin
     3 tablespoons chopped toasted pistachios
        Pepper

1. Place feta on plate and freeze until slightly firm, about 15 minutes.

2. Cook oil, lemon zest, and shallot in Dutch oven over medium-low heat until shallot is softened, about 5 minutes. Off heat, discard zest and stir in lemon juice. Add spinach, cover, and let sit until just beginning to wilt, about 30 seconds.

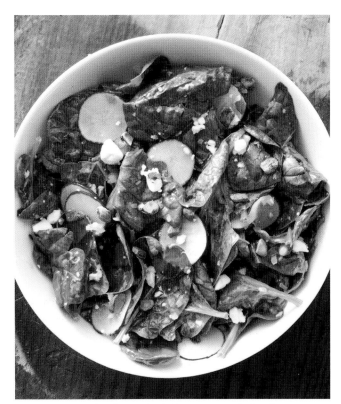

Curly-leaf spinach wilts perfectly for a warm salad and retains some bite without overcooking.

3. Transfer spinach mixture and liquid left in pot to large bowl. Add radishes, pistachios, and feta and gently toss to coat. Season with pepper to taste. Serve.

PER SERVING
Cal 120 • **Total Fat** 10g • **Sat Fat** 2.5g • **Chol** 5mg
Sodium 105mg • **Total Carbs** 4g • **Fiber** 2g • **Total Sugar** 1g
Added Sugar 0g • **Protein** 3g • **Total Carbohydrate Choices** <0.5

VARIATIONS
Warm Spinach Salad with Apple, Blue Cheese, and Pecans
SERVES 6

WHY THIS RECIPE WORKS Spinach pairs well with nuts, fruit, and pungent cheeses, and in this warm salad, the classic pairing of apples, pecans, and blue cheese works perfectly. For the warm dressing, we heat oil with orange zest and shallot until the shallot is softened, then we remove the zest and add white vinegar and a little orange juice. Once we add the dressing to the spinach and allow it to wilt, the apple, pecans, and blue cheese are added. Do not substitute flat-leaf or baby spinach here. Be sure to cook the spinach just until it begins to wilt; any longer and the leaves will overcook and clump.

1½ ounces blue cheese, crumbled (⅓ cup)
  3 tablespoons extra-virgin olive oil
  1 (3-inch) strip orange zest plus 1 tablespoon juice
  1 shallot, minced
  1 teaspoon white vinegar
 10 ounces curly-leaf spinach, stemmed and torn into bite-size pieces
  ½ Fuji, Gala, or Golden Delicious apple, cored and cut into ½-inch pieces
  3 tablespoons chopped toasted pecans
    Pepper

1. Place blue cheese on plate and freeze until slightly firm, about 15 minutes.

2. Cook oil, orange zest, and shallot in Dutch oven over medium-low heat until shallot is softened, about 5 minutes. Off heat, discard zest and stir in orange juice and vinegar. Add spinach, cover, and let sit until just beginning to wilt, about 30 seconds.

3. Transfer spinach mixture and liquid left in pot to large bowl. Add apple, pecans, and blue cheese and gently toss to coat. Season with pepper to taste. Serve.

PER SERVING
Cal 130 • **Total Fat** 12g • **Sat Fat** 2.5g • **Chol** 5mg
Sodium 120mg • **Total Carbs** 5g • **Fiber** 2g • **Total Sugar** 2g
Added Sugar 0g • **Protein** 3g • **Total Carbohydrate Choices** <0.5

Warm Spinach Salad with Strawberries, Goat Cheese, and Almonds
SERVES 6

WHY THIS RECIPE WORKS For another take on warm spinach salad, we turned to the winning combo of thinly sliced strawberries and mild goat cheese. For the warm dressing, tangy grapefruit zest and juice keep things bright when paired with extra-virgin olive oil and shallot. For crunch we added toasted sliced almonds. Do not substitute flat-leaf or baby spinach here. Be sure to cook the spinach just until it begins to wilt; any longer and the leaves will overcook and clump.

1½ ounces goat cheese, crumbled (⅓ cup)
  3 tablespoons extra-virgin olive oil
  1 (3-inch) strip grapefruit zest plus 1½ tablespoons juice
  1 shallot, minced

10 ounces curly-leaf spinach, stemmed and torn into bite-size pieces

8 ounces strawberries, hulled and sliced thin (1¼ cups)

3 tablespoons toasted sliced almonds

Pepper

1. Place goat cheese on plate and freeze until slightly firm, about 15 minutes.

2. Cook oil, grapefruit zest, and shallot in Dutch oven over medium-low heat until shallot is softened, about 5 minutes. Off heat, discard zest and stir in grapefruit juice. Add spinach, cover, and let sit until just beginning to wilt, about 30 seconds.

3. Transfer spinach mixture and liquid left in pot to large bowl. Add strawberries, almonds, and goat cheese and gently toss to coat. Season with pepper to taste. Serve.

PER SERVING

Cal 120 • **Total Fat** 10g • **Sat Fat** 2g • **Chol** 5mg
Sodium 70mg • **Total Carbs** 6g • **Fiber** 2g • **Total Sugar** 3g
Added Sugar 0g • **Protein** 4g • **Total Carbohydrate Choices** 0.5

NOTES FROM THE TEST KITCHEN

Buying Salad Greens

Not only is there a dizzying array of greens available at the supermarket now, but in a good market you can buy the same greens in more than one way: full heads, prewashed in a bag, in a clamshell, and loose in bulk bins. Which is the right choice for you? A sturdy lettuce like romaine can be washed and stored for up to a week, making it a good option for many nights' worth of salads. Bags of prewashed baby spinach, arugula, and mesclun mix offer great convenience, but be sure to turn over the bags and inspect the greens as closely as you can; the sell-by date alone doesn't ensure quality, so if you see moisture in the bag or hints of blackened leaf edges, move on.

Don't buy bags of already-cut lettuce that you can otherwise buy as whole heads, like romaine, Bibb, or red leaf. Precut lettuce will be inferior in quality because the leaves begin to spoil once they are cut (bagged hearts of romaine are fine). Endive and radicchio are always sold in heads and, because they are sturdy and will last a while, they are nice to have on hand to complement other greens and to add more interest to a salad. When planning a special salad for company, for the best results you should buy the greens either the day of the party or the day before.

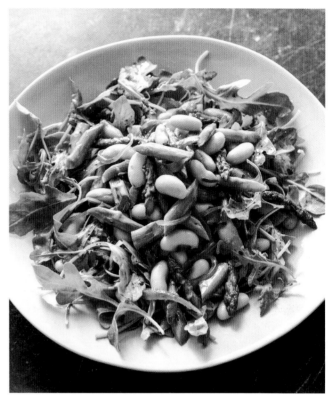

Slicing asparagus on the bias increases the surface area so it cooks quickly when sautéed.

Asparagus and Arugula Salad with Cannellini Beans

SERVES 6

WHY THIS RECIPE WORKS To incorporate asparagus into a bright, fresh salad, we found that choosing the right cooking method was key. Steaming produced bland, mushy spears, but sautéing the asparagus over high heat delivered deep flavor and tender texture. We sliced the spears on a bias to expose as much of the inner fibers to the cooking surface as possible. With olive oil in a hot pan, we browned some red onion before adding the asparagus pieces. Just 4 minutes of cooking was enough to produce uniformly tender pieces. Creamy cannellini beans provided a subtly nutty and smooth contrast to the asparagus; plus, they gave our salad extra protein and fiber. While the asparagus mixture cooled, we made a simple vinaigrette of balsamic, olive oil, salt, and pepper. For the greens, we knew peppery arugula would hold up well against the other bold flavors, so we dressed and plated it before tossing the asparagus in the dressing as well. Look for asparagus spears no thicker than ½ inch for this recipe.

5 tablespoons extra-virgin olive oil
½ red onion, sliced thin
1 pound asparagus, trimmed and cut into 1-inch lengths
  on bias
  Salt and pepper
1 (15-ounce) can no-salt-added cannellini beans, rinsed
2 tablespoons plus 2 teaspoons balsamic vinegar
6 ounces (6 cups) baby arugula

1. Heat 2 tablespoons oil in 12-inch nonstick skillet over high heat until just smoking. Add onion and cook until lightly browned, about 1 minute. Add asparagus, ¼ teaspoon salt, and ¼ teaspoon pepper and cook, stirring occasionally, until asparagus is browned and crisp-tender, about 4 minutes. Transfer to bowl, stir in beans, and let cool slightly.

2. Whisk remaining 3 tablespoons oil, vinegar, ¼ teaspoon salt, and ⅛ teaspoon pepper together in small bowl. Gently toss arugula with 2 tablespoons dressing until coated. Season with pepper to taste. Divide arugula among individual plates. Gently toss asparagus mixture with remaining dressing and arrange over arugula. Serve.

PER SERVING
Cal 170 • **Total Fat** 12g • **Sat Fat** 1.5g • **Chol** 0mg
Sodium 220mg • **Total Carbs** 12g • **Fiber** 4g • **Total Sugar** 4g
Added Sugar 0g • **Protein** 5g • **Total Carbohydrate Choices** 1

VARIATION
Asparagus, Red Pepper, and Spinach Salad with Goat Cheese
SERVES 6

WHY THIS RECIPE WORKS We liked the idea of baby spinach tossed with a simple vinaigrette and topped with a mix of bell pepper strips and asparagus. Since raw vegetables are not always appealing in a salad like this, we briefly sautéed the pepper matchsticks and the asparagus pieces before dressing and arranging them over the dressed spinach. Crumbled tangy goat cheese was the finishing touch. Look for asparagus spears no thicker than ½ inch for this recipe.

5 tablespoons extra-virgin olive oil
1 red bell pepper, stemmed, seeded, and cut into
  2-inch-long matchsticks
1 pound asparagus, trimmed and cut into 1-inch
  lengths on bias
  Salt and pepper

1 shallot, sliced thin
1 tablespoon plus 1 teaspoon sherry vinegar
1 garlic clove, minced
6 ounces (6 cups) baby spinach
2 ounces goat cheese, crumbled (½ cup)

1. Heat 1 tablespoon oil in 12-inch nonstick skillet over high heat until just smoking. Add bell pepper and cook until lightly browned, about 2 minutes. Add asparagus, ¼ teaspoon salt, and ⅛ teaspoon pepper and cook, stirring occasionally, until asparagus is browned and almost tender, about 2 minutes. Stir in shallot and cook until softened and asparagus is crisp-tender, about 1 minute. Transfer to bowl and let cool slightly.

2. Whisk remaining ¼ cup oil, vinegar, garlic, ¼ teaspoon salt, and ⅛ teaspoon pepper together in small bowl. Gently toss spinach with 2 tablespoons dressing until coated. Season with pepper to taste. Divide spinach among individual plates. Gently toss asparagus mixture with remaining dressing and arrange over spinach. Sprinkle with goat cheese. Serve.

PER SERVING
Cal 160 • **Total Fat** 14g • **Sat Fat** 3g • **Chol** 5mg
Sodium 260mg • **Total Carbs** 6g • **Fiber** 3g • **Total Sugar** 3g
Added Sugar 0g • **Protein** 4g • **Total Carbohydrate Choices** 0.5

Kale Salad with Sweet Potatoes and Pomegranate Vinaigrette
SERVES 8

WHY THIS RECIPE WORKS We love the earthy flavor of uncooked kale, but the texture of raw kale can be a little tough. Many recipes call for tossing it with dressing and letting it tenderize in the fridge overnight, but this method didn't deliver the tender leaves we were after, and the long sitting time wasn't very convenient. Luckily, we found another technique that worked better and faster: massaging. Squeezing and massaging the kale broke down the cell walls in much the same way that heat would, darkening the leaves and turning them silky. Nutritious roasted sweet potatoes, shredded radicchio, crunchy pecans, a sprinkling of Parmesan cheese, and a pomegranate vinaigrette made our kale salad heartier. Tuscan kale (also known as dinosaur or Lacinato kale) is more tender than curly-leaf and red kale; if using curly-leaf or red kale, increase the massaging time to 5 minutes. Do not use baby kale. You can find pomegranate molasses in the international aisle of most well-stocked supermarkets.

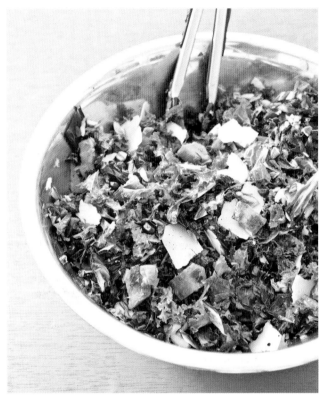

Caramelized sweet potatoes and a tangy pomegranate vinaigrette nicely complement earthy kale.

SALAD

1½ pounds sweet potatoes, peeled and cut into ½-inch pieces

2 teaspoons extra-virgin olive oil

Pepper

12 ounces Tuscan kale, stemmed and sliced crosswise into ½-inch-wide strips (7 cups)

½ head radicchio (5 ounces), cored and sliced thin

⅓ cup pecans, toasted and chopped

½ ounce Parmesan cheese, shaved

VINAIGRETTE

2 tablespoons water

1½ tablespoons pomegranate molasses

1 small shallot, minced

1 tablespoon cider vinegar

Salt and pepper

¼ cup extra-virgin olive oil

1. FOR THE SALAD Adjust oven rack to middle position and heat oven to 400 degrees. Toss sweet potatoes with oil and season with pepper. Arrange potatoes in single layer in rimmed baking sheet and roast until browned, 25 to 30 minutes, stirring potatoes halfway through roasting. Transfer to plate and let cool for 20 minutes. Meanwhile, vigorously squeeze and massage kale with hands until leaves are uniformly darkened and slightly wilted, about 1 minute.

2. FOR THE VINAIGRETTE Whisk water, pomegranate molasses, shallot, vinegar, ¼ teaspoon salt, and ¼ teaspoon pepper together in large bowl. While whisking constantly, drizzle in oil until completely emulsified.

3. Add potatoes, kale, and radicchio to bowl with vinaigrette and gently toss to coat. Season with pepper to taste. Sprinkle with pecans and Parmesan. Serve.

PER SERVING

Cal 190 • **Total Fat** 12g • **Sat Fat** 1.5g • **Chol** 0mg
Sodium 150mg • **Total Carbs** 18g • **Fiber** 4g • **Total Sugar** 5g
Added Sugar 1g • **Protein** 4g • **Total Carbohydrate Choices** 1

MASSAGING KALE

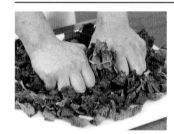

Vigorously squeeze and massage kale with hands over counter or in large bowl until leaves are uniformly darkened and slightly wilted, about 1 minute for flat-leaf kale (or 5 minutes for curly-leaf or red kale).

Mediterranean Chopped Salad
SERVES 6

WHY THIS RECIPE WORKS A Mediterranean salad always sounds like a healthy choice, but in a restaurant you're apt to wind up with a pile of watery iceberg lettuce topped with a few vegetables, stale feta cheese, olives, and a fat-laden, creamy dressing. Here we give Mediterranean chopped salad a fresh makeover with a bright vinaigrette that allows all the other components to shine, hearty romaine lettuce, and the right mix of other ingredients. To keep the tomatoes and cucumber crisp, we toss them with a small amount of salt and let them sit to draw out their moisture. Then we combine the tomato mixture, nutty chickpeas, olives, and onion with the vinaigrette for 5 minutes to give their flavors a chance to meld. Just these few extra steps deliver a nutritious and fresh-tasting chopped salad.

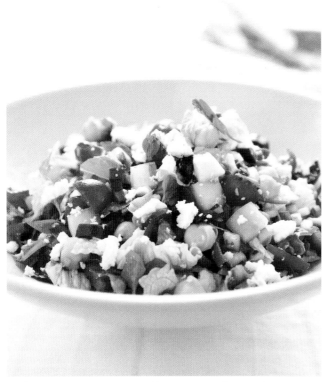

To draw excess moisture out of tomatoes and cucumbers, we lightly salt and drain them before tossing everything together.

12 ounces cherry tomatoes, quartered
1 cucumber, peeled, halved lengthwise, seeded, and cut into ½-inch pieces
  Salt and pepper
3 tablespoons extra-virgin olive oil
3 tablespoons red wine vinegar
1 garlic clove, minced
1 (15-ounce) can no-salt-added chickpeas, rinsed
⅓ cup pitted kalamata olives, chopped
¼ cup finely chopped red onion
1 romaine lettuce heart (6 ounces), cut into ½-inch pieces
3 ounces feta cheese, crumbled (¾ cup)
½ cup chopped fresh parsley

1. Toss tomatoes and cucumber with ½ teaspoon salt in colander and let drain for 15 to 30 minutes.

2. Whisk oil, vinegar, and garlic together in large bowl. Add tomato mixture, chickpeas, olives, and onion and gently toss to coat. Let sit at room temperature until flavors meld, about 5 minutes.

3. Add lettuce, feta, and parsley and gently toss to coat. Season with pepper to taste. Serve.

PER SERVING
Cal 180 • **Total Fat** 10g • **Sat Fat** 2.5g • **Chol** 10mg
Sodium 330mg • **Total Carbs** 13g • **Fiber** 3g • **Total Sugar** 3g
Added Sugar 0g • **Protein** 6g • **Total Carbohydrate Choices** 1

VARIATIONS
Fennel, Cucumber, and Apple Chopped Salad
SERVES 6

WHY THIS RECIPE WORKS This fresh take on a chopped salad forgoes the usual olives and feta, letting lots of chopped apple, fennel, and cucumber take center stage. Certainly, hearty chopped romaine can stand up to this combination, especially when tossed with a white wine vinaigrette and topped with goat cheese.

1 cucumber, peeled, halved lengthwise, seeded, and cut into ½-inch pieces
  Salt and pepper
3 tablespoons extra-virgin olive oil
3 tablespoons white wine vinegar
2 Fuji, Gala, or Golden Delicious apples, cored and cut into ¼-inch pieces
1 fennel bulb, stalks discarded, bulb halved, cored, and cut into ¼-inch pieces
¼ cup finely chopped red onion
1 romaine lettuce heart (6 ounces), cut into ½-inch pieces
¼ cup chopped fresh tarragon
3 ounces goat cheese, crumbled (¾ cup)

1. Toss cucumber with ½ teaspoon salt in colander and let drain for 15 to 30 minutes.

2. Whisk oil and vinegar together in large bowl. Add cucumber, apples, fennel, and onion and gently toss to coat. Let sit at room temperature until flavors meld, about 5 minutes.

3. Add lettuce and tarragon and gently toss to coat. Season with pepper to taste and sprinkle with goat cheese. Serve.

PER SERVING
Cal 160 • **Total Fat** 10g • **Sat Fat** 3g • **Chol** 5mg
Sodium 230mg • **Total Carbs** 14g • **Fiber** 3g • **Total Sugar** 9g
Added Sugar 0g • **Protein** 4g • **Total Carbohydrate Choices** 1

All About Seeds

Similar to nuts, seeds are fantastic ingredients to have on hand to add to virtually any dish. A plant-based source of protein, just a small handful provides good healthy fats plus fiber, minerals, and other nutrients. For optimal flavor, toast them in a dry 12-inch nonstick skillet over medium heat until the seeds are golden and fragrant.

Pepitas

Hulled pumpkin seed kernels, also known as pepitas, are actually one of the most flavorful seeds out there in addition to being high in important nutrients (a quarter cup contains 8 to 9 grams of protein). When toasted (which is how we like them best), they have a nutty, slightly sweet flavor that makes them the perfect addition to many dishes. They add a wonderful textural crunch when mixed into salads or sprinkled over your favorite fall soup. A handful sprinkled over yogurt is also a big winner.

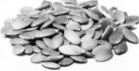

Sesame Seeds

Sesame seeds can be grayish ivory, brown, red, or black and are used in both savory and sweet recipes. Their nutty, subtle honey quality suits granola, bread, and sweets. We like their subtle texture in Sesame-Lemon Cucumber Salad (page 103).

Sunflower Seeds

Sunflower seeds are mildly sweet and creamy. Remove the black-and-white shells and eat the seeds out of hand or toss into salads or slaws. Instead of pine nuts, we reached for sunflower seeds to make the pesto for our Pasta with Kale Pesto, Tomatoes, and Chicken (page 161).

Radish, Orange, and Avocado Chopped Salad
SERVES 6

WHY THIS RECIPE WORKS Radishes are the star of this colorful and healthy salad—a great choice as they are both filling and low in calories and carbohydrates while also adding vital nutrients. Here we pair them with orange sections, cucumber, creamy chunks of avocado, and pungent chopped red onion. Lime juice ensures that the vinaigrette can stand up to all these ingredients, but what really makes this salad shine is the addition of sharp, shredded Manchego cheese (a little goes a long way), minced cilantro, and pepitas. You can substitute Parmesan for the Manchego cheese. Use the large holes of a box grater to shred the Manchego.

1 cucumber, peeled, halved lengthwise, seeded, and cut into ½-inch pieces
  Salt and pepper
2 oranges
3 tablespoons extra-virgin olive oil
3 tablespoons lime juice (2 limes)
1 garlic clove, minced
10 radishes, trimmed, halved, and sliced thin
½ avocado, cut into ½-inch pieces
¼ cup finely chopped red onion
1 romaine lettuce heart (6 ounces), cut into ½-inch pieces
2 ounces Manchego cheese, shredded (½ cup)
½ cup minced fresh cilantro
¼ cup roasted unsalted pepitas

1. Toss cucumber with ½ teaspoon salt in colander and let drain for 15 to 30 minutes.

2. Cut away peel and pith from oranges. Quarter oranges, then slice crosswise into ½-inch-thick pieces. Whisk oil, lime juice, and garlic together in large bowl. Add cucumber, orange pieces, radishes, avocado, and onion and gently toss to coat. Let sit at room temperature until flavors meld, about 5 minutes.

3. Add lettuce, Manchego, and cilantro and gently toss to coat. Season with pepper to taste and sprinkle with pepitas. Serve.

PER SERVING
Cal 200 • **Total Fat** 16g • **Sat Fat** 4.5g • **Chol** 5mg
Sodium 230mg • **Total Carbs** 11g • **Fiber** 3g • **Total Sugar** 6g
Added Sugar 0g • **Protein** 5g • **Total Carbohydrate Choices** 1

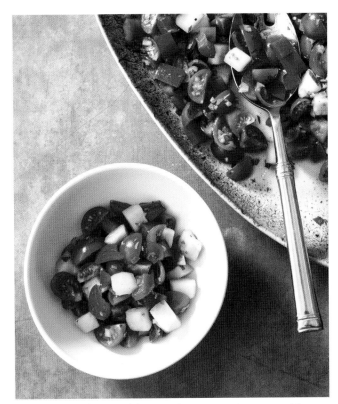

Borrowing the flavors of the popular summertime soup, this refreshing low-carb, low-cal gazpacho salad is easy to make.

Gazpacho Salad
SERVES 6

WHY THIS RECIPE WORKS If you love traditional gazpacho, then you'll love this crisp and colorful salad that mimics its key flavor components and is super low in calories—yet still satisfying. Salting and draining the tomatoes and cucumbers for 15 to 30 minutes before tossing them with the other ingredients ensures that you don't end up with a soupy salad. We prefer the flavor of sherry vinegar in this salad, but white wine vinegar can be substituted.

  1 pound cherry tomatoes, quartered
  1 cucumber, peeled, halved lengthwise, seeded, and cut into ½-inch pieces
    Salt and pepper
  5 teaspoons extra-virgin olive oil
  4 teaspoons sherry vinegar
  1 shallot, minced

  1 garlic clove, minced
  1 red bell pepper, stemmed, seeded, and cut into ½-inch pieces
  ¼ cup minced fresh cilantro

  1. Toss tomatoes and cucumber with ½ teaspoon salt in colander and let drain for 15 to 30 minutes.

  2. Whisk oil, vinegar, shallot, and garlic together in large bowl. Add tomato mixture, bell pepper, and cilantro and gently toss to coat. Season with pepper to taste and let sit until flavors meld, about 15 minutes. Serve.

PER SERVING
Cal 60 • **Total Fat** 4g • **Sat Fat** 0.5g • **Chol** 0mg
Sodium 150mg • **Total Carbs** 5g • **Fiber** 2g • **Total Sugar** 3g
Added Sugar 0g • **Protein** 1g • **Total Carbohydrate Choices** <0.5

Roasted Beet and Carrot Salad with Cumin and Pistachios
SERVES 6

WHY THIS RECIPE WORKS Beets and carrots are a winning combination, and roasting them brings out their earthy sweetness. Wrapping the beets in foil allowed them to cook gently, without missing out on the distinct, concentrated flavor of roasting. Steaming them in foil and then slicing the beets also helped to minimize "bleeding" of any liquid. To turn the beets and carrots into a salad, we tossed them with an equally earthy vinaigrette while they were still hot, which allowed them to absorb maximum flavor. Cumin added warmth to the dressing and shallot gave it a subtle, oniony bite. Pistachios lent nice color and crunch. Adding the nuts with lemon zest and chopped parsley just before serving resulted in a bright, well-balanced salad. You can use either golden or red beets (or a mix of both) in this recipe. To ensure even cooking, use beets that are of similar size—roughly 2 to 3 inches in diameter.

  1 pound beets, trimmed
  1 pound carrots, peeled and sliced ¼ inch thick on bias
  2½ tablespoons extra-virgin olive oil
    Salt and pepper
  1 tablespoon grated lemon zest plus 3 tablespoons juice
  1 small shallot, minced
  ½ teaspoon ground cumin
  ½ cup shelled pistachios, toasted and chopped
  2 tablespoons minced fresh parsley

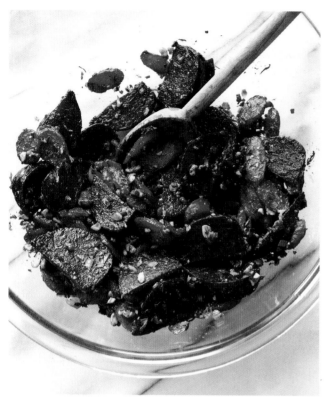

We toss roasted carrots and beets in the dressing while they're still warm so they absorb maximum flavor.

1. Adjust oven racks to middle and lowest positions. Place rimmed baking sheet on lower rack and heat oven to 450 degrees. Wrap beets individually in aluminum foil and place on second rimmed baking sheet. Toss carrots with 1 tablespoon oil, ¼ teaspoon salt, and ½ teaspoon pepper in bowl.

2. Working quickly, arrange carrots in single layer on hot sheet, then return to oven on lower rack. Place sheet with beets on upper rack. Roast until carrots are tender and well browned on 1 side, 20 to 25 minutes, and beets are tender and tip of paring knife inserted into beets meets little resistance (you will need to unwrap beets to test them), 35 to 45 minutes.

3. Carefully open foil packets and let beets sit until cool enough to handle. Carefully rub off beet skins using paper towel. Halve beets lengthwise, then slice into ½-inch-thick wedges, and, if large, halve crosswise.

4. Whisk lemon juice, shallot, cumin, ¼ teaspoon salt, and ⅛ teaspoon pepper together in large bowl until combined. While whisking constantly, drizzle in remaining 1½ tablespoons oil until completely emulsified. Add beets and carrots, gently toss to coat,

and let cool to room temperature, about 20 minutes. (Beet mixture can be refrigerated for up to 24 hours; bring to room temperature before continuing.)

5. Add pistachios, parsley, and lemon zest and gently toss to coat. Season with pepper to taste. Serve.

PER SERVING

Cal 170 • **Total Fat** 11g • **Sat Fat** 1.5g • **Chol** 0mg
Sodium 280mg • **Total Carbs** 15g • **Fiber** 5g • **Total Sugar** 8g
Added Sugar 0g • **Protein** 4g • **Total Carbohydrate Choices** 1

Green Bean Salad with Cilantro Sauce

SERVES 8

WHY THIS RECIPE WORKS To dress up a simple green bean salad, we came up with a fresh take on pesto by swapping out the traditional basil for bright, grassy cilantro. A single scallion brightened the green color of the sauce, and walnuts and garlic cloves, briefly toasted in a skillet, added nutty depth. The fruity flavor of extra-virgin olive oil complemented the other flavors in the dressing nicely. Finally, a touch of lemon juice rounded out the flavors and helped to loosen the sauce. We blanched and shocked the beans to set their vibrant green color and ensure that they were evenly cooked. Don't worry about drying the beans before tossing them with the sauce; any water that clings to the beans will help to thin out the sauce.

¼ cup walnuts
2 garlic cloves, unpeeled
2½ cups fresh cilantro leaves and stems, trimmed (2 bunches)
4 teaspoons lemon juice
1 scallion, sliced thin
Salt and pepper
½ cup extra-virgin olive oil
2 pounds green beans, trimmed

1. Cook walnuts and garlic in 8-inch skillet over medium heat, stirring often, until toasted and fragrant, 5 to 7 minutes; transfer to bowl. Let garlic cool slightly, then peel.

2. Process walnuts, garlic, cilantro, lemon juice, scallion, ½ teaspoon salt, and ⅛ teaspoon pepper in food processor until smooth, about 1 minute, scraping down sides of bowl as needed. With processor running, slowly add oil until incorporated; transfer to large bowl.

3. Bring 4 quarts water to boil in large pot. Fill large bowl halfway with ice and water. Add green beans and 1 tablespoon salt to boiling water and cook until crisp-tender, 3 to 5 minutes. Drain green beans, transfer to prepared ice bath, and let sit until chilled, about 2 minutes.

4. Drain green beans, transfer to bowl with cilantro sauce, and gently toss to coat. (Salad can be refrigerated for up to 4 hours; bring to room temperature before serving.) Season with pepper to taste. Serve.

PER SERVING

Cal 180 • **Total Fat** 16g • **Sat Fat** 2g • **Chol** 0mg
Sodium 190mg • **Total Carbs** 8g • **Fiber** 3g • **Total Sugar** 3g
Added Sugar 0g • **Protein** 3g • **Total Carbohydrate Choices** 0.5

TRIMMING ENDS FROM GREEN BEANS

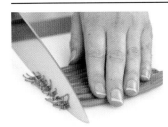

Instead of trimming ends from one green bean at a time, streamline process by lining up beans on cutting board and trimming stem ends with just one slice.

Brussels Sprout Salad with Pecorino and Pine Nuts
SERVES 6

WHY THIS RECIPE WORKS We think it is good to have many recipes in your repertoire using Brussels sprouts because they are so nutrient dense. To make Brussels sprouts shine in a salad, we needed to get rid of some of their vegetal rawness. Rather than cooking the sprouts, we sliced them very thin and then marinated them in a bright vinaigrette made with lemon juice and Dijon mustard. The 30-minute soak in the acidic dressing softened and seasoned the sprouts, bringing out and balancing their flavor. Toasted pine nuts and shredded Pecorino Romano, added to the salad just before serving, provided a layer of crunch and nutty richness. For the best texture, slice the sprouts as thinly as possible by hand. Use the large holes of a box grater to shred the Pecorino Romano.

2 tablespoons lemon juice
1 tablespoon Dijon mustard
1 small shallot, minced
1 garlic clove, minced
  Salt and pepper
¼ cup extra-virgin olive oil
1 pound Brussels sprouts, trimmed, halved, and sliced very thin
1 ounce Pecorino Romano cheese, shredded (⅓ cup)
¼ cup pine nuts, toasted

1. Whisk lemon juice, mustard, shallot, garlic, and ⅛ teaspoon salt in large bowl until combined. While whisking constantly, drizzle in oil until completely emulsified. Add Brussels sprouts, gently toss to coat, and let sit for at least 30 minutes or up to 2 hours.

2. Stir in Pecorino and pine nuts. Season with pepper to taste. Serve.

PER SERVING

Cal 170 • **Total Fat** 15g • **Sat Fat** 2.5g • **Chol** 5mg
Sodium 190mg • **Total Carbs** 8g • **Fiber** 3g • **Total Sugar** 2g
Added Sugar 0g • **Protein** 5g • **Total Carbohydrate Choices** 0.5

SLICING BRUSSELS SPROUTS FOR SALAD

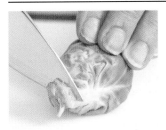 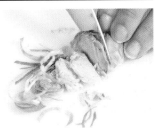

1. Peel off any loose or discolored leaves and slice off bottom of stem end, leaving leaves attached.

2. Halve Brussels sprouts through stem end, then slice very thin.

Brussels Sprout and Kale Salad with Herbs and Peanuts
SERVES 4

WHY THIS RECIPE WORKS Raw Brussels sprouts and kale leaves may sound like an odd combination for a salad, but these two highly nutritious vegetables are perfect together; since the uncooked leaves hold up well for hours, they're ideal for picnics and making ahead. To keep our slaw crisp and light, we left the Brussels sprouts raw and marinated them in the dressing to soften them just slightly. A vigorous massage tenderized the kale leaves in just a minute. A simple cider and coriander vinaigrette, fresh cilantro and mint, chopped peanuts, plus a squeeze of lime juice gave this slaw a refreshing Southeast Asian profile. Tuscan kale (also known as dinosaur or Lacinato kale) is more tender than curly-leaf and red kale; if using curly-leaf or red kale, increase the massaging time to 5 minutes. Do not use baby kale. For the best texture, slice the sprouts as thinly as possible by hand.

- ⅓ cup cider vinegar
- 2 tablespoons extra-virgin olive oil
- 1 tablespoon lime juice
- ½ teaspoon ground coriander
  Salt and pepper
- 1 pound Brussels sprouts, trimmed, halved, and sliced very thin
- 8 ounces Tuscan kale, stemmed and sliced into ¼-inch-wide strips (4½ cups)
- ¼ cup dry-roasted, unsalted peanuts, chopped
- 1 tablespoon chopped fresh cilantro
- 1 tablespoon chopped fresh mint

1. Whisk vinegar, oil, lime juice, coriander, ¼ teaspoon salt, and ¼ teaspoon pepper together in large bowl. Add Brussels sprouts and gently toss to coat. Cover and let sit for at least 30 minutes or up to 2 hours.

2. Vigorously squeeze and massage kale with hands until leaves are uniformly darkened and slightly wilted, about 1 minute. Add kale, peanuts, cilantro, and mint to bowl with Brussels sprouts and gently toss to coat. Season with pepper to taste. Serve.

PER SERVING

Cal 190 • **Total Fat** 12g • **Sat Fat** 2g • **Chol** 0mg
Sodium 190mg • **Total Carbs** 15g • **Fiber** 6g • **Total Sugar** 4g
Added Sugar 0g • **Protein** 7g • **Total Carbohydrate Choices** 1

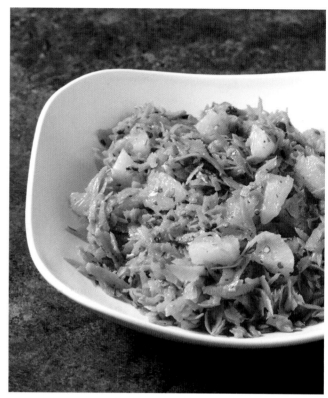

Full of fiber and vitamins, raw carrots are the star of this colorful, low-calorie side salad.

Moroccan-Style Carrot Salad
SERVES 6

WHY THIS RECIPE WORKS In this side salad, nutrient-rich carrots take center stage. The classic Moroccan salad combines grated carrots with olive oil, citrus, and warm spices like cumin and cinnamon. We tried grating the carrots both with a coarse grater and with a food processor and found that the coarse grater worked better. To complement the earthy carrots, we added orange segments, reserving some of the orange juice to add to the dressing. We balanced the sweet orange juice with a squeeze of lemon juice and small amounts of cumin, cayenne, and cinnamon. The musty aroma and slight nuttiness of the cumin nicely complemented the carrots. To add color and freshness, we stirred in some minced cilantro before serving.

- 2 oranges
- 1 tablespoon lemon juice
- ¾ teaspoon ground cumin
- ⅛ teaspoon cayenne pepper
- ⅛ teaspoon ground cinnamon

Salt and pepper
1 pound carrots, peeled and shredded
3 tablespoons minced fresh cilantro
3 tablespoons extra-virgin olive oil

1. Cut away peel and pith from oranges. Holding fruit over bowl, use paring knife to slice between membranes to release segments. Cut segments in half crosswise and let drain in fine-mesh strainer set over large bowl, reserving juice.

2. Whisk lemon juice, cumin, cayenne, cinnamon, and ½ teaspoon salt into bowl with reserved orange juice. Add orange segments and carrots and gently toss to coat. Let sit until liquid starts to pool in bottom of bowl, 3 to 5 minutes.

3. Drain salad in fine-mesh strainer then return to bowl. (Salad can be refrigerated for up to 1 hour; bring to room temperature before serving.) Stir in cilantro and oil and season with pepper to taste. Serve.

PER SERVING

Cal 110 • **Total Fat** 7g • **Sat Fat** 1g • **Chol** 0mg
Sodium 190mg • **Total Carbs** 12g • **Fiber** 3g • **Total Sugar** 7g
Added Sugar 0g • **Protein** 1g • **Total Carbohydrate Choices** 1

Sesame-Lemon Cucumber Salad
SERVES 4

WHY THIS RECIPE WORKS Cucumbers can make for a cool, crisp salad, but they often turn soggy from their own moisture. For a cucumber salad with good crunch, we found that weighting salted cucumbers forced more water from them than salting alone. After many tests, we determined that 1 to 3 hours worked best: Even after 12 hours, the cucumbers gave up no more water than they had after 3 hours. For a bit of zip, we liked pairing the cucumbers with a rice vinegar and lemon juice dressing; sesame oil and seeds added nutty flavor. This salad is best served within 1 hour of being dressed.

3 cucumbers, peeled, halved lengthwise, seeded, and sliced ¼ inch thick
    Salt and pepper
¼ cup rice vinegar
2 tablespoons toasted sesame oil
1 tablespoon lemon juice
1 tablespoon sesame seeds, toasted
⅛ teaspoon red pepper flakes, plus extra for seasoning

1. Toss cucumbers with 1 tablespoon salt in colander set over large bowl. Weight cucumbers with 1 gallon-size zipper-lock bag filled with water; drain for 1 to 3 hours. Rinse and pat dry.

2. Whisk vinegar, oil, lemon juice, sesame seeds, and pepper flakes together in large bowl. Add cucumbers and gently toss to coat. Season with pepper to taste. Serve at room temperature or chilled.

PER SERVING

Cal 90 • **Total Fat** 8g • **Sat Fat** 1g • **Chol** 0mg
Sodium 290mg • **Total Carbs** 4g • **Fiber** 1g • **Total Sugar** 2g
Added Sugar 0g • **Protein** 1g • **Total Carbohydrate Choices** <0.5

VARIATION
Yogurt-Mint Cucumber Salad
SERVES 4

WHY THIS RECIPE WORKS This refreshing take on a cool cucumber salad features a creamy, protein-rich dressing thanks to a full cup of low-fat yogurt in addition to olive oil. Since cucumbers and mint are a classic pairing, we added a whopping ¼ cup of minced fresh mint to the dressing along with cumin and garlic—all of which ensured that the salad was brightly flavored. This salad is best served within 1 hour of being dressed.

3 cucumbers, peeled, halved lengthwise, seeded, and sliced ¼ inch thick
1 small red onion, halved and sliced thin
    Salt and pepper
1 cup plain low-fat yogurt
¼ cup minced fresh mint
2 tablespoons extra-virgin olive oil
1 garlic clove, minced
½ teaspoon ground cumin

1. Toss cucumbers and onion with 1 tablespoon salt in colander set over large bowl. Weight cucumber-onion mixture with 1 gallon-size zipper-lock bag filled with water; drain for 1 to 3 hours. Rinse and pat dry.

2. Whisk yogurt, mint, oil, garlic, and cumin together in large bowl. Add cucumber-onion mixture and gently toss to coat. Season with pepper to taste. Serve at room temperature or chilled.

PER SERVING

Cal 130 • **Total Fat** 8g • **Sat Fat** 1.5g • **Chol** 5mg
Sodium 340mg • **Total Carbs** 10g • **Fiber** 2g • **Total Sugar** 7g
Added Sugar 0g • **Protein** 5g • **Total Carbohydrate Choices** 1

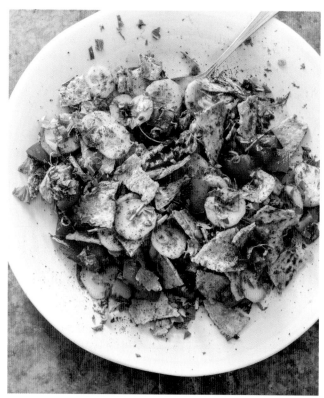

Tangy sumac adds bright flavor while baked whole-wheat pita chips add crunch to this traditional Mediterranean salad.

Fattoush
SERVES 6

WHY THIS RECIPE WORKS Fattoush is an eastern Mediterranean salad that combines fresh produce and herbs, toasted pita bread, and bright, tangy sumac. Our goal was to balance the sweetly acidic flavor of sumac with the fresh vegetables, while also preventing the pita from becoming soggy. Sumac, a commonly used spice across the Mediterranean, traditionally lends a citrusy punch to fattoush, so we opted to use an ample amount in the dressing. We did not seed and salt the cucumbers and tomatoes in this recipe to make use of the flavorful seeds and juice of the tomatoes. In order to make the whole-wheat pita pieces moisture-resistant, we brushed their craggy sides with plenty of olive oil before baking them. The oil prevented the pita from absorbing moisture from the salad and becoming soggy while still allowing them to pick up flavor from the lemony dressing. You can find sumac in most well-stocked supermarkets. The success of this recipe depends on ripe, in-season tomatoes.

2 (6½-inch) whole-wheat pita breads
7 tablespoons extra-virgin olive oil
  Pepper
3 tablespoons lemon juice
4 teaspoons ground sumac
¼ teaspoon minced garlic
1 pound ripe tomatoes, cored and cut into ¾-inch pieces
1 English cucumber, peeled and sliced ⅛ inch thick
1 cup baby arugula, chopped
½ cup chopped fresh cilantro
½ cup chopped fresh mint
4 scallions, sliced thin

1. Adjust oven rack to middle position and heat oven to 375 degrees. Using kitchen shears, cut around perimeter of each pita and separate into 2 thin rounds. Cut each round in half. Place pitas smooth side down on wire rack set in rimmed baking sheet. Brush 3 tablespoons oil on surface of pitas. (Pitas do not need to be uniformly coated. Oil will spread during baking.) Season with pepper. Bake until pitas are crisp and pale golden brown, 10 to 14 minutes. Let cool to room temperature.

2. Whisk lemon juice, sumac, and garlic together in large bowl and let sit for 10 minutes. Whisk in remaining ¼ cup oil.

3. Break pitas into ½-inch pieces. Add pita pieces, tomatoes, cucumber, arugula, cilantro, mint, and scallions to bowl with dressing and gently toss to coat. Season with pepper to taste. Serve immediately.

PER SERVING

Cal 230 • **Total Fat** 17g • **Sat Fat** 2.5g • **Chol** 0mg
Sodium 170mg • **Total Carbs** 19g • **Fiber** 4g • **Total Sugar** 4g
Added Sugar 0g • **Protein** 4g • **Total Carbohydrate Choices** 1

French Potato Salad with Dijon and Fines Herbes
SERVES 6

WHY THIS RECIPE WORKS: This satisfying French take on potato salad utilizes unpeeled potatoes for more fiber and nutrients and dresses them with fruity extra-virgin olive oil and fresh herbs. The potatoes (small red potatoes are traditional) should be tender but not mushy, and the flavor of the vinaigrette should permeate the relatively bland potatoes. To eliminate torn skins and broken slices, a common pitfall in boiling skin-on red potatoes, we sliced the potatoes before boiling them. To evenly infuse the potatoes

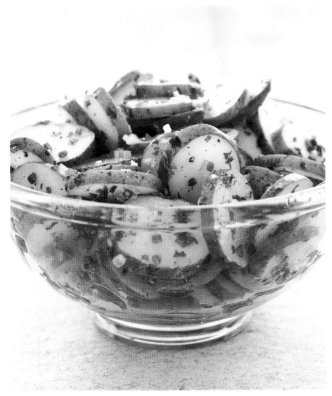

1. Place potatoes in large saucepan, add water to cover by 1 inch, and bring to boil. Add salt, reduce to simmer, and cook until potatoes are tender and paring knife can be slipped in and out of potatoes with little resistance, about 6 minutes.

2. While potatoes are cooking, lower skewered garlic into simmering water and blanch for 45 seconds. Run garlic under cold running water, then remove from skewer and mince.

3. Reserve ¼ cup cooking water, then drain potatoes and arrange in tight single layer on rimmed baking sheet. Whisk minced garlic, oil, vinegar, mustard, pepper, and reserved potato cooking water together in bowl, then drizzle over potatoes. Let potatoes sit until flavors meld, about 10 minutes. (Potatoes can be refrigerated for up to 8 hours; bring to room temperature before continuing.)

4. Transfer potatoes to large bowl. Sprinkle shallot, chervil, parsley, chives, and tarragon over potatoes and gently toss to coat using rubber spatula. Serve.

PER SERVING

Cal 190 • **Total Fat** 10g • **Sat Fat** 1.5g • **Chol** 0mg
Sodium 260mg • **Total Carbs** 25g • **Fiber** 3g • **Total Sugar** 2g
Added Sugar 0g • **Protein** 3g • **Total Carbohydrate Choices** 1.5

To infuse potatoes with great flavor, we drizzle them with a mustard vinaigrette while still warm, then add lots of fresh herbs.

with the garlicky mustard vinaigrette, we spread the warm potatoes on a baking sheet and poured the vinaigrette over the top. Gently folding in the herbs just before serving added fresh flavor and helped keep the potatoes intact. If fresh chervil isn't available, substitute an additional ½ tablespoon of minced parsley and an additional ½ teaspoon of tarragon. Use small red potatoes measuring 1 to 2 inches in diameter.

2 pounds small red potatoes, unpeeled, sliced ¼ inch thick
2 tablespoons salt
1 garlic clove, peeled and threaded on skewer
¼ cup extra-virgin olive oil
1½ tablespoons white wine or champagne vinegar
2 teaspoons Dijon mustard
½ teaspoon pepper
1 small shallot, minced
1 tablespoon minced fresh chervil
1 tablespoon minced fresh parsley
1 tablespoon minced fresh chives
1 teaspoon minced fresh tarragon

NOTES FROM THE TEST KITCHEN

The Best Supermarket Extra-Virgin Olive Oil

If you are aiming to use less oil, the quality of the oil really matters. Extra-virgin oils range wildly in price, color, and quality, so it's hard to know which to buy. While many things can affect the quality and flavor of olive oil, the type of olive, the time of harvest (earlier means greener, more bitter, and pungent; later, more mild and buttery), and the processing are the most important factors. The best-quality olive oil comes from olives pressed as quickly as possible without heat (which coaxes more oil from the olives at the expense of flavor). Our favorite supermarket extra-virgin olive oil, **California Olive Ranch Everyday Extra Virgin Olive Oil** ($9.99 for 500 ml), is a standout for its "fruity," "fragrant" flavor. In fact, its flavor rivaled that of our favorite high-end extra-virgin oil.

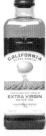

Roasted Winter Squash Salad with Za'atar and Parsley
SERVES 6

WHY THIS RECIPE WORKS The sweet, nutty flavor of roasted butternut squash pairs best with flavors that are bold enough to balance that sweetness. To fill this role in our roasted butternut squash salad, we chose the traditional eastern Mediterranean spice blend za'atar (a lively combination of toasted sesame seeds, thyme, and sumac). We found that using high heat and placing the oven rack in the lowest position produced perfectly browned squash with a firm center in about 30 minutes. Dusting the za'atar over the hot squash worked much like toasting the spice, boosting its flavor. For a foil to the tender squash, we considered a host of nuts before landing on toasted pumpkin seeds (pepitas). They provided the textural accent the dish needed and reinforced the squash's flavor. Pomegranate seeds added a burst of tartness and color. You can find za'atar in the spice aisle of most well-stocked supermarkets. You can substitute chopped red grapes or small blueberries for the pomegranate seeds.

- 3 pounds butternut squash, peeled, seeded, and cut into ½-inch pieces (8 cups)
- ¼ cup extra-virgin olive oil
  Salt and pepper
- 1½ teaspoons za'atar
- 1 small shallot, minced
- 2 tablespoons lemon juice
- ¾ cup fresh parsley leaves
- ⅓ cup roasted unsalted pepitas
- ½ cup pomegranate seeds

1. Adjust oven rack to lowest position and heat oven to 450 degrees. Toss squash with 1 tablespoon oil and season with pepper. Arrange squash in single layer on rimmed baking sheet and roast until well browned and tender, 30 to 35 minutes, stirring halfway through roasting. Sprinkle squash with za'atar and let cool for 15 minutes. (Squash can be refrigerated for up to 24 hours; bring to room temperature before continuing.)

2. Whisk shallot, lemon juice, ¼ teaspoon salt, and remaining 3 tablespoons oil together in large bowl. Add squash, parsley, and pepitas and gently toss to coat. Sprinkle with pomegranate seeds. Serve.

PER SERVING
Cal 230 • **Total Fat** 13g • **Sat Fat** 2g • **Chol** 0mg
Sodium 110mg • **Total Carbs** 27g • **Fiber** 5g • **Total Sugar** 7g
Added Sugar 0g • **Protein** 4g • **Total Carbohydrate Choices** 2

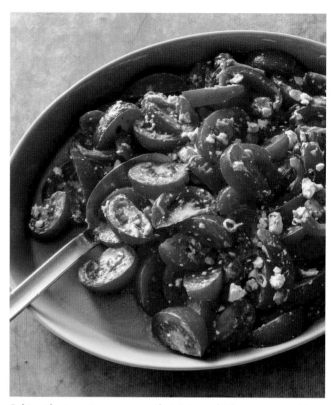

Salting the tomatoes seasons their juice, which we use to add flavor to the salad dressing.

Tomato Salad with Feta and Cumin-Yogurt Dressing
SERVES 6

WHY THIS RECIPE WORKS Juicy summer tomatoes are full of vitamins and make a great salad, so we set out to create one with complementary flavors and a creamy dressing that was big on flavor. Tomatoes exude lots of liquid when cut, so to get rid of some of the tomato juice without losing all its valuable flavor, we lightly salted the tomatoes. This also seasoned them and their juice at the same time. We reserved a measured amount of the flavorful juice to add to the dressing so as to not water down the salad. Greek yogurt laid the foundation for the creamy dressing, and we boosted its tang with lemon juice and the reserved tomato juice. To that we added fresh oregano, cumin, and garlic, but some tasters found the cumin and garlic too harsh. A quick zap in the microwave was all it took to effectively bloom the spice and cook the garlic, successfully mellowing their flavors. We tossed the tomatoes with the dressing, finishing with just the right amount of briny feta to add richness and another layer of flavor. The success of this recipe depends on ripe, in-season tomatoes.

2½ pounds ripe tomatoes, cored and cut into
    ½-inch-thick wedges
¼ teaspoon salt
3 tablespoons extra-virgin olive oil
1 garlic clove, minced
1 teaspoon ground cumin
¼ cup plain 2 percent Greek yogurt
1 scallion, sliced thin
1 tablespoon lemon juice
1 tablespoon minced fresh oregano
2 ounces feta cheese, crumbled (½ cup)

1. Toss tomatoes with salt and let drain in colander set over large bowl for 15 to 20 minutes. Pour off all but 1 tablespoon juice and reserve juice in bowl.

2. Combine oil, garlic, and cumin in separate bowl and microwave until fragrant, about 30 seconds; let cool slightly. Whisk oil mixture, yogurt, scallion, lemon juice, and oregano into reserved tomato juice until combined. Add tomatoes and feta and gently toss to coat. Serve immediately.

PER SERVING

Cal 130 • **Total Fat** 10g • **Sat Fat** 2.5g • **Chol** 10mg
Sodium 170mg • **Total Carbs** 9g • **Fiber** 2g • **Total Sugar** 6g
Added Sugar 0g • **Protein** 4g • **Total Carbohydrate Choices** 0.5

Cherry Tomato Salad with Feta and Olives

SERVES 6

WHY THIS RECIPE WORKS Cherry tomatoes can make a great salad, but they exude liquid when cut. To get rid of some of the tomato juice, we added a small amount of salt to draw out the tomatoes' liquid, before whirling them in a salad spinner to separate the seeds and juice from the flesh. We then reduced the tomato juice to a flavorful concentrate (adding garlic, oregano, shallot, olive oil, and vinegar) and reunited it with the tomatoes. Just a little feta cheese went a long way to add richness. If cherry tomatoes are unavailable, substitute grape tomatoes cut in half along the equator. If you don't have a salad spinner, wrap the bowl tightly with plastic wrap after the salted tomatoes have sat for 30 minutes and gently shake to remove seeds and excess liquid. Strain the liquid and proceed with the recipe as directed. If you have less than ½ cup of juice after spinning, proceed with the recipe using the entire amount of juice and reduce it to 3 tablespoons as directed (the cooking time will be shorter).

Buying and Storing Fresh Tomatoes

Buying tomatoes at the height of summer won't guarantee juicy, flavorful fruit, but keeping these guidelines in mind will help.

Choose Locally Grown Tomatoes

The best way to ensure a flavorful tomato is to buy local, if at all possible. The shorter the distance a tomato has to travel, the riper it can be when it's picked. And commercial tomatoes are engineered to be sturdier, with thicker walls and less of the flavorful juice and seeds.

Looks Aren't Everything

When selecting tomatoes, oddly shaped tomatoes are fine, and even cracked skin is OK. Avoid tomatoes that are overly soft or leaking juice. Choose tomatoes that smell fruity and feel heavy. And consider trying heirloom tomatoes; grown from naturally pollinated plants and seeds, they are some of the best local tomatoes you can find.

Buy Supermarket Tomatoes on the Vine

If supermarket tomatoes are your only option, look for tomatoes sold on the vine. Although this does not mean that they were fully ripened on the vine, they are better than regular supermarket tomatoes, which are picked when still green and blasted with ethylene gas to develop texture and color.

Storing Tomatoes

Once you've brought your tomatoes home, proper storage is important to preserve their fresh flavor and texture for as long as possible. Here are the rules we follow in the test kitchen:

- Never refrigerate tomatoes; the cold damages enzymes that produce flavor compounds, and it ruins their texture, turning the flesh mealy. Even when cut, tomatoes should be kept at room temperature (wrap them tightly in plastic wrap).
- If the vine is still attached, leave it on and store the tomatoes stem end up. Tomatoes off the vine should be stored stem side down. We have found that this prevents moisture from escaping and bacteria from entering and thus prolongs shelf life.
- To quickly ripen hard tomatoes, store them in a paper bag with a banana or apple, both of which emit ethylene gas, which hastens ripening.

1½ pounds cherry tomatoes, quartered
¼ teaspoon salt
1 shallot, minced
1 tablespoon red wine vinegar
2 garlic cloves, minced
2 teaspoons minced fresh oregano
1 small cucumber, peeled, halved lengthwise, seeded, and cut into ½-inch pieces
½ cup pitted kalamata olives, chopped
2 ounces feta cheese, crumbled (½ cup)
3 tablespoons chopped fresh parsley
2 tablespoons extra-virgin olive oil

1. Toss tomatoes with salt in bowl and let sit for 30 minutes. Transfer tomatoes to salad spinner and spin until seeds and excess liquid have been removed, 45 to 60 seconds, stopping to redistribute tomatoes several times during spinning; set tomatoes aside. Strain ½ cup of tomato liquid through fine-mesh strainer into liquid measuring cup; discard remaining liquid.

2. Combine tomato liquid, shallot, vinegar, garlic, and oregano in small saucepan and bring to simmer over medium heat; cook until reduced to 3 tablespoons, 6 to 8 minutes. Transfer to large bowl and let cool to room temperature, about 5 minutes. Add drained tomatoes, cucumber, olives, feta, parsley, and oil and gently toss to coat. Serve immediately.

PER SERVING
Cal 100 • **Total Fat** 8g • **Sat Fat** 2g • **Chol** 10mg
Sodium 210mg • **Total Carbs** 7g • **Fiber** 2g • **Total Sugar** 4g
Added Sugar 0g • **Protein** 3g • **Total Carbohydrate Choices** 0.5

VARIATION
Cherry Tomato Salad with Basil and Fresh Mozzarella
In dressing, substitute balsamic vinegar for red wine vinegar and omit garlic and oregano. Omit cucumber, olives, feta, and parsley. Instead, add 1½ cups roughly torn fresh basil leaves and 8 ounces fresh mozzarella, cut into ½-inch pieces and patted dry with paper towels, to tomatoes with dressing.

PER SERVING
Cal 180 • **Total Fat** 13g • **Sat Fat** 6g • **Chol** 25mg
Sodium 190mg • **Total Carbs** 6g • **Fiber** 2g • **Total Sugar** 4g
Added Sugar 0g • **Protein** 8g • **Total Carbohydrate Choices** <0.5

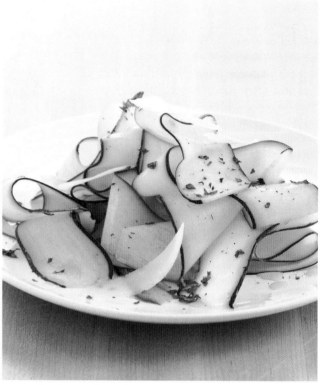

Dressed with just olive oil, lemon juice, mint, and Parmesan, delicate zucchini ribbons make a light and summery side salad.

Zucchini Ribbon Salad with Shaved Parmesan
SERVES 4

WHY THIS RECIPE WORKS This elegant alternative to a lettuce-based salad is also a unique way to serve zucchini without losing its crunchy texture or fresh flavor by cooking. Slicing the zucchini into thin ribbons using a peeler or mandoline maximized its surface area for dressing to cling to. We dressed the zucchini simply with a touch of olive oil and lemon juice so that the bright flavors of the vegetable weren't overshadowed by a heavy dressing. Minced mint leaves enhanced the refreshing quality of the zucchini, while shaved Parmesan cheese provided savory body without weighing the ribbons down. The success of this dish depends on using small, in-season zucchini, good olive oil, and high-quality Parmesan.

4 zucchini (6 ounces each), trimmed and sliced lengthwise into ribbons
¼ teaspoon pepper
3 tablespoons extra-virgin olive oil

2 tablespoons lemon juice

2 ounces Parmesan cheese, shaved

2 tablespoons minced fresh mint

Gently toss zucchini with pepper, then arrange attractively on serving platter. Drizzle with oil and lemon juice, then sprinkle with Parmesan and mint. Serve immediately.

PER SERVING

Cal 190 • **Total Fat** 15g • **Sat Fat** 3.5 • **Chol** 10g

Sodium 270mg • **Total Carbs** 7g • **Fiber** 2g • **Total Sugar** 2

Added Sugar 0g • **Protein** 9 g • **Total Carbohydrate Choices** 1

MAKING ZUCCHINI RIBBONS

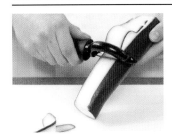

Using a vegetable peeler or mandoline, slice zucchini lengthwise into very thin ribbons.

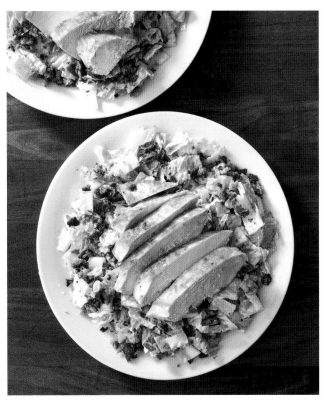

To make a supercreamy Caesar salad dressing, we rely on a combination of Greek yogurt and mayonnaise.

Chicken Caesar Salad
SERVES 4

WHY THIS RECIPE WORKS Many people looking to lighten their diet assume that having salad for dinner is a safe bet. But consider one of the most celebrated dinner salads of all: the chicken Caesar. Its crisp romaine lettuce, juicy grilled chicken, and garlic croutons may not seem all that bad, but layer on Parmesan cheese and a dressing made with eggs and oil, and the fat and salt can add up quickly. We knew that we could do better. Tasters found that the flavor of fat-enriched mayonnaise gave them the classic creamy notes they wanted, but an all-mayo dressing was a nutritional no-go. Luckily, we found a healthy ingredient that bulked up our dressing, and gave it a pleasant tang and extra body: Greek yogurt. With those two ingredients as our base, along with the classic flavorings of Caesar dressing, we emulsified in olive oil for richness, and had a dressing that tasters declared as good as the full-fat original. We simply seared the chicken in olive oil, letting the natural browning provide intense chicken-y flavor. Instead of choosing a low-fat crouton, which tasters found dry and flavorless, we created a pangrattato, or garlicky bread crumb topping. The crumbs found their way into every part of the salad, bringing crunch with them—and as a bonus we used much less bread than needed to make croutons. Now we had a healthy, delicious chicken Caesar salad that no one would suspect of skimping on a thing. We prefer a whole-wheat baguette to make the bread crumbs in this salad, but you can substitute hearty whole-wheat sandwich bread in a pinch.

SALAD

  2 ounces whole-wheat baguette, cut into 1-inch pieces (²/₃ cup)

  2 tablespoons extra-virgin olive oil

  ¼ teaspoon garlic powder

    Salt and pepper

  1 tablespoon grated Parmesan cheese

  4 (6-ounce) boneless, skinless chicken breasts, trimmed of all visible fat

  3 romaine lettuce hearts (18 ounces), cut into ½-inch pieces

DRESSING

⅓ cup mayonnaise

¼ cup plain 2 percent Greek yogurt

4 teaspoons lemon juice

1 tablespoon water

2 teaspoons Dijon mustard

1 teaspoon Worcestershire sauce

1 anchovy fillet, rinsed and minced to paste

1 small garlic clove, minced

3 tablespoons extra-virgin olive oil

3 tablespoons grated Parmesan cheese
   Pepper

1. FOR THE SALAD Pulse bread in food processor into coarse crumbs measuring ⅛ to ¼ inch, about 10 pulses. Combine crumbs, 1 tablespoon oil, garlic powder, and pinch pepper in 12-inch non-stick skillet. Cook over medium heat, stirring often, until crumbs are crisp and golden, about 10 minutes. Off heat, stir in Parmesan. Set aside to cool.

2. Pat chicken dry with paper towels and sprinkle with ⅛ tea-spoon salt and ⅛ teaspoon pepper. Heat remaining 1 tablespoon oil in now-empty skillet over medium-high heat until just smok-ing. Cook chicken until golden brown and registers 160 degrees, about 6 minutes per side. Transfer chicken to cutting board, tent with aluminum foil, and let rest for 5 to 10 minutes. Slice chicken crosswise into ½-inch-thick slices.

3. FOR THE DRESSING Whisk mayonnaise, yogurt, lemon juice, water, mustard, Worcestershire, anchovy, and garlic in large bowl until combined. While whisking constantly, drizzle in oil until completely emulsified. Stir in Parmesan and season with pepper to taste. Add lettuce and gently toss to coat. Divide salad among individual plates, sprinkle with bread crumbs, and top with chicken. Serve.

PER SERVING

Cal 590 • **Total Fat** 38g • **Sat Fat** 7g • **Chol** 135mg
Sodium 570mg • **Total Carbs** 14g • **Fiber** 2g • **Total Sugar** 5g
Added Sugar 0g • **Protein** 46g • **Total Carbohydrate Choices** 1

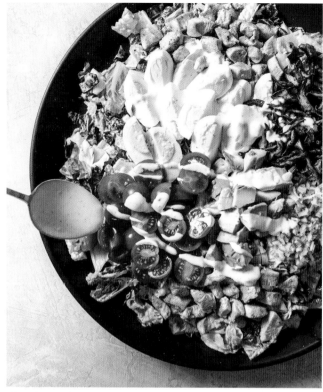

Shiitake mushrooms sautéed with smoked paprika and chili powder provide our Cobb salad with smoky bacon flavor.

Cobb Salad
SERVES 4

WHY THIS RECIPE WORKS Stunning presentation aside, Cobb salad has all the markers of a powerhouse meal, including eggs, avoca-dos, tomato, and lean chicken—we just had to do something about all that sodium-laden bacon and cheese. We were sad to sacrifice bacon's smoky flavor until we tried sautéing shiitake mushrooms with smoked paprika and chili powder. Now we had smokiness and even some umami meatiness minus the preservatives. Using romaine instead of the often-used iceberg upped the nutritional ante, and radicchio contributed beautiful color and more texture. For the dressing, we mashed just a bit of blue cheese with butter-milk then whisked in mayo and sour cream, white wine vinegar, and garlic powder for an impressively flavorful lower-fat dressing. We tossed some with our greens and drizzled the rest over our still-classic, yet mindfully updated, Cobb salad.

8 ounces boneless, skinless chicken breasts, trimmed of all visible fat and cut into ½-inch pieces
Salt and pepper
2 teaspoons canola oil
3 large eggs
10 ounces shiitake mushrooms, stemmed and sliced thin
⅛ teaspoon smoked paprika
⅛ teaspoon chili powder
⅓ cup finely chopped red onion
2 teaspoons lemon juice
⅓ cup buttermilk
1 ounce strong blue cheese, such as Roquefort or Stilton, crumbled (¼ cup)
⅓ cup mayonnaise
⅓ cup low-fat sour cream
1 tablespoon white wine vinegar
¼ teaspoon garlic powder
2 romaine lettuce hearts (12 ounces), cut into ½-inch pieces
½ small head radicchio (3 ounces), cored and cut into ½-inch pieces
1 avocado, halved, pitted, and cut into ½-inch pieces
6 ounces cherry tomatoes, halved

1. Pat chicken dry with paper towels and sprinkle with ⅛ teaspoon salt and ⅛ teaspoon pepper. Heat 1 teaspoon oil in 12-inch nonstick skillet over medium-high heat until shimmering. Add chicken and cook, stirring occasionally, until cooked through, 4 to 6 minutes. Transfer to plate and let cool. Do not clean skillet.

2. Meanwhile, bring 1 inch water to rolling boil in medium saucepan over high heat. Place eggs in steamer basket. Transfer basket to saucepan. Cover, reduce heat to medium-low, and cook eggs for 13 minutes.

3. When eggs are almost finished cooking, combine 2 cups ice cubes and 2 cups cold water in medium bowl. Using tongs or spoon, transfer eggs to prepared ice bath and let sit while finishing salad.

4. Heat remaining 1 teaspoon oil in now-empty skillet over medium heat until shimmering. Add mushrooms and ⅛ teaspoon salt, cover, and cook until mushrooms have released their liquid, 4 to 6 minutes. Uncover and increase heat to medium-high. Stir in paprika, chili powder, and ⅛ teaspoon pepper and cook until mushrooms are golden, 4 to 6 minutes. Transfer to second plate and let cool. Toss onion with lemon juice and set aside.

5. Mash buttermilk and blue cheese together with fork in small bowl until mixture resembles cottage cheese with small curds. Stir in mayonnaise, sour cream, 3 tablespoons water, vinegar, garlic powder, and ¼ teaspoon pepper until combined.

6. Peel eggs, then quarter. Gently toss lettuce and radicchio with ½ cup dressing in bowl until well coated. Transfer to serving platter and mound in even layer. Arrange eggs, cooled mushrooms, onion, avocado, and tomatoes in single mounds over greens, leaving space at both ends. Arrange half of chicken in each open space at ends of platter. Drizzle remaining dressing over salad. Serve.

PER SERVING

Cal 450 • **Total Fat** 32g • **Sat Fat** 7g • **Chol** 195mg
Sodium 490mg • **Total Carbs** 17g • **Fiber** 6g • **Total Sugar** 7g
Added Sugar 0g • **Protein** 25g • **Total Carbohydrate Choices** 1

NOTES FROM THE TEST KITCHEN

All About Avocados

Most famous as the star of guacamole, avocados are one of the only fruits that have an abundance of heart-healthy monounsaturated fat. Because they are rich in fats, avocados enable your body to better absorb fat-soluble vitamins that may be in other foods eaten with it. In addition, avocados are a great source of fiber and plenty of vitamins and minerals. Here are our tips for buying and storing avocados.

Buying Avocados

Although there are many varieties of avocado, in the United States small, rough-skinned Hass avocados are the most common, and we prefer them in the test kitchen. When they're ripe, their skin turns from green to dark purply black, and the fruit yields to a gentle squeeze. When selecting avocados, a good test is to try to flick the small stem off the avocado. If it comes off easily and you can see green underneath it, the avocado is ripe. If you see brown underneath after prying it off, the avocado is not usable. If it does not come off easily, the avocado is still unripe.

Ripening and Storing Avocados

At room temperature, rock-hard avocados generally ripen within two days, but they may ripen unevenly. Once ripe, they will last two days, on average, if kept at room temperature. Avocados may take up to four days to ripen in the refrigerator, but they will ripen more evenly. Ripe avocados last about five days when refrigerated, though some discoloration may occur. Store them toward the front of the refrigerator, on the middle or bottom shelf, where temperatures are more moderate.

All About Vinegars

Bright, acidic vinegar is essential to making many salad dressings. We also frequently reach for vinegar to add acidity and flavor to sauces, stews, soups, and bean dishes. Because different vinegars have distinctly different flavors, you will want to stock several varieties in your pantry.

Balsamic Vinegar

Traditional Italian balsamic vinegars are aged for years to develop complex flavor—but they're very pricey. They're best saved to drizzle over finished dishes. Our recommended best buy for high-end balsamic is **Oliviers & Co. Premium Balsamic Vinegar of Modena**. For vinaigrettes and glazes, we use commercial balsamic vinegars, which are younger wine vinegars with added sugar and coloring. Our favorite everyday balsamic is **Bertolli Balsamic Vinegar of Modena**.

Red Wine Vinegar

Use this slightly sweet, sharp vinegar for bold vinaigrettes. With its high acidity level, it works well with potent flavors. We prefer red wine vinegars made from a blend of wine and Concord grapes; our winning brand is **Laurent du Clos**.

White Wine Vinegar

This vinegar's refined, fruity bite is perfect for light vinaigrettes. We also use it in dishes like potato salad where the color of red wine vinegar would detract from the presentation. **Napa Valley Naturals Organic White Wine Vinegar** is our favorite.

Sherry Vinegar

Sherry vinegar is a Spanish condiment with complex savory flavors. It adds fruity depth to vegetable salads as well as gazpachos. Our favorite is **Napa Valley Naturals Reserve**.

Cider Vinegar

This vinegar has a bite and a fruity sweetness perfect for vinaigrettes; it works well in salads tossed with apple or dried fruits. Our favorite is **Heinz Filtered Apple Cider Vinegar**.

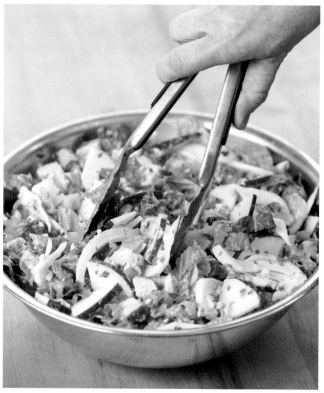

This bright and fresh main-dish salad combines lean poached chicken with crisp vegetables and sweet apples.

Fennel, Apple, and Chicken Chopped Salad
SERVES 4

WHY THIS RECIPE WORKS All too often, chopped salads wind up tasting mediocre and doused in dressing. We were set on creating a simple version that was fresh and flavorful. We settled on a mix of flavors and textures, selecting cucumber, fennel, apples, and romaine. Red onion added a bit of sharpness, and a modest amount of crumbled goat cheese offered a creamy textural contrast. We lightly salted the cucumber to remove excess moisture, allowing it to drain in a colander. Poaching the chicken in a steamer basket enabled us to use no extra fat. Once the chicken cooled, we cut the breasts into chunks and combined the pieces with the other salad ingredients. We decided to whisk the goat cheese into the dressing in place of some of the oil, and also found that marinating the heartier ingredients in the dressing for just five minutes before adding the romaine infused every component with flavor while still keeping it fresh and light. Use any sweet apple here, such as Fuji, Jonagold, Pink Lady, Jonathan, Macoun, or Gala.

- 1 cucumber, peeled, halved lengthwise, seeded, and sliced ½ inch thick
  Salt and pepper
- 1 pound boneless, skinless chicken breasts, trimmed of all visible fat and pounded to ¾-inch thickness
- 3 ounces goat cheese, crumbled (¾ cup)
- ¼ cup cider vinegar
- ¼ cup minced fresh tarragon
- 1 tablespoon extra-virgin olive oil
- 2 Fuji, Gala, or Golden Delicious apples, cored, quartered, and sliced crosswise ¼ inch thick
- 1 fennel bulb, stalks discarded, bulb halved, cored, and sliced ¼ inch thick
- ½ cup finely chopped red onion
- 1 romaine lettuce heart (6 ounces), cut into ½-inch pieces

1. Toss cucumber with ½ teaspoon salt in colander and let drain for 15 to 30 minutes.

2. Whisk 4 quarts water and 2 tablespoons salt in Dutch oven until salt is dissolved. Arrange breasts, skinned side up, in steamer basket, making sure not to overlap them. Submerge steamer basket in water.

3. Heat pot over medium heat, stirring liquid occasionally to even out hot spots, until water registers 175 degrees, 15 to 20 minutes. Turn off heat, cover pot, remove from burner, and let sit until meat registers 160 degrees, 17 to 22 minutes. Transfer chicken to paper towel–lined plate and refrigerate until cool, about 30 minutes. (Chicken can be refrigerated for up to 2 days.)

4. Whisk goat cheese, vinegar, tarragon, and oil together in large bowl. Pat chicken dry with paper towels and cut into ½-inch pieces. Add chicken, cucumber, apples, fennel, and onion to dressing and gently toss to coat. Let sit at room temperature until flavors meld, about 5 minutes. Add lettuce and gently toss to coat. Season with pepper to taste. Serve.

PER SERVING
Cal 310 • **Total Fat** 11g • **Sat Fat** 4.5g • **Chol** 95mg
Sodium 410mg • **Total Carbs** 22g • **Fiber** 5g • **Total Sugar** 14g
Added Sugar 0g • **Protein** 32g • **Total Carbohydrate Choices** 1.5

PREPARING FENNEL

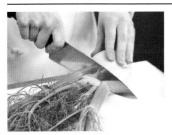

1. Cut off stalks and feathery fronds.

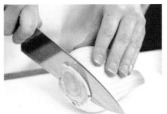

2. Trim very thin slice from base and remove any tough or blemished outer layers from bulb.

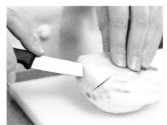

3. Cut bulb in half through base, then use small, sharp knife to remove pyramid shaped core.

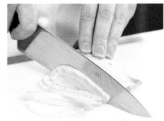

4. Slice each half into thin strips and, if called for in a recipe, chop strips crosswise.

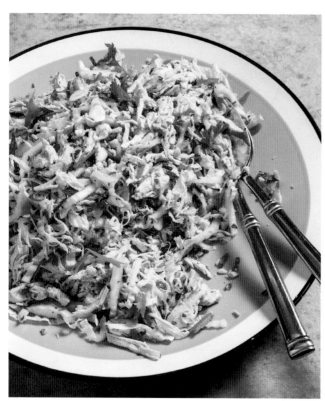

To minimize the added fat in this salad, we poach the chicken in water before adding it to flavorful Asian-inspired ingredients.

Warm Cabbage Salad with Chicken
SERVES 6

WHY THIS RECIPE WORKS This healthy salad features lean poached chicken, a flavorful Asian dressing, and crisp shredded cabbage. With poaching, not only could we cook the chicken without any oil, but the method ensured it was moist and tender by cooking it evenly and gently. For the fragrant dressing, we heated canola oil along with garlic, rice vinegar, fish sauce, and chili-garlic sauce and then warmed the shredded chicken in this mixture before tossing it with the shredded cabbage mixture. Be careful not to simmer the dressing for very long before adding the chicken in step 2 or it will over-reduce. If you like a spicier salad, add the full 2 teaspoons of Asian chili-garlic sauce.

DRESSING AND CHICKEN
Salt
1½ pounds boneless, skinless chicken breasts, trimmed of all visible fat and pounded to 1-inch thickness
3 tablespoons canola oil
1 tablespoon grated fresh ginger
2 garlic cloves, minced
5 tablespoons rice vinegar
2 tablespoons fish sauce
1–2 teaspoons Asian chili-garlic sauce

SALAD
½ head napa cabbage, cored and sliced thin (5½ cups)
2 carrots, peeled and shredded
4 scallions, sliced thin on bias
½ cup fresh cilantro leaves
½ cup minced fresh mint
3 tablespoons coarsely chopped dry-roasted unsalted peanuts

1. FOR THE DRESSING AND CHICKEN Whisk 4 quarts water and 2 tablespoons salt in Dutch oven until salt is dissolved. Arrange breasts, skinned side up, in steamer basket, making sure not to overlap them. Submerge steamer basket in water.

2. Heat pot over medium heat, stirring liquid occasionally to even out hot spots, until water registers 175 degrees, 15 to 20 minutes. Turn off heat, cover pot, remove from burner, and let sit until meat registers 160 degrees, 17 to 22 minutes. Transfer chicken to paper towel–lined plate and refrigerate until cool, about 30 minutes. (Chicken can be refrigerated for up to 2 days.)

3. Pat chicken dry with paper towels and shred into bite-size pieces with 2 forks. Heat oil in 12-inch skillet over medium heat until shimmering. Add ginger and garlic and cook until fragrant, about 30 seconds. Whisk in vinegar, fish sauce, and chili-garlic sauce and bring to simmer. Add chicken and cook until heated through, about 1 minute.

4. FOR THE SALAD Combine all ingredients in large bowl. Add chicken mixture and gently toss to coat. Serve immediately.

PER SERVING
Cal 270 • **Total Fat** 12g • **Sat Fat** 1.5g • **Chol** 85mg
Sodium 380mg • **Total Carbs** 8g • **Fiber** 3g • **Total Sugar** 3g
Added Sugar 0g • **Protein** 29g • **Total Carbohydrate Choices** 0.5

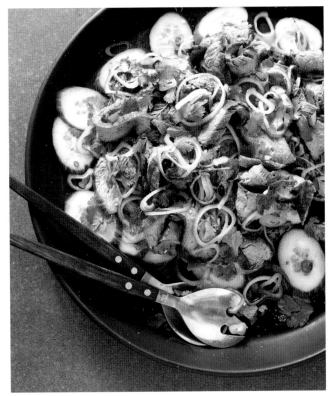

Grilled lean flank steak adds good protein to this low-carb main dish salad.

Thai Grilled-Steak Salad
SERVES 6

WHY THIS RECIPE WORKS A steak salad is a great way to enjoy a smaller amount of meat at dinner. We were inspired by Thai grilled beef salad, which combines charred steak with nutrient-rich herbs and a bright, bracing dressing. We grilled flank steak over a modified two-level fire, which charred the beef but kept the inside juicy. We also made our own toasted rice powder, a traditional ingredient that gave the salad a fuller body. It's integral to the texture and flavor of the dish. Toasted rice powder (*kao kua*) can also be found in many Asian markets; if using, substitute 1 tablespoon kao kua for the ground white rice. If a fresh Thai chile is unavailable, substitute half of a serrano chile.

 1 teaspoon paprika
 1 teaspoon cayenne pepper
 1 tablespoon white rice
 3 tablespoons lime juice (2 limes)
 2 tablespoons fish sauce

 2 tablespoons water
 1 (1½-pound) flank steak, trimmed of all visible fat
 ¼ teaspoon salt
 ¼ teaspoon white pepper
1½ cups fresh mint leaves, torn
1½ cups fresh cilantro leaves
 4 shallots, sliced thin
 1 Thai chile, stemmed and sliced into thin rounds
 1 English cucumber, sliced ¼ inch thick on bias

1. Heat paprika and cayenne in 8-inch skillet over medium heat and cook, shaking skillet, until fragrant, about 1 minute. Transfer to small bowl. Return now-empty skillet to medium-high heat, add rice, and toast, stirring frequently, until deep golden brown, about 5 minutes. Transfer to second small bowl and let cool for 5 minutes. Grind rice with spice grinder, mini food processor, or mortar and pestle until it resembles fine meal, 10 to 30 seconds (you should have about 1 tablespoon rice powder).

2. Whisk lime juice, fish sauce, water, and ¼ teaspoon toasted paprika mixture together in large bowl; set aside.

3A. FOR A CHARCOAL GRILL Open bottom vent completely. Light large chimney starter filled with charcoal briquettes (6 quarts). When top coals are partially covered with ash, pour evenly over half of grill. Set cooking grate in place, cover, and open lid vent completely. Heat grill until hot, about 5 minutes.

3B. FOR A GAS GRILL Turn all burners to high, cover, and heat grill until hot, about 15 minutes. Leave primary burner on high and turn off other burner(s).

4. Clean and oil cooking grate. Pat steak dry with paper towels, then sprinkle with salt and white pepper. Place steak over hotter part of grill and cook until beginning to char and beads of moisture appear on outer edges of meat, 5 to 6 minutes. Flip steak and continue to cook on second side until charred and meat registers 120 to 125 degrees (for medium-rare), about 5 minutes. Transfer steak to cutting board, tent with aluminum foil, and let rest for 5 to 10 minutes (or let cool completely, about 1 hour).

5. Slice steak about ¼ inch thick against grain on bias. Whisk lime juice mixture to recombine, then add steak, mint, cilantro, shallots, chile, and half of rice powder and gently toss to coat. Line serving platter with cucumber slices. Place steak mixture on top of cucumbers and serve, passing remaining toasted paprika mixture and remaining rice powder separately.

PER SERVING
Cal 220 • **Total Fat** 8g • **Sat Fat** 3g • **Chol** 80mg
Sodium 400mg • **Total Carbs** 11g • **Fiber** 3g • **Total Sugar** 3g
Added Sugar 0g • **Protein** 27g • **Total Carbohydrate Choices** 1

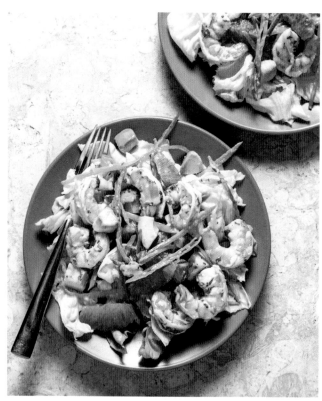

For this bright salad, we poach the shrimp off the heat, which allows them to cook through evenly without turning rubbery.

Shrimp Salad with Avocado and Grapefruit
SERVES 4

WHY THIS RECIPE WORKS We wanted to translate an appetizer favorite, shrimp cocktail, into a fresh summertime salad. In order to avoid overcooking the shrimp, we gently poached them off the heat and then shocked them in an ice bath. Using a blender made the dressing a breeze. In addition to using buttery avocado in the dressing, we also tossed whole avocado chunks with the shrimp, along with crunchy snow peas and fragrant mint. Bibb lettuce made an attractive base for the other ingredients and provided additional texture. If your grapefruit tastes especially tart, add ¼ teaspoon additional honey to the dressing. If you are short on grapefruit juice, substitute water. Be ready to serve the salad shortly after making the dressing; the avocado will begin to discolor the dressing within an hour or so.

1 lemon, halved
1 bay leaf
½ teaspoon peppercorns
1 pound extra-large shrimp (21 to 25 per pound), peeled, deveined, and tails removed
1 grapefruit
1 avocado, halved, pitted, and cut into ½-inch pieces
3 tablespoons lime juice
1½ teaspoons grated fresh ginger
½ teaspoon honey
¼ teaspoon pepper
⅛ teaspoon salt
2 ounces snow peas, strings removed and sliced thin lengthwise
1 tablespoon chopped fresh mint
2 small heads Bibb lettuce (12 ounces), leaves separated and torn into bite-size pieces
2 tablespoons extra-virgin olive oil

1. Place 3 cups water in medium saucepan. Squeeze lemon halves into water, then add spent halves, bay leaf, and peppercorns. Bring to boil over high heat and cook for 2 minutes.

2. Off heat, add shrimp. Cover and let steep until shrimp are firm and pink, about 7 minutes. Fill large bowl halfway with ice and water. Drain shrimp, discarding lemon halves and bay leaf, and transfer to prepared ice bath. Let sit until chilled, about 2 minutes. Transfer shrimp to paper towel–lined plate. (Shrimp can be refrigerated for up to 24 hours.)

3. Cut away peel and pith from grapefruit. Holding fruit over fine-mesh strainer set in bowl, use paring knife to slice between membranes to release segments. Measure out and reserve ¼ cup juice; discard remaining juice. Process reserved grapefruit juice, one-quarter of avocado, 2 tablespoons lime juice, ginger, honey, pepper, and salt in blender until smooth; transfer dressing to large bowl.

4. Add shrimp, grapefruit segments, snow peas, mint, and remaining avocado to bowl with dressing and gently toss to coat. Combine lettuce, oil, and remaining 1 tablespoon lime juice in separate bowl and gently toss to coat. Arrange lettuce on individual plates and top with shrimp mixture. Drizzle with any dressing remaining in bowl and serve.

PER SERVING
Cal 260 • **Total Fat** 15g • **Sat Fat** 2.5g • **Chol** 105mg **Sodium** 210mg • **Total Carbs** 18g • **Fiber** 4g • **Total Sugar** 8g **Added Sugar** 1g • **Protein** 15g • **Total Carbohydrate Choices** 1

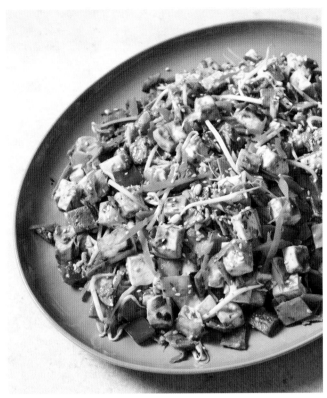

High in protein and low in saturated fat, tofu is the appealing centerpiece of this crunchy salad.

Tofu Salad with Vegetables
SERVES 6

WHY THIS RECIPE WORKS All too often tofu is a supporting player and not the star of the show. We wanted to develop a recipe that was all about the tofu. After all, it's a great source of protein, creamy but low in saturated fat, and it marries well with lots of different flavors. Tasters unanimously chose soft tofu for its creamy, custard-like texture. To drain the tofu of excess moisture, we simply cut it into cubes and placed them on multiple layers of paper towels to drain. While tofu would be the star, we needed other vegetables to fill out our salad. Tasters liked carrots, snow peas, and bell peppers for both their crisp textures and bright colors. Bean sprouts, which are often used in Asian cooking, added a nice crunch and clean flavor. For the dressing, we favored a blend of peanut butter, hoisin sauce, lime juice, sesame oil, and garlic, a combination that created the right balance of salty, acidic, and savory. A little chili-garlic sauce added a touch of heat. To achieve the ideal consistency, we found that 3 tablespoons of hot water thinned the dressing out perfectly for coating the tofu and vegetables. Broiling the tofu gave it some light charring and extra flavor. We gently tossed it with our vegetables and the remaining dressing. Thinly sliced scallions, minced cilantro, and toasted sesame seeds gave our salad just the right finishing touches. We prefer the texture of soft tofu in this recipe; however, firm tofu may be substituted.

DRESSING
- 3 tablespoons unsalted creamy peanut butter
- 3 tablespoons hot water
- ¼ cup hoisin sauce
- 4 teaspoons lime juice
- 2 teaspoons toasted sesame oil
- 1 garlic clove, minced
- ¾ teaspoon Asian chili-garlic sauce
- ½ teaspoon salt

SALAD
- 28 ounces soft tofu, cut into ¾-inch pieces
- 8 ounces snow peas, strings removed and cut into ½-inch pieces
- 1 red or yellow bell pepper, stemmed, seeded, and cut into ½-inch pieces
- 4 ounces (2 cups) bean sprouts
- 2 carrots, peeled and shredded
- 2 scallions, sliced thin on bias
- 3 tablespoons minced fresh cilantro
- 1 tablespoon toasted sesame seeds
  Pepper

1. FOR THE DRESSING Whisk peanut butter and water in large bowl until smooth, then whisk in hoisin, lime juice, sesame oil, garlic, chili-garlic sauce, and salt until combined; set aside.

2. FOR THE SALAD Position oven rack 6 inches from broiler element and heat broiler. Line rimmed baking sheet with aluminum foil. Spread tofu on paper–towel lined baking sheet and let drain for 20 minutes. Gently press dry with paper towels.

3. Gently toss tofu with half of dressing in separate bowl and spread in even layer on prepared sheet. Broil tofu until spotty brown, 5 to 6 minutes.

4. Add snow peas, bell pepper, bean sprouts, carrots, and scallions to bowl with remaining dressing and gently toss to coat. Gently fold in tofu, cilantro, and sesame seeds. Season with pepper to taste and let sit until flavors meld, about 15 minutes. Serve.

PER SERVING
Cal 220 • **Total Fat** 12g • **Sat Fat** 1g • **Chol** 0mg
Sodium 260mg • **Total Carbs** 14g • **Fiber** 4g • **Total Sugar** 6g
Added Sugar 0g • **Protein** 15g • **Total Carbohydrate Choices** 1

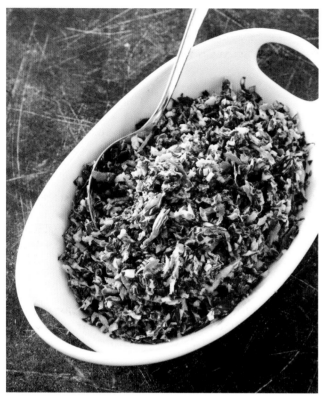

Salting, rinsing, and draining shredded cabbage eliminates extra water so it doesn't dilute the dressing.

Buttermilk Coleslaw
SERVES 10

WHY THIS RECIPE WORKS Cabbage slaws have a tendency to be nothing more than watery, bland piles of the shredded greens drowning in a heavy dressing. We wanted our cabbage to have more flavor and a pickle-crisp crunch, and we wanted a lighter dressing. We first salted and drained the cabbage to reduce the excess moisture, which would dilute the salad's texture and flavor. We then tossed the cabbage with shredded carrots for additional color and crunch. For the dressing, we combined buttermilk, mayo, and sour cream to achieve its characteristic creamy consistency, while scallions, parsley, vinegar, and mustard provided flavorful seasoning.

- 1 head red or green cabbage (2 pounds), cored and sliced thin
  Salt and pepper
- 1 cup buttermilk
- ¼ cup mayonnaise
- ¼ cup low-fat sour cream
- 3 scallions, sliced thin
- 3 tablespoons minced fresh parsley or cilantro
- 2 teaspoons cider vinegar, plus extra for seasoning
- 1 teaspoon Dijon mustard
- 2 carrots, peeled and shredded

1. Toss cabbage with 1 teaspoon salt in colander and let sit until wilted, about 1 hour. Rinse cabbage under cold water, drain, and thoroughly pat dry with paper towels.

2. Whisk buttermilk, mayonnaise, sour cream, scallions, parsley, vinegar, mustard, ¼ teaspoon salt, and ¼ teaspoon pepper together in large bowl until smooth. Add dried cabbage and carrots and gently toss to coat. Cover and refrigerate until flavors meld, about 1 hour or up to 24 hours. Season with pepper and extra vinegar to taste. Serve.

PER 1-CUP SERVING

Cal 90 • **Total Fat** 4.5g • **Sat Fat** 1g • **Chol** 5mg
Sodium 190mg • **Total Carbs** 9g • **Fiber** 3g • **Total Sugar** 5g
Added Sugar 0g • **Protein** 3g • **Total Carbohydrate Choices** 0.5

SHREDDING CABBAGE

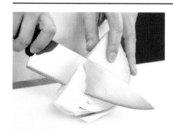

1. Cut cabbage into quarters, then trim and discard hard core.

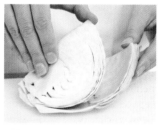

2. Separate cabbage into small stacks of leaves that flatten when pressed.

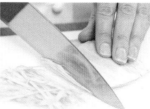

3. Use chef's knife to cut each stack of cabbage leaves into thin shreds.

Mediterranean Tuna Salad
SERVES 6

WHY THIS RECIPE WORKS A brownbag staple, tuna salad too often turns out bland or overridden with mayonnaise. We found the key to great tuna salad is to first thoroughly drain the chunked tuna. Next, we decided to ditch the mayonnaise. Instead, we relied on the vibrant flavors of good-quality extra-virgin olive oil, lemon juice, and Dijon mustard to make a luscious base to bind our salad together. We added red onion and garlic to the mix and let it sit to temper the alliums' harsh bite. Red bell pepper, crunchy celery, and kalamata olives turned this lunchtime basic into a sophisticated, protein-rich meal. Good-quality olive oil and canned tuna are crucial for this recipe. The salad is great served over a bed of lettuce or as part of an open-faced sandwich.

- 3 tablespoons lemon juice, plus extra for seasoning
- 2 teaspoons Dijon mustard
  Pepper
- 5 tablespoons extra-virgin olive oil
- ¼ cup minced red onion
- 1 garlic clove, minced
- 4 (5-ounce) cans solid white tuna in water, drained and flaked
- 2 celery ribs, minced
- 1 red bell pepper, stemmed, seeded, and chopped fine
- ¼ cup pitted kalamata olives, minced
- ¼ cup minced fresh parsley

Whisk lemon juice, mustard, and ½ teaspoon pepper in large bowl until combined. While whisking constantly, drizzle in oil until completely emulsified. Stir in red onion and garlic and let sit

Buying Canned Tuna

Most large seafood producers cook their fish twice: once before it's canned, then again when it's heated inside the sealed can to kill bacteria. This leads to fish that's lost much of its natural flavor, moisture, and meaty bite. Our favorite canned tuna, **Wild Planet Wild Albacore Tuna,** packs raw tuna into cans by hand and then cooks its tuna just once, preserving the fresh flavor and meaty texture of the fish. If you're watching your sodium intake, check labels when shopping; some brands pack tuna in broths that contain sodium, and even those packed in water have varying amounts of salt added.

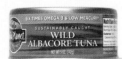

for 5 minutes. Add tuna, celery, bell pepper, olives, and parsley and gently toss to coat. (Salad can be refrigerated for up to 24 hours.) Season with extra lemon juice and pepper to taste. Serve.

PER ⅔-CUP SERVING
Cal 200 • **Total Fat** 14g • **Sat Fat** 2g • **Chol** 25mg
Sodium 300mg • **Total Carbs** 3g • **Fiber** 1g • **Total Sugar** 1g
Added Sugar 0g • **Protein** 15g • **Total Carbohydrate Choices** <0.5

VARIATION
Mediterranean Tuna Salad with Carrots, Radishes, and Cilantro

Substitute 6 thinly sliced radishes for celery, 2 peeled and shredded carrots for bell pepper, and minced fresh cilantro for parsley.

PER ⅔-CUP SERVING
Cal 200 • **Total Fat** 14g • **Sat Fat** 2g • **Chol** 25mg
Sodium 310mg • **Total Carbs** 4g • **Fiber** 1g • **Total Sugar** 2g
Added Sugar 0g • **Protein** 15g • **Total Carbohydrate Choices** <0.5

Classic Chicken Salad
SERVES 6

WHY THIS RECIPE WORKS Recipes for chicken salad are only as good as the chicken itself. To ensure juicy, flavorful meat, our ideal method is to poach 1½ pounds boneless, skinless chicken breasts in a steamer basket set within a Dutch oven with 4 quarts of salted water that we then heat to 175 degrees. (The chicken absorbs very little of the salt in the water.) We then turn off the heat, cover the pot, and let the chicken sit until it reaches 160 degrees. This yields such incomparably moist chicken that a mere ⅓ cup of mayo was enough. This salad tastes great served over a bed of lettuce or as part of an open-faced sandwich.

- Salt and pepper
- 1½ pounds boneless, skinless chicken breasts, trimmed of all visible fat and pounded to ¾-inch thickness
- ⅓ cup mayonnaise
- 2 tablespoons lemon juice
- 1 teaspoon extra-virgin olive oil
- ¼ teaspoon celery seeds
- 2 celery ribs, chopped fine
- 2 scallions, minced
- 2 tablespoons minced fresh parsley or tarragon

1. Whisk 4 quarts water and 2 tablespoons salt in Dutch oven until salt is dissolved. Arrange breasts, skinned side up, in steamer basket, making sure not to overlap them. Submerge steamer basket in water.

2. Heat pot over medium heat, stirring liquid occasionally to even out hot spots, until water registers 175 degrees, 15 to 20 minutes. Turn off heat, cover pot, remove from burner, and let sit until meat registers 160 degrees, 17 to 22 minutes. Transfer chicken to paper towel–lined plate and refrigerate until cool, about 30 minutes.

3. Whisk mayonnaise, lemon juice, oil, celery seeds, ¼ teaspoon salt, and ¼ teaspoon pepper in large bowl until combined. Pat chicken dry with paper towels and cut into ½-inch pieces. Add chicken, celery, scallions, and parsley to mayonnaise mixture and gently toss to coat. (Salad can be refrigerated for up to 2 days.) Season with pepper to taste. Serve.

PER ¾-CUP SERVING

Cal 230 • Total Fat 13g • Sat Fat 2g • Chol 85mg
Sodium 290mg • Total Carbs 1g • Fiber 0g • Total Sugar 0g
Added Sugar 0g • Protein 26g • Total Carbohydrate Choices <0.5

Chicken Salad with Fennel, Lemon, and Parmesan
SERVES 6

WHY THIS RECIPE WORKS To give chicken salad another flavor dimension, we added Parmesan, bright lemon zest and juice, fragrant fennel, and fresh basil. This recipe tastes great served over a bed of lettuce or as part of an open-faced sandwich.

  Salt and pepper
1½ pounds boneless, skinless chicken breasts, trimmed of all visible fat and pounded to ¾-inch thickness
⅓ cup mayonnaise
¼ cup grated Parmesan cheese
 1 teaspoon extra-virgin olive oil
½ teaspoon grated lemon zest plus 3 tablespoons juice
¼ teaspoon celery seeds
 1 fennel bulb, stalks discarded, bulb halved, cored, and chopped fine
 2 tablespoons finely chopped red onion
 2 tablespoons minced fresh basil

---

1. Whisk 4 quarts water and 2 tablespoons salt in Dutch oven until salt is dissolved. Arrange breasts, skinned side up, in steamer basket, making sure not to overlap them. Submerge steamer basket in water.

2. Heat pot over medium heat, stirring liquid occasionally to even out hot spots, until water registers 175 degrees, 15 to 20 minutes. Turn off heat, cover pot, remove from burner, and let sit until meat registers 160 degrees, 17 to 22 minutes. Transfer chicken to paper towel–lined plate and refrigerate until cool, about 30 minutes.

3. Whisk mayonnaise, Parmesan, oil, lemon zest and juice, celery seeds, ¼ teaspoon salt, and ¼ teaspoon pepper in large bowl until combined. Pat chicken dry with paper towels and cut into ½-inch pieces. Add chicken, fennel, onion, and basil to mayonnaise mixture and gently toss to coat. (Salad can be refrigerated for up to 2 days.) Season with pepper to taste. Serve.

PER ¾-CUP SERVING

Cal 260 • Total Fat 14g • Sat Fat 3g • Chol 90mg
Sodium 380mg • Total Carbs 4g • Fiber 1g • Total Sugar 2g
Added Sugar 0g • Protein 28g • Total Carbohydrate Choices <0.5

Curried Chicken Salad with Raisins and Almonds
SERVES 6

WHY THIS RECIPE WORKS For a sweet and spicy chicken salad, we combine our chicken with golden raisins, warm curry powder, crunchy almonds, and fresh cilantro. This recipe tastes great served over a bed of lettuce or as part of an open-faced sandwich.

  Salt and pepper
1½ pounds boneless, skinless chicken breasts, trimmed of all visible fat and pounded to ¾-inch thickness
⅓ cup mayonnaise
 2 tablespoons lemon juice
 2 teaspoons curry powder
 1 teaspoon extra-virgin olive oil
¼ teaspoon celery seeds
 2 celery ribs, chopped fine
 2 scallions, minced
⅓ cup golden raisins
 3 tablespoons toasted sliced almonds
 2 tablespoons minced fresh cilantro

1. Whisk 4 quarts water and 2 tablespoons salt in Dutch oven until salt is dissolved. Arrange breasts, skinned side up, in steamer basket, making sure not to overlap them. Submerge steamer basket in water.

2. Heat pot over medium heat, stirring liquid occasionally to even out hot spots, until water registers 175 degrees, 15 to 20 minutes. Turn off heat, cover pot, remove from burner, and let sit until meat registers 160 degrees, 17 to 22 minutes. Transfer chicken to paper towel–lined plate and refrigerate until cool, about 30 minutes.

3. Whisk mayonnaise, lemon juice, curry powder, oil, celery seeds, ¼ teaspoon salt, and ¼ teaspoon pepper together in large bowl until combined. Pat chicken dry with paper towels and cut into ½-inch pieces. Add chicken, celery, scallions, raisins, almonds, and cilantro to mayonnaise mixture and gently toss to coat. (Salad can be refrigerated for up to 2 days.) Season with pepper to taste. Serve.

PER ¾-CUP SERVING

Cal 280 • **Total Fat** 14g • **Sat Fat** 2g • **Chol** 85mg
Sodium 290mg • **Total Carbs** 9g • **Fiber** 2g • **Total Sugar** 7g
Added Sugar 0g • **Protein** 27g • **Total Carbohydrate Choices** 1

Spicy Chipotle Chicken Salad with Corn
SERVES 6

WHY THIS RECIPE WORKS For a Tex-Mex spin on chicken salad, we added chipotle chile for spice, vibrant lime juice, convenient frozen corn, and fresh cilantro. This recipe tastes great served over a bed of lettuce or as part of an open-faced sandwich.

> Salt and pepper
> 1½ pounds boneless, skinless chicken breasts, trimmed of all visible fat and pounded to ¾-inch thickness
> ⅓ cup mayonnaise
> 3 tablespoons lime juice (2 limes)
> 2 teaspoons minced canned chipotle chile in adobo sauce
> 1 teaspoon extra-virgin olive oil
> 1 red bell pepper, stemmed, seeded, and chopped fine
> ⅓ cup frozen corn, thawed
> 2 scallions, minced
> 2 tablespoons minced fresh cilantro

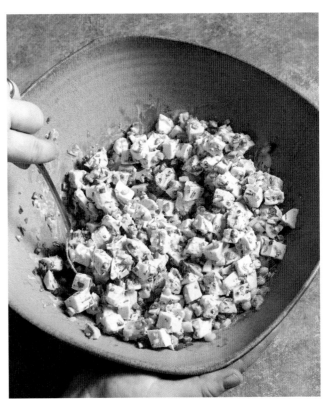

Poaching chicken breasts in water in a steamer basket results in tender, moist white meat that's perfect for chicken salad.

1. Whisk 4 quarts water and 2 tablespoons salt in Dutch oven until salt is dissolved. Arrange breasts, skinned side up, in steamer basket, making sure not to overlap them. Submerge steamer basket in water.

2. Heat pot over medium heat, stirring liquid occasionally to even out hot spots, until water registers 175 degrees, 15 to 20 minutes. Turn off heat, cover pot, remove from burner, and let sit until meat registers 160 degrees, 17 to 22 minutes. Transfer chicken to paper towel–lined plate and refrigerate until cool, about 30 minutes.

3. Whisk mayonnaise, lime juice, chipotle, oil, ¼ teaspoon salt, and ¼ teaspoon pepper in large bowl until combined. Pat chicken dry with paper towels and cut into ½-inch pieces. Add chicken, bell pepper, corn, scallions, and cilantro to mayonnaise mixture and gently toss to coat. (Salad can be refrigerated for up to 2 days.) Season with pepper to taste. Serve.

PER ¾-CUP SERVING

Cal 240 • **Total Fat** 13g • **Sat Fat** 2g • **Chol** 85mg
Sodium 280mg • **Total Carbs** 4g • **Fiber** 1g • **Total Sugar** 1g
Added Sugar 0g • **Protein** 26g • **Total Carbohydrate Choices** <0.5

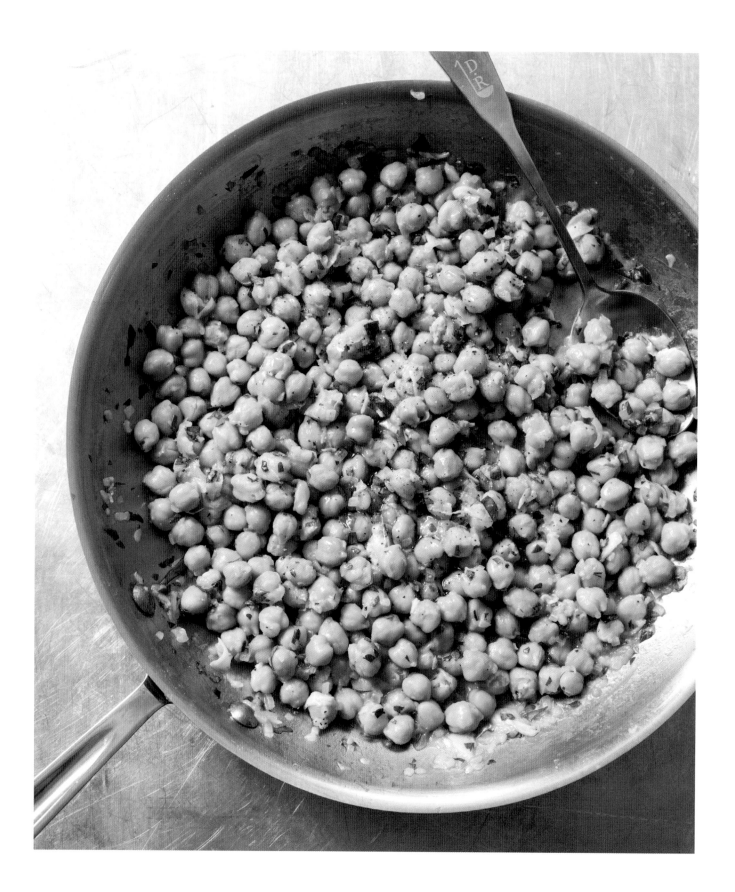

RICE, GRAIN, AND BEAN SIDES

Photo: Chickpeas with Garlic and Parsley

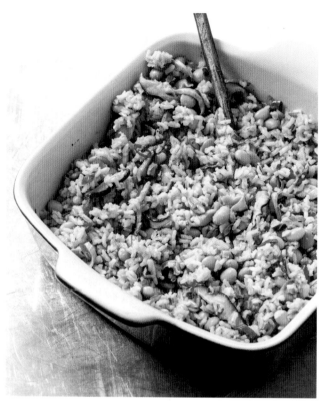

For perfectly cooked brown rice, we use the oven and bake the rice in a flavor-packed broth until tender.

Baked Brown Rice with Shiitakes and Edamame
SERVES 6

WHY THIS RECIPE WORKS Baking brown rice in the oven is a handy trick that delivers perfectly cooked rice every time, making it easy to turn to more nutritious brown rice as a side dish option. Here we set out to bulk up rice with add-ins that would complement the hearty flavor and texture of brown rice while also adding nutrients. A combination of sautéed shiitake mushrooms, scallions, and fresh ginger made for a simple, refreshing upgrade. Once the rice was tender, we sprinkled edamame over the top and then added scallion greens, rice vinegar, and a touch of sesame oil. Medium-grain or short-grain brown rice can be substituted for the long-grain rice.

1 cup long-grain brown rice, rinsed
1 tablespoon canola oil
4 ounces shiitake mushrooms, stemmed and sliced thin
4 scallions, white parts minced, green parts sliced thin on bias

2 teaspoons grated fresh ginger
2 cups low-sodium vegetable broth
½ teaspoon salt
1 cup frozen edamame, thawed
1 tablespoon unseasoned rice vinegar, plus extra for seasoning
1 teaspoon toasted sesame oil

1. Adjust oven rack to middle position and heat oven to 375 degrees. Spread rice in 8-inch square baking dish.

2. Heat canola oil in medium saucepan over medium heat until shimmering. Add mushrooms, scallion whites, and ginger and cook, stirring occasionally, until softened, 5 to 7 minutes. Stir in broth and salt. Cover pot, increase heat to high, and bring to boil. Once boiling, stir to combine, then immediately pour mixture over rice. Cover dish tightly with aluminum foil and bake until rice is tender and liquid is absorbed, 50 to 60 minutes.

3. Remove dish from oven and uncover. Sprinkle edamame over rice, cover, and let sit for 5 minutes. Add scallion greens, vinegar, and sesame oil and fluff gently with fork to combine. Season with vinegar to taste. Serve.

PER ¾-CUP SERVING

Cal 180 • **Total Fat** 6g • **Sat Fat** 1g • **Chol** 0mg
Sodium 240mg • **Total Carbs** 28g • **Fiber** 3g • **Total Sugar** 2g
Added Sugar 0g • **Protein** 5g • **Total Carbohydrate Choices** 2

Brown Rice with Tomatoes and Chickpeas
SERVES 8

WHY THIS RECIPE WORKS This nutty and protein-packed brown rice dish is built entirely in a 12-inch skillet for convenience. To ensure that our brown rice took on plenty of rich flavor, we began with a traditional base of chopped onion and chopped bell peppers. Once both were nicely browned, we stirred in the rice along with three aromatic powerhouses: minced garlic, crumbled saffron threads, and a pinch of cayenne pepper. A generous amount of broth was enough to both cook the rice and add some extra flavor to our mix-ins during cooking. We added nutrient-rich canned chickpeas to the skillet halfway through cooking so they could soften slightly while the rice finished cooking. A simple mix of quartered grape tomatoes, bright sliced scallions, and citrusy minced cilantro, united by some olive oil and fresh lime juice, made for a vibrant finishing touch.

12 ounces grape tomatoes, quartered

5 scallions, sliced thin

¼ cup minced fresh cilantro

4 teaspoons extra-virgin olive oil

1 tablespoon lime juice

Salt and pepper

2 red bell peppers, stemmed, seeded, and chopped fine

1 onion, chopped fine

1 cup long-grain brown rice, rinsed

4 garlic cloves, minced

Pinch saffron threads, crumbled

Pinch cayenne pepper

3¼ cups unsalted chicken broth

1 (15-ounce) can no-salt-added chickpeas, rinsed

1. Combine tomatoes, scallions, cilantro, 2 teaspoons oil, lime juice, ⅛ teaspoon salt, and ⅛ teaspoon pepper in bowl; set aside for serving.

2. Heat remaining 2 teaspoons oil in 12-inch skillet over medium heat until shimmering. Add bell peppers, onion, and ¼ teaspoon salt and cook until softened and lightly browned, 8 to 10 minutes. Stir in rice, garlic, saffron, and cayenne and cook until fragrant, about 30 seconds.

3. Stir in broth, scraping up any browned bits, and bring to simmer. Reduce heat to medium-low, cover, and cook, stirring occasionally, for 25 minutes.

4. Stir in chickpeas and ⅛ teaspoon salt, cover, and cook until rice is tender and broth is almost completely absorbed, 25 to 30 minutes. Season with pepper to taste. Serve, topping individual portions with tomato mixture.

PER ¾-CUP SERVING

Cal 180 • **Total Fat** 3.5g • **Sat Fat** 0.5g • **Chol** 0mg
Sodium 210mg • **Total Carbs** 30g • **Fiber** 4g • **Total Sugar** 4g
Added Sugar 0g • **Protein** 6g • **Total Carbohydrate Choices** 2

Wild Rice Pilaf with Scallions and Almonds
SERVES 6

WHY THIS RECIPE WORKS Properly cooked wild rice is chewy yet tender and pleasingly rustic—not crunchy or gluey. To balance the wild rice's strong flavor, we started by adding some long-grain white rice. To properly cook wild rice and white rice together in one pilaf, the wild rice needed a jump-start. We simmered it in plenty of liquid and then drained. In the now-empty pot, we sautéed onion and briefly toasted the white rice in the oil, then added the

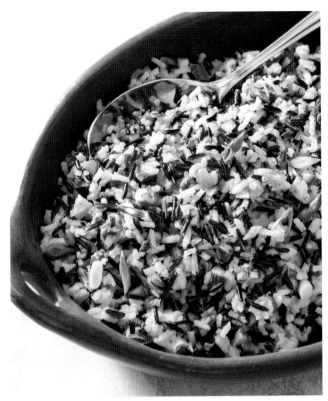

Wild rice can be tricky to cook, but our stovetop method makes it foolproof.

parcooked wild rice and chicken broth and simmered until both rices were fully cooked. Almonds, scallions, and lime juice were the final finishes. To make this dish vegetarian, substitute vegetable broth for the chicken broth.

½ cup wild rice, picked over and rinsed

2 bay leaves

3 tablespoons extra-virgin olive oil

1 onion, chopped fine

Salt and pepper

½ cup long-grain white rice, rinsed

1½ cups unsalted chicken broth

4 sprigs fresh thyme

¾ cup whole almonds, toasted and chopped coarse

3 scallions, sliced thin

1 tablespoon lime juice

1. Bring 1½ cups water, wild rice, and bay leaves to boil in medium saucepan over medium-high heat. Reduce heat to low, cover, and simmer for 25 minutes. Discard bay leaves. Drain rice and set aside. Wipe saucepan dry.

2. Heat oil in now-empty saucepan over medium heat until shimmering. Add onion and ½ teaspoon salt and cook until softened, about 5 minutes. Add white rice and cook, stirring frequently, until grain edges begin to turn translucent, about 3 minutes.

3. Stir in wild rice, broth, and thyme sprigs and bring to simmer. Reduce heat to low, cover, and cook until rice is tender and broth is absorbed, 16 to 18 minutes. Off heat, lay clean dish towel underneath lid and let rice sit for 10 minutes.

4. Discard thyme sprigs. Add almonds, scallions, and lime juice to pilaf and fluff gently with fork to combine. Season with pepper to taste. Serve.

PER ⅔-CUP SERVING

Cal 300 • **Total Fat** 17g • **Sat Fat** 1.5g • **Chol** 0mg
Sodium 230mg • **Total Carbs** 32g • **Fiber** 4g • **Total Sugar** 3g
Added Sugar 0g • **Protein** 9g • **Total Carbohydrate Choices** 2

NOTES FROM THE TEST KITCHEN

Getting to Know Whole Grains

Whole grains are an important part of the diabetic diet because of the protein and fiber they deliver (in addition to other nutrients). Whole grains are considered whole because the bran, germ, and endosperm are present in the same proportions as when the grain was growing. Once processed, a whole grain must still offer the same nutrients as found in the original form to be considered whole grain. The bran contains most of the fiber, while the germ contains some B vitamins, protein, minerals, and healthy fats. The endosperm contains starchy carbohydrates, proteins, and traces of vitamins and minerals. Refining grains diminishes their nutritional quality. Because different types of whole grains offer different ratios of nutrients, it's best to consume a variety.

PER ¼ CUP UNCOOKED	PROTEIN	FIBER
Bulgur	4g	6g
Farro	6g	4g
Quinoa	6g	3g
Long-Grain Brown Rice	4g	2g
Wild Rice	6g	2g
Wheat Berries	6g	6g

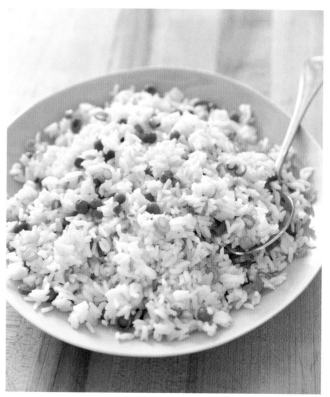

We toast the rice grains first to give our basmati pilaf nutty flavor and then use less cooking water to help keep the rice firm.

Basmati Rice Pilaf with Herbs and Toasted Almonds
SERVES 6

WHY THIS RECIPE WORKS We wanted to create a basmati rice pilaf with interesting flavors that would pair well with any number of entrées. Rinsing the rice before cooking removed excess starch and ensured fluffy grains. Toasting the rice gave it a nutty quality, and garlic, turmeric, and cinnamon brought big flavors. Instead of following the traditional ratio of 1 cup of rice to 2 cups of water, we found that using less liquid made for a firmer texture that tasters liked. As soon as the grains absorbed the water, we removed the saucepan from the heat and placed a dish towel under the pan's lid to absorb excess moisture so the rice could finish steaming in the residual heat. We then stirred in herbs and heart-healthy almonds. Long-grain white, jasmine, or Texmati rice can be substituted for the basmati.

1 tablespoon extra-virgin olive oil
1 small onion, chopped fine
Salt and pepper

1 cup basmati rice, rinsed
2 garlic cloves, minced
½ teaspoon ground turmeric
¼ teaspoon ground cinnamon
1½ cups water
¼ cup minced fresh parsley, chives, or basil
¼ cup sliced almonds, toasted

1. Heat oil in large saucepan over medium heat until shimmering. Add onion and ½ teaspoon salt and cook until softened, about 5 minutes. Add rice, garlic, turmeric, and cinnamon and cook, stirring frequently, until grain edges begin to turn translucent, about 3 minutes.

2. Stir in water and bring to simmer. Reduce heat to low, cover, and simmer gently until rice is tender and water is absorbed, 16 to 18 minutes.

3. Off heat, lay clean dish towel underneath lid and let pilaf sit for 10 minutes. Add parsley and almonds to pilaf and fluff gently with fork to combine. Season with pepper to taste. Serve.

PER ⅔-CUP SERVING

Cal 150 • **Total Fat** 4.5g • **Sat Fat** 0g • **Chol** 0mg
Sodium 200mg • **Total Carbs** 25g • **Fiber** 2g • **Total Sugar** 1g
Added Sugar 0g • **Protein** 3g • **Total Carbohydrate Choices** 2

VARIATION

Basmati Rice Pilaf with Peas, Scallions, and Lemon

Substitute 1 teaspoon grated lemon zest and ⅛ teaspoon red pepper flakes for turmeric and cinnamon. Substitute ½ cup thawed frozen peas, 2 thinly sliced scallions, and 1 tablespoon lemon juice for the parsley and almonds.

PER ⅔-CUP SERVING

Cal 140 • **Total Fat** 2.5g • **Sat Fat** 0g • **Chol** 0mg
Sodium 200mg • **Total Carbs** 26g • **Fiber** 2g • **Total Sugar** 1g
Added Sugar 0g • **Protein** 3g • **Total Carbohydrate Choices** 2

RINSING RICE AND GRAINS

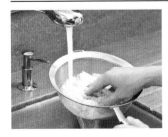

In some recipes, rinsing helps rid rice and grains of excess starch. To rinse, place rice or grains in fine-mesh strainer and run under cool water until water runs clear, occasionally stirring lightly with your hand. Let drain briefly.

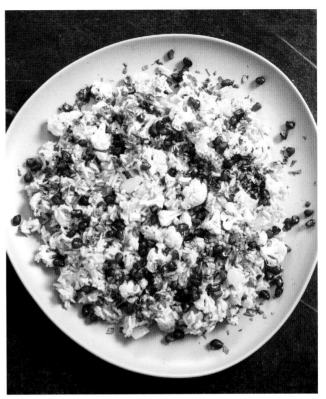

Roasting cauliflower florets quickly ups their flavor and makes a nutritious addition to basmati rice.

Spiced Basmati Rice with Cauliflower and Pomegranate
SERVES 6

WHY THIS RECIPE WORKS For a rice side dish with some nutritional punch, we wanted to pair aromatic basmati rice with sweet, earthy roasted cauliflower. We tossed small cauliflower florets with ground black pepper for heat and cumin for depth, then roasted at a high temperature for a short time to caramelize and crisp the florets without rendering them limp and mushy. To cook the rice, we first toasted it in a flavorful mixture of sautéed onion, garlic, and spices, then simmered it until tender and fluffy. To serve, we topped the spiced rice with our roasted cauliflower and finished the dish with nutritious crunchy pomegranate seeds and a mix of fresh herbs. Long-grain white, jasmine, or Texmati rice can be substituted for the basmati.

½ head cauliflower (1 pound), cored and
  cut into ¾-inch florets
2 tablespoons extra-virgin olive oil
  Salt and pepper

¼ teaspoon ground cumin

½ onion, chopped coarse

¾ cup basmati rice, rinsed

2 garlic cloves, minced

¼ teaspoon ground cinnamon

¼ teaspoon ground turmeric

1¼ cups water

¼ cup pomegranate seeds

1 tablespoon chopped fresh cilantro

1 tablespoon chopped fresh mint

1. Adjust oven rack to lowest position and heat oven to 475 degrees. Toss cauliflower with 1 tablespoon oil, ⅛ teaspoon salt, ¼ teaspoon pepper, and ⅛ teaspoon cumin. Arrange cauliflower in single layer on rimmed baking sheet and roast until just tender, 8 to 10 minutes; set aside.

2. Heat remaining 1 tablespoon oil in large saucepan over medium heat until shimmering. Add onion and ¼ teaspoon salt and cook until softened and lightly browned, 5 to 7 minutes. Add rice, garlic, cinnamon, turmeric, and remaining ⅛ teaspoon cumin and cook, stirring frequently, until grain edges begin to turn translucent, about 3 minutes.

3. Stir in water and bring to simmer. Reduce heat to low, cover, and simmer gently until rice is tender and water is absorbed, 16 to 18 minutes.

4. Off heat, lay clean dish towel underneath lid and let pilaf sit for 10 minutes. Add cauliflower to pilaf and fluff gently with fork to combine. Season with pepper to taste. Transfer to serving platter and sprinkle with pomegranate seeds, cilantro, and mint. Serve.

PER 1-CUP SERVING

Cal 150 • **Total Fat** 5g • **Sat Fat** 1g • **Chol** 0mg
Sodium 170mg • **Total Carbs** 23g • **Fiber** 3g • **Total Sugar** 3g
Added Sugar 0g • **Protein** 3g • **Total Carbohydrate Choices** 1.5

NOTES FROM THE TEST KITCHEN

Storing Rice, Grains, and Beans

To prevent rice, grains, and beans from spoiling in the pantry, store them in airtight containers; if you can, keep rice and grains in the freezer. This is especially important for whole grains, which turn rancid with oxidation. Use rice and grains within six months. Beans can keep for up to a year, but you will get the best results if you use beans within the first month or two of purchase.

Barley with Lemon and Herbs
SERVES 6

WHY THIS RECIPE WORKS Barley is a fiber powerhouse, a plus for those on a diabetic diet. This side dish is super simple, fragrant with fresh herbs and a bright, lemony vinaigrette. For grains that are distinct and boast a tender chew, we cook barley like pasta—boiled in a large volume of salted water and then drained—which rids the grains of much of their sticky starch that would otherwise cause them to clump. Once cooked, we briefly cool the grains on a rimmed baking sheet to help them dry thoroughly, and then toss them with an acid-heavy dressing (1:1 oil to acid instead of the typical 3:1 ratio), aromatics, and herbs for a flavorful, hearty side. Do not substitute hulled, hull-less, quick-cooking, or presteamed barley for the pearled barley in this recipe. The cooking time for pearled barley will vary from brand to brand (our preferred brand, Bob's Red Mill, is one of the longer-cooking brands), so start checking for doneness after about 25 minutes. This dish can be served warm or at room temperature.

1½ cups pearled barley

Salt and pepper

3 tablespoons extra-virgin olive oil

1 teaspoon grated lemon zest plus 3 tablespoons juice

2 tablespoons minced shallot

1 teaspoon Dijon mustard

6 scallions, sliced thin on bias

¼ cup minced fresh mint

¼ cup minced fresh cilantro

1. Bring 4 quarts water to boil in large pot. Add barley and 1 teaspoon salt and cook, adjusting heat to maintain gentle boil, until barley is tender with slight chew, 25 to 45 minutes.

2. Meanwhile, whisk oil, lemon zest and juice, shallot, mustard, ¼ teaspoon salt, and ½ teaspoon pepper in large bowl.

3. Drain barley well. Transfer to parchment paper–lined rimmed baking sheet and spread into even layer. Let sit until no longer steaming, 5 to 7 minutes. Add barley to bowl with dressing and toss to coat. Add scallions, mint, and cilantro and gently toss to combine. Season with pepper to taste. Serve.

PER ¾-CUP SERVING

Cal 250 • **Total Fat** 8g • **Sat Fat** 1g • **Chol** 0mg
Sodium 150mg • **Total Carbs** 41g • **Fiber** 9g • **Total Sugar** 1g
Added Sugar 0g • **Protein** 5g • **Total Carbohydrate Choices** 3

All About Grains

Most supermarkets sell many different types of grains. Note that whole grains are both healthier and more filling than refined grains. Here are some of the test kitchen's favorites.

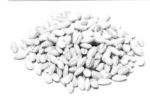

Barley

While barley might be most familiar as a key ingredient in beer, it is a nutritious high-fiber, high-protein cereal grain with a nutty flavor that is similar to that of brown rice. It is great in soups and in salads, as risotto, and as a simple side dish. Barley is available in multiple forms: Hulled barley, which is sold with the hull removed and the fiber-rich bran intact, is considered a whole grain and is higher in nutrients compared with pearled barley, which is hulled barley that has been polished to remove the bran (while it's not technically a whole grain, it offers many whole grain benefits). There is a quick-cooking barley, which is available as kernels or flakes. Hulled barley takes a long time to cook and should be soaked prior to cooking. Pearled barley cooks much more quickly, making it a more versatile choice when you are adding it to soups or making risotto or a simple pilaf. Use it as a stand-in for dishes where you might ordinarily use rice, such as stir-fries or curries.

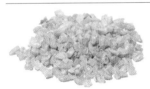

Bulgur

Bulgur is made from parboiled or steamed wheat kernels/berries that are dried and then cracked. The result of this process is a relatively fast-cooking, highly nutritious grain that can be used in a variety of applications. Bulgur is perfect for tabbouleh and salads because it requires little more than a soak to become tender and flavorful. We especially like soaking it in flavorful liquids, such as lemon or lime juice, to imbue the whole grain with bright flavor. Coarse-grind bulgur, which requires simmering, is our top choice for making pilaf. Note that medium-grind bulgur can work in either application if you make adjustments to soaking or cooking times. On the other hand, cracked wheat, which is often sold alongside bulgur, is not precooked and cannot be substituted for bulgur. Be sure to rinse bulgur, regardless of grain size, to remove excess starches that can turn the grain gluey.

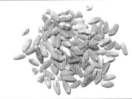

Farro

These hulled whole-wheat kernels boast a sweet, nutty flavor and a chewy bite. In Italy, the grain is available in three sizes—farro piccolo, farro medio, and farro grande—but the midsize type is most common in the United States. Although we often turn to the absorption method for quicker-cooking grains, farro takes better to the pasta method because the abundance of water cooks the grains more evenly. When cooked, the grains will be tender but have a slight chew, similar to al dente pasta.

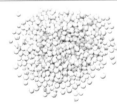

Quinoa

Quinoa originated in the Andes mountains of South America, and while it is generally treated as a grain, it is actually the seed of the goosefoot plant. Sometimes referred to as a "super grain," quinoa is high in protein, and its protein is complete, which means it possesses all of the amino acids in the balanced amounts that our bodies require. Beyond its nutritional prowess, we love quinoa for its addictive crunchy texture, nutty taste, and ease of preparation. Cooked as a pilaf or for a salad, it can be ready in about 20 minutes. Unless labeled "prewashed," quinoa should always be rinsed before cooking to remove its protective layer (called saponin), which is unpleasantly bitter.

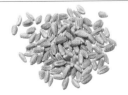

Wheat berries

Wheat berries, often erroneously referred to as "whole wheat," are whole, unprocessed kernels of wheat. Since none of the grain has been removed, wheat berries are an excellent source of nutrition. Compared to other forms of wheat (cracked wheat, bulgur, and flour), wheat berries require a relatively long cooking time. In the test kitchen, we like to toast the dry wheat berries until they are fragrant, and then simmer them for about an hour until they are tender but still retain a good bite.

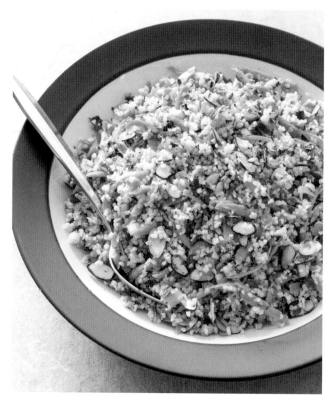

This nutritious no-cook bulgur salad is easy to prepare and superflavorful thanks to fresh herbs and a lemony dressing.

Bulgur Salad with Carrots and Almonds
SERVES 8

WHY THIS RECIPE WORKS Bulgur is known for its nutty flavor and versatility, acting as a nutritious, hearty medium for delivering big, bold flavors. To transform this whole grain into a satisfying salad, we started by softening the bulgur in a mixture of water, lemon juice, and salt for an hour and a half, until it had the perfect chew and was thoroughly seasoned. Fresh mint, cilantro, and scallions made the salad crisp and bright, and cumin and cayenne added depth of flavor to our simple lemon vinaigrette. Sweet shredded carrots nicely accented the rich, nutty taste of the bulgur, and toasted almonds provided complementary crunch. We also decided to develop another version of our salad with sweet, juicy grapes and tangy feta. When shopping, do not confuse bulgur with cracked wheat, which has a much longer cooking time and will not work in this recipe.

1½ cups medium-grind bulgur, rinsed
1 cup water
6 tablespoons lemon juice (2 lemons)
Salt and pepper
⅓ cup extra-virgin olive oil
½ teaspoon ground cumin
⅛ teaspoon cayenne pepper
4 carrots, peeled and shredded
3 scallions, sliced thin
½ cup sliced almonds, toasted
⅓ cup chopped fresh mint
⅓ cup chopped fresh cilantro

1. Combine bulgur, water, ¼ cup lemon juice, and ¼ teaspoon salt in bowl. Cover and let sit at room temperature until grains are softened and liquid is fully absorbed, about 1½ hours.

2. Whisk remaining 2 tablespoons lemon juice, oil, cumin, cayenne, and ¼ teaspoon salt together in large bowl. Add bulgur, carrots, scallions, almonds, mint, and cilantro and gently toss to combine. Season with pepper to taste. Serve.

PER ¾-CUP SERVING
Cal 230 • **Total Fat** 13g • **Sat Fat** 1.5g • **Chol** 0mg
Sodium 180mg • **Total Carbs** 26g • **Fiber** 6g • **Total Sugar** 2g
Added Sugar 0g • **Protein** 5g • **Total Carbohydrate Choices** 2

VARIATION
Bulgur Salad with Grapes and Feta
SERVES 6

WHY THIS RECIPE WORKS For the perfect salty-sweet combination, we paired juicy red grapes with briny feta, which provided this nutrient-dense whole grain with plenty of interesting flavor and texture. Slivered almonds provided additional crunch and protein, and a substantial amount of fresh mint contributed freshness and bright color. When shopping, do not confuse bulgur with cracked wheat, which has a much longer cooking time and will not work in this recipe.

1½ cups medium-grind bulgur, rinsed
1 cup water
5 tablespoons lemon juice (2 lemons)
Salt and pepper
¼ cup extra-virgin olive oil
¼ teaspoon ground cumin
Pinch cayenne pepper
4 ounces seedless red grapes, quartered (⅔ cup)
½ cup slivered almonds, toasted
2 ounces feta cheese, crumbled (½ cup)
2 scallions, sliced thin
¼ cup chopped fresh mint

1. Combine bulgur, water, ¼ cup lemon juice, and ¼ teaspoon salt in bowl. Cover and let sit at room temperature until grains are softened and liquid is fully absorbed, about 1½ hours.

2. Whisk remaining 1 tablespoon lemon juice, oil, cumin, and cayenne together in large bowl. Add bulgur, grapes, ⅓ cup almonds, ⅓ cup feta, scallions, and mint and gently toss to combine. Season with pepper to taste. Sprinkle with remaining almonds and remaining feta before serving.

PER ¾-CUP SERVING

Cal 230 • **Total Fat** 12g • **Sat Fat** 2.5g • **Chol** 5mg
Sodium 150mg • **Total Carbs** 25g • **Fiber** 5g • **Total Sugar** 3g
Added Sugar 0g • **Protein** 6g • **Total Carbohydrate Choices** 1.5

Tabbouleh
SERVES 4

WHY THIS RECIPE WORKS Tabbouleh, a salad made of bulgur, parsley, and tomatoes, is a great choice for those with diabetes because of its balance of a healthy whole grain and vegetables. We found that salting the tomatoes rid them of excess moisture, and soaking the bulgur in lemon juice and some of the drained tomato liquid, rather than in water, allowed it to absorb lots of flavor as it softened. Scallions added the right amount of oniony flavor, and parsley, mint, and a bit of cayenne rounded out the dish. Adding the herbs and vegetables while the bulgur was still soaking gave the components time to mingle. Do not confuse bulgur with cracked wheat, which has a much longer cooking time and will not work in this recipe.

    3 tomatoes, cored and cut into ½-inch pieces
       Salt and pepper
    ½ cup medium-grind bulgur, rinsed
    ¼ cup lemon juice (2 lemons)
    6 tablespoons extra-virgin olive oil
    ⅛ teaspoon cayenne pepper
 1½ cups minced fresh parsley
    ½ cup minced fresh mint
    2 scallions, sliced thin

1. Toss tomatoes with ¼ teaspoon salt in fine-mesh strainer set over bowl and let drain, tossing occasionally, for 30 minutes; reserve 2 tablespoons drained tomato juice. Combine bulgur, 2 tablespoons lemon juice, and reserved tomato juice in bowl and let sit until grains begin to soften, 30 to 40 minutes.

2. Whisk remaining 2 tablespoons lemon juice, oil, cayenne, and ¼ teaspoon salt together in large bowl. Add tomatoes, bulgur, parsley, mint, and scallions and gently toss to combine. Cover and

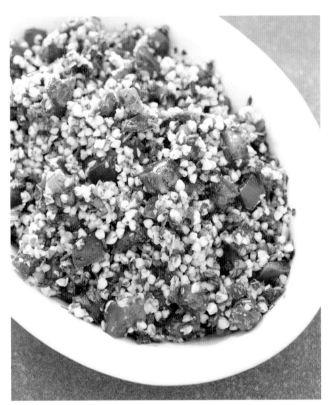

To give our tabbouleh great flavor, we soak the bulgur in juice drained from the tomatoes and lemon juice instead of water.

let sit at room temperature until flavors have melded and grains are softened, about 1 hour. Before serving, toss salad to recombine and season with pepper to taste.

PER 1-CUP SERVING

Cal 280 • **Total Fat** 22g • **Sat Fat** 3g • **Chol** 0mg
Sodium 320mg • **Total Carbs** 21g • **Fiber** 5g • **Total Sugar** 3g
Added Sugar 0g • **Protein** 4g • **Total Carbohydrate Choices** 1.5

VARIATION
Spiced Tabbouleh

Add ¼ teaspoon ground cinnamon and ¼ teaspoon ground allspice to dressing with cayenne.

PER 1-CUP SERVING

Cal 290 • **Total Fat** 22g • **Sat Fat** 3g • **Chol** 0mg
Sodium 320mg • **Total Carbs** 21g • **Fiber** 5g • **Total Sugar** 3g
Added Sugar 0g • **Protein** 4g • **Total Carbohydrate Choices** 1.5

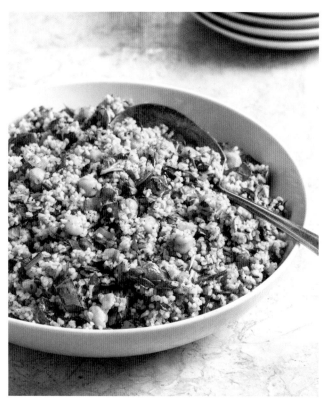

Fragrant spice blends like za'atar are a great way to punch up flavor without adding salt.

Bulgur with Chickpeas, Spinach, and Za'atar
SERVES 8

WHY THIS RECIPE WORKS This dish combines creamy, nutty chickpeas and hearty bulgur with the clean, vegetal punch of fresh spinach. One great way to boost flavor without salt is by using spice blends; here we chose the aromatic eastern Mediterranean blend *za'atar*, with its fragrant wild herbs, toasted sesame seeds, and tangy sumac. We found that incorporating the za'atar at two distinct points in the cooking process brought out its most complex flavor. First, to release its deep, earthy flavors, we bloomed half of the za'atar in an aromatic base of onion and garlic before adding the bulgur, chickpeas, and cooking liquid. We added the remainder of the za'atar and the spinach off the heat: The residual heat was enough to perfectly soften the spinach and to highlight the za'atar's more delicate aromas. When shopping for za'atar, look for a blend that doesn't include salt. Do not confuse bulgur with cracked wheat, which has a much longer cooking time and will not work in this recipe.

3 tablespoons extra-virgin olive oil
1 onion, chopped fine
   Salt and pepper
3 garlic cloves, minced
2 tablespoons za'atar
1 cup medium-grind bulgur, rinsed
1 (15-ounce) can no-salt-added chickpeas, rinsed
¾ cup low-sodium vegetable broth
¾ cup water
3 ounces (3 cups) baby spinach, chopped
1 tablespoon lemon juice

1. Heat 2 tablespoons oil in large saucepan over medium heat until shimmering. Add onion and ½ teaspoon salt and cook until softened, about 5 minutes. Stir in garlic and 1 tablespoon za'atar and cook until fragrant, about 30 seconds.

2. Stir in bulgur, chickpeas, broth, and water and bring to simmer. Reduce heat to low, cover, and simmer gently until bulgur is tender, 16 to 18 minutes.

3. Off heat, lay clean dish towel underneath lid and let bulgur sit for 10 minutes. Add spinach, lemon juice, remaining 1 tablespoon za'atar, and remaining 1 tablespoon oil and fluff gently with fork to combine. Season with pepper to taste. Serve.

PER ¾-CUP SERVING
Cal 160 • **Total Fat** 6g • **Sat Fat** 1g • **Chol** 0mg
Sodium 180mg • **Total Carbs** 21g • **Fiber** 4g • **Total Sugar** 1g
Added Sugar 0g • **Protein** 5g • **Total Carbohydrate Choices** 1.5

Couscous with Tomato, Scallion, and Lemon
SERVES 6

WHY THIS RECIPE WORKS Couscous is a supersimple, versatile side dish that is hands-off and quick to come together. For a healthier option, we chose to use whole-wheat couscous, which has more fiber. Toasting the couscous before adding liquid helped bring out its nutty flavor. After just 12 minutes, the grains were perfectly cooked. Once we had fluffed the couscous with a fork, we boosted its flavor profile with lemon, tomato, and scallion, keeping the dish light and fresh. Do not use Israeli couscous in this recipe; its larger size requires a different cooking method.

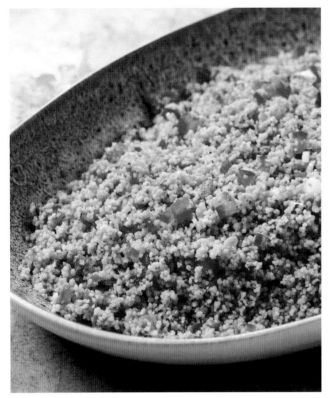

We treat quick-cooking whole-wheat couscous like a grain and toast it before adding any liquid to bring out its nutty flavor.

1 cup whole-wheat couscous
2 tablespoons extra-virgin olive oil
1 onion, chopped fine
  Salt and pepper
2 garlic cloves, minced
1 teaspoon grated lemon zest plus 1½ teaspoons lemon juice
⅛ teaspoon cayenne pepper
¾ cup water
¾ cup unsalted chicken broth
1 tomato, cored, seeded, and chopped fine
1 scallion, sliced thin

1. Toast couscous in medium saucepan over medium-high heat, stirring often, until a few grains begin to brown, about 3 minutes. Transfer couscous to large bowl and set aside.

2. Heat 1 tablespoon oil in now-empty saucepan over medium heat until shimmering. Add onion and ½ teaspoon salt and cook until softened, about 5 minutes. Stir in garlic, lemon zest, and cayenne and cook until fragrant, about 30 seconds. Stir in water and broth and bring to boil.

3. Once boiling, immediately pour broth mixture over couscous, cover tightly with plastic wrap, and let sit until grains are tender, about 12 minutes.

4. Add remaining 1 tablespoon oil, lemon juice, tomato, and scallion and fluff gently with fork to combine. Season with pepper to taste and serve.

PER ¾-CUP SERVING

Cal 170 • **Total Fat** 5g • **Sat Fat** 0.5g • **Chol** 0mg
Sodium 210mg • **Total Carbs** 28g • **Fiber** 5g • **Total Sugar** 3g
Added Sugar 0g • **Protein** 6g • **Total Carbohydrate Choices** 2

VARIATIONS
Couscous with Carrots, Chickpeas, and Herbs
SERVES 8

WHY THIS RECIPE WORKS For a warm, spicier couscous side, we bloomed coriander and ginger in a saucepan with oil, garlic, carrots, and onion before adding our liquid and grains and letting the grains sit until tender. Parsley and lemon juice added a hit of freshness before serving. Do not use Israeli couscous in this recipe; its larger size requires a different cooking method.

1 cup whole-wheat couscous
2 tablespoons extra-virgin olive oil
2 carrots, peeled and chopped fine
1 onion, chopped fine
  Salt and pepper
2 garlic cloves, minced
½ teaspoon ground coriander
½ teaspoon ground ginger
¾ cup water
¾ cup unsalted chicken broth
1 (15-ounce) can no-salt-added chickpeas, rinsed
¼ cup minced fresh parsley, cilantro, and/or mint
1½ teaspoons lemon juice

1. Toast couscous in medium saucepan over medium-high heat, stirring often, until a few grains begin to brown, about 3 minutes. Transfer couscous to large bowl and set aside.

2. Heat 1 tablespoon oil in now-empty saucepan over medium heat until shimmering. Add carrots, onion, and ½ teaspoon salt and cook until softened, 6 to 8 minutes. Stir in garlic, coriander, and ginger and cook until fragrant, about 30 seconds. Stir in water, broth, and chickpeas and bring to boil.

3. Once boiling, immediately pour broth mixture over couscous, cover tightly with plastic wrap, and let sit until grains are tender, about 12 minutes.

4. Add remaining 1 tablespoon oil, parsley, and lemon juice and fluff gently with fork to combine. Season with pepper to taste and serve.

PER ¾-CUP SERVING

Cal 170 • **Total Fat** 4g • **Sat Fat** 0.5g • **Chol** 0mg
Sodium 180mg • **Total Carbs** 28g • **Fiber** 5g • **Total Sugar** 3g
Added Sugar 0g • **Protein** 6g • **Total Carbohydrate Choices** 2

Couscous with Saffron, Raisins, and Toasted Almonds
SERVES 6

WHY THIS RECIPE WORKS Just a tiny bit of saffron, along with cinnamon and cayenne, worked wonders transforming couscous into a flavorful side. Raisins added just a touch of sweetness and plumped up nicely when cooked with the grains. Sliced almonds provided a slight crunch to our cooked couscous, and a squeeze of lemon juice brightened all the flavors. Do not use Israeli couscous in this recipe; its larger size requires a different cooking method.

 1 **cup whole-wheat couscous**
 2 **tablespoons extra-virgin olive oil**
 1 **onion, chopped fine**
    Salt and pepper
⅛ **teaspoon saffron threads, crumbled**
⅛ **teaspoon ground cinnamon**
⅛ **teaspoon cayenne pepper**
¾ **cup water**
¾ **cup unsalted chicken broth**
½ **cup raisins**
¼ **cup sliced almonds, toasted**
1½ **teaspoons lemon juice**

1. Toast couscous in medium saucepan over medium-high heat, stirring often, until a few grains begin to brown, about 3 minutes. Transfer couscous to large bowl and set aside.

2. Heat 1 tablespoon oil in now-empty saucepan over medium heat until shimmering. Add onion and ½ teaspoon salt and cook until softened, about 5 minutes. Stir in saffron, cinnamon, and cayenne and cook until fragrant, about 30 seconds. Stir in water, broth, and raisins and bring to boil.

3. Once boiling, immediately pour broth mixture over couscous, cover tightly with plastic wrap, and let sit until grains are tender, about 12 minutes.

4. Add remaining 1 tablespoon oil, almonds, and lemon juice and fluff gently with fork to combine. Season with pepper to taste and serve.

PER ¾-CUP SERVING

Cal 230 • **Total Fat** 7g • **Sat Fat** 1g • **Chol** 0mg
Sodium 220mg • **Total Carbs** 36g • **Fiber** 5g • **Total Sugar** 14g
Added Sugar 0g • **Protein** 6g • **Total Carbohydrate Choices** 2.5

Farro Salad with Asparagus, Snap Peas, and Tomatoes
SERVES 8

WHY THIS RECIPE WORKS Whole-grain farro is versatile, nutritious, and makes a great base for a grain side. We wondered if we could bypass the traditional step of soaking the grains overnight and then cooking them slowly in favor of a simpler, quicker method. We learned that boiling the grains in plenty of salted water and then draining them yielded nicely firm but tender farro—no soaking necessary. To make sure this salad looked as good as it tasted, we briefly boiled bite-size pieces of asparagus and snap peas to bring out their vibrant color and crisp-tender bite. A lemon-dill dressing complemented the earthy farro. Cherry tomatoes and feta offered a full-flavored finish. We prefer the flavor and texture of whole farro; pearled farro can be used, but the texture may be softer. Do not use quick-cooking or presteamed farro (read the ingredient list on the package to determine this) in this recipe. The cooking time for farro can vary greatly among different brands, so we recommend beginning to check for doneness after 10 minutes.

 6 **ounces asparagus, trimmed and cut into 1-inch lengths**
 6 **ounces sugar snap peas, strings removed, halved crosswise**
    Salt and pepper
1½ **cups whole farro**
 3 **tablespoons extra-virgin olive oil**
 2 **tablespoons lemon juice**
 2 **tablespoons minced shallot**
 1 **teaspoon Dijon mustard**
 6 **ounces cherry tomatoes, halved**
 2 **ounces feta cheese, crumbled (½ cup)**
 3 **tablespoons chopped fresh dill**

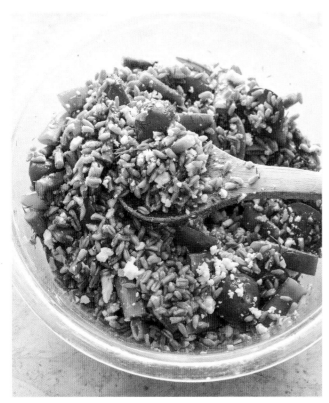

Cooking farro in plenty of boiling water ensures tender grains that are ready to be paired with fresh vegetables and herbs.

1. Bring 4 quarts water to boil in large pot. Add asparagus, snap peas, and 1 teaspoon salt and cook until crisp-tender, about 3 minutes. Using slotted spoon, transfer vegetables to large plate and let cool completely, about 15 minutes.

2. Return water to boil, add farro, and cook until grains are tender with slight chew, 15 to 30 minutes. Drain farro well. Transfer to parchment paper–lined rimmed baking sheet and spread into even layer. Let cool completely, about 15 minutes.

3. Whisk oil, lemon juice, shallot, mustard, and ¼ teaspoon pepper together in large bowl. Add vegetables, farro, tomatoes, ¼ cup feta, and dill and gently toss to combine. Season with pepper to taste. Transfer to serving platter and sprinkle with remaining ¼ cup feta. Serve.

PER ¾-CUP SERVING
Cal 210 • **Total Fat** 8g • **Sat Fat** 2g • **Chol** 5mg
Sodium 120mg • **Total Carbs** 31g • **Fiber** 4g • **Total Sugar** 4g
Added Sugar 0g • **Protein** 7g • **Total Carbohydrate Choices** 2

VARIATION
Farro Salad with Cucumber, Yogurt, and Mint
SERVES 8

WHY THIS RECIPE WORKS This *tzatziki*-inspired farro salad boasts a bit of creaminess from protein-rich Greek yogurt. Fresh mint and cucumber provide additional texture and fragrance. We prefer the flavor and texture of whole farro; pearled farro can be used, but the texture may be softer. Do not use quick-cooking or presteamed farro (read the ingredient list on the package to determine this) in this recipe. The cooking time for farro can vary greatly among different brands, so we recommend beginning to check for doneness after 10 minutes.

1½ cups whole farro
    Salt and pepper
  3 tablespoons extra-virgin olive oil
  2 tablespoons lemon juice
  2 tablespoons minced shallot
  2 tablespoons plain 2 percent Greek yogurt
  1 English cucumber, halved lengthwise, seeded, and cut into ¼-inch pieces
  6 ounces cherry tomatoes, halved
  1 cup baby arugula
  3 tablespoons chopped fresh mint

1. Bring 4 quarts water to boil in large pot. Add farro and 1 teaspoon salt and cook until grains are tender with slight chew, 15 to 30 minutes. Drain farro well. Transfer to parchment paper–lined rimmed baking sheet and spread into even layer. Let cool completely, about 15 minutes.

2. Whisk oil, lemon juice, shallot, yogurt, ¼ teaspoon salt, and ¼ teaspoon pepper together in large bowl. Add farro, cucumber, tomatoes, arugula, and mint and gently toss to combine. Season with pepper to taste. Serve.

PER ¾-CUP SERVING
Cal 190 • **Total Fat** 7g • **Sat Fat** 1g • **Chol** 0mg
Sodium 100mg • **Total Carbs** 30g • **Fiber** 4g • **Total Sugar** 3g
Added Sugar 0g • **Protein** 5g • **Total Carbohydrate Choices** 2

All About Cooking Grains

The types of grains and the best methods for cooking them can vary tremendously. Some grains, such as bulgur, cook in minutes, and others, such as barley or wheat berries, take much longer. Here in the test kitchen we have homed in on three basic methods for cooking grains. We then determined which are best for each type of grain. While some grains, such as bulgur, take well to any cooking method, others will turn out best when cooked with a specific method.

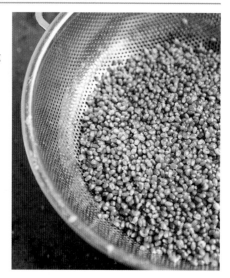

PILAF-STYLE DIRECTIONS Rinse (see page 127) and then dry grain on towel. Heat 1 tablespoon oil in medium saucepan (preferably nonstick) over medium-high heat until shimmering. Stir in grain and toast until lightly golden and fragrant, 2 to 3 minutes. Stir in water and ¼ teaspoon salt. Bring mixture to simmer, then reduce heat to low, cover, and continue to simmer until grain is tender and has absorbed all of water, following cooking times given below. Off heat, let grain stand for 10 minutes, then fluff with fork.

BOILING DIRECTIONS Bring water to boil in large saucepan. Stir in grain and salt. Return to boil, then reduce to simmer and cook until grain is tender, following cooking times given in chart below. Drain.

MICROWAVE DIRECTIONS Rinse grain (see page 127). Combine water, grain, 1 tablespoon oil, and ¼ teaspoon salt in bowl. Cover and cook following times given below. Remove from microwave and fluff with fork. Cover bowl with plastic wrap, poke several vent holes with tip of knife, and let sit until completely tender, about 5 minutes.

TYPE OF GRAIN	COOKING METHOD	AMOUNT OF GRAIN	AMOUNT OF WATER	AMOUNT OF SALT	COOKING TIME
Pearled Barley	Pilaf-Style	1 cup	1⅔ cups	¼ teaspoon	20 to 40 minutes
	Boiled	1 cup	4 quarts	1 teaspoon	25 to 45 minutes
	Microwave	X	X	X	X
Bulgur (medium-to coarse-grind)	Pilaf-Style*	1 cup	1½ cups	¼ teaspoon	16 to 18 minutes
	Boiled	1 cup	4 quarts	1 teaspoon	5 minutes
	Microwave	1 cup	1 cup	¼ teaspoon	5 to 10 minutes
Farro	Pilaf-Style	X	X	X	X
	Boiled	1 cup	4 quarts	1 teaspoon	15 to 30 minutes
	Microwave	X	X	X	X
Wheat Berries	Pilaf-Style	X	X	X	X
	Boiled	1 cup	4 quarts	½ teaspoon	1 hour to 1 hour 10 minutes
	Microwave	X	X	X	X

* For bulgur pilaf, do not rinse, and skip the toasting step, adding the grain to the pot with the liquid.
X = Not recommended

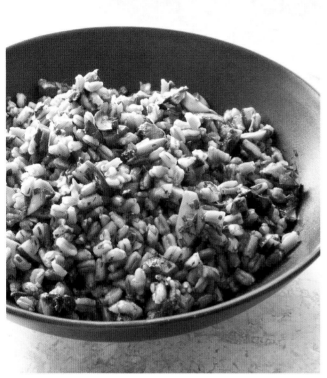

Meaty mushrooms and nutty farro combine to make a hearty and healthy whole-grain side dish.

Warm Farro with Mushrooms and Thyme
SERVES 6

WHY THIS RECIPE WORKS We wanted to pair earthy, hearty mushrooms with equally hearty farro. To start, we used the pasta method (an abundance of water) to boil our farro, which ensured the grains cooked evenly and required only half an hour. We then moved on to the mushrooms, sautéing them with shallot and thyme until the moisture evaporated and the mushrooms achieved some browning. Scraping up the browned bits in the pan with sherry rounded things out with sweetness and acidity before we added the farro. We prefer the flavor and texture of whole farro; pearled farro can be used, but the texture may be softer. Do not use quick-cooking or presteamed farro (read the ingredient list on the package to determine this) in this recipe. The cooking time for farro can vary greatly among different brands, so we recommend beginning to check for doneness after 10 minutes.

1½ cups whole farro
  Salt and pepper
3 tablespoons extra-virgin olive oil
12 ounces cremini mushrooms, trimmed and chopped coarse
1 shallot, minced
1½ teaspoons minced fresh thyme or ½ teaspoon dried
3 tablespoons dry sherry
3 tablespoons minced fresh parsley
1½ teaspoons sherry vinegar, plus extra for seasoning

1. Bring 4 quarts water to boil in large pot. Add farro and 1 teaspoon salt and cook until grains are tender with slight chew, 15 to 30 minutes. Drain farro, return to now-empty pot, and cover to keep warm.

2. Heat 2 tablespoons oil in 12-inch skillet over medium heat until shimmering. Add mushrooms, shallot, thyme, and ¼ teaspoon salt and cook, stirring occasionally, until moisture has evaporated and vegetables start to brown, 8 to 10 minutes. Stir in sherry, scraping up any browned bits, and cook until skillet is almost dry.

3. Add farro and remaining 1 tablespoon oil and cook until heated through, about 2 minutes. Off heat, stir in parsley and vinegar. Season with pepper and extra vinegar to taste and serve.

PER ⅔-CUP SERVING
Cal 250 • **Total Fat** 9g • **Sat Fat** 1g • **Chol** 0mg
Sodium 135mg • **Total Carbs** 39g • **Fiber** 4g • **Total Sugar** 4g
Added Sugar 0g • **Protein** 7g • **Total Carbohydrate Choices** 2.5

VARIATION
Warm Farro with Fennel and Parmesan
SERVES 6

WHY THIS RECIPE WORKS To give farro a different flavor profile, we quickly sautéed fennel to give it a subtle sweetness, then paired it with garlic and thyme. After we tossed the fennel with our cooked farro, a sprinkle of Parmesan provided some richness and a slightly salty bite. We prefer the flavor and texture of whole farro; pearled farro can be used, but the texture may be softer. Do not use quick-cooking or presteamed farro (read the ingredient list on the package to determine this) in this recipe. The cooking time for farro can vary greatly among different brands, so we recommend beginning to check for doneness after 10 minutes.

1½ cups whole farro
   Salt and pepper
3 tablespoons extra-virgin olive oil
1 onion, chopped fine
1 small fennel bulb, stalks discarded, bulb halved, cored, and chopped fine
3 garlic cloves, minced
1 teaspoon minced fresh thyme or ¼ teaspoon dried
1 ounce Parmesan cheese, grated (½ cup)
¼ cup minced fresh parsley
2 teaspoons sherry vinegar, plus extra for seasoning

1. Bring 4 quarts water to boil in large pot. Add farro and 1 teaspoon salt and cook until grains are tender with slight chew, 15 to 30 minutes. Drain farro, return to now-empty pot, and cover to keep warm.

2. Heat 2 tablespoons oil in 12-inch skillet over medium heat until shimmering. Add onion, fennel, and ¼ teaspoon salt and cook until softened, 6 to 8 minutes. Stir in garlic and thyme and cook until fragrant, about 30 seconds. Add farro and remaining 1 tablespoon oil and cook until heated through, about 2 minutes. Off heat, stir in Parmesan, parsley, and vinegar. Season with pepper and extra vinegar to taste. Serve.

PER ⅔-CUP SERVING

Cal 280 • **Total Fat** 10g • **Sat Fat** 1.5g • **Chol** 5mg
Sodium 240mg • **Total Carbs** 41g • **Fiber** 6g • **Total Sugar** 4g
Added Sugar 0g • **Protein** 9g • **Total Carbohydrate Choices** 3

Creamy Parmesan Polenta
SERVES 6

WHY THIS RECIPE WORKS Polenta makes a perfect foil for rich stews and braises, or it can be topped with sautéed vegetables for a simple, satisfying dinner. However, it's often loaded with butter, creamy cheese, and salt, making it a super-indulgent dish high in saturated fat and sodium. We wanted a diabetic-friendly polenta with deep corn flavor and a smooth, rich consistency. From the outset, we knew that the right type of cornmeal was essential. Coarse-ground degerminated cornmeal gave us the soft but hearty texture and sweet, nutty flavor we were looking for. Adding a pinch of baking soda to the pot helped to soften the cornmeal's endosperm, which cut down on the cooking time. The baking soda also encouraged the granules to break down and release their starch in a uniform way, creating a silky, creamy consistency with minimal stirring. While many recipes are heavy-handed with the salt, we relied on good-quality Parmesan cheese to contribute

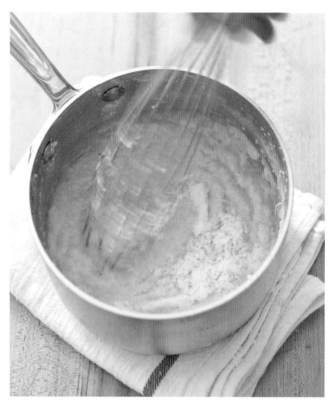

A pinch of baking soda is the trick to perfectly creamy, smooth polenta that cooks quickly and doesn't require constant stirring.

saltiness as well as a complementary nutty flavor. Olive oil and fresh parsley, stirred in at the last minute, ensured a satisfying, rich flavor and silkiness. If the polenta bubbles or sputters even slightly after the first 10 minutes, the heat is too high and you may need a flame tamer.

5 cups water
   Salt and pepper
   Pinch baking soda
1 cup coarse-ground cornmeal
1 ounce Parmesan cheese, grated (½ cup)
¼ cup minced fresh parsley or basil
1 tablespoons extra-virgin olive oil

1. Bring water to boil in large saucepan over medium-high heat. Stir in ½ teaspoon salt and baking soda. While whisking constantly, slowly pour cornmeal into water in steady stream. Bring mixture to boil, stirring constantly, then reduce heat to lowest setting and cover.

2. After 5 minutes, whisk polenta to smooth out any lumps that may have formed. (Make sure to scrape down sides and bottom of saucepan.) Cover and continue to cook, without stirring, until polenta grains are tender but slightly al dente, about 25 minutes. (Polenta should be loose and barely hold its shape; it will continue to thicken as it cools.)

3. Off heat, stir in Parmesan, parsley, and oil and season with pepper to taste. Cover and let sit for 5 minutes. Serve.

PER ¾-CUP SERVING

Cal 100 • **Total Fat** 4g • **Sat Fat** 1g • **Chol** 5mg
Sodium 300mg • **Total Carbs** 14g • **Fiber** 2g • **Total Sugar** 0g
Added Sugar 0g • **Protein** 4g • **Total Carbohydrate Choices** 1

MAKING A FLAME TAMER

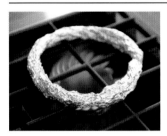

A flame tamer keeps polenta, risotto, and sauces from simmering too briskly. To make one, crumble a sheet of heavy-duty aluminum foil and shape into a 1-inch-thick ring of even thickness the size of your burner.

NOTES FROM THE TEST KITCHEN

Sorting Out Polenta

In the supermarket, cornmeal can be labeled as anything from yellow grits to corn semolina. Forget the names. When shopping for the right product to make polenta, there are three things to consider: "instant" or "quick-cooking" versus the traditional style; degerminated versus whole-grain meal; and grind size.

Instant and quick-cooking cornmeals are parcooked and comparatively bland—leave them on the shelf. Though we love the full corn flavor of whole-grain cornmeal, it remains slightly gritty no matter how long you cook it. We prefer degerminated cornmeal, in which the hard hull and germ are removed from each kernel (check the back label or ingredient list to see if your cornmeal is degerminated; if it's not explicitly labeled as such, you can assume it's whole-grain).

As for grind, we found that coarser grains brought the most desirable and pillowy texture to our Creamy Parmesan Polenta. However, grind coarseness can vary dramatically from brand to brand since there are no standards to ensure consistency—one manufacturer's "coarse" may be another's "fine." To identify coarse polenta as really coarse, the grains should be about the size of couscous.

Quinoa Pilaf with Lemon and Thyme
SERVES 6

WHY THIS RECIPE WORKS Quinoa is a nutritionally dense alternative to rice that is easier to prepare. It has an appealingly nutty flavor and a crunchy texture, but often turns into a mushy mess with washed-out flavor and an underlying bitterness. We wanted a simple quinoa pilaf with light, distinct grains and great flavor. We found that most recipes for quinoa pilaf turn out woefully overcooked quinoa because they call for far too much liquid. We reduced the water to ensure tender grains with a satisfying bite. We also toasted the quinoa in a dry saucepan to develop its natural nutty flavor before simmering. We enlivened our pilaf with some sautéed onion and finished it with herbs and a squeeze of lemon juice. Be sure to rinse the quinoa in a fine-mesh strainer before using; rinsing removes the quinoa's bitter protective coating (called saponin).

1½ cups prewashed white quinoa, rinsed
 2 tablespoons extra-virgin olive oil
 1 onion, minced
½ teaspoon salt
¼ teaspoon pepper
1¾ cups water
 1 (2-inch) strip lemon zest plus 2 teaspoons juice
 1 teaspoon minced fresh thyme or ¼ teaspoon dried
 2 tablespoons minced fresh parsley

1. Toast quinoa in medium saucepan over medium-high heat, stirring often, until quinoa is very fragrant and makes continuous popping sound, 5 to 7 minutes; transfer to bowl.

2. Heat oil in now-empty saucepan over medium heat until shimmering. Add onion, salt, and pepper and cook until softened, about 5 minutes. Stir in water, lemon zest, thyme, and quinoa and bring to simmer. Reduce heat to low, cover, and cook until grains are just tender and liquid is absorbed, 18 to 20 minutes, stirring once halfway through cooking.

3. Off heat, lay clean dish towel underneath lid and let pilaf sit for 10 minutes. Discard lemon zest. Add lemon juice and parsley and fluff gently with fork to combine. Serve.

PER ⅔-CUP SERVING

Cal 210 • **Total Fat** 7g • **Sat Fat** 1g • **Chol** 0mg
Sodium 200mg • **Total Carbs** 29g • **Fiber** 3g • **Total Sugar** 2g
Added Sugar 0g • **Protein** 6g • **Total Carbohydrate Choices** 2

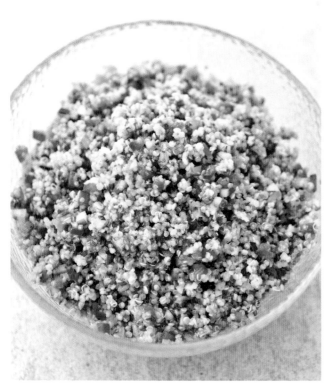

Protein- and fiber-rich quinoa makes a healthy side that is easily dressed up with fresh cilantro and crisp bell pepper.

Quinoa Salad with Red Bell Pepper and Cilantro
SERVES 4

WHY THIS RECIPE WORKS For an easy quinoa side dish, we toasted the grains to bring out their nutty flavor before adding our liquid. Once they had absorbed all the water, we transferred them to a baking sheet to expedite cooling before tossing them with crunchy bell pepper, onion, jalapeño, and fresh cilantro. To make a bright, flavorful dressing, we whisked together lime juice, mustard, garlic, and cumin. To make this dish spicier, include the chile's seeds. After 12 minutes of cooking, there will still be a little bit of water in the pan, but this will evaporate as the quinoa cools. Be sure to rinse the quinoa in a fine-mesh strainer before using; rinsing removes the quinoa's bitter protective coating (called saponin).

1 cup prewashed white quinoa, rinsed
1½ cups water
   Salt and pepper
2 tablespoons lime juice
1 tablespoon extra-virgin olive oil

2 teaspoons Dijon mustard
1 small garlic clove, minced
½ teaspoon ground cumin
½ red bell pepper, chopped fine
½ jalapeño chile, stemmed, seeded, and minced
2 tablespoons finely chopped red onion
1 tablespoon minced fresh cilantro

1. Toast quinoa in medium saucepan over medium-high heat, stirring often, until quinoa is very fragrant and makes continuous popping sound, 5 to 7 minutes. Stir in water and ¼ teaspoon salt and bring to simmer. Reduce heat to low, cover, and cook until quinoa is nearly tender and most of liquid is absorbed, about 12 minutes.

2. Transfer quinoa to parchment paper–lined rimmed baking sheet and spread into even layer. Let sit until tender and cool, about 20 minutes.

3. Whisk lime juice, oil, mustard, garlic, and cumin together in large bowl. Add quinoa, bell pepper, jalapeño, onion, and cilantro and gently toss to combine. Season with pepper to taste and serve.

PER ¾-CUP SERVING
Cal 200 • **Total Fat** 6g • **Sat Fat** 1g • **Chol** 0mg
Sodium 230mg • **Total Carbs** 29g • **Fiber** 3g • **Total Sugar** 2g
Added Sugar 0g • **Protein** 6g • **Total Carbohydrate Choices** 2

Wheat Berry Salad with Roasted Red Pepper, Feta, and Arugula
SERVES 6

WHY THIS RECIPE WORKS Wheat berries are whole, unprocessed kernels of wheat. Since none of the grain has been removed, they are an excellent source of healthy fiber. Thanks to their earthy flavor, chewy exterior, and tender interior, they're ideal for a satisfying salad. We tossed them in a tangy vinaigrette of sherry vinegar, garlic, cumin, and cayenne. To our bold pair of ingredients— roasted red peppers and feta cheese—we added peppery arugula to balance the sweetness of the peppers and fresh cilantro for brightness. Canned chickpeas rounded out this healthy side dish. If using quick-cooking or presteamed wheat berries (read the ingredient list on the package to determine this), you will need to decrease the cooking time in step 1.

1 cup wheat berries
   Salt
2 tablespoons extra-virgin olive oil

2 tablespoons sherry vinegar

2 garlic cloves, minced

½ teaspoon ground cumin

⅛ teaspoon cayenne pepper

1 (15-ounce) can no-salt-added chickpeas, rinsed

½ cup jarred roasted red peppers, rinsed, patted dry, and chopped

2 ounces feta cheese, crumbled (½ cup)

¼ cup minced fresh cilantro

2 ounces (2 cups) baby arugula, chopped coarse

1. Bring 4 quarts water to boil in large pot. Add wheat berries and ½ teaspoon salt and cook until tender with slight chew, 60 to 70 minutes.

2. Whisk oil, vinegar, garlic, cumin, and cayenne together in large bowl. Drain wheat berries, add to bowl with dressing, and gently toss to coat. Let cool slightly, about 15 minutes.

3. Stir in chickpeas, red peppers, feta, and cilantro. Add arugula and gently toss to combine. Serve.

PER 1-CUP SERVING

Cal 230 • **Total Fat** 7g • **Sat Fat** 2 • **Chol** 10mg
Sodium 170mg • **Total Carbs** 32g • **Fiber** 6g • **Total Sugar** 2g
Added Sugar 0g • **Protein** 8g • **Total Carbohydrate Choices** 2

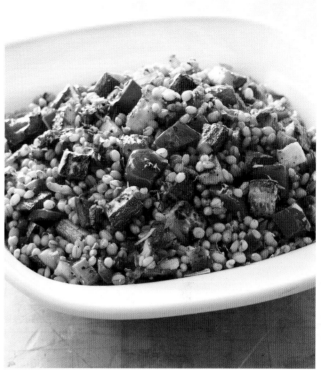

Nutritious vegetables bulk up simple wheat berries without adding too many carbs to this vibrant side dish.

Warm Wheat Berries with Zucchini, Red Bell Pepper, and Oregano

SERVES 6

WHY THIS RECIPE WORKS Warm wheat berries with vegetables is an excellent choice for a diabetes-friendly side dish. In order to bulk up the dish without adding too many carbohydrates, we turned to crisp-tender zucchini, red onion, and sweet red bell pepper. Browning the vegetables gave them great flavor; but we found that sautéing them in batches was essential to achieving the deep sear we were after. We cooked the wheat berries using the pasta method to ensure even cooking, and then allowed the warm wheat berries to soak in a bold oregano vinaigrette while the vegetables were cooking. If using quick-cooking or presteamed wheat berries (read the ingredient list on the package to determine this), you will need to decrease the wheat berry cooking time in step 1.

1½ cups wheat berries

Salt and pepper

2 tablespoons extra-virgin olive oil

3 tablespoons red wine vinegar

1 tablespoon grated lemon zest

1 tablespoon minced fresh oregano or 1½ teaspoons dried

1 garlic clove, minced

1 zucchini, cut into ½-inch pieces

1 red onion, chopped

1 red bell pepper, stemmed, seeded, and cut into ½-inch pieces

1. Bring 4 quarts water to boil in large pot. Add wheat berries and ½ teaspoon salt and cook until tender with slight chew, 60 to 70 minutes.

2. Whisk 1 tablespoon oil, vinegar, lemon zest, oregano, and garlic together in large bowl. Drain wheat berries, add to bowl with dressing, and gently toss to coat.

3. Heat 2 teaspoons oil in 12-inch nonstick skillet over medium-high heat until just smoking. Add zucchini and ¼ teaspoon salt and cook, stirring occasionally, until deep golden brown and beginning to char in spots, 6 to 8 minutes; transfer to bowl with wheat berries.

4. Return now-empty skillet to medium-high heat and add remaining 1 teaspoon oil, onion, bell pepper, and ¼ teaspoon salt. Cook, stirring occasionally, until onion is charred at edges and pepper skin is charred and blistered, 8 to 10 minutes. Add wheat berry–zucchini mixture to skillet and cook until heated through, about 2 minutes. Season with pepper to taste. Serve.

PER ⅔-CUP SERVING

Cal 220 • **Total Fat** 5g • **Sat Fat** 0.5g • **Chol** 0mg
Sodium 210mg • **Total Carbs** 38g • **Fiber** 7g • **Total Sugar** 2g
Added Sugar 0g • **Protein** 7g • **Total Carbohydrate Choices** 2.5

NOTES FROM THE TEST KITCHEN

Getting to Know Lentils

Lentils come in dozens of sizes and colors and the differences in flavor and color are considerable. Because they are thin-skinned, they require no soaking, which makes them a versatile legume. In the test kitchen, we evaluated the most commonly available types of lentils in terms of taste, texture, and appearance. Here's what we found.

Brown and Green Lentils These larger lentils are what you'll find in every supermarket. They are a uniform drab brown or green. Tasters commented on their "mild yet light and earthy flavor"; some found their texture "creamy," while others complained that they were "chalky." But everyone agreed that they held their shape and were tender inside. This is an all-purpose lentil, great in soups and salads or simmered, then tossed with olive oil and herbs.

Lentilles du Puy These dark green French lentils from the city of Le Puy are smaller than the more common brown and green varieties. They are a dark olive green, almost black. Tasters praised these for their "rich, earthy, complex flavor" and "firm yet tender texture." This is the kind to use if you are looking for lentils that will keep their shape (and look beautiful on the plate) when cooked, so they're perfect for salads and dishes where the lentils take center stage.

Red and Yellow Lentils Split, very colorful, and skinless, these small orange-red or golden-yellow lentils completely disintegrate when cooked. If you are looking for lentils that will quickly break down into a thick puree, these are the ones to use (see Dal, page 145).

Lentil Salad with Olives, Mint, and Feta
SERVES 4

WHY THIS RECIPE WORKS Lentils, like beans, are high in fiber and protein, which can help stabilize blood sugar for those on a diabetic diet. For a Greek-inspired lentil salad, we needed to ensure that the lentils would stay intact through cooking. French green lentils were the perfect choice, since they hold their shape well. A salt soak softened their skins, leading to fewer blowouts. Cooking the lentils in the oven heated them gently and uniformly, and we boosted their flavor by adding garlic and a bay leaf. A simple, tart vinaigrette perfectly balanced the lentils. Mint, shallot, and kalamata olives brought the salad to life; a sprinkle of feta finished the dish. *Lentilles du Puy*, also called French green lentils, are our first choice for this recipe, but brown, black, or regular green lentils are fine, too (note that cooking times will vary depending on the type used). Salt-soaking helps keep the lentils intact, but if you don't have time, they'll still taste good. You will need a medium ovensafe saucepan for this recipe.

Salt and pepper
1 cup lentilles du Puy, picked over and rinsed
5 garlic cloves, lightly crushed and peeled
1 bay leaf
5 tablespoons extra-virgin olive oil
3 tablespoons white wine vinegar
½ cup pitted kalamata olives, chopped coarse
½ cup chopped fresh mint
1 large shallot, minced
1 ounce feta cheese, crumbled (¼ cup)

1. Dissolve 1 teaspoon salt in 4 cups warm water (about 110 degrees) in bowl. Add lentils and soak at room temperature for 1 hour. Drain well.

2. Adjust oven rack to middle position and heat oven to 325 degrees. Combine lentils, 4 cups water, garlic, bay leaf, and ½ teaspoon salt in medium ovensafe saucepan. Cover, transfer saucepan to oven, and cook until lentils are tender but remain intact, 40 to 60 minutes.

3. Drain lentils well; discard garlic and bay leaf. Whisk oil and vinegar together in large bowl. Add lentils, olives, mint, and shallot and gently toss to combine. Season with pepper to taste. Transfer to serving dish and sprinkle with feta. Serve.

PER ¾-CUP SERVING

Cal 350 • **Total Fat** 21g • **Sat Fat** 3.5g • **Chol** 5mg
Sodium 200mg • **Total Carbs** 31g • **Fiber** 8g • **Total Sugar** 2g
Added Sugar 0g • **Protein** 12g • **Total Carbohydrate Choices** 2

Lentil Salad with Hazelnuts and Goat Cheese

Omit olives. Substitute 3 tablespoons red wine vinegar for white wine vinegar and add 2 teaspoons Dijon mustard to oil and vinegar. Substitute ¼ cup chopped fresh parsley for mint and ¼ cup crumbled goat cheese for feta. Sprinkle salad with ¼ cup coarsely chopped toasted hazelnuts with the feta.

PER ¾-CUP SERVING

Cal 390 • **Total Fat** 24g • **Sat Fat** 4g • **Chol** 5mg
Sodium 170mg • **Total Carbs** 31g • **Fiber** 8g • **Total Sugar** 2g
Added Sugar 0g • **Protein** 13g • **Total Carbohydrate Choices** 2

Lentil Salad with Carrots and Cilantro

Omit shallot and feta. Toss 2 carrots, peeled and cut into 2-inch-long matchsticks, with 1 teaspoon ground cumin, ½ teaspoon ground cinnamon, and ⅛ teaspoon cayenne pepper in bowl; cover and microwave until carrots are tender but still crisp, 2 to 4 minutes. Substitute 3 tablespoons lemon juice for white wine vinegar, carrots for olives, and ¼ cup chopped fresh cilantro for mint.

PER ¾-CUP SERVING

Cal 330 • **Total Fat** 19g • **Sat Fat** 2.5g • **Chol** 0mg
Sodium 105mg • **Total Carbs** 33g • **Fiber** 8g • **Total Sugar** 3g
Added Sugar 0g • **Protein** 11g • **Total Carbohydrate Choices** 2

Lentil Salad with Spinach, Walnuts, and Parmesan

Place 4 ounces baby spinach and 2 tablespoons water in bowl; cover and microwave until spinach is wilted and volume is halved, about 4 minutes. Remove bowl from microwave and keep covered for 1 minute. Drain spinach thoroughly in colander, then chop coarse. Return spinach to colander and press with rubber spatula to release remaining liquid. Substitute 2 tablespoons sherry vinegar for white wine vinegar, spinach for olives and mint, and ¼ cup coarsely grated Parmesan cheese for feta. Sprinkle salad with 2 tablespoons coarsely chopped toasted walnuts before serving.

PER ¾-CUP SERVING

Cal 380 • **Total Fat** 23g • **Sat Fat** 3.5g • **Chol** 5mg
Sodium 230mg • **Total Carbs** 31g • **Fiber** 8g • **Total Sugar** 2g
Added Sugar 0g • **Protein** 15g • **Total Carbohydrate Choices** 2

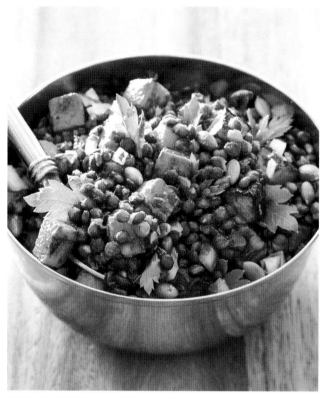

Brining lentils for a salad thoroughly seasons them and helps them hold their shape after cooking.

Spiced Lentil Salad with Winter Squash
SERVES 6

WHY THIS RECIPE WORKS To make a satisfying, nutritious lentil dish, adding roasted winter squash worked perfectly, allowing a hearty serving that didn't tip the scales in terms of carbohydrates or calories. To accentuate the delicate butternut squash flavor, we tossed the squash with balsamic vinegar and extra-virgin olive oil and roasted it in a hot oven. Putting the rack in the lowest position encouraged deep, even browning. We opted for French lentils, which hold their shape well during cooking and have a robust flavor, and soaked them in a saltwater solution to season them throughout and ensure fewer blowouts. Warm spices bloomed in oil infused the dish with more flavor. For the dressing, we used balsamic vinegar and Dijon mustard. Parsley and red onion gave the dish freshness, and pepitas added texture. *Lentilles du Puy* (also called French green lentils) are our first choice for this recipe but brown, or regular green lentils are fine, too (note that cooking times will vary depending on the type used). Salt-soaking helps keep the lentils intact, but if you don't have time, they'll still taste good. You will need a medium ovensafe saucepan for this recipe.

Salt and pepper

1 cup lentilles du Puy, picked over and rinsed

1 pound butternut squash, peeled, seeded, and cut into ½-inch pieces (3 cups)

5 tablespoons extra-virgin olive oil

2 tablespoons balsamic vinegar

1 garlic clove, minced

½ teaspoon ground coriander

¼ teaspoon ground cumin

¼ teaspoon ground ginger

⅛ teaspoon ground cinnamon

1 teaspoon Dijon mustard

½ cup fresh parsley leaves

¼ cup finely chopped red onion

1 tablespoon roasted, unsalted pepitas

1. Dissolve 1 teaspoon salt in 4 cups warm water (about 110 degrees) in bowl. Add lentils and soak at room temperature for 1 hour. Drain well.

2. Adjust oven racks to middle and lowest positions and heat oven to 450 degrees. Toss squash with 1 tablespoon oil, 1½ teaspoons vinegar, ¼ teaspoon salt, and ¼ teaspoon pepper. Arrange squash in single layer on rimmed baking sheet and roast on lower rack until well browned and tender, 20 to 25 minutes, stirring halfway through roasting. Let cool slightly. Reduce oven temperature to 325 degrees.

3. Cook 1 tablespoon oil, garlic, coriander, cumin, ginger, and cinnamon in medium ovensafe saucepan over medium heat until fragrant, about 1 minute. Stir in 4 cups water and lentils. Cover, transfer saucepan to upper rack in oven, and cook until lentils are tender but remain intact, 40 to 60 minutes.

4. Drain lentils well. Whisk remaining 3 tablespoons oil, remaining 1½ tablespoons vinegar, and mustard together in large bowl. Add squash, lentils, parsley, and onion and gently toss to combine. Season with pepper to taste. Transfer to serving platter and sprinkle with pepitas. Serve.

PER ¾-CUP SERVING

Cal 250 • **Total Fat** 13g • **Sat Fat** 2g • **Chol** 0mg
Sodium 180mg • **Total Carbs** 28g • **Fiber** 6g • **Total Sugar** 3g
Added Sugar 0g • **Protein** 8g • **Total Carbohydrate Choices** 2

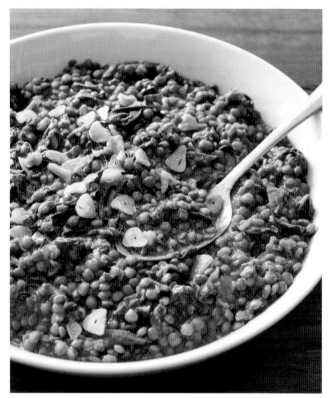

This lentil side dish has plenty of flavor thanks to garlic-infused olive oil and a sprinkle of crisp garlic chips.

Lentils with Spinach and Garlic Chips
SERVES 4

WHY THIS RECIPE WORKS The combination of lentils and spinach is a classic, but can often translate into a drab, mushy side dish. Here, tender yet firm lentils and perfectly wilted spinach are studded with garlic chips for an unmistakably bold dish. We started by frying sliced garlic in olive oil; the crunchy golden garlic chips added a nice textural contrast to the final dish and infused the cooking oil with garlic flavor. Tasters preferred the clean flavor of lentils cooked in water over those cooked in broth. Allowing sturdy curly-leaf spinach to wilt in the pot with the lentils was simple and avoided using extra dishes; the mineral-y flavor of the spinach complemented the earthy lentils perfectly. As a finishing touch, we stirred in some red wine vinegar for brightness. It's important to cook the garlic until just golden—if it becomes too dark, it will have an unpleasant bitter taste. If you can't find curly-leaf spinach, you can substitute flat-leaf spinach; do not substitute baby spinach. Green or brown lentils are our first choice for this recipe, but it will work with any type of lentil except red or yellow (note that cooking times will vary depending on the type used).

2 tablespoons extra-virgin olive oil

4 garlic cloves, sliced thin

1 onion, chopped fine

Salt and pepper

1 teaspoon ground coriander

1 teaspoon ground cumin

2½ cups water

1 cup green or brown lentils, picked over and rinsed

8 ounces curly-leaf spinach, stemmed and chopped coarse

1 tablespoon red wine vinegar

1. Cook oil and garlic in large saucepan over medium-low heat, stirring often, until garlic turns crisp and golden but not brown, about 5 minutes. Using slotted spoon, transfer garlic to paper towel–lined plate; set aside for serving.

2. Add onion and ¼ teaspoon salt to fat left in saucepan and cook over medium heat until softened and lightly browned, 5 to 7 minutes. Stir in coriander and cumin and cook until fragrant, about 30 seconds.

3. Stir in water and lentils and bring to simmer. Reduce heat to low, cover, and cook, stirring occasionally, until lentils are mostly tender but still intact, 30 to 50 minutes.

4. Stir in spinach, 1 handful at a time, and cook, stirring occasionally, until spinach is wilted and lentils are completely tender, about 8 minutes. Stir in vinegar and ⅛ teaspoon salt and season with pepper to taste. Transfer to serving dish, sprinkle with toasted garlic, and serve.

PER ¾-CUP SERVING

Cal 250 • **Total Fat** 8g • **Sat Fat** 1g • **Chol** 0mg
Sodium 270mg • **Total Carbs** 33g • **Fiber** 9g • **Total Sugar** 2g
Added Sugar 0g • **Protein** 9g • **Total Carbohydrate Choices** 2

Dal (Spiced Red Lentils)
SERVES 4

WHY THIS RECIPE WORKS Dals are spiced lentil stews common throughout India. We wanted our dal to be simple yet still have complex flavors so we created a blend of warm spices with a subtle layer of heat. Blooming the spices in oil deepened their flavors and onion, garlic, and ginger rounded out the aromatics. Getting a porridge-like consistency required cooking red lentils with just the right amount of water: 3 cups water to 1 cup lentils. Before serving, we added cilantro for color and freshness, diced tomato for acidity, and a bit of butter for richness. Do not substitute other types of lentils here; red lentils have a very different texture.

SPICE MIXTURE

½ teaspoon ground coriander

½ teaspoon ground cumin

¼ teaspoon ground cinnamon

¼ teaspoon ground turmeric

⅛ teaspoon ground cardamom

⅛ teaspoon red pepper flakes

LENTILS

1 tablespoon canola oil

4 garlic cloves, minced

1½ teaspoons grated fresh ginger

1 onion, chopped fine

Salt and pepper

3 cups water

1 cup red lentils, picked over and rinsed

12 ounces plum tomatoes, cored, seeded, and chopped

½ cup minced fresh cilantro

1 tablespoon unsalted butter

1. **FOR THE SPICE MIXTURE** Combine all spices in smal bowl.

2. **FOR THE LENTILS** Cook spice mixture, oil, garlic, and ginger in large saucepan over medium heat, stirring occasionally, until fragrant, about 1 minute. Stir in onion and ¼ teaspoon salt and cook until softened, about 5 minutes.

3. Stir in water and lentils, bring to simmer, and cook until lentils are tender and resemble thick, coarse puree, 20 to 25 minutes. Off heat, stir in tomatoes, cilantro, butter, and ⅛ teaspoon salt. Season with pepper to taste and serve.

PER ¾-CUP SERVING

Cal 260 • **Total Fat** 8g • **Sat Fat** 2g • **Chol** 10mg
Sodium 240mg • **Total Carbs** 36g • **Fiber** 9g • **Total Sugar** 6g
Added Sugar 0g • **Protein** 14g • **Total Carbohydrate Choices** 2.5

VARIATION
Dal with Coconut Milk
The addition of coconut milk provides a lush, creamy texture and rich flavor.

Omit butter. Substitute 1 cup light coconut milk for 1 cup water.

PER ¾-CUP SERVING

Cal 280 • **Total Fat** 9g • **Sat Fat** 4g • **Chol** 0mg
Sodium 240mg • **Total Carbs** 37g • **Fiber** 9g • **Total Sugar** 6g
Added Sugar 0g • **Protein** 14g • **Total Carbohydrate Choices** 2.5

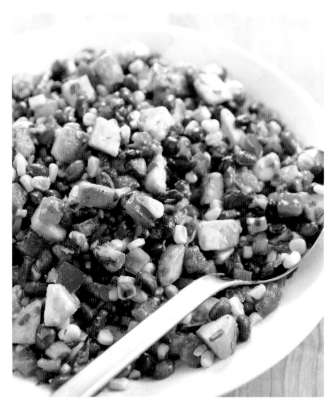

Canned black beans and avocado provide a fiber-rich base for an easy and flavorful salad.

Southwestern Black Bean Salad
SERVES 4

WHY THIS RECIPE WORKS For an easy, light, summertime bean salad, we combined fiber-rich black beans with fresh corn, bright tomato, and creamy avocado. Toasting the corn in a skillet until golden brown brought out its natural sweetness. Chipotle chile, cilantro, and lime juice provided the perfect Southwestern flavor profile to this easy-to-prepare salad. Fresh corn is important for the flavor of the salad—don't substitute frozen or canned corn.

  2 scallions, sliced thin
  3 tablespoons lime juice (2 limes)
  2 tablespoons extra-virgin olive oil
1½ teaspoons minced canned chipotle chile in adobo sauce
     Salt and pepper
  2 ears corn, kernels cut from cobs
  1 (15-ounce) can no-salt-added black beans, rinsed
  1 tomato, cored and chopped
  1 avocado, halved, pitted, and cut into ½-inch pieces
  3 tablespoons minced fresh cilantro

1. Whisk scallions, lime juice, 1 tablespoon oil, chipotle, ¼ teaspoon salt, and ¼ teaspoon pepper together in large bowl.

2. Heat remaining 1 tablespoon oil in medium skillet over medium-high heat until just smoking. Add corn and ⅛ teaspoon salt and cook, stirring occasionally, until golden brown, 6 to 8 minutes. Transfer corn, beans, and tomato to bowl with dressing and gently toss to coat. Gently fold in avocado and cilantro. Season with pepper to taste and serve.

PER ¾-CUP SERVING
Cal 260 • **Total Fat** 16g • **Sat Fat** 2g • **Chol** 0mg
Sodium 230mg • **Total Carbs** 26g • **Fiber** 9g • **Total Sugar** 4g
Added Sugar 0g • **Protein** 7g • **Total Carbohydrate Choices** 2

Cuban Black Beans
SERVES 8

WHY THIS RECIPE WORKS For our Cuban black beans, we started with dried beans and brined them to ensure the perfect texture. Just two slices of bacon provided the perfect meaty base for our beans, to which we added onions, garlic, bell pepper, and seasonings. We then transferred the pot to the oven, where we stirred it every half hour until the beans were perfectly cooked. Removing the lid allowed the bean mixture to thicken to a desirable consistency. A hefty handful of cilantro and a splash of lime juice perked up all the flavors before serving.

     Salt and pepper
  1 pound dried black beans (2½ cups) picked over and rinsed
  2 slices bacon, chopped fine
  2 onions, chopped
  1 red bell pepper, stemmed, seeded, and chopped
  1 teaspoon ground cumin
  6 garlic cloves, minced
  2 teaspoons minced fresh oregano or ¾ teaspoon dried
 ¼ teaspoon red pepper flakes
3½ cups water
  2 bay leaves
 ⅛ teaspoon baking soda
 ¼ cup minced fresh cilantro
  1 tablespoon lime juice

1. Dissolve 1½ tablespoons salt in 2 quarts cold water in large container. Add beans and soak at room temperature for at least 8 hours or up to 1 day. Drain and rinse well.

2. Adjust oven rack to lower-middle position and heat oven to 300 degrees. Cook bacon in Dutch oven over medium heat until crisp, 5 to 7 minutes. Stir in onions, bell pepper, cumin, and ½ teaspoon salt and cook until softened, 5 to 7 minutes. Stir in garlic, oregano, and red pepper flakes and cook until fragrant, about 30 seconds. Stir in water, scraping up any browned bits. Stir in beans, bay leaves, and baking soda and bring to simmer.

3. Cover, transfer pot to oven, and bake, stirring every 30 minutes, until beans are tender, about 1½ hours. Remove lid and continue to bake until liquid has thickened, 15 to 30 minutes, stirring halfway through cooking.

4. Discard bay leaves. Let beans sit for 10 minutes. Stir in cilantro and lime juice. Season with pepper to taste and serve.

PER ¾-CUP SERVING

Cal 240 • **Total Fat** 3g • **Sat Fat** 1g • **Chol** 5mg
Sodium 240mg • **Total Carbs** 40g • **Fiber** 6g • **Total Sugar** 8g
Added Sugar 0g • **Protein** 13g • **Total Carbohydrate Choices** 2.5

NOTES FROM THE TEST KITCHEN

Choose No-Salt-Added Canned Beans

It's no secret that canned products are full of sodium, and beans are no exception. Canned beans, depending on the type, can have up to or even over 400 milligrams of sodium per half-cup serving, which doesn't leave a lot of room for any other sodium in your meal. Though draining and rinsing beans reduces sodium by about 41 percent (just draining can reduce sodium by 36 percent), we wanted even less sodium. So in these recipes, we use unsalted (or "no salt added") canned beans, and we always drain and rinse them. Note that unsalted beans still contain naturally occurring sodium, so they're not completely salt-free. You can also find low-sodium beans (which means they must contain 140 milligrams of sodium or less per serving), but we prefer the cleaner flavor of the unsalted variety, which also gives better control of the sodium.

Black-Eyed Peas with Walnuts and Pomegranate
SERVES 4

WHY THIS RECIPE WORKS For a black-eyed pea side dish that would boast big flavor and also be simple to prepare, we looked to Egyptian cuisine for inspiration. In Egypt, black-eyed peas are a pantry staple, and their delicate skins, creamy interiors, and fairly mild

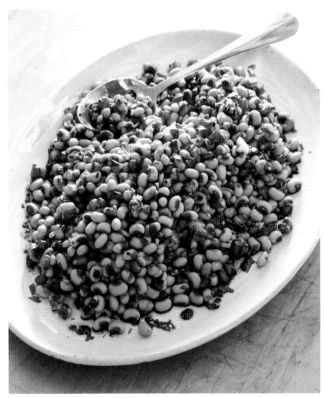

Creamy black-eyed peas pair well with a tart dressing and healthy crunchy add-ins.

flavor make them a great base for a tart dressing and crunchy additions. To simplify preparation, we used canned black-eyed peas, which have great flavor and texture. We turned to other common Egyptian salad additions like walnuts and pomegranate seeds for their flavor and texture contrasts, along with scallions and parsley for fresh notes. We created a punchy dressing by using equal parts lemon juice and pomegranate molasses, which offered balanced acidity and tang.

> 2 tablespoons extra-virgin olive oil
> 2 tablespoons lemon juice
> 2 tablespoons pomegranate molasses
> ¼ teaspoon ground coriander
> ¼ teaspoon ground cumin
> ⅛ teaspoon ground fennel seed
>   Salt and pepper
> 2 (15-ounce) cans no-salt-added black-eyed peas, rinsed
> ½ cup pomegranate seeds
> ½ cup minced fresh parsley
> ⅓ cup walnuts, toasted and chopped
> 4 scallions, sliced thin

Whisk oil, lemon juice, pomegranate molasses, coriander, cumin, fennel seed, ¼ teaspoon salt, and ⅛ teaspoon pepper together in large bowl until smooth. Add peas, pomegranate seeds, parsley, walnuts, and scallions and toss to combine. Season with ⅛ teaspoon salt and pepper to taste.

PER ¾-CUP SERVING

Cal 260 • **Total Fat** 14g • **Sat Fat** 1.5g • **Chol** 0mg
Sodium 250mg • **Total Carbs** 29g • **Fiber** 7g • **Total Sugar** 8g
Added Sugar 4g • **Protein** 9g • **Total Carbohydrate Choices** 2

RELEASING POMEGRANATE SEEDS

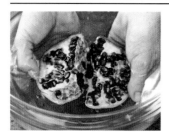

To release the kernels with less mess, halve the pomegranate and submerge it in a bowl of water. As you gently pull it apart, the seeds will sink, separating from the bitter pith and membrane that hold them.

Easy Greek-Style Chickpea Salad
SERVES 6

WHY THIS RECIPE WORKS Greek salad is a crowd pleaser, so we wanted to take the salad's key flavors and transform them into a heartier chickpea-based salad. We started by making a vinaigrette of lemon juice, oil, and garlic, then tossed in the chickpeas with cucumber, red onion, fresh mint and parsley, and briny feta and olives. This low-calorie, protein-rich salad comes together quickly.

    3 tablespoons lemon juice
    1 tablespoon extra-virgin olive oil
    1 tablespoon Dijon mustard
    1 small garlic clove, minced
      Salt and pepper
    2 (15-ounce) cans no-salt-added chickpeas, rinsed
    1 cucumber, peeled, halved lengthwise, seeded, and cut into ½-inch pieces
    ½ small red onion, chopped fine
    ¼ cup minced fresh mint
    1 tablespoon minced fresh parsley
    1 ounce feta cheese, crumbled (¼ cup)
    2 tablespoons chopped pitted kalamata olives

Whisk lemon juice, oil, mustard, garlic, and ¼ teaspoon salt together in large bowl. Add chickpeas, cucumber, onion, mint, parsley, feta, and olives and gently toss to combine. Season with pepper to taste and serve.

PER ⅔-CUP SERVING

Cal 120 • **Total Fat** 4g • **Sat Fat** 1g • **Chol** 5mg
Sodium 240mg • **Total Carbs** 15g • **Fiber** 4g • **Total Sugar** 2g
Added Sugar 0g • **Protein** 6g • **Total Carbohydrate Choices** 1

VARIATION
North African-Style Chickpea Salad
SERVES 6

WHY THIS RECIPE WORKS For a chickpea salad with a North African flavor profile, we added cumin and paprika to our dressing for extra warmth. Shredded carrot added color and texture, raisins provided some sweetness, and fresh mint tied everything together.

    2 tablespoons extra-virgin olive oil
 1½ tablespoons lemon juice
    1 small garlic clove, minced
    ½ teaspoon ground cumin
    ½ teaspoon paprika
      Salt and pepper
    2 (15-ounce) cans no-salt-added chickpeas, rinsed
    1 carrot, peeled and shredded
    ½ cup raisins
    2 tablespoons minced fresh mint

Whisk oil, lemon juice, garlic, cumin, paprika, and ½ teaspoon salt together in large bowl. Add chickpeas, carrot, raisins, and mint and gently toss to combine. Season with pepper to taste and serve.

PER ⅔-CUP SERVING

Cal 190 • **Total Fat** 5g • **Sat Fat** 0.5g • **Chol** 0mg
Sodium 230mg • **Total Carbs** 27g • **Fiber** 4g • **Total Sugar** 11g
Added Sugar 0g • **Protein** 6g • **Total Carbohydrate Choices** 2

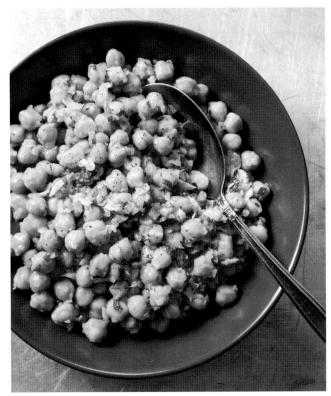

Convenient canned chickpeas are a good source of protein and don't require extended cooking.

Chickpeas with Garlic and Parsley
SERVES 4

WHY THIS RECIPE WORKS With their buttery, nutty flavor and creamy texture, chickpeas can make a terrific side dish when sautéed simply with a few flavorful ingredients. In search of flavors that would easily transform our canned chickpeas, we reached for garlic and red pepper flakes. Instead of mincing the garlic, we cut it into thin slices and sautéed them in extra-virgin olive oil to mellow their flavor. The thin slivers maintained their presence in the finished dish. We softened chopped onion along with this aromatic base, then added the chickpeas with chicken broth, which imparted a rich, savory backbone to the dish without overpowering it. As final touches, fresh parsley and lemon juice gave the chickpeas a burst of freshness.

3 tablespoons extra-virgin olive oil
4 garlic cloves, sliced thin
⅛ teaspoon red pepper flakes
1 onion, chopped fine
   Salt and pepper
2 (15-ounce) cans no-salt-added chickpeas, rinsed
1 cup unsalted chicken broth
2 tablespoons minced fresh parsley
2 teaspoons lemon juice

1. Cook 2 tablespoons oil, garlic, and pepper flakes in 12-inch skillet over medium heat, stirring frequently, until garlic turns golden but not brown, about 3 minutes. Stir in onion and ¼ teaspoon salt and cook until softened and lightly browned, 5 to 7 minutes. Stir in chickpeas and broth and bring to simmer. Reduce heat to medium-low, cover, and cook until chickpeas are heated through and flavors meld, about 7 minutes.

2. Uncover, increase heat to high, and continue to cook until nearly all liquid has evaporated, about 3 minutes. Off heat, stir in parsley and lemon juice. Season with pepper to taste and drizzle with remaining 1 tablespoon oil. Serve.

PER ¾-CUP SERVING
Cal 260 • **Total Fat** 12g • **Sat Fat** 1.5g • **Chol** 0mg
Sodium 210mg • **Total Carbs** 27g • **Fiber** 6g • **Total Sugar** 3g
Added Sugar 0g • **Protein** 9g • **Total Carbohydrate Choices** 2

VARIATIONS
Chickpeas with Bell Peppers, Scallions, and Basil
Add 1 chopped red bell pepper to skillet with onion. Substitute 2 tablespoons chopped fresh basil and 2 thinly sliced scallions for parsley.

PER ¾-CUP SERVING
Cal 270 • **Total Fat** 12g • **Sat Fat** 1.5g • **Chol** 0mg
Sodium 210mg • **Total Carbs** 29g • **Fiber** 7g • **Total Sugar** 4g
Added Sugar 0g • **Protein** 10g • **Total Carbohydrate Choices** 2

Chickpeas with Smoked Paprika and Cilantro
Omit red pepper flakes. Add ½ teaspoon smoked paprika to skillet before chickpeas and cook until fragrant, about 30 seconds. Substitute minced fresh cilantro for parsley and sherry vinegar for lemon juice.

PER ¾-CUP SERVING
Cal 260 • **Total Fat** 12g • **Sat Fat** 1.5g • **Chol** 0mg
Sodium 210mg • **Total Carbs** 27g • **Fiber** 6g • **Total Sugar** 3g
Added Sugar 0g • **Protein** 9g • **Total Carbohydrate Choices** 2

Chickpeas with Saffron, Mint, and Yogurt
Omit red pepper flakes. Add ⅛ teaspoon crumbled saffron threads to skillet before chickpeas and cook until fragrant, about 30 seconds.

Add ⅓ cup raisins to skillet with chickpeas. Substitute minced fresh mint for parsley, then stir in ¼ cup low-fat plain yogurt before serving.

PER ¾-CUP SERVING
Cal 310 • **Total Fat** 12g • **Sat Fat** 1.5g • **Chol** 0mg
Sodium 230mg • **Total Carbs** 38g • **Fiber** 7g • **Total Sugar** 13g
Added Sugar 0g • **Protein** 10g • **Total Carbohydrate Choices** 2.5

White Bean Salad with Bell Peppers
SERVES 4

WHY THIS RECIPE WORKS This well-balanced, ultraflavorful white bean salad is the perfect way to add great fiber and protein to a meal. We used classic Spanish flavors and ingredients to give the salad an identity. Cannellini beans worked perfectly, since they have a savory, buttery flavor that tasters enjoyed. We steeped the beans in a garlicky broth, which infused them with flavor. While the beans sat, we had enough time to rid our shallots of any harsh flavors by marinating them briefly in nutty, complex sherry vinegar. Red bell pepper offered sweetness and crunch. Parsley provided grassy, herby flavor, and chives gave the salad some subtle onion notes, rounding out the dish nicely. Our simple salad was easy to put together yet had surprisingly complex flavor.

- ¼ cup extra-virgin olive oil
- 3 garlic cloves, peeled and smashed
- 2 (15-ounce) cans no-salt-added cannellini beans, rinsed
  Salt and pepper
- 1 small shallot, minced
- 2 teaspoons sherry vinegar
- 1 red bell pepper, stemmed, seeded, and cut into
  ¼-inch pieces
- ¼ cup chopped fresh parsley
- 2 teaspoons chopped fresh chives

1. Cook 1 tablespoon oil and garlic in medium saucepan over medium heat, stirring frequently, until garlic turns golden but not brown, about 3 minutes. Stir in beans, 2 cups water, and 1 teaspoon salt and bring to simmer. Remove from heat, cover, and let sit for 20 minutes.

2. Meanwhile, combine shallot and vinegar in large bowl and let sit for 20 minutes. Drain beans and discard garlic. Add beans, remaining 3 tablespoons oil, bell pepper, parsley, chives, and ¼ teaspoon salt to shallot mixture. Gently toss to combine and season with pepper to taste. Let sit for 20 minutes. Serve.

PER ¾-CUP SERVING
Cal 250 • **Total Fat** 15g • **Sat Fat** 2g • **Chol** 0mg
Sodium 270mg • **Total Carbs** 22g • **Fiber** 6g • **Total Sugar** 3g
Added Sugar 0g • **Protein** 7g • **Total Carbohydrate Choices** 1.5

VARIATION
White Bean Salad with Oranges and Celery
Omit chives. Substitute 2 oranges, peel and pith removed, quartered, and sliced ¼-inch thick for bell pepper. Add ½ cup thinly sliced celery to shallot mixture with beans.

PER ¾-CUP SERVING
Cal 270 • **Total Fat** 15g • **Sat Fat** 2g • **Chol** 0mg
Sodium 270mg • **Total Carbs** 28g • **Fiber** 7g • **Total Sugar** 8g
Added Sugar 0g • **Protein** 8g • **Total Carbohydrate Choices** 2

Sicilian White Beans and Escarole
SERVES 6

WHY THIS RECIPE WORKS Combining the buttery texture of cannellini beans with tender, slightly bitter escarole results in a well-balanced and simple side dish that has good protein and doesn't tip the scales in terms of carbohydrates. Canned beans made this dish simple, and their texture was a perfect counterpoint to the greens. Sautéed onions gave the dish a rich, deep flavor base without requiring too much time at the stove. Red pepper flakes lent a slight heat without overwhelming the other ingredients, and a combination of broth and water provided a flavorful backbone. We added the escarole and beans along with the liquid, and then cooked the greens just until the leaves were wilted before cranking up the heat so the liquid would quickly evaporate. This short stint on the heat prevented the beans from breaking down and becoming mushy. Once we took the pot off the heat, we stirred in lemon juice for a bright finish and drizzled on some extra olive oil for richness. Chicory can be substituted for the escarole; however, its flavor is stronger.

2 tablespoons extra-virgin olive oil

2 onions, chopped fine

Salt and pepper

4 garlic cloves, minced

⅛ teaspoon red pepper flakes

1 head escarole (1 pound), trimmed and sliced 1 inch thick

1 (15-ounce) can no-salt-added cannellini beans, rinsed

1 cup unsalted chicken broth

1 cup water

2 teaspoons lemon juice

1. Heat 1 tablespoon oil in Dutch oven over medium heat until shimmering. Add onions and ¼ teaspoon salt and cook until softened and lightly browned, 5 to 7 minutes. Stir in garlic and pepper flakes and cook until fragrant, about 30 seconds.

2. Stir in escarole, beans, broth, and water and bring to simmer. Cook, stirring occasionally, until escarole is wilted, about 5 minutes. Increase heat to high and cook until liquid is nearly evaporated, 10 to 15 minutes. Stir in lemon juice and season with pepper to taste. Drizzle with remaining 1 tablespoon oil and serve.

PER ⅔-CUP SERVING

Cal 110 • **Total Fat** 5g • **Sat Fat** 0.5g • **Chol** 0mg
Sodium 150mg • **Total Carbs** 13g • **Fiber** 5g • **Total Sugar** 2g
Added Sugar 0g • **Protein** 4g • **Total Carbohydrate Choices** 1

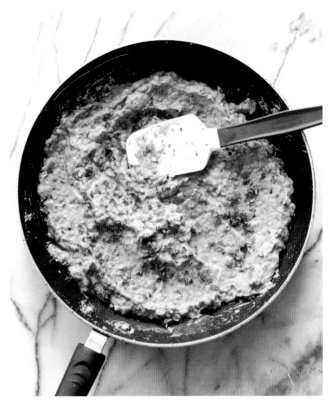

Pureeing canned red kidney beans with water turns them smooth and creamy.

Refried Beans
SERVES 8

WHY THIS RECIPE WORKS Store-bought refried beans can be loaded with calories and stabilizers. Since it is easy to make a big batch yourself, we recommend it if you're trying to eat more healthfully. After a quick spin in the food processor with a little water to smooth them out, high-fiber canned kidney beans were ready for flavorings. We sautéed chopped onion, a jalapeño, garlic, and cumin, then folded the beans into this fragrant mixture until the flavors melded. A little additional olive oil and chopped cilantro added richness and bright flavor with few added calories per serving. To make this dish spicier, include the chile seeds.

3 (15-ounce) cans no-salt-added red kidney beans, rinsed

1 cup water

2 tablespoons extra-virgin olive oil

1 onion, chopped fine

1 large jalapeño chile, stemmed, seeded, and minced

Salt

2 garlic cloves, minced

1 teaspoon ground cumin

¼ cup minced fresh cilantro

1. Process beans and water in food processor until smooth, about 2 minutes, scraping down sides of bowl as needed.

2. Heat 1 tablespoon oil in medium saucepan over medium heat until shimmering. Add onion, jalapeño, and ½ teaspoon salt and cook until softened, about 5 minutes. Stir in garlic and cumin and cook until fragrant. Stir in bean mixture.

3. Reduce heat to low and cook, stirring often, until beans have thickened and flavors meld, about 10 minutes. Off heat, stir in cilantro and remaining 1 tablespoon oil. Serve.

PER ½-CUP SERVING

Cal 120 • **Total Fat** 3.5g • **Sat Fat** 0g • **Chol** 0mg
Sodium 180mg • **Total Carbs** 17g • **Fiber** 9g • **Total Sugar** 2g
Added Sugar 0g • **Protein** 7g • **Total Carbohydrate Choices** 1

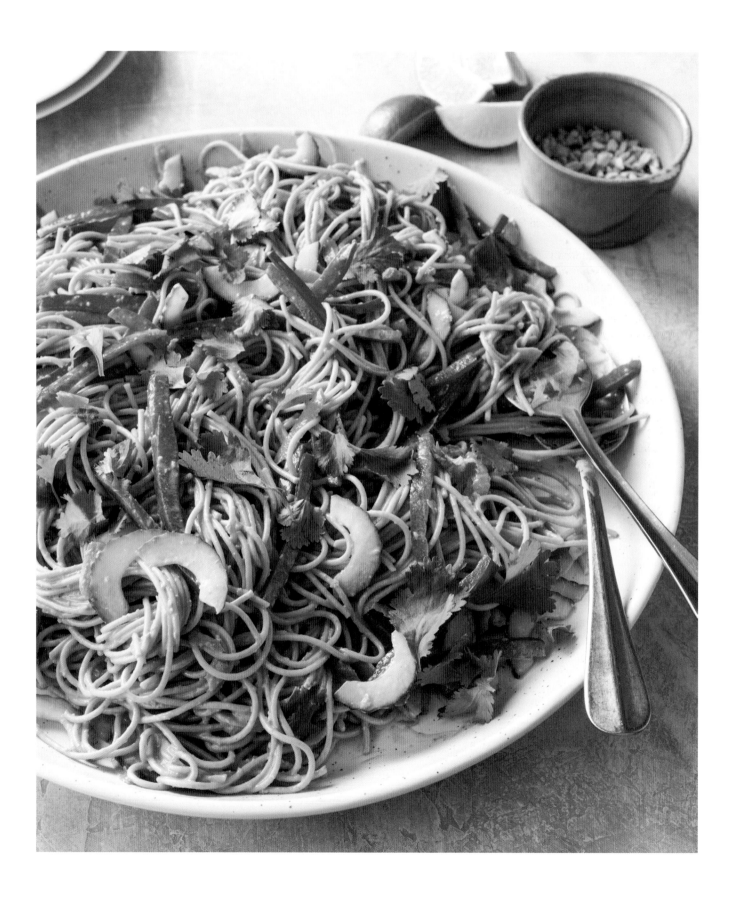

PASTA

Photo: Peanut Noodle Salad

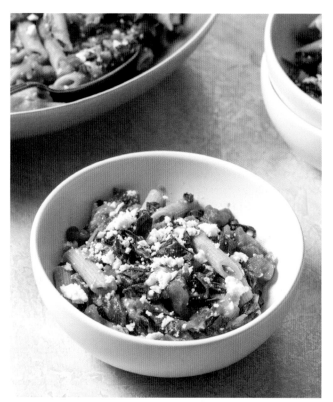

A few robust ingredients give our fresh tomato sauce plenty of flavor in a short amount of time.

Penne with Fresh Tomato Sauce, Spinach, and Feta

SERVES 4

WHY THIS RECIPE WORKS For a quick but complex tomato sauce that didn't rely on canned tomatoes, we looked to Greece for inspiration. Mint and feta paired well with fresh tomatoes, and baby spinach added savory depth. The success of this recipe depends on ripe, in-season tomatoes. The skillet will be quite full when stirring in the spinach in step 1 (stir gently to start), but will become more manageable as the spinach wilts. Other 100 percent whole-wheat pasta shapes can be substituted for the penne, but the cup amounts may vary (see page 164 for more information).

2 tablespoons extra-virgin olive oil
2 garlic cloves, minced
3 pounds ripe tomatoes, cored, peeled, seeded, and cut into ½-inch pieces
5 ounces (5 cups) baby spinach
8 ounces (2¼ cups) 100 percent whole-wheat penne
   Salt and pepper

4 ounces feta cheese, crumbled (1 cup)
2 tablespoons chopped fresh mint or oregano
1 tablespoon lemon juice

1. Cook oil and garlic in 12-inch skillet over medium heat, stirring often, until garlic turns golden, about 3 minutes. Stir in tomatoes and cook until they begin to lose their shape, about 8 minutes. Stir in spinach, 1 handful at a time, and cook until spinach is wilted and tomatoes have made chunky sauce, 2 minutes.

2. Meanwhile, bring 4 quarts water to boil in large pot. Add pasta and 1 teaspoon salt and cook, stirring often, until al dente. Reserve ½ cup cooking water, then drain pasta and return it to pot.

3. Stir ¾ cup feta, mint, lemon juice, ⅛ teaspoon salt, and ⅛ teaspoon pepper into sauce. Add sauce to pasta and toss to combine. Season with pepper to taste and adjust consistency with reserved cooking water as needed. Sprinkle with remaining ¼ cup feta and serve.

PER 1½-CUP SERVING
Cal 390 • **Total Fat** 15g • **Sat Fat** 5g • **Chol** 25mg
Sodium 420mg • **Total Carbs** 50g • **Fiber** 11g • **Total Sugar** 10g
Added Sugar 0g • **Protein** 15g • **Total Carbohydrate Choices** 3

PEELING TOMATOES

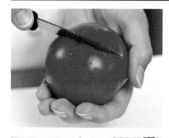

1. Cut out stem and core of each tomato, then score small X at base.

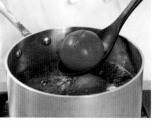

2. Lower tomatoes into boiling water and simmer until skins loosen, 30 to 60 seconds.

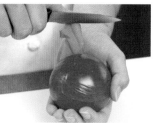

3. Use paring knife to remove strips of loosened skin starting at X at base of each tomato.

Fusilli with Zucchini, Tomatoes, and Pine Nuts
SERVES 6

WHY THIS RECIPE WORKS The combination of pasta and summer squash results in a light, flavorful dish that's full of color. Because summer squash contains so much liquid, we salted and drained it to keep our sauce from ending up watery. The skin helps to keep the squash pieces intact. The lightly salted squash also browned beautifully; just 5 minutes in a hot skillet provided a nice char and plenty of extra flavor. To accompany the squash, we chose halved grape tomatoes, fresh basil, and pine nuts and then finished the sauce with balsamic vinegar. A combination of zucchini and summer squash makes for a more colorful dish, but either may be used exclusively if desired. Cherry tomatoes can be substituted for the grape tomatoes. We prefer using kosher salt because residual grains can be easily wiped away from the squash; if using table salt, be sure to reduce all of the salt amounts in the recipe by half. For a milder dish, use the smaller amount of red pepper flakes. Other 100 percent whole-wheat pasta shapes can be substituted for the fusilli, but the cup amounts may vary (see page 164 for more information).

 2 pounds zucchini and/or summer squash, halved lengthwise and sliced ½ inch thick
   Kosher salt and pepper
 3 tablespoons extra-virgin olive oil
 3 garlic cloves, minced
⅛–½ teaspoon red pepper flakes
 12 ounces (4½ cups) 100 percent whole-wheat fusilli
 12 ounces grape tomatoes, halved
 ½ cup chopped fresh basil
 2 tablespoons balsamic vinegar
 ¼ cup grated Parmesan cheese
 ¼ cup pine nuts, toasted

1. Toss squash with 1 tablespoon salt in colander and let drain for 30 minutes. Pat squash dry with paper towels and carefully wipe away any residual salt.

2. Heat ½ tablespoon oil in 12-inch nonstick skillet over high heat until just smoking. Add half of squash and cook, turning once, until golden brown and slightly charred, 5 to 7 minutes, reducing heat if squash begins to scorch; transfer to large plate. Repeat with ½ tablespoon oil and remaining squash; transfer to plate.

3. Heat 1 tablespoon oil in now-empty skillet over medium heat until shimmering. Add garlic and pepper flakes and cook until fragrant, about 30 seconds. Stir in squash and cook until heated through, about 30 seconds.

4. Meanwhile, bring 4 quarts water to boil in large pot. Add pasta and 2 teaspoons salt and cook, stirring often, until al dente. Reserve ½ cup cooking water, then drain pasta and return it to pot. Add squash mixture, tomatoes, basil, vinegar, and remaining 1 tablespoon oil and toss to combine. Adjust consistency with reserved cooking water as needed. Sprinkle individual portions with Parmesan and pine nuts.

PER 1½-CUP SERVING
Cal 340 • Total Fat 14g • Sat Fat 2g • Chol 5mg
Sodium 220mg • Total Carbs 44g • Fiber 8g • Total Sugar 7g
Added Sugar 0g • Protein 12g • Total Carbohydrate Choices 3

Fusilli with Skillet-Roasted Cauliflower, Garlic, and Walnuts
SERVES 6

WHY THIS RECIPE WORKS When done right, careful control of heat can transform cauliflower from a mild-mannered vegetable to an intensely flavored, sweet, and nutty foil for pasta. Cutting the cauliflower into small florets created plenty of exposed surface area to maximize flavorful browning and caramelization. Starting the cauliflower in a cold covered pan allowed the florets to gradually steam in their own moisture before we removed the lid and let them turn golden brown. We found that cream-based sauces muted the nutty cauliflower flavor so we focused on a simple lemony dressing, using both lemon juice for brightness and zest to bolster its flavor without making the dish overly acidic. We rounded out the sauce with fresh parsley and some Parmesan and topped each serving with toasted walnuts to add a pleasing crunch. Other 100 percent whole-wheat pasta shapes can be substituted for the fusilli, but the cup amounts may vary (see page 164 for more information).

 ¼ cup extra-virgin olive oil
 1 head cauliflower (2 pounds), cored and cut into ½-inch florets
   Salt and pepper
 3 garlic cloves, minced
 1 teaspoon grated lemon zest plus 1–2 tablespoons juice
 ¼ teaspoon red pepper flakes
 12 ounces (4½ cups) 100 percent whole-wheat fusilli
 1 ounce Parmesan cheese, grated (½ cup)
 2 tablespoons chopped fresh parsley
 ¼ cup walnuts, toasted and chopped coarse

1. Combine 2 tablespoons oil and cauliflower florets in 12-inch nonstick skillet and sprinkle with ½ teaspoon salt and ¼ teaspoon pepper. Cover skillet and cook over medium-high heat until florets start to brown and edges just start to become translucent (do not lift lid), about 5 minutes. Remove lid and continue to cook, stirring every 2 minutes, until florets turn golden brown in many spots, about 12 minutes.

2. Push cauliflower to sides of skillet. Add 1 tablespoon oil, garlic, lemon zest, and pepper flakes to center and cook, stirring with rubber spatula, until fragrant, about 30 seconds. Stir garlic mixture into cauliflower and continue to cook, stirring occasionally, until cauliflower is tender but still firm, about 3 minutes.

3. Meanwhile, bring 4 quarts water to boil in large pot. Add pasta and 1 teaspoon salt and cook, stirring often, until al dente. Reserve 1 cup cooking water, then drain pasta and return it to pot.

4. Add cauliflower mixture, ¼ cup Parmesan, parsley, ½ cup reserved cooking water, 1 tablespoon lemon juice, and remaining 1 tablespoon oil to pasta and toss to combine. Season with extra lemon juice to taste and adjust consistency with reserved cooking water as needed. Sprinkle individual portions with walnuts and remaining ¼ cup Parmesan. Serve.

PER 1½-CUP SERVING
Cal 360 • **Total Fat** 16g • **Sat Fat** 2.5g • **Chol** 5mg
Sodium 390mg • **Total Carbs** 44g • **Fiber** 10g • **Total Sugar** 4g
Added Sugar 0g • **Protein** 13g • **Total Carbohydrate Choices** 3

RESERVING PASTA COOKING WATER

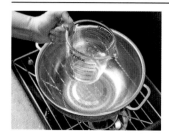

To remind yourself to reserve pasta water, place measuring cup in colander in sink before cooking pasta.

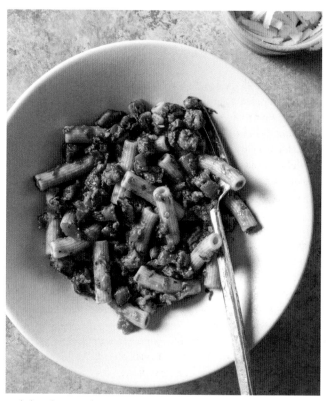

Lightly salting and microwaving eggplant draws out moisture and helps it brown without absorbing too much oil.

Pasta alla Norma with Olives and Capers
SERVES 6

WHY THIS RECIPE WORKS With its lively combination of tender eggplant, robust sauce, al dente pasta, and milky ricotta salata, *pasta alla Norma* sings with each bite—appropriate, given that it was named for the title character of an opera. For our version, we microwaved salted eggplant on coffee filters to draw out its moisture, which collapsed the air pockets in the eggplant so less oil would be absorbed, before browning. A secret ingredient, anchovies, gave our tomato sauce a deep, savory flavor without any fishiness. Although not traditional, capers and chopped kalamatas provided potency without tipping the salt into unhealthy territory. Finally, ricotta salata added a bit of tang. If you can't find ricotta salata you can substitute French feta, Pecorino Romano, or Cotija (a firm, crumbly Mexican cheese). We prefer to use kosher salt in this recipe because it clings best to the eggplant in step 1; if using table salt, reduce salt amounts by half. To give this dish a little extra kick, add additional pepper flakes. Other 100 percent whole-wheat pasta shapes can be substituted for the rigatoni, but the cup amounts may vary (see page 164 for more information).

1½ pounds eggplant, cut into ½-inch pieces
    Kosher salt and pepper
3½ tablespoons extra-virgin olive oil
  4 garlic cloves, minced
  2 anchovy fillets, rinsed and minced
¼ teaspoon red pepper flakes
  1 (28-ounce) can no-salt-added crushed tomatoes
½ cup pitted kalamata olives, chopped coarse
  6 tablespoons minced fresh parsley
  2 tablespoons capers, rinsed
12 ounces (3⅓ cups) 100 percent whole-wheat rigatoni
  2 ounces ricotta salata, shredded (½ cup)

1. Line large plate with double layer of coffee filters and lightly spray with vegetable oil spray. Toss eggplant with ½ teaspoon salt, then spread out over coffee filters. Microwave eggplant, uncovered, until dry to touch and slightly shriveled, about 10 minutes, tossing halfway through cooking. Let cool slightly.

2. Transfer eggplant to large bowl, drizzle with 1 tablespoon oil, and gently toss to coat. Heat 1 tablespoon oil in 12-inch nonstick skillet over medium-high heat until shimmering. Add eggplant and cook, stirring occasionally, until well browned and fully tender, about 10 minutes; transfer to clean plate.

3. Let skillet cool slightly, about 3 minutes. Add 1 tablespoon oil, garlic, anchovies, and pepper flakes to now-empty skillet and cook over medium heat, stirring often, until garlic is lightly golden and fragrant, about 1 minute. Stir in tomatoes, increase heat to medium-high, and simmer, stirring occasionally, until slightly thickened, 8 to 10 minutes. Add eggplant and cook, stirring occasionally, until eggplant is heated through and flavors meld, 3 to 5 minutes. Stir in olives, parsley, capers, and remaining ½ tablespoon oil.

4. Meanwhile, bring 4 quarts water to boil in large pot. Add pasta and 2 teaspoons salt and cook, stirring often, until al dente. Reserve ½ cup cooking water, then drain pasta and return it to pot. Add sauce and toss to combine. Season with salt and pepper to taste and adjust consistency with reserved cooking water as needed. Serve with ricotta salata.

PER 1½-CUP SERVING

Cal 370 • **Total Fat** 13g • **Sat Fat** 2.5g • **Chol** 10mg
Sodium 440mg • **Total Carbs** 50g • **Fiber** 12g • **Total Sugar** 9g
Added Sugar 0g • **Protein** 12g • **Total Carbohydrate Choices** 3

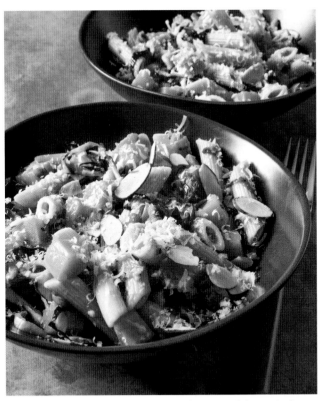

Just a bit of mascarpone cheese stirred in toward the end of cooking provides this hearty pasta dish with rich creaminess.

Penne with Butternut Squash and Sage
SERVES 6

WHY THIS RECIPE WORKS We wanted a pasta dish that put butternut squash center stage. Sautéing the squash first amplified its mild flavor and ensured that it took on rich, caramelized flavor that fit well with hearty whole-wheat penne. We then built a sauce in the same pan we used to brown the squash, and after a short braise we had perfectly cooked and deeply flavorful squash with a silky texture. A modest amount of mascarpone gave the sauce a velvety texture, and scallions provided a pungent note that contrasted nicely with the sweet earthiness of the squash. A final sprinkling of sliced almonds added a crunch of protein. Fresh sage is a natural pairing with squash, and crucial to the flavor of this dish; do not substitute dried sage. You can substitute cream cheese for the mascarpone. When simmering the squash in step 3, do not stir too frequently or the squash will begin to fall apart. Other 100 percent whole-wheat pasta shapes can be substituted for the penne, but the cup amounts may vary (see page 164 for more information).

3 tablespoons extra-virgin olive oil

1 pound butternut squash, peeled, seeded, and cut into ½-inch pieces (2½ cups)

1 small head radicchio (6 ounces), halved, cored, and sliced thin

6 scallions, sliced thin

3 garlic cloves, minced

⅛ teaspoon ground nutmeg

Salt and pepper

¾ cup dry white wine

1½ cups unsalted chicken broth

2 ounces Parmesan cheese, grated (1 cup)

1 ounce (2 tablespoons) mascarpone cheese

2 tablespoons minced fresh sage

1 tablespoon lemon juice

12 ounces (3½ cups) 100 percent whole-wheat penne

¼ cup sliced almonds, toasted

1. Heat 1 tablespoon oil in 12-inch nonstick skillet over medium heat until shimmering. Add squash and cook, stirring frequently, until spotty brown, 10 to 15 minutes; transfer to bowl. Add radicchio and 1 tablespoon oil to now-empty skillet and cook over medium heat, stirring occasionally, until wilted and beginning to brown, about 1 minute. Transfer to small bowl.

2. Add remaining 1 tablespoon oil, scallions, garlic, nutmeg, and ½ teaspoon salt to now-empty skillet and cook over medium heat until scallions are softened, 1 to 2 minutes. Stir in wine, scraping up any browned bits, and cook until reduced by half, about 2 minutes.

3. Stir in broth and squash and bring to simmer. Reduce heat to low and cook until squash is tender and sauce has thickened slightly, 10 to 15 minutes. Off heat, gently stir in ½ cup Parmesan, mascarpone, sage, and lemon juice.

4. Meanwhile, bring 4 quarts water to boil in large pot. Add pasta and 1 teaspoon salt and cook, stirring often, until al dente. Reserve ½ cup cooking water, then drain pasta and return it to pot. Add squash mixture and radicchio and gently toss to combine. Adjust consistency with reserved cooking water as needed. Sprinkle individual portions with almonds and remaining ½ cup Parmesan. Serve.

PER 1½-CUP SERVING

Cal 390 • **Total Fat** 15g • **Sat Fat** 3.5g • **Chol** 15mg
Sodium 440mg • **Total Carbs** 48g • **Fiber** 9g • **Total Sugar** 4g
Added Sugar 0g • **Protein** 14g • **Total Carbohydrate Choices** 3

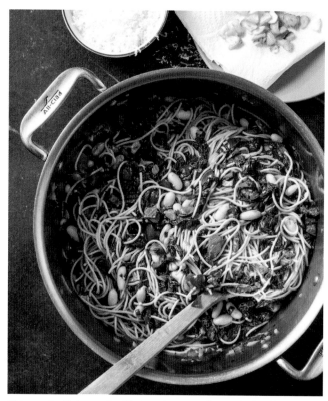

This rustic dish gets its fiber and protein from whole-wheat pasta, curly spinach, and creamy cannellini beans.

Spaghetti with Spinach, Beans, Tomatoes, and Garlic Chips
SERVES 6

WHY THIS RECIPE WORKS Whole-wheat pasta, hearty greens, and savory beans are humble ingredients on their own; when combined, they make a rustic, full-flavored Italian dish. We wanted to retain the complex flavor of this satisfying dish but make it an easy and quick midweek meal. To start, we opted to use spinach, as it requires only a quick braise. This meant that we could easily infuse it with aromatic flavors like onion, garlic, spicy red pepper flakes, and chicken broth. The spinach, beans, and sauce had to cook with the pasta for only a few minutes to blend harmoniously. Whole-wheat pasta stood up to the bold flavors of the sauce and complemented the earthiness of the greens. To brighten up our dish we added diced tomatoes, and for a salty bite, chopped kalamata olives and grated Parmesan cheese. For a spicier dish, use the larger amount of pepper flakes.

3 tablespoons extra-virgin olive oil

8 garlic cloves, peeled (5 sliced thin lengthwise, 3 minced)

1 onion, chopped fine

¼–½ teaspoon red pepper flakes

1¼ pounds curly spinach, stemmed and cut into 1-inch pieces

¾ cup unsalted chicken broth

1 (14.5-ounce) can no-salt-added diced tomatoes, drained
Salt and pepper

1 (15-ounce) can no-salt-added cannellini beans, rinsed

¾ cup pitted kalamata olives, chopped coarse

12 ounces 100 percent whole-wheat spaghetti

1 ounce Parmesan cheese, grated (½ cup)

1. Cook oil and sliced garlic in 12-inch straight-sided sauté pan over medium heat, stirring often, until garlic turns golden but not brown, about 3 minutes. Using slotted spoon, transfer garlic to paper towel–lined plate; set aside.

2. Add onion to oil left in pan and cook over medium heat until softened and lightly browned, 5 to 7 minutes. Stir in minced garlic and pepper flakes and cook until fragrant, about 30 seconds. Add half of spinach and cook, tossing occasionally, until starting to wilt, about 2 minutes. Add remaining spinach, broth, tomatoes, and ⅛ teaspoon salt and bring to simmer. Reduce heat to medium, cover (pan will be very full), and cook, tossing occasionally, until spinach is completely wilted, about 10 minutes (mixture will be somewhat soupy). Off heat, stir in beans and olives.

3. Meanwhile, bring 4 quarts water to boil in large pot. Add pasta and 1 teaspoon salt and cook, stirring often, until just shy of al dente. Reserve ½ cup cooking water, then drain pasta and return it to pot. Add spinach mixture and cook over medium heat, tossing to combine, until pasta absorbs most of liquid, about 2 minutes.

4. Off heat, stir in Parmesan. Season with pepper to taste and adjust consistency with reserved cooking water as needed. Sprinkle individual portions with garlic chips. Serve.

PER 1½-CUP SERVING

Cal 360 • **Total Fat** 11g • **Sat Fat** 1.5g • **Chol** 5mg
Sodium 360mg • **Total Carbs** 50g • **Fiber** 11g • **Total Sugar** 3g
Added Sugar 0g • **Protein** 15g • **Total Carbohydrate Choices** 3

Cooking Pasta 101

Cooking pasta seems simple, but perfect pasta takes some finesse. Here's how we do it in the test kitchen.

USE PLENTY OF WATER

To prevent sticking, you'll need 4 quarts of water to cook up to 1 pound of dried pasta. Pasta leaches starch as it cooks; without plenty of water to dilute it, the starch will coat the noodles and they will stick. Use a pot with at least a 6-quart capacity so that the water won't boil over.

SALT THE WATER

Adding salt to the pasta cooking water is essential; it seasons and flavors the pasta, allowing you to add only a minimal amount of sodium to the final dish. Add 1 teaspoon of salt per 4 quarts of water. Be sure to add the salt with the pasta, not before, so it will dissolve and not stain the pot.

SKIP THE OIL

Adding oil to cooking water just creates a slick on the surface of the water, doing nothing to prevent pasta from sticking. And when you drain the pasta, the oil prevents the pasta sauce from adhering. To prevent pasta from sticking, simply stir the pasta for a minute or two when you add it to the boiling water, then stir occasionally while it's cooking.

CHECK OFTEN FOR DONENESS

The instructions given on the box are almost always too long and will result in overcooked pasta. Tasting is the best way to check for doneness. We typically prefer pasta cooked al dente, when it still has a little bite left in the center.

RESERVE SOME WATER

Reserve about ½ cup of cooking water before draining the pasta—the water is flavorful and can loosen a thick sauce.

DON'T RINSE

Drain the pasta in a colander, but don't rinse the pasta (the exceptions are lasagna noodles [pages 167–169] and the pasta for Peanut Noodle Salad [page 171]), where we rinse in order to cool down); it washes away starch. Let a little water cling to the cooked pasta to help the sauce adhere.

KEEP IT HOT

If you're using a large serving bowl for the pasta, place it under the colander while draining the pasta. The hot water heats up the bowl, which keeps the pasta warm longer.

All About Parmesan

Produced using traditional methods for the past 800 years in one government-designated area of northern Italy, this hard cow's-milk cheese has a distinctive buttery, nutty, and slightly sharp taste. We frequently reach for it to sprinkle on top of pasta dishes or to add a rich, salty flavor to sauces, soups, and stews.

BUYING PARMESAN

We love authentic Italian Parmigiano-Reggiano in the test kitchen (note that it is not vegetarian because it is made with animal rennet). To ensure that you're buying a properly aged cheese, examine the condition of the rind. It should be a few shades darker than the straw-colored interior and should penetrate about ½ inch deep (younger or improperly aged cheeses will have a paler, thinner rind). And closely scrutinize the center of the cheese. Those small white spots found on many samples are actually good things—they signify the presence of calcium phosphate crystals, which are formed only after the cheese has been aged for the proper amount of time.

STORING PARMESAN

We found that the best way to preserve Parmesan's flavor and texture is to wrap it in parchment paper, then aluminum foil. However, if you have just a small piece of cheese, tossing it in a zipper-lock bag works almost as well; just be sure to squeeze out as much air as possible before sealing the bag.

PARMESAN VERSUS PECORINO ROMANO

Parmesan and Pecorino Romano have similar textures and flavors, and often you'll see one as an alternative to the other in recipes. We have found that Parmesan and Pecorino Romano generally can be used interchangeably, especially when the amount called for is moderate. However, when Parmesan is called for in larger quantities, stick with the Parmesan, as Pecorino Romano can be fairly pungent.

CAN YOU PREGRATE YOUR OWN PARMESAN?

We've never been tempted by tasteless powdered Parmesan cheese. But what about grating your own? We found that tasters were hard-pressed to detect any difference between freshly grated Parmesan and cheese that had been grated and stored for up to three weeks. So go ahead and grate your Parmesan ahead; refrigerate in an airtight container.

Linguine with Meatless "Meat" Sauce
SERVES 6

WHY THIS RECIPE WORKS We wanted to create a vegetarian version of a savory, unctuous tomato-meat sauce. The typical Italian American meat sauce gets most of its savory depth from browning the ground beef. As the beef cooks, it releases juices that reduce and form a flavor-packed fond on the bottom of the pot. By zeroing in on the specific qualities meat brings to a meat sauce, we were able to replicate them in our meatless version. To achieve a deep savory flavor, we browned cremini mushrooms and tomato paste to maximize these sources of umami. Extra-virgin olive oil did double duty, enriching the sauce and helping toast the classic Italian aromatics: garlic, dried oregano, and red pepper flakes. We bulked up the sauce with chopped chickpeas that had been rinsed of their excess starch. To thin the sauce without watering down its flavor, we added vegetable broth. Make sure to rinse the chickpeas after pulsing them in the food processor or the sauce will be too thick.

  5 ounces cremini mushrooms, trimmed
  3 tablespoons extra-virgin olive oil
    Salt
  1 small onion, chopped
  3 garlic cloves, minced
  ½ teaspoon dried oregano
  ⅛ teaspoon red pepper flakes
  2 tablespoons no-salt-added tomato paste
  1 (14-ounce) can no-salt-added crushed tomatoes
  1 cup low-sodium vegetable broth
  1 cup no-salt-added canned chickpeas, rinsed
 12 ounces 100 percent whole-wheat linguine
  2 tablespoons chopped fresh basil
  1 ounce Parmesan cheese, grated (½ cup)

1. Pulse mushrooms in food processor until chopped into ⅛- to ¼-inch pieces, 7 to 10 pulses, scraping down sides of bowl as needed. (Do not clean workbowl.)

2. Heat 2 tablespoons oil in Dutch oven over medium-high heat until shimmering. Add mushrooms and ½ teaspoon salt and cook, stirring occasionally, until mushrooms are browned and fond has formed on bottom of pot, about 8 minutes.

3. While mushrooms cook, pulse onion in food processor until finely chopped, 7 to 10 pulses, scraping down sides of bowl as needed. (Do not clean workbowl.) Transfer onion to pot with mushrooms and cook, stirring occasionally, until onion is soft and translucent, about 5 minutes. Combine remaining 1 tablespoon oil, garlic, oregano, and pepper flakes in bowl.

4. Add tomato paste to pot and cook, stirring constantly, until mixture is rust-colored, 1 to 2 minutes. Reduce heat to medium and push vegetables to sides of pot. Add garlic mixture to center and cook, stirring constantly, until fragrant, about 30 seconds. Stir in tomatoes and broth; bring to simmer over high heat. Reduce heat to low and simmer sauce for 5 minutes, stirring occasionally.

5. While sauce simmers, pulse chickpeas in food processor until chopped into ¼-inch pieces, 5 to 7 pulses. Transfer chickpeas to fine-mesh strainer and rinse under cold running water until water runs clear; drain well. Add chickpeas to pot and simmer until sauce is slightly thickened, about 15 minutes.

6. Meanwhile, bring 4 quarts water to boil in large pot. Add pasta and 1 teaspoon salt and cook, stirring often, until al dente. Reserve ½ cup cooking water, then drain pasta and return it to pot. Add sauce and toss to combine. Adjust consistency with reserved cooking water as needed. Stir in 1 tablespoon basil. Sprinkle individual portions with Parmesan and remaining 1 tablespoon basil. Serve.

PER 1-CUP SERVING

Cal 350 • **Total Fat** 10g • **Sat Fat** 2g • **Chol** 5mg
Sodium 380mg • **Total Carbs** 49g • **Fiber** 9g • **Total Sugar** 5g
Added Sugar 0g • **Protein** 13g • **Total Carbohydrate Choices** 3

Pasta with Kale Pesto, Tomatoes, and Chicken

SERVES 6

WHY THIS RECIPE WORKS For a luscious, creamy, bold-flavored pesto pasta dish that we could feel good about eating, we took a closer look at what goes into a classic pesto. Though we love pine nuts in pesto, we opted for roasted sunflower seeds for a slight twist on the classic. To give our pesto more body, we deviated from traditional basil and added kale and spinach to the mix as well. Sautéed chicken breast and cherry tomatoes gave our dish more bulk and added protein to make it hearty. Other 100 percent whole-wheat pasta shapes can be substituted for the farfalle, but the cup amounts may vary (see page 164 for more information).

1¼ ounces curly kale, stemmed and chopped (¾ cup)
½ cup fresh basil leaves
½ cup baby spinach
3 tablespoons roasted sunflower seeds
1½ tablespoons water
1 garlic clove, minced
   Salt and pepper
¼ cup plus 1 teaspoon extra-virgin olive oil

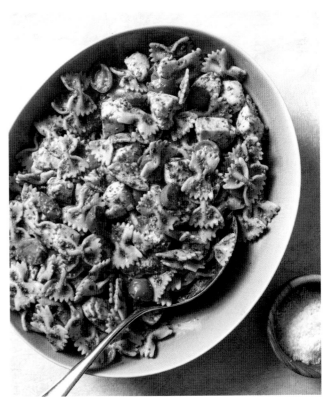

We supercharge traditional pesto by combining kale, spinach, and roasted sunflower seeds along with the basil.

1 ounce Parmesan cheese, grated (½ cup)
1½ pounds boneless, skinless chicken breast, trimmed of all visible fat and cut into 1-inch pieces
12 ounces cherry tomatoes, halved
12 ounces (4½ cups) 100 percent whole-wheat farfalle

1. Process kale, basil, spinach, sunflower seeds, water, garlic, and ¼ teaspoon salt in food processor until smooth, about 30 seconds, scraping down sides of bowl as needed. With processor running, slowly add ¼ cup oil until incorporated. Transfer mixture to bowl, stir in ¼ cup Parmesan, and season with pepper to taste. (Pesto can be refrigerated with plastic wrap pressed flush to surface for up to 3 days.)

2. Pat chicken dry with paper towels and season with ¼ teaspoon salt and ¼ teaspoon pepper. Heat remaining 1 teaspoon oil in 12-inch nonstick skillet over medium-high heat until shimmering. Add chicken to skillet and cook, stirring occasionally, until lightly browned all over and cooked through, about 5 minutes. Add cherry tomatoes to skillet and cook until softened slightly, about 2 minutes.

3. Meanwhile, bring 4 quarts water to boil in large pot. Add pasta and 1 teaspoon salt and cook, stirring often, until al dente. Reserve ½ cup cooking water, then drain pasta and return it to pot. Add pesto and chicken-tomato mixture and toss to combine. Season with pepper to taste and adjust consistency with reserved cooking water as needed. Sprinkle individual portions with remaining ¼ cup Parmesan. Serve.

PER 1⅓-CUP SERVING

Cal 470 • Total Fat 18g • Sat Fat 3g • Chol 85mg
Sodium 400mg • Total Carbs 39g • Fiber 7g • Total Sugar 3g
Added Sugar 0g • Protein 36g • Total Carbohydrate Choices 2.5

Penne with Chicken and Pan-Roasted Broccoli

SERVES 6

WHY THIS RECIPE WORKS Often, restaurant versions of pasta with chicken and broccoli are laden with bland sauce that merely covers up the overcooked ingredients. Instead of steaming, we chose to skillet-roast the broccoli, knowing that browning the vegetable would equal a big punch of flavor. We added sliced garlic, lemon zest, fresh thyme, and red pepper flakes for additional layers of aromatic flavor. We browned chunks of boneless, skinless chicken breast and then finished cooking them in our wine- and broth-based sauce. Parmesan cheese and a sprinkling of fresh parsley rounded out the seasoning and added a fresh finish to the dish. Be sure to peel the broccoli stalks completely or they will be tough. You will need a 12-inch nonstick skillet with a tight-fitting lid for this recipe. Other 100 percent whole-wheat pasta shapes can be substituted for the penne, but the cup amounts may vary (see page 164 for more information).

2 tablespoons extra-virgin olive oil
1 pound broccoli, florets cut into 1½-inch pieces, stems trimmed, peeled, and cut on bias into ¼-inch-thick slices about 1½ inches long
8 garlic cloves, peeled (4 sliced thin, 4 minced)
1 tablespoon grated lemon zest
⅛–¼ teaspoon red pepper flakes
   Salt and pepper
3 tablespoons water
1 pound boneless, skinless chicken breasts, trimmed of all visible fat and cut into 1-inch pieces

3 shallots, minced
2 teaspoons minced fresh thyme
2 tablespoons all-purpose flour
2 cups unsalted chicken broth
1 cup dry white wine
12 ounces (3½ cups) 100 percent whole-wheat penne
1 ounce Parmesan cheese, grated (½ cup)
2 tablespoons minced fresh parsley

1. Heat 1 tablespoon oil in 12-inch nonstick skillet over medium-high heat until just smoking. Add broccoli stems in even layer and cook, without stirring, until browned on bottoms, about 2 minutes. Add florets to skillet and toss to combine; cook, without stirring, until bottom sides of florets just begin to brown, 1 to 2 minutes longer.

2. Stir in sliced garlic, 1 teaspoon lemon zest, pepper flakes, and ¼ teaspoon pepper and cook until fragrant, about 30 seconds. Stir in water and cover skillet; cook until broccoli is bright green but still crisp, about 2 minutes. Uncover and continue to cook until water has evaporated and broccoli is crisp-tender, about 2 minutes. Transfer broccoli to medium bowl and set aside.

3. Heat remaining 1 tablespoon oil in now-empty skillet over high heat until just smoking. Add chicken and ¼ teaspoon salt and cook, stirring occasionally, until lightly browned but not fully cooked, about 3 minutes; transfer to separate bowl.

4. Reduce heat to medium, add shallots and ⅛ teaspoon salt to now-empty skillet, and cook until just softened, 2 to 3 minutes. Stir in minced garlic and thyme and cook until fragrant, about 30 seconds.

5. Stir in flour and cook for 1 minute. Slowly whisk in broth and wine and bring to simmer, scraping up any browned bits. Cook, stirring occasionally, until sauce has thickened, about 12 minutes. Return chicken and any accumulated juices to skillet. Cook until chicken is cooked through, about 1 minute. Off heat, stir in remaining 2 teaspoons lemon zest.

6. Meanwhile, bring 4 quarts water to boil in large pot. Add pasta and 1 teaspoon salt and cook, stirring often, until al dente. Reserve ½ cup of cooking water, drain pasta, then return to pot. Add chicken-sauce mixture, broccoli, Parmesan, and parsley and toss to combine. Adjust consistency with reserved cooking water as needed. Serve.

PER 1½-CUP SERVING

Cal 420 • Total Fat 10g • Sat Fat 2g • Chol 60mg
Sodium 400mg • Total Carbs 47g • Fiber 9g • Total Sugar 4g
Added Sugars 0g • Protein 30g • Total Carbohydrate Choices 3

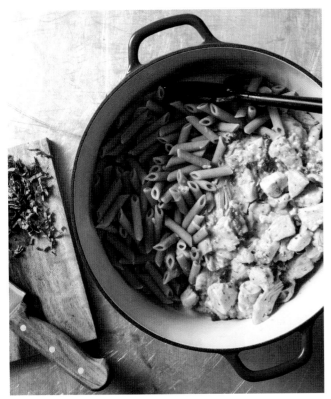

Frozen artichokes are lower in sodium than canned or marinated ones and are full of fiber.

Lemony Penne with Chicken, Sun-Dried Tomatoes, and Artichokes

SERVES 6

WHY THIS RECIPE WORKS For a light and bright pasta dish, we turned to a Mediterranean-inspired flavor profile of lemon, sun-dried tomatoes, and artichoke hearts. We started by cooking lean chicken breast, which only took a few minutes since it was cut into small pieces. We then built a flavorful sauce by sautéing a base of leeks before adding white wine and chicken broth for extra flavor; garlic and fresh thyme provided an aromatic backdrop. Chewy sun-dried tomatoes were a welcome textural contrast and their rich, sweet flavor stood up well to the whole-wheat pasta. We used convenient frozen artichokes, as they are lower in sodium than canned or marinated varieties. Lemon zest and a full ¼ cup of lemon juice added a citrusy pop, while Parmesan cheese enhanced the dish's seasoning. Shredded basil was the perfect fresh finish and drove home the summery flavors. Other 100 percent whole-wheat pasta shapes can be substituted for the penne, but the cup amounts may vary (see page 164 for more information).

1 pound boneless, skinless chicken breasts, trimmed of all visible fat and cut into 1-inch pieces
  Salt and pepper
1 tablespoon extra-virgin olive oil
1 leek, white and light green parts only, halved lengthwise, sliced thin, and washed thoroughly
6 garlic cloves, minced
2 teaspoons minced fresh thyme
2 tablespoons all-purpose flour
2 cups unsalted chicken broth
1 cup dry white wine
9 ounces frozen artichoke hearts, thawed
⅓ cup oil-packed sun-dried tomatoes, patted dry and sliced thin
1½ ounces Parmesan cheese, grated (¾ cup)
2 teaspoons grated lemon zest plus ¼ cup juice (2 lemons)
12 ounces (3½ cups) 100 percent whole-wheat penne
2 tablespoons shredded fresh basil

1. Pat chicken dry with paper towels and sprinkle with ¼ teaspoon salt and ¼ teaspoon pepper. Heat 1½ teaspoons oil in 12-inch nonstick skillet over high heat until just smoking. Add chicken and cook, stirring occasionally, until lightly browned but not fully cooked, about 3 minutes; transfer to bowl.

2. Add remaining 1½ teaspoons oil to now-empty skillet and heat over medium heat until shimmering. Add leek and ⅛ teaspoon salt and cook until just beginning to soften, about 2 minutes. Stir in garlic and thyme and cook until fragrant, about 30 seconds. Stir in flour and cook for 1 minute.

3. Slowly whisk in broth and wine and bring to simmer, scraping up any browned bits. Cook, stirring occasionally, until sauce has thickened, about 12 minutes.

4. Return chicken and any accumulated juices to skillet along with artichokes and sun-dried tomatoes. Cook until chicken is cooked through, about 1 minute. Off heat, stir in Parmesan and lemon zest and juice.

5. Meanwhile, bring 4 quarts water to boil in large pot. Stir in pasta and 1 teaspoon salt and cook, stirring often, until al dente. Reserve ½ cup pasta water, then drain pasta and return it to pot. Add chicken-sauce mixture and basil and gently toss to combine. Adjust consistency with reserved cooking water as needed. Serve.

PER 1½-CUP SERVING
Cal 430 • **Total Fat** 9g • **Sat Fat** 2g • **Chol** 60mg
Sodium 400mg • **Total Carbs** 51g • **Fiber** 11g • **Total Sugar**s 4g
Added Sugar 0g • **Protein** 30g • **Total Carbohydrate Choices** 3.5

Measuring Less Than a Pound of Pasta

It's easy enough to measure out a pound of pasta, as most packages are sold in this quantity. But in this book, recipes call for less than 1 pound of pasta. Obviously, you can weigh out partial pounds of pasta using a scale or judge by how full the box is, but we think it's easier to measure shaped pasta using a dry measuring cup, and strand pasta by determining the diameter.

PASTA TYPE	8 OUNCES	12 OUNCES
Elbow Macaroni	1¾ cups	2¾ cups
Rigatoni	2¼ cups	3⅓ cups
Penne	2¼ cups	3½ cups
Orecchiette	2½ cups	3¾ cups
Farfalle, Fusilli, Rotini	3 cups	4½ cups
Medium Shells	3¼ cups	4¾ cups

When 8 ounces of uncooked strand pasta are bunched together into a tight circle, the diameter measures about 1¼ inches. When 12 ounces of uncooked strand pasta are bunched together into a tight circle, the diameter measures about 1½ inches.

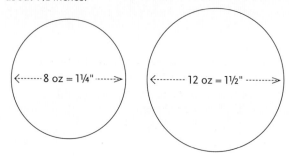

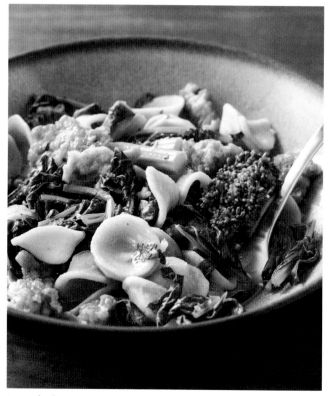

Lean chicken sausage gives this pasta dish meaty richness and protein without too much fat.

Orecchiette with Broccoli Rabe and Sausage
SERVES 6

WHY THIS RECIPE WORKS To create a more nutritionally balanced version of the classic orecchiette with broccoli rabe and sausage, we opted for whole-wheat pasta instead of the classic refined variety, upping the fiber content and making an already hearty meal even more satiating. Just 8 ounces of sausage was plenty to provide meaty, umami flavor without making the dish too rich. Broccoli rabe's bitterness was balanced out by the sausage, along with a hefty dose of garlic and a pinch of red pepper flakes. Stirring in Parmesan cheese at the end provided a boost of salty flavor without the need to add additional salt. You can substitute Asiago for Parmesan in this recipe. Other 100 percent whole-wheat pasta shapes can be substituted for the orecchiette, but the cup amounts may vary (see chart at left for more information).

¼ cup extra-virgin olive oil
8 ounces sweet Italian chicken sausage, casings removed
6 garlic cloves, minced

¼ teaspoon red pepper flakes
1 pound broccoli rabe, trimmed and cut into 1½-inch pieces
  Salt and pepper
12 ounces (3¾ cups) 100 percent whole-wheat orecchiette
1 ounce Parmesan or Asiago cheese, grated (½ cup)

1. Heat oil in 12-inch nonstick skillet over medium heat until shimmering. Add sausage, breaking up pieces with wooden spoon, and cook until lightly browned, 5 to 7 minutes. Stir in garlic and pepper flakes and cook until fragrant, about 30 seconds; set skillet aside.

2. Meanwhile, bring 4 quarts water to boil in large pot. Add broccoli rabe and 1 teaspoon salt and cook, stirring often, until crisp-tender, about 2 minutes. Using slotted spoon, transfer broccoli rabe to skillet with sausage.

3. Return water to boil, add pasta, and cook, stirring often, until al dente. Reserve 1 cup cooking water, then drain pasta and return it to pot. Add sausage–broccoli rabe mixture, Parmesan, ⅓ cup reserved cooking water, and ¼ teaspoon salt and toss to combine. Season with pepper to taste and adjust consistency with remaining ⅔ cup reserved cooking water as needed. Serve.

PER 1½-CUP SERVING
Cal 380 • **Total Fat** 16g • **Sat Fat** 3.5g • **Chol** 15mg
Sodium 490mg • **Total Carbs** 46g • **Fiber** 7g • **Total Sugar** 2g
Added Sugar 0g • **Protein** 19g • **Total Carbohydrate Choices** 3

Spaghetti and Meatballs
SERVES 6

WHY THIS RECIPE WORKS The obvious way to cut some of the fat and calories found in meatballs is to swap in ground turkey for the traditional mixture of ground beef, pork, and veal. To ensure the meatballs didn't dry out, we used an egg yolk and a splash of milk in our panade, with one slice of whole-wheat bread instead of the traditional white. Parmesan cheese provided plenty of saltiness, and utilizing fresh basil both in the meatballs and as a garnish emphasized its fresh flavor. Chilling the meatballs before browning them helped them to stay together during cooking. Whole-wheat spaghetti was the perfect fiber-rich bed for these leaner, crowd-pleasing meatballs. Do not use ground turkey breast here (also labeled 99 percent fat-free) or the meatballs will taste dry and grainy. The meatballs and sauce can be prepared through step 4 and refrigerated in an airtight container for up to 3 days or frozen for up to 2 months. Thaw (if necessary) and gently reheat in a covered pot over medium-low heat.

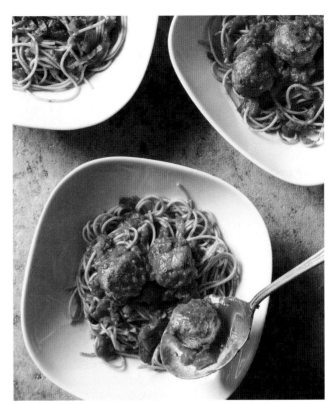

We make this classic comfort food leaner by choosing ground turkey instead of traditional, fattier ground meats.

MEATBALLS
1 (1¼-ounce) slice 100 percent whole-wheat sandwich bread, crusts removed, torn into pieces
1½ tablespoons 1 percent low-fat milk
¼ cup grated Parmesan cheese
3 tablespoons chopped fresh basil
1 large egg yolk
2 garlic cloves, minced
  Salt and pepper
1½ pounds ground turkey
1 tablespoon extra-virgin olive oil

PASTA AND SAUCE
1 onion, chopped fine
  Salt
4 garlic cloves, minced
½ teaspoon minced fresh oregano
⅛ teaspoon red pepper flakes
1 (28-ounce) can no-salt-added crushed tomatoes
1 (14.5-ounce) can no-salt-added diced tomatoes
12 ounces 100 percent whole-wheat spaghetti
3 tablespoons shredded fresh basil

1. FOR THE MEATBALLS Mash bread and milk together in bowl to smooth paste. Stir in Parmesan, basil, egg yolk, garlic, ½ teaspoon salt, and ¼ teaspoon pepper. Add turkey and combine with hands until mixture is uniformly smooth. Gently form mixture into 1½-inch round meatballs (18 meatballs) and place on large plate. Refrigerate until firm, about 1 hour.

2. Heat oil in 12-inch nonstick skillet over medium heat until just smoking. Brown meatballs on all sides, about 10 minutes. Transfer meatballs to paper towel–lined plate, leaving fat in skillet.

3. FOR THE PASTA AND SAUCE Add onion and ¼ teaspoon salt to fat left in skillet and cook over medium heat until browned, about 8 minutes. Stir in garlic, oregano, and red pepper flakes and cook until fragrant, about 30 seconds. Stir in crushed tomatoes and diced tomatoes with their juices. Bring to simmer, reduce heat to medium-low, and cook until sauce has thickened slightly, about 20 minutes.

4. Add meatballs to sauce and bring to simmer. Cover and cook, turning meatballs occasionally, until cooked through, about 10 minutes.

5. Meanwhile, bring 4 quarts water to boil in large pot. Add pasta and 1 teaspoon salt and cook, stirring often, until al dente. Reserve ½ cup cooking water, then drain pasta and return it to pot.

6. Add basil and several large spoonfuls of sauce (without meatballs) to the pasta and toss to combine. Adjust consistency with reserved cooking water as needed. Divide pasta between six individual bowls. Top each bowl with 3 meatballs and additional sauce. Serve.

PER 1½-CUP SERVING OF PASTA WITH 3 MEATBALLS
Cal 430 • **Total Fat** 7g • **Sat Fat** 3g • **Chol** 80mg
Sodium 490mg • **Total Carbs** 49g • **Fiber** 10g • **Total Sugar** 9g
Added Sugar 0g • **Protein** 40g • **Total Carbohydrate Choices** 3

NOTES FROM THE TEST KITCHEN

Buying Canned Tomatoes

Since canned tomatoes are processed at the height of freshness, they deliver more flavor than off-season fresh tomatoes. But with all the options at the supermarket, it's not always clear what you should buy. And to make matters more confusing, canned tomatoes are also quite high in sodium; just ½ cup of canned diced tomatoes can contain around 250 milligrams of sodium. Because we wanted to limit sodium as much as possible in the recipes in this book, we opted for no-salt-added canned tomatoes, just as we do with canned beans (page 147) and store-bought broths (page 59). Doing so allows us to better control the sodium in our dishes.

Rigatoni with Turkey Ragu
SERVES 6

WHY THIS RECIPE WORKS A classic Bolognese-style sauce uses multiple types of ground and cured meats and often simmers with rich heavy cream, all of which result in a dish with too much saturated fat and sodium. We set out to create a lighter version of Bolognese that was still packed with rich, meaty flavor. We traded the classic ground beef and pork for turkey and added meaty flavor with the addition of a mix of dried porcini and cremini mushrooms. In place of additional salt, we added 2 minced anchovy fillets, which provided a more complex, umami boost of flavor. We simmered our turkey and vegetable base in red wine and milk to lighten up the sauce. Using whole-wheat rigatoni was the final piece of the puzzle; the short, tubular shape made it perfect for grabbing lots of meaty sauce, and the earthy flavor of the pasta stood up to our flavorful sauce. Do not use ground turkey breast here (also labeled 99 percent fat-free) or the turkey will taste dry and grainy. Other 100 percent whole-wheat pasta shapes can be substituted for the rigatoni, but the cup amounts may vary (see page 164 for more information).

- 1 onion, chopped coarse
- 1 carrot, chopped coarse
- 1 celery rib, chopped coarse
- 6 ounces cremini mushrooms, trimmed and quartered
- 1 ounce dried porcini mushrooms, rinsed and chopped coarse
- 1 (28-ounce) can no-salt-added whole peeled tomatoes
- 1 tablespoon extra-virgin olive oil
  Salt and pepper
- 2 garlic cloves, minced
- 1 tablespoon no-salt-added tomato paste
- 2 anchovy fillets, minced
- 1 pound ground turkey
- 1 cup 1 percent low-fat milk
- ½ cup dry red wine
- 12 ounces (3⅓ cups) 100 percent whole-wheat rigatoni

1. Pulse onion, carrot, and celery in food processor until finely chopped, about 10 pulses; transfer to large bowl. Pulse cremini and porcini mushrooms in now-empty processor until finely chopped, about 5 pulses; transfer to bowl with onion mixture.

2. Pulse tomatoes with their juice in now-empty processor until mostly smooth, about 8 pulses. Transfer to separate bowl.

3. Heat oil in 12-inch skillet over medium heat until just shimmering. Add vegetable mixture, ¼ teaspoon salt, and ⅛ teaspoon pepper and cook until softened and lightly browned, 8 to 10 minutes. Stir in garlic and cook until fragrant, about 30 seconds. Stir in tomato paste and anchovies and cook for 1 minute.

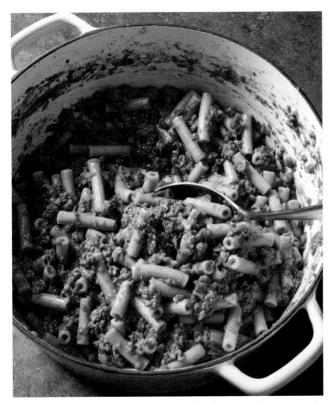

To create a meatier sauce using ground turkey, we add umami-rich anchovies and both dried and fresh mushrooms.

4. Stir in turkey and cook, breaking up meat with wooden spoon, until no longer pink and mixture begins to look dry, about 4 minutes. Stir in milk and bring to simmer, scraping up any browned bits. Cook until milk is nearly evaporated, 8 to 10 minutes.

5. Stir in wine and simmer until nearly evaporated, about 10 minutes. Stir in processed tomato mixture and simmer until sauce has thickened, 15 to 20 minutes.

6. Meanwhile, bring 4 quarts water to boil in large pot. Add pasta and 1 teaspoon salt and cook, stirring often, until al dente. Reserve ½ cup of cooking water, then drain pasta and return it to pot. Add sauce and toss to combine. Adjust consistency with reserved cooking water as needed. Serve.

PER 1½-CUP SERVING

Cal 380 • **Total Fat** 6g • **Sat Fat** 2g • **Chol** 35mg
Sodium 390mg • **Total Carbs** 49g • **Fiber** 9g • **Total Sugar** 10g
Added Sugar 0g • **Protein** 32g • **Total Carbohydrate Choices** 3

Spinach Lasagna
SERVES 12

WHY THIS RECIPE WORKS Classic spinach lasagna, with its rich béchamel sauce and layers of melted cheese, can pack more calories and fat than traditional lasagna with a tomato-based meat sauce. We wanted a spinach lasagna highlighted by a delicate, creamy sauce and tender noodles that was appropriate for a diabetes diet. We decided on convenient frozen spinach, as it helped cut down the cooking time. To cut a significant amount of saturated fat from the sauce, we replaced the butter commonly used in making a roux with a far lesser amount of heart-healthy olive oil. For richness and a quintessential creamy texture, we turned to a combination of cheeses (ricotta and mozzarella). Baked pasta dishes often emerge from the oven with mushy noodles and a dried-out sauce, so to avoid these pitfalls, we undercooked the pasta slightly (not quite al dente, but still a little raw and firm). This way, the pasta could finish cooking in the sauce as the lasagna baked in the oven. Using plenty of milk and simmering only to thicken slightly allowed us to easily stir in additional ingredients. The fluidity of the sauce helped prevent it from drying up as it thickened further while the casserole baked.

- 1 pound (2 cups) whole-milk ricotta cheese
- 10 ounces whole-milk mozzarella cheese, shredded (2½ cups)
- 2 ounces Parmesan cheese, grated (1 cup)
- 1 large egg, lightly beaten
  Salt and pepper
- 2 tablespoons extra-virgin olive oil
- 1 onion, chopped fine
- 8 garlic cloves, minced
- ¼ cup all-purpose flour
- 5 cups 1 percent low-fat milk
- 2 bay leaves
- ½ teaspoon ground nutmeg
- 30 ounces frozen spinach, thawed, squeezed dry, and chopped coarse
- 16 100 percent whole-wheat lasagna noodles

1. Stir ricotta, 1½ cups mozzarella, ½ cup Parmesan, egg, ½ teaspoon pepper, and ¼ teaspoon salt in bowl until well combined; cover and refrigerate until needed.

2. Heat oil in large saucepan over medium heat until shimmering. Add onion and cook until softened, about 5 minutes. Stir in garlic and cook until fragrant, about 30 seconds. Stir in flour and cook for 1 minute. Slowly whisk in milk and bay leaves. Bring to simmer and cook, stirring occasionally, until sauce has thickened slightly, about 10 minutes.

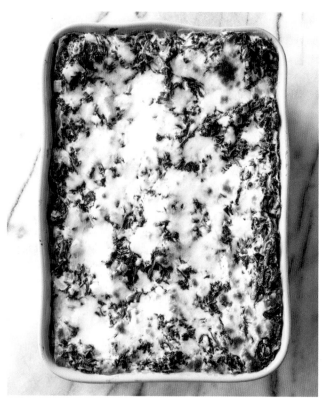

Using olive oil and milk in the creamy white sauce for spinach lasagna cuts down on saturated fat.

3. Off heat, discard bay leaves. Whisk in nutmeg and remaining ½ cup Parmesan. Stir in spinach, breaking up any clumps, until well combined. Cover and set aside.

4. Adjust oven rack to middle position and heat oven to 375 degrees. Lightly coat 13 by 9-inch baking dish with vegetable oil spray. Bring 4 quarts water to boil in large pot. Add noodles and 1 teaspoon salt and cook, stirring often, until almost al dente. Drain and rinse noodles under cold water until cool. Lay pasta out over clean kitchen towels.

5. Spread 1 cup spinach sauce over bottom of baking dish. Place 4 noodles on top of sauce and spread ¼ cup of ricotta mixture evenly down center of each noodle. Spoon 1 cup more spinach sauce evenly over ricotta. Repeat layering two more times.

6. For final layer, place remaining 4 noodles on top, spread remaining 2 cups spinach sauce over noodles, and sprinkle with remaining 1 cup mozzarella. Spray large sheet of aluminum foil lightly with vegetable oil spray, then cover lasagna.

7. Place lasagna on foil-lined rimmed baking sheet and bake until sauce is bubbling, 40 to 45 minutes. Uncover lasagna and continue to bake until cheese is melted and beginning to brown, about 20 minutes. Let cool for 10 to 20 minutes before serving.

PER 3¼ BY 3-INCH SERVING

Cal 360 • **Total Fat** 16g • **Sat Fat** 8g • **Chol** 55mg
Sodium 550mg • **Total Carbs** 35g • **Fiber** 5g • **Total Sugar** 8g
Added Sugar 0g • **Protein** 22g • **Total Carbohydrate Choices** 2

Turkey and Cheese Lasagna
SERVES 12

WHY THIS RECIPE WORKS Lasagna is notoriously fatty, thanks to rich tomato-meat sauce and generous portion sizes. We wanted a delicious meat and cheese lasagna that would satisfy the most discerning of tastes, while still being diabetic friendly. For the cheese layer, we stuck with tradition and combined ricotta, Parmesan, fresh basil, and an egg to help thicken and bind the mixture. As for the sauce, we substituted lean ground turkey for more traditional ground beef, allowing us to slash the saturated fat and calorie counts further. For an even healthier take on this Italian-American comfort food, we reached for whole-wheat noodles instead of the classic curly-edge ones. After layering the ingredients, we covered the pan for the first part of the baking time, and then uncovered it to create a bubbling lasagna with a beautifully browned cheese topping. Be sure to use ground turkey, not ground turkey breast (also labeled 99 percent fat-free), in this recipe.

  1 pound (2 cups) whole-milk ricotta cheese
 12 ounces whole-milk mozzarella cheese, shredded (3 cups)
  1 ounce Parmesan cheese, grated (½ cup)
  1 cup chopped fresh basil
  1 large egg, lightly beaten
    Salt and pepper
1½ teaspoons extra-virgin olive oil
  1 onion, chopped fine
  6 garlic cloves, minced
  ¼ teaspoon dried oregano
  ⅛ teaspoon red pepper flakes
  1 pound ground turkey

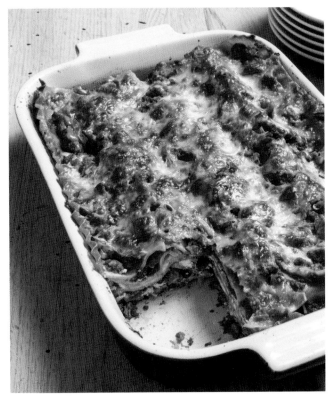

We love the hearty flavor and firm texture that whole-wheat noodles bring to our lasagnas.

1 (28-ounce) can no-salt-added crushed tomatoes
1 (28-ounce) can no-salt-added diced tomatoes
16 100 percent whole-wheat lasagna noodles

1. Mix ricotta, 2 cups mozzarella, Parmesan, ½ cup basil, egg, ¼ teaspoon salt, and ½ teaspoon pepper in bowl until well combined; cover and refrigerate until needed.

2. Heat oil in Dutch oven over medium heat until shimmering. Add onion and cook until softened, about 5 minutes. Stir in garlic, oregano, and red pepper flakes and cook until fragrant, about 30 seconds.

3. Add ground turkey and cook, breaking up meat with wooden spoon, until no longer pink, about 5 minutes. Stir in tomatoes with their juices and ¼ teaspoon salt and bring to simmer. Cook, stirring occasionally, until sauce has thickened slightly, about 15 minutes. Off heat, stir in remaining ½ cup basil, cover, and set aside.

4. Adjust oven rack to middle position and heat oven to 375 degrees. Lightly coat 13 by 9-inch baking dish with vegetable oil spray. Bring 4 quarts water to boil in large pot. Add noodles and 1 teaspoon salt and cook, stirring often, until almost al dente. Drain and rinse noodles under cold water until cool. Lay pasta out over clean kitchen towels.

5. Spread 1½ cups meat sauce over bottom of baking dish. Place 4 noodles on top of sauce and spread ¼ cup ricotta mixture evenly down center of each noodle. Spoon 1½ cups more sauce evenly over ricotta. Repeat layering two more times.

6. For final layer, place remaining 4 noodles on top and spread remaining 2 cups sauce over noodles. Sprinkle with remaining 1 cup mozzarella. Spray large sheet of aluminum foil lightly with vegetable oil spray, then cover lasagna.

7. Place lasagna on foil-lined rimmed baking sheet and bake until sauce is bubbling, 40 to 45 minutes. Uncover lasagna and continue to bake until cheese is melted and beginning to brown, about 20 minutes. Let cool for 10 to 20 minutes before serving.

PER 3¼ BY 3-INCH SERVING

Cal 350 • **Total Fat** 14g • **Sat Fat** 8g • **Chol** 70mg
Sodium 460mg • **Total Carbs** 32g • **Fiber** 5g • **Total Sugar** 6g
Added Sugar 0g • **Protein** 27g • **Total Carbohydrate Choices** 2

NOTES FROM THE TEST KITCHEN

Whole-Wheat Pasta

Whole-wheat pasta is a great way to incorporate more whole grains into your diet. Though it is not lower in carbs compared to traditional white pasta, it does boast fiber and protein (our winning spaghetti has a substantial 6 grams of fiber and 7 grams of protein per 2-ounce serving) plus vitamins and minerals. Whole-wheat pasta can also provide a heartier texture and nuttier flavor to dishes. We had good luck using **Bionaturae Organic 100% Whole Wheat Spaghetti** and **Bionaturae Organic 100% Whole Wheat Lasagne**, which have a pleasant chew and are made from 100 percent whole- wheat flour for optimal nutritional benefits.

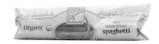
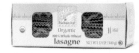

Noodles with Mustard Greens and Shiitake-Ginger Sauce

SERVES 6

WHY THIS RECIPE WORKS Noodles and greens are a common pairing in Asia. We thought this partnership was a great way to create a diabetes-friendly pasta dish that was delicate yet filling. We set out to develop a recipe that married the spicy bite of mustard greens with classic, neutral-flavored rice noodles. Typically made from rice flour and water, these noodles are available fresh, frozen, or dried and come in a variety of shapes and thicknesses. For a healthier approach to this Asian-inspired dish, we opted for brown rice noodles. We created a highly aromatic, flavorful broth from Asian pantry staples to bring the noodles to life. First, we browned meaty shiitake mushrooms to get plenty of flavor out of them, and then we added water and mirin along with rice vinegar, soy sauce, garlic, and fresh ginger. Dried shiitake mushrooms, sesame oil, and chili-garlic sauce rounded out the Asian flavor profile. After this mixture simmered and reduced, we had a sauce that was light and brothy but super savory—perfect for flavoring and cooking the mustard greens. We finished our noodle bowl by topping each portion with the broth-infused vegetable mixture, followed by scallions for freshness and sesame seeds for a little textural contrast.

- 8 ounces (⅛-inch-wide) brown rice noodles
- 2 tablespoons toasted sesame oil
- 1 tablespoon canola oil
- 8 ounces shiitake mushrooms, stemmed and sliced thin
- 2 cups water
- ¼ cup mirin
- 3 tablespoons rice vinegar
- 2 tablespoons low-sodium soy sauce
- 1 tablespoon grated fresh ginger
- 2 garlic cloves, minced
- ½ ounce dried shiitake mushrooms, rinsed and minced
- 1 teaspoon Asian chili-garlic sauce
- 1 pound mustard greens, stemmed and chopped into 1-inch pieces
- 4 ounces frozen shelled edamame
- 3 scallions, sliced thin
- 2 teaspoons sesame seeds, toasted
  Pepper

1. Bring 3 quarts water to boil in large saucepan. Place noodles in large bowl and pour boiling water over noodles. Stir and let soak until noodles are soft and pliable but not fully tender, about 8 minutes, stirring once halfway through soaking. Drain noodles and

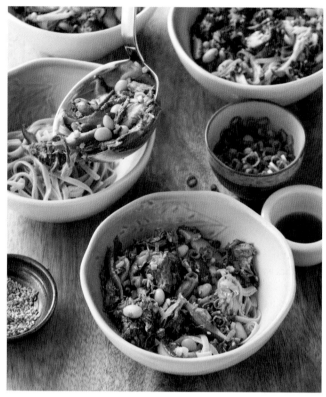

Brown rice noodles and a hefty amount of mustard greens provide these Asian-inspired noodles with plenty of fiber.

rinse under cold running water until water runs clear. Drain noodles well, then toss with 2 teaspoons sesame oil. Portion noodles into 6 individual serving bowls; set aside.

2. Heat canola oil in Dutch oven over medium-high heat until shimmering. Add fresh mushrooms and cook, stirring occasionally, until softened and lightly browned, about 5 minutes. Stir in water, mirin, vinegar, soy sauce, ginger, garlic, dried mushrooms, chili-garlic sauce, and 1 teaspoon sesame oil. Bring to simmer and cook until liquid has reduced by half, 8 to 10 minutes.

3. Stir in mustard greens and edamame, return to simmer, and cook, stirring often, until greens are nearly tender, 5 to 7 minutes.

4. Divide mustard green–mushroom mixture and sauce among noodle bowls. Top with scallions and sesame seeds and drizzle with remaining 1 tablespoon sesame oil. Season with pepper to taste and serve.

PER 1⅓-CUP SERVING

Cal 290 • **Total Fat** 9g • **Sat Fat** 1.5g • **Chol** 0mg
Sodium 250mg • **Total Carbs** 43g • **Fiber** 7g • **Total Sugar** 7g
Added Sugar 0g • **Protein** 9g • **Total Carbohydrate Choices** 3

Peanut Noodle Salad
SERVES 6

WHY THIS RECIPE WORKS With crisp vegetables and tender noodles coated in a velvety, mildly spicy peanut sauce, this flavorful salad offers a refreshing change of pace—but a peek at the fat and calorie counts reveals that it can be a nutritional nightmare. Scaling back on the peanut butter helped cut calories and saturated fat, but we made sure there was still plenty of nutty flavor. A bit of toasted sesame oil, which we added to our cooked noodles to prevent them from sticking, further amped up the nuttiness of the dish. Rinsing the cooked pasta with cold water kept it from overcooking and helped to remove some of the starch so it wouldn't become pasty. And putting more emphasis on the vegetables in this dish—we reduced the pasta from 1 pound to 12 ounces and doubled the amount of carrot and bell pepper—promised a peanut noodle salad that was lower in carbs but still satisfying. Chopped peanuts sprinkled over the top emphasized the nutty flavor profile and gave the dish an added crunch. Minced cilantro provided a fresh, clean finish. Use a milder hot sauce, such as the test kitchen's favorite, Frank's RedHot Original Cayenne Pepper Sauce, in this recipe. If using a hotter sauce, such as Tabasco, reduce the amount to ½ teaspoon.

½ cup natural unsweetened unsalted creamy peanut butter
3 tablespoons low-sodium soy sauce
3 tablespoons rice vinegar
1 tablespoon grated fresh ginger
2 garlic cloves, minced
1 teaspoon hot sauce
½ cup hot water
12 ounces 100 percent whole-wheat spaghetti
   Salt and pepper
1 tablespoon toasted sesame oil
2 red bell peppers, stemmed, seeded, and sliced thin
2 carrots, peeled and shredded
½ English cucumber, halved lengthwise, seeded, and sliced thin
¼ cup roasted unsalted peanuts, chopped coarse
⅓ cup fresh cilantro leaves
   Lime wedges

1. Whisk peanut butter, soy sauce, vinegar, ginger, garlic, and hot sauce together in large bowl until well combined. Whisking constantly, add hot water 1 tablespoon at a time, until dressing has consistency of heavy cream (you may not need all of water).

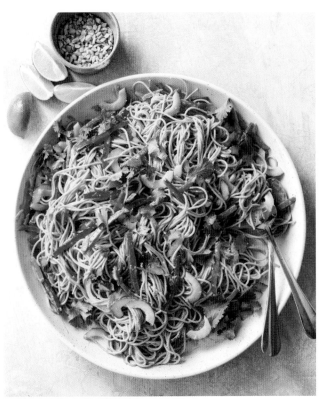

Upping the amount of vegetables and using less spaghetti helps to keep the carb count of this noodle dish in check.

2. Bring 4 quarts water to boil in large pot. Add pasta and 1 teaspoon salt and cook, stirring often, until tender. Reserve ¾ cup cooking water, then drain pasta and rinse with cold water until cool. Drain pasta well and toss with sesame oil. Transfer pasta to large bowl with peanut butter mixture and toss to combine.

3. Stir in bell peppers, carrots, cucumber, ¼ teaspoon salt, and pepper to taste and toss until combined. Add reserved cooking water as needed to adjust consistency. Sprinkle each portion with 2 teaspoons chopped peanuts. Sprinkle with cilantro and serve with lime wedges.

PER 1½-CUP SERVING

Cal 400 • **Total Fat** 18g • **Sat Fat** 3g • **Chol** 0mg
Sodium 490mg • **Total Carbs** 47g • **Fiber** 9g • **Total Sugar** 7g
Added Sugar 1g • **Protein** 15g • **Total Carbohydrate Choices** 3

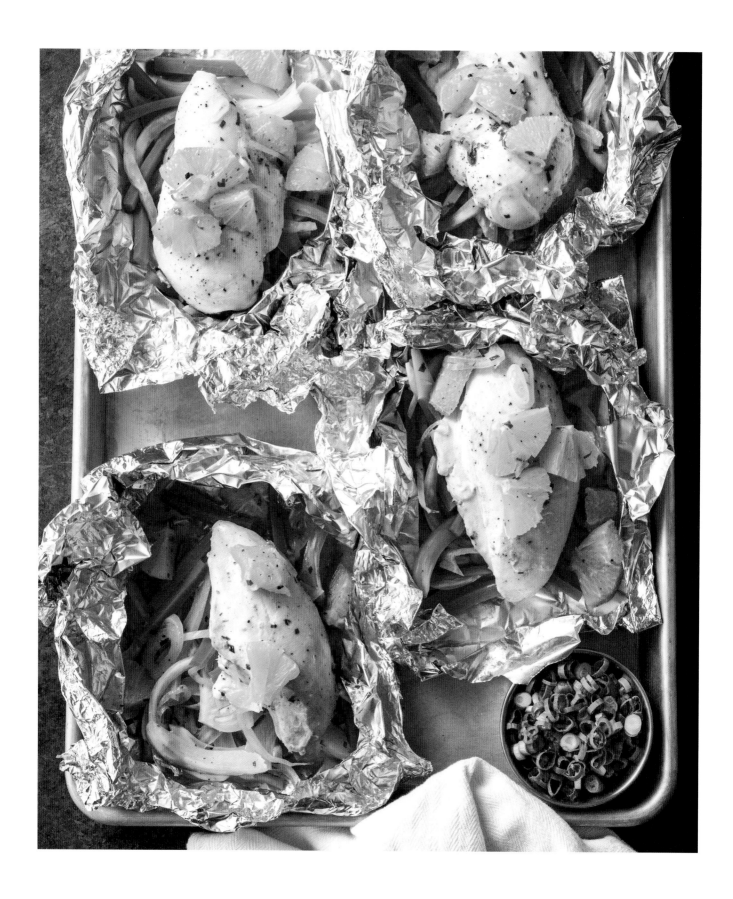

POULTRY

Photo: Chicken Baked in Foil with Fennel, Carrots, and Orange

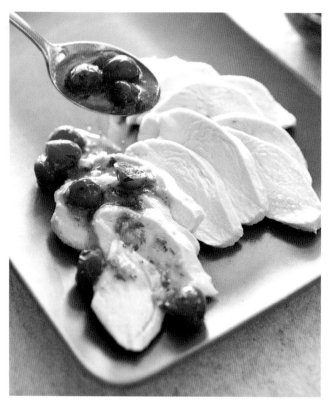

To keep lean chicken breast juicy and flavorful, we poach it in a brine of water, low-sodium soy sauce, and garlic.

Poached Chicken Breasts with Warm Tomato-Ginger Vinaigrette
SERVES 4

WHY THIS RECIPE WORKS While poached chicken may sound like bland diet food, we actually love this method as it is very forgiving and an easy path to moist, succulent chicken every time. First, we created a flavorful poaching liquid; soy sauce adds great flavor with minimal effect on the final sodium count. Allowing the chicken to gently poach in the residual heat, elevated in a steamer basket, ensured even cooking. We then paired the poached chicken with a bold vinaigrette and added halved cherry tomatoes to give the finished dish even more substance. Parsley may be substituted for the cilantro in the vinaigrette. You can omit the tomato-ginger vinaigrette and instead serve with any of the sauces on page 206.

CHICKEN
4 (6-ounce) boneless, skinless chicken breasts, trimmed of all visible fat
½ cup low-sodium soy sauce
6 garlic cloves, smashed and peeled

VINAIGRETTE
2 tablespoons extra-virgin olive oil
1 small shallot, minced
1 teaspoon grated fresh ginger
Pinch ground cumin
Pinch ground fennel
6 ounces cherry tomatoes, halved
Salt and pepper
1 tablespoon chopped fresh cilantro
1½ teaspoons red wine vinegar

1. FOR THE CHICKEN Pound chicken breasts to uniform thickness as needed. Whisk 4 quarts water, soy sauce, and garlic together in Dutch oven. Arrange breasts, skinned side up, in steamer basket, making sure not to overlap them. Submerge steamer basket in water.

2. Heat pot over medium heat, stirring liquid occasionally to even out hot spots, until water registers 175 degrees, 15 to 20 minutes. Turn off heat, cover pot, remove from burner, and let sit until chicken registers 160 degrees, 17 to 22 minutes. Transfer breasts to plate, tent with aluminum foil, and let rest while preparing vinaigrette.

3. FOR THE VINAIGRETTE Heat 1 tablespoon oil in 10-inch nonstick skillet over medium heat until shimmering. Add shallot, ginger, cumin, and fennel and cook until fragrant, about 15 seconds. Stir in tomatoes and ⅛ teaspoon salt and cook, stirring frequently, until tomatoes have softened, 3 to 5 minutes. Off heat, stir in cilantro, vinegar, and remaining 1 tablespoon oil. Season with pepper to taste. Spoon vinaigrette evenly over each breast before serving.

PER SERVING
Cal 280 • **Total Fat** 12g • **Sat Fat** 2g • **Chol** 125mg
Sodium 240mg • **Total Carbs** 3g • **Fiber** 1g • **Total Sugar** 2g
Added Sugar 0g • **Protein** 39g • **Total Carbohydrate Choices** 0

POUNDING CHICKEN BREASTS

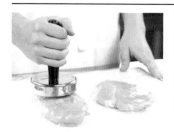

To create chicken breasts of even thickness, simply pound the thicker end of each breast until they are all of uniform thickness. Though some breasts will still be larger in size, at least they will cook at the same rate.

Pan-Seared Chicken Breasts with Leek and White Wine Pan Sauce

SERVES 4

WHY THIS RECIPE WORKS Simple pan-seared chicken breasts are an easy choice when aiming to eat more healthfully, but it can get tiresome to eat them again and again unless you can vary the flavorings. A great way to do that is to make a simple pan sauce using the fond left behind in the skillet. Here we turned to a classic leek and white wine sauce that is easy to execute and super flavorful thanks to the wine and just a tablespoon of butter, which we swirl in at the end along with fragrant tarragon and a little whole-grain mustard. You can omit the leek and white wine pan sauce and instead make any of the sauces on page 206.

CHICKEN

- 4 (6-ounce) boneless, skinless chicken breasts, trimmed of all visible fat
- Salt and pepper
- 1 tablespoon canola oil

PAN SAUCE

- 1 leek, white and light green parts only, halved lengthwise, sliced ¼ inch thick, and washed thoroughly
- Salt and pepper
- 1 teaspoon all-purpose flour
- ¾ cup unsalted chicken broth
- ½ cup dry white wine or dry vermouth
- 1 tablespoon unsalted butter, chilled
- 2 teaspoons chopped fresh tarragon
- 1 teaspoon whole-grain mustard

1. FOR THE CHICKEN Pound chicken breasts to uniform thickness as needed. Pat dry with paper towels and sprinkle with ¼ teaspoon salt and ⅛ teaspoon pepper. Heat oil in 12-inch skillet over medium-high heat until just smoking. Cook breasts, turning as needed, until well browned and register 160 degrees, about 10 minutes. Transfer breasts to plate, tent with aluminum foil, and let rest while preparing sauce.

2. FOR THE PAN SAUCE Pour off all but 2 teaspoons fat from skillet. (If necessary, add oil to equal 2 teaspoons.) Add leek and ⅛ teaspoon salt and cook over medium heat until softened and lightly browned, 5 to 7 minutes. Stir in flour and cook for 1 minute. Slowly whisk in broth and wine, scraping up any browned bits and smoothing out any lumps. Bring to simmer and cook sauce until thickened and measures about ¾ cup, 3 to 5 minutes.

3. Off heat, whisk in butter until combined, then whisk in tarragon, mustard, and any accumulated chicken juices. Season with pepper to taste. Spoon sauce evenly over each breast before serving.

PER SERVING

Cal 310 • **Total Fat** 11g • **Sat Fat** 3g • **Chol** 130mg
Sodium 350mg • **Total Carbs** 5g • **Fiber** 1g • **Total Sugar** 1g
Added Sugar 0g • **Protein** 39g • **Total Carbohydrate Choices** <0.5

NOTES FROM THE TEST KITCHEN

Parsing Poultry Parts

Chicken is one of the leanest meats and different cuts of chicken are essentially similar in their ratios of healthy fats to unhealthy fats but different in their relative total fat and total protein content. There are differences, too, between the taste of dark meat and light meat and between skinless chicken and chicken with skin (and the bones in bone-in chicken pieces can make it hard to figure out how many ounces you're actually eating). We've assembled a chart of the most common cuts we used in the recipes in this book.

	CAL	UNSAT FAT	SAT FAT
6 Ounces Boneless, Skinless Chicken Breast	204	4g	1g
6-Ounce Bone-In, Skinless Split Chicken Breast	163	4g	1g
6-Ounce Bone-In, Skin-On Split Chicken Breast	234	13g	3.5g
3 Ounces Boneless, Skinless Chicken Thigh	102	4g	1g
5-Ounce Bone-In, Skinless Chicken Thigh	103	4g	1g
5-Ounce Bone-In, Skin-On Chicken Thigh	266	20g	5g
4-Ounce Bone-In, Skinless Chicken Drumstick	76	2g	1g
4-Ounce Bone-In, Skin-On Chicken Drumstick	122	7g	2g
4 Ounces Ground Chicken	150	9g	2.5g
4 Ounces Boneless, Skinless Turkey Cutlet	120	1g	0g
4 Ounces Ground Turkey	120	2g	2g

Chicken Piccata
SERVES 4

WHY THIS RECIPE WORKS Chicken piccata is a simple Italian dish that highlights the incredibly tender texture of chicken cutlets (as opposed to whole chicken breast) as well as the fresh, clean flavor of lemon. The problem with most recipes, however, is that the chicken turns out rubbery and the sauce bland, with little lemon flavor. In addition, this dish often relies on an abundance of butter, turning what should be a light, fresh dish into a heavy one. To start, we decided to flour the chicken on just one side to keep it from becoming gummy and starchy. After sautéing the chicken in a little canola oil, we built a simple sauce by first cooking capers and garlic in the fat left behind and then deglazing the pan with broth and wine; we then simmered it all with strips of lemon zest, which infused the sauce with bold lemon flavor. We returned the chicken to the skillet to let it heat through in the sauce. Once our chicken was perfectly done, we gave our sauce its finishing touch by whisking in lemon juice and just a bit of butter to add richness and body. Make sure that the cutlets do not overcook—they take only about 4 minutes to cook through completely. If you can't find chicken cutlets at the supermarket, you can make your own by slicing four 6-ounce boneless, skinless chicken breasts in half horizontally. To make slicing the chicken easier, put it in the freezer for 15 minutes. Serve with lemon wedges.

¼ cup plus 1 teaspoon all-purpose flour
8 (3-ounce) chicken cutlets, ¼ inch thick, trimmed of all visible fat
⅛ teaspoon salt
⅛ teaspoon pepper
2 tablespoons canola oil
2 tablespoons capers, rinsed
2 garlic cloves, minced
1 cup unsalted chicken broth
½ cup dry white wine
4 (2-inch) strips lemon zest plus 4 teaspoons juice
1 tablespoon unsalted butter, chilled

1. Spread ¼ cup flour in shallow dish. Pat chicken cutlets dry with paper towels and sprinkle with salt and pepper. Working with 1 cutlet at a time, lightly dredge one side in flour, shaking off excess.

2. Heat 1 tablespoon oil in 12-inch skillet over medium heat until shimmering. Place 4 cutlets floured side down in skillet and cook until golden brown on first side, about 3 minutes. Flip cutlets and cook until no longer pink, about 1 minute. Transfer

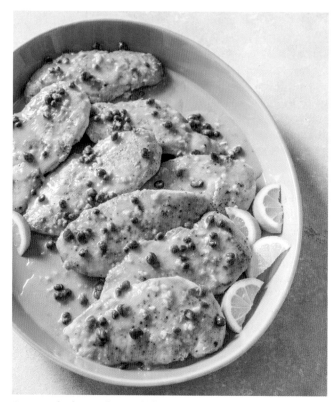

Coating chicken cutlets with flour on just one side prevents this classic Italian dish from becoming too heavy and starchy.

cutlets to large plate and tent with aluminum foil. Repeat with remaining 1 tablespoon oil and remaining 4 cutlets; transfer to plate and tent with foil.

3. Add capers and garlic to oil left in skillet and cook over medium heat until fragrant, about 30 seconds. Stir in remaining 1 teaspoon flour and cook for 1 minute. Slowly whisk in broth, wine, and lemon zest, scraping up any browned bits and smoothing out any lumps. Bring to simmer and cook sauce until thickened slightly and measures about ½ cup, 10 to 15 minutes.

4. Discard lemon zest. Nestle chicken into sauce along with any accumulated juices and cook until heated through, about 30 seconds. Transfer chicken to serving dish. Off heat, whisk lemon juice and butter into sauce until combined. Spoon sauce evenly over each cutlet before serving.

PER SERVING
Cal 340 • **Total Fat** 14g • **Sat Fat** 3g • **Chol** 130mg
Sodium 280mg • **Total Carbs** 5g • **Fiber** 1g • **Total Sugar** 1g
Added Sugar 0g • **Protein** 40g • **Total Carbohydrate Choices** <0.5

Capers 101

Capers are sun-dried pickled flower buds from the spiny shrub *Capparis spinosa*, and their unique flavor is most commonly found in French and Italian cooking. Capers pack an acidic punch with a lingering sweetness that is both floral and pungent. Capers range in size from tiny nonpareils to large caperberries, and they develop flavor from being cured, either in a brine (sometimes with vinegar) or packed in salt. Because of this, they tend to be high in sodium, so we always rinse them to remove some of the sodium. And because they pack so much distinct, briny flavor, just a tablespoon or two is all you need. Brined capers are the most commonly available, and we've found that we prefer the smaller nonpareil capers for their compact size and slight crunch. Our favorite brand is **Reese**.

PREPARING CHICKEN CUTLETS

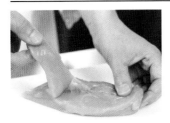

1. If small strip of meat (tenderloin) is loosely attached to underside of breast, pull it off and reserve for another use.

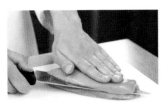

2. Lay chicken smooth side up on cutting board. With your hand on top of chicken, carefully slice it in half horizontally to yield 2 pieces between ⅜ and ½ inch thick.

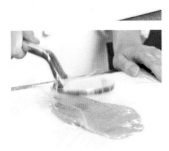

3. Lay each cutlet between 2 sheets of plastic wrap and pound with meat pounder or small skillet until roughly ¼ inch thick.

Almond-Crusted Chicken Breasts
SERVES 4

WHY THIS RECIPE WORKS One way to dress up a humble chicken breast for a weeknight dinner is to coat it with a layer of nuts, which offer more nutrients and a welcome crunch without all the carbs that a traditional breaded chicken breast would rack up. But many recipes go overboard on the coating. Looking for a way to keep the rich, nutty flavor of this dish intact, we found that instead of white bread crumbs we could swap in a half cup of whole-wheat panko bread crumbs for a good portion of the coating. As an added benefit, this move actually improved the texture of the coating by making it more crisp. Grinding the almonds to fine crumbs helped the nutty coating stick to the chicken, and toasting them with the panko in canola oil, along with chopped shallot and minced garlic, contributed some richness without making things greasy. Before breading the chicken, we brushed it with a mixture of yogurt and egg yolk, which further ensured the coating stayed in place while also helping the chicken stay moist and tender.

½ cup slivered almonds
2 tablespoons canola oil
1 large shallot, minced
¼ teaspoon salt
1 garlic clove, minced
1 teaspoon minced fresh thyme or ¼ teaspoon dried
½ cup 100 percent whole-wheat panko bread crumbs
¼ teaspoon pepper
2 tablespoons minced fresh parsley
1 tablespoon plain low-fat yogurt
1 large egg yolk
½ teaspoon grated lemon zest, plus lemon wedges for serving
4 (6-ounce) boneless, skinless chicken breasts, trimmed of all visible fat

1. Adjust oven rack to middle position and heat oven to 300 degrees. Set wire rack in rimmed baking sheet and lightly spray with canola oil spray. Process almonds in food processor until finely chopped, 20 to 30 seconds.

2. Heat oil in 12-inch nonstick skillet over medium heat until shimmering. Add shallot and salt and cook until softened, 1 to 2 minutes. Stir in garlic and thyme and cook until fragrant, about 30 seconds. Reduce heat to medium-low, add almonds, panko, and pepper and cook, stirring frequently, until well browned and crisp, about 8 minutes. Transfer almond mixture to shallow dish and let cool for 10 minutes. Stir in parsley.

3. Whisk yogurt, egg yolk, and lemon zest together in second shallow dish. Pound chicken breasts to uniform thickness as needed. Pat chicken breasts dry with paper towels and brush skinned side of breasts evenly with yogurt mixture. Working with 1 breast at a time, dredge coated side in nut mixture, pressing gently to adhere.

4. Transfer breasts crumb side up to prepared sheet and bake until chicken registers 160 degrees, 20 to 25 minutes, rotating sheet halfway through baking. Serve with lemon wedges.

PER SERVING

Cal 390 • **Total Fat** 19g • **Sat Fat** 2.5g • **Chol** 170mg
Sodium 240mg • **Total Carbs** 12g • **Fiber** 3g • **Total Sugar** 2g
Added Sugar 0g • **Protein** 43g • **Total Carbohydrate Choices** 1

NOTES FROM THE TEST KITCHEN

Tasting Boneless, Skinless Chicken Breasts

Americans roast plenty of whole chickens, but they cook even more chicken breasts. The lean white meat portions account for 60 percent of the chicken sold in stores, and the vast majority of those are the boneless, skinless variety.

Our investigation of boneless, skinless chicken breasts homed in on processing. And it was only when we asked the manufacturer of our winner, **Bell & Evans**, to walk us through its methods that we uncovered a good, albeit peculiar, reason for our findings: Once a Bell & Evans whole chicken is broken down into parts, the breasts are "aged" on the bone in chilled containers for as long as 12 hours before the bones (and skin) are removed. This aging period, it turns out, actually improves tenderness. While four to six hours of chilling before boning is effective—and 12 hours is ideal—many companies skip the aging process altogether. Why? Building time into the process costs money. Instead, some opt for shortcut tenderizing methods like electrical stimulation of the carcass, which forces the breast muscle to contract and relax, releasing its energy.

Tasters noticed the difference, lauding Bell & Evans breasts for being "mega-juicy and tender" and deeming the texture of breasts that came from an electrically stimulated carcass "unremarkable." Its $6.99 per pound price tag makes Bell & Evans relatively pricey, but we think the premium results more than justify the premium expense.

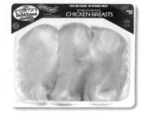

Parmesan-Crusted Chicken Breasts with Warm Bitter Greens and Fennel Salad
SERVES 4

WHY THIS RECIPE WORKS Chicken cutlets are often dripping with oil, smothered with handfuls of cheese, and served over a mountain of pasta. For a modern, healthier twist, we served flavorful cutlets with a fresh salad. Instead of a thick layer of cheese, we added a smaller amount of grated Parmesan to our whole-wheat breading, boosting the flavor with Italian seasonings. A nonstick skillet helped us use a moderate amount of oil while still browning the cutlets perfectly. To bring in some tomato flavor, we used our skillet to soften fennel and cherry tomatoes before tossing them with radicchio, frisée, and baby arugula in a simple vinaigrette for a warm, gently wilted salad. The slight bitterness of the greens paired well with the sweet fennel and juicy chicken.

½ cup all-purpose flour
2 large eggs
½ cup 100 percent whole-wheat panko bread crumbs
1 ounce Parmesan cheese, grated (½ cup)
½ teaspoon garlic powder
½ teaspoon dried oregano
4 (6-ounce) boneless, skinless chicken breasts, trimmed of all visible fat
5 tablespoons extra-virgin olive oil
1 tablespoon white wine vinegar
1½ teaspoons minced shallot
½ teaspoon Dijon mustard
Salt and pepper
2 fennel bulbs, stalks discarded, bulbs halved, cored, and sliced thin
1 pound cherry tomatoes, halved
½ head radicchio (5 ounces), cored and sliced thin
1 head frisée (6 ounces), trimmed and cut into bite-size pieces
3 ounces (3 cups) baby arugula

1. Adjust oven rack to middle position and heat oven to 200 degrees. Set wire rack in rimmed baking sheet. Spread flour in shallow dish. Beat eggs in second shallow dish. Combine panko, Parmesan, garlic powder, and oregano in third shallow dish. Pound chicken breasts to uniform thickness as needed, then pat dry with paper towels. Working with 1 breast at a time, dredge in flour, dip in egg, then coat with panko mixture, pressing gently to adhere.

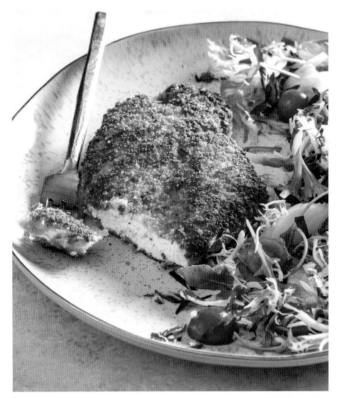

For an easy, great-tasting chicken dinner, we coat cutlets in a mix of panko and Parmesan cheese and serve them with a salad.

2. Heat 3 tablespoons oil in 12-inch nonstick skillet over medium heat until shimmering. Add 2 breasts and cook until chicken is tender, golden brown, and crisp, 3 to 4 minutes per side. Transfer to prepared sheet and keep warm in oven. Repeat with remaining 2 breasts; transfer to prepared sheet in oven.

3. Whisk 1 tablespoon oil, vinegar, shallot, mustard, ¼ teaspoon salt, and pinch pepper together in large bowl. Wipe skillet clean with paper towels. Heat remaining 1 tablespoon oil in skillet over medium heat until shimmering. Add fennel and cook until softened and lightly browned, 5 to 7 minutes. Add tomatoes and cook until beginning to soften, about 2 minutes. Transfer to bowl with vinaigrette along with radicchio, frisée, and arugula and gently toss to combine. Season with pepper to taste. Serve with chicken.

PER SERVING

Cal 570 • **Total Fat** 27g • **Sat Fat** 5g • **Chol** 220mg
Sodium 490mg • **Total Carbs** 30g • **Fiber** 8g • **Total Sugar** 9g
Added Sugar 0g • **Protein** 51g • **Total Carbohydrate Choices** 2

Pan-Seared Chicken Breasts with Warm Mediterranean Grain Pilaf
SERVES 4

WHY THIS RECIPE WORKS Here we pair lean, boneless, skinless chicken breasts rubbed with a little cumin, salt, and pepper with a bulgur side dish packed with vegetables and bold flavors. Since fine-grind bulgur takes only 5 minutes to cook, we were able to engineer this recipe to use just one pan. After cooking the chicken in a skillet, we sautéed frozen artichoke hearts, a great source of fiber, until they were nicely browned. Next, we steamed the bulgur directly in the skillet to take advantage of all that flavorful fond, which seasoned our grain side nicely. To finish, we simply stirred cherry tomatoes, feta cheese, parsley, olives, and a little lemon juice into the bulgur after steaming. When shopping, do not confuse bulgur with cracked wheat, which has a much longer cooking time and will not work in this recipe. Do not use coarse- or medium-grind bulgur in this recipe.

½ teaspoon ground cumin
   Salt and pepper
4 (6-ounce) boneless, skinless chicken breasts, trimmed of all visible fat
¼ cup extra-virgin olive oil
9 ounces frozen artichoke hearts, thawed and patted dry
1½ cups water
1 cup fine-grind bulgur
10 ounces cherry tomatoes, halved
3 ounces feta cheese, crumbled (¾ cup)
¾ cup minced fresh parsley
⅓ cup pitted kalamata olives, chopped
1 tablespoon lemon juice, plus lemon wedges for serving

1. Combine cumin, ¼ teaspoon salt, and ⅛ teaspoon pepper in bowl. Pound chicken breasts to uniform thickness as needed. Pat dry with paper towels and sprinkle with cumin mixture. Heat 1 tablespoon oil in 12-inch skillet over medium-high heat until just smoking. Cook breasts, turning as needed, until golden brown and register 160 degrees, about 10 minutes. Transfer breasts to plate, tent with aluminum foil, and let rest while preparing pilaf.

2. Heat 1 tablespoon oil in now-empty skillet over medium-high heat until shimmering. Add artichoke hearts and cook, without stirring, until spotty brown, about 2 minutes. Stir in water, scraping up any browned bits, and bring to boil. Stir in bulgur and ⅛ teaspoon salt. Off heat, cover and let sit until grains are softened and liquid is fully absorbed, about 5 minutes.

3. Add tomatoes, feta, parsley, olives, lemon juice, and remaining 2 tablespoons oil to pilaf and gently fluff with fork to combine. Season with pepper to taste. Serve chicken with pilaf and lemon wedges.

PER SERVING

Cal 560 • **Total Fat** 25g • **Sat Fat** 6g • **Chol** 145mg
Sodium 600mg • **Total Carbs** 37g • **Fiber** 10g • **Total Sugar** 3g
Added Sugar 0g • **Protein** 48g • **Total Carbohydrate Choices** 2.5

How Much Sodium Is in Brined Food?

There are a number of foods that we typically poach or soak in a saltwater solution, or brine, before cooking. The salt in the brine doesn't just season the food; in the case of meat, poultry, and fish, it improves juiciness and tenderness. It also helps dried beans cook faster and gives them a creamier texture and more tender skin (see Ultimate Beef Chili, page 79). That said, we've often wondered just how much sodium ends up in brined food, especially when considering the nutritional parameters of certain diets like that required for diabetes. To find out, we sent cooked samples of boneless, skinless chicken breasts that we brined for our standard recommended times to an independent lab for sodium analysis. We also analyzed plain water–soaked samples so that we could then subtract any naturally occurring sodium. Here's how much sodium brining adds to each food. (Note: The Dietary Guidelines for Americans recommend less than 2,300 milligrams daily for people under 51 and less than 1,500 milligrams for those 51 and older.)

Much to our surprise, we found that very little brining salt actually ends up in the final product. So we won't shy away from brining in certain recipes, as we believe the culinary benefits are certainly worth the scant amount of sodium it contributes. For example:

6 Ounces Cooked Boneless, Skinless Chicken Breast

BRINING FORMULA 2 quarts water, ¼ cup salt, 1 hour

ADDED SODIUM 270 milligrams

SALT EQUIVALENT Less than ⅛ teaspoon

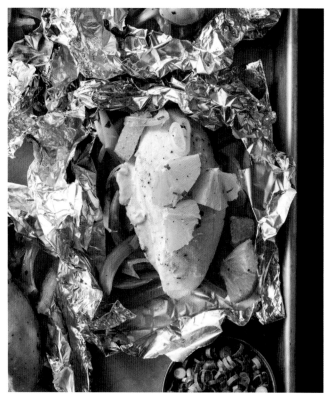

Steaming chicken in a foil packet with flavorful vegetables is a healthy way to cook the lean meat and keep it moist and juicy.

Chicken Baked in Foil with Fennel, Carrots, and Orange
SERVES 4

WHY THIS RECIPE WORKS Steaming in a pouch (we use aluminum foil) is an excellent way to cook delicate chicken breasts. Besides being healthy, this method is fast and convenient, and it keeps everything moist. We solved the bland problem by adding vegetables and fruits that are first tossed with a little olive oil and bold seasonings like tarragon and shallot. The result is moist, perfectly cooked chicken with highly flavorful vegetables. To prevent overcooking, open each packet promptly after baking.

2 oranges
2 tablespoons extra-virgin olive oil
1 shallot, sliced thin
1 teaspoon minced fresh tarragon
   Salt and pepper
2 carrots, peeled and cut into 2-inch-long matchsticks
1 fennel bulb, stalks discarded, bulb halved, cored, and sliced thin

4 (6-ounce) boneless, skinless chicken breasts, trimmed of all visible fat

2 scallions, sliced thin

1. Adjust oven rack to middle position and heat oven to 450 degrees. Cut eight 12-inch square sheets of aluminum foil.

2. Cut away peel and pith from oranges. Quarter oranges, then slice crosswise into ½-inch-thick pieces; transfer to bowl. Combine oil, shallot, tarragon, ¼ teaspoon salt, and ⅛ teaspoon pepper in separate medium bowl. Toss oranges with half of oil mixture. Add carrots and fennel to remaining oil mixture and toss to coat. Pound chicken breasts to uniform thickness as needed. Pat breasts dry with paper towels and sprinkle with ¼ teaspoon salt and ⅛ teaspoon pepper.

3. Arrange carrot-fennel mixture evenly in center of four pieces of foil. Lay breasts over vegetables then spoon orange mixture over top.

4. Place remaining pieces of foil on top and fold edges over several times to seal. Place packets on rimmed baking sheet and bake until chicken registers 160 degrees, about 25 minutes. (To test doneness of chicken, you will need to open one packet.)

5. Carefully open packets, allowing steam to escape away from you, and let cool briefly. Smooth out edges of foil and, using spatula, gently slide chicken, vegetables, and any accumulated juices onto individual plates. Sprinkle with scallions and serve.

PER SERVING

Cal 340 • **Total Fat** 12g • **Sat Fat** 2g • **Chol** 125mg
Sodium 420mg • **Total Carbs** 17g • **Fiber** 5g • **Total Sugar** 11g
Added Sugar 0g • **Protein** 40g • **Total Carbohydrate Choices** 1

VARIATION
Chicken Baked in Foil with Tomatoes and Zucchini
SERVES 4

WHY THIS RECIPE WORKS This variation relies on zucchini and tomatoes as a succulent chicken topping. To be sure the zucchini did not shed too much moisture, we first tossed it with a bit of salt to draw out the water. A pungent olive oil, garlic, oregano, red pepper flake, and pepper mixture united this dish. To prevent overcooking, open each packet promptly after baking.

2 zucchini, sliced ¼ inch thick
   Salt and pepper
2 tablespoons extra-virgin olive oil
2 garlic cloves, minced
1 teaspoon minced fresh oregano or ¼ teaspoon dried
⅛ teaspoon red pepper flakes

3 plum tomatoes, cored, seeded, and cut into ½-inch pieces
4 (6-ounce) boneless, skinless chicken breasts, trimmed of all visible fat
¼ cup chopped fresh basil
   Lemon wedges

1. Toss zucchini with ¼ teaspoon salt in colander and let drain for 30 minutes. Spread zucchini out on several layers of paper towels and pat dry; transfer to bowl. Adjust oven rack to middle position and heat oven to 450 degrees. Cut eight 12-inch square sheets of aluminum foil.

2. Combine oil, garlic, oregano, pepper flakes, and ⅛ teaspoon pepper in medium bowl. Toss zucchini with half of oil mixture in separate bowl. Add tomatoes to remaining oil mixture and toss to coat. Pound chicken breasts to uniform thickness as needed. Pat breasts dry with paper towels and sprinkle with ¼ teaspoon salt and ⅛ teaspoon pepper.

3. Arrange zucchini evenly in center of four pieces of foil. Lay breasts over zucchini then spoon tomato mixture over top.

4. Place remaining pieces of foil on top and fold edges over several times to seal. Place packets on rimmed baking sheet and bake until chicken registers 160 degrees, about 25 minutes. (To test doneness of chicken, you will need to open one packet.)

5. Carefully open packets, allowing steam to escape away from you, and let cool briefly. Smooth out edges of foil and, using spatula, gently slide chicken, vegetables, and any accumulated juices onto individual plates. Sprinkle with basil and serve with lemon wedges.

PER SERVING

Cal 300 • **Total Fat** 12g • **Sat Fat** 2g • **Chol** 125mg
Sodium 310mg • **Total Carbs** 6g • **Fiber** 2g • **Total Sugar** 3g
Added Sugar 0g • **Protein** 40g • **Total Carbohydrate Choices** <0.5

MAKING A FOIL PACKET

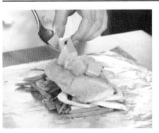 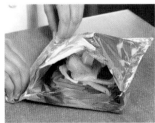

1. Arrange vegetables in center of sheet of aluminum foil. Lay chicken on top of vegetables and spoon topping over chicken.

2. Place second piece of foil on top of chicken and fold edges of foil together several times to create well-sealed packet.

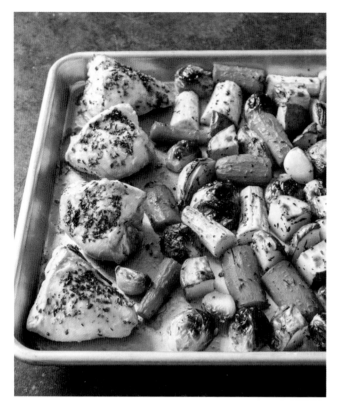

Tossing the vegetables with the chicken juices at the end of cooking amped up the flavor and kept everything moist.

One-Pan Roasted Chicken Breasts with Root Vegetables

SERVES 4

WHY THIS RECIPE WORKS Cooking vegetables and chicken together on the same sheet pan is a helpful and healthful technique which turns out an easy, go-to weeknight dinner. The chicken juices mix with the roasting vegetables, creating extra layers of flavor throughout the dish. We chose bone-in, skin-on breasts (we removed the skin before serving) to prevent drying out while roasting. We arranged the vegetables on two-thirds of the sheet and the breasts on the opposite end; this allowed the vegetables to get direct heat and roast in the same time it took to cook the chicken through.

- 12 ounces Brussels sprouts, trimmed and halved
- 12 ounces red potatoes, unpeeled, cut into 1-inch pieces
- 8 ounces parsnips, peeled and cut into 2-inch lengths, thick ends halved lengthwise
- 4 carrots, peeled and cut into 2-inch lengths, thick ends halved lengthwise
- 4 shallots, peeled and halved lengthwise
- 6 garlic cloves, peeled
- 3 tablespoons extra-virgin olive oil
- 4 teaspoons minced fresh thyme or 1½ teaspoons dried
- 2 teaspoons minced fresh rosemary or ¾ teaspoon dried
  Salt and pepper
- 2 (12-ounce) bone-in split chicken breasts, trimmed of all visible fat and halved crosswise
  Lemon wedges

1. Adjust oven rack to upper-middle position and heat oven to 475 degrees. Combine Brussels sprouts, potatoes, parsnips, carrots, shallots, garlic, 2 tablespoons oil, 2 teaspoons thyme, 1 teaspoon rosemary, ¼ teaspoon salt, and ¼ teaspoon pepper in bowl. Combine remaining 1 tablespoon oil, remaining 2 teaspoons thyme, remaining 1 teaspoon rosemary, ¼ teaspoon salt, and ⅛ teaspoon pepper in separate bowl.

2. Pound chicken breast pieces to uniform thickness as needed, then pat dry with paper towels. Using your fingers, gently loosen skin covering each breast piece, then rub oil mixture evenly under skin.

3. Spread vegetables cut side down in single layer over three-quarters of rimmed baking sheet. Place chicken pieces skin side up on empty portion of sheet. Roast until vegetables are browned and tender and chicken registers 160 degrees, 25 to 35 minutes, rotating sheet halfway through roasting. Discard chicken skin. Toss vegetables with any accumulated chicken juices. Serve with lemon wedges.

PER SERVING

Cal 410 • **Total Fat** 14g • **Sat Fat** 2.5g • **Chol** 80mg
Sodium 430mg • **Total Carbs** 43g • **Fiber** 10g • **Total Sugar** 11g
Added Sugar 0g • **Protein** 32g • **Total Carbohydrate Choices** 3

PREPPING BRUSSELS SPROUTS

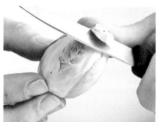 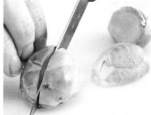

1. Peel off any loose or discolored leaves and slice off bottom of stem end, leaving leaves attached.

2. Cut sprouts in half through stem end so that leaves stay intact.

One-Pan Roasted Chicken Breasts with Butternut Squash and Kale
SERVES 4

WHY THIS RECIPE WORKS In order to combine sturdy squash, dark leafy greens, and chicken in a single pan, we'd need to get them to cook at the same rate. Halving bone-in split breasts assisted in even cooking as did starting the chicken and squash before the kale. A simple sage marinade seasoned both the chicken and vegetables. In just 25 minutes, we had crisp-skinned chicken, tender but not mushy squash, and lightly crispy kale. A sprinkling of unsweetened dried cherries added fiber and a sweet-tart chew to the mix. We topped our chicken with a drizzle of light, creamy yogurt sauce accented with orange zest and garlic to bring the dish into harmony. Both curly and Lacinato kale will work in this recipe.

5 tablespoons extra-virgin olive oil
2 tablespoons minced fresh sage
   Salt and pepper
¾ cup plain low-fat yogurt
1 tablespoon water
7 garlic cloves, peeled (6 halved, 1 minced)
1 teaspoon grated orange zest
2 pounds butternut squash, peeled, seeded, and cut into 1-inch pieces (6 cups)
8 shallots, peeled and halved lengthwise
2 teaspoons paprika
2 (12-ounce) bone-in split chicken breasts, trimmed of all visible fat and halved crosswise
8 ounces kale, stemmed and cut into 2-inch pieces
½ cup unsweetened dried cherries

1. Adjust oven rack to upper-middle position and heat oven to 475 degrees. Combine oil, sage, ½ teaspoon salt, and ½ teaspoon pepper in bowl. Combine yogurt, water, minced garlic, orange zest, and 1 tablespoon oil mixture in separate bowl. Season with pepper to taste and refrigerate sauce until ready to serve.

2. Combine squash, shallots, halved garlic cloves, and 3 tablespoons oil mixture in large bowl; set aside. Stir paprika into remaining oil mixture. Pound chicken breast pieces to uniform thickness as needed, then pat dry with paper towels. Using your fingers, gently loosen skin covering each breast piece, then rub remaining oil mixture evenly under skin.

3. Spread vegetable mixture in single layer over three-quarters of rimmed baking sheet. Place chicken pieces skin side up on empty portion of sheet and roast for 15 minutes.

4. Meanwhile, vigorously squeeze and massage kale with hands in now-empty bowl until leaves are uniformly darkened and slightly wilted, about 1 minute. Rotate sheet, stir kale and cherries into vegetables, and roast until vegetables are browned and tender and chicken registers 160 degrees, 10 to 20 minutes, stirring vegetables halfway through roasting.

5. Discard chicken skin. Toss vegetables with any accumulated chicken juices. Serve, passing yogurt sauce separately.

PER SERVING

Cal 580 • **Total Fat** 23g • **Sat Fat** 4g • **Chol** 100mg
Sodium 420mg • **Total Carbs** 56g • **Fiber** 9g • **Total Sugar** 19g
Added Sugar 0g • **Protein** 40g • **Total Carbohydrate Choices** 4

One-Pan Roasted Chicken Breasts with Cauliflower, Shallots, and Tomatoes
SERVES 4

WHY THIS RECIPE WORKS A sheet pan full of roast chicken, cauliflower, and tomatoes is the promise of a satisfying, nutritious meal with minimal cleanup. We used halved bone-in split chicken breasts, which cook more quickly than a whole chicken, and rubbed the meat with seasoned oil. Cutting the cauliflower into wedges provided a flat side for good contact with the baking sheet. Grape tomatoes added nice color and juicy bursts of acidity. Tossing the vegetables with the chicken juices at the end added flavor and moisture.

1 head cauliflower (2 pounds), cored and cut into 8 wedges through stem end
6 shallots, peeled and halved lengthwise
¼ cup extra-virgin olive oil
2 tablespoons chopped fresh sage or 2 teaspoons dried
   Salt and pepper
2 garlic cloves, minced
1 teaspoon grated lemon zest, plus lemon wedges for serving
2 (12-ounce) bone-in split chicken breasts, trimmed of all visible fat and halved crosswise
8 ounces grape tomatoes
1 tablespoon chopped fresh parsley

1. Adjust oven rack to upper-middle position and heat oven to 475 degrees. Combine cauliflower, shallots, 2 tablespoons oil, 1 tablespoon sage, ¼ teaspoon salt, and ½ teaspoon pepper in bowl. Combine garlic, lemon zest, remaining 2 tablespoons oil, remaining 1 tablespoon sage, ¼ teaspoon salt, and ⅛ teaspoon pepper in separate bowl.

2. Pound chicken breast pieces to uniform thickness as needed, then pat dry with paper towels. Using your fingers, gently loosen skin covering each breast piece, then rub oil mixture evenly under skin.

3. Spread vegetables cut side down in single layer over three-quarters of rimmed baking sheet. Place chicken pieces skin side up on empty portion of sheet and roast for 15 minutes. Rotate sheet, spread tomatoes over vegetables, and roast until vegetables are browned and tender and chicken registers 160 degrees, 10 to 20 minutes. Discard chicken skin. Toss vegetables with parsley and any accumulated chicken juices. Serve with lemon wedges.

PER SERVING

Cal 360 • **Total Fat** 18g • **Sat Fat** 3g • **Chol** 100mg
Sodium 390mg • **Total Carbs** 15g • **Fiber** 4g • **Total Sugar** 7g
Added Sugar 0g • **Protein** 34g • **Total Carbohydrate Choices** 1

NOTES FROM THE TEST KITCHEN

Buying Chicken

Here is what you should know before you head to the meat counter.

Boneless, Skinless Breasts and Cutlets Boneless, skinless chicken breasts are the weeknight warrior of the meat world, as they are quick to prepare and can adapt to almost any flavor profile. They're also a great choice for those paying close attention to nutrition labels as they're low in fat and high in protein. Try to pick a package with breasts of similar size, and pound them to an even thickness so they will cook at the same rate. You can buy cutlets ready to go at the grocery store, but we don't recommend it. These cutlets are usually ragged and of various sizes; it's better to cut your own cutlets from breasts.

Bone-In Parts You can buy a whole chicken or chicken parts at the supermarket, but sometimes it's hard to tell by looking at the package if the chicken has been properly butchered. If you have extra time, buy a whole chicken and butcher it yourself.

Whole Chickens Whole chickens come in various sizes. Broilers and fryers are younger chickens that weigh 2½ to 4½ pounds. A roaster (or "oven-stuffer roaster") is an older chicken and usually clocks in between 5 and 7 pounds. Stewing chickens, which are older laying hens, are best used for stews since the meat is tougher and more stringy. A 3½-to 4-pound bird will feed four people.

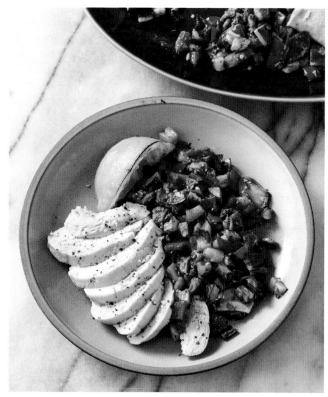

To prevent the vegetables from becoming soggy, we roast them in an even layer on a baking sheet before adding the chicken.

One-Pan Roasted Chicken Breasts with Ratatouille
SERVES 4

WHY THIS RECIPE WORKS Roasted chicken and ratatouille is simplicity on a plate: the flavors of summer in perfect balance. It's also a great option for a weeknight dinner. Despite its simple nature, the preparation can be onerous, requiring multiple pans and cooking stages for the ratatouille alone. Seeking an easier method, we turned to a sheet pan. Not only would its large surface area accommodate both the chicken and the vegetables, but exposing the vegetables to dry heat would prevent them from becoming soggy—a hallmark of bad ratatouille. We selected bone-in chicken breasts, which gave us juicy, tender meat without being too fussy or producing too much grease, and pounded them to an even thickness to ensure they cooked at the same rate. We chopped eggplant, zucchini, and red bell pepper into bite-size pieces and tossed them with canned tomatoes (ideal for year-round cooking), seasoning them with garlic and plenty of thyme to drive home the authentic flavor. We started by roasting the vegetables alone first to achieve nice browning on the eggplant and ensure all the vegetables had plenty of time to become tender. Halfway through roasting, we stirred the vegetables, added the chicken, and added lemon wedges to roast for a flavor boost. Just 15 minutes later, our chicken was ready, the ratatouille was tender and moist but not wet, and we even had juicy roasted lemon wedges to squeeze over everything.

- 1 (14.5-ounce) can no-salt-added diced tomatoes, drained
- 12 ounces eggplant, cut into ½-inch pieces
- 1 small zucchini (6 ounces), cut into ½-inch pieces
- 1 red bell pepper, stemmed, seeded, and cut into ½-inch pieces
- 2 tablespoons extra-virgin olive oil
- 4 garlic cloves, halved
- 1 tablespoon minced fresh thyme or 1½ teaspoons dried
  Salt and pepper
- 2 (12-ounce) bone-in split chicken breasts, trimmed of all visible fat and halved crosswise
- 1 lemon, quartered
- 2 tablespoons minced fresh parsley

1. Adjust oven rack to upper-middle position and heat oven to 475 degrees. Lightly grease rimmed baking sheet with canola oil spray. Toss tomatoes, eggplant, zucchini, bell pepper, oil, garlic, 1 teaspoon thyme, ¼ teaspoon salt, and ¼ teaspoon pepper together in bowl. Spread vegetables in even layer over prepared sheet and roast until beginning to wilt, about 15 minutes.

2. Combine remaining 2 teaspoons thyme, ¼ teaspoon salt, and ⅛ teaspoon pepper in bowl. Pound chicken breast pieces to uniform thickness as needed. Pat dry with paper towels and sprinkle with thyme mixture.

3. Using spatula, stir vegetables, then clear one-quarter of sheet and redistribute vegetables into even layer. Place chicken pieces skin side up and lemon wedges cut side down on now-empty portion of sheet. Roast until vegetables are browned and tender and chicken registers 160 degrees, about 15 minutes, rotating sheet hallway through roasting. Discard chicken skin. Toss vegetables with parsley and any accumulated chicken juices. Serve with lemon wedges.

PER SERVING

Cal 290 • **Total Fat** 11g • **Sat Fat** 2g • **Chol** 100mg
Sodium 370mg • **Total Carbs** 14g • **Fiber** 5g • **Total Sugar** 7g
Added Sugar 0g • **Protein** 33g • **Total Carbohydrate Choices** 1

Pomegranate-Glazed Chicken Breasts with Farro Salad
SERVES 4

WHY THIS RECIPE WORKS Pomegranate molasses is a powerhouse of an ingredient. Used sparingly, it can transform mild-tasting chicken breasts with its sweet-tart flavor and lustrous sheen. Applying the glaze to the chicken in stages allowed each layer to thicken and brown before we added another coating. A little cinnamon further increased the dish's complexity. Roasting the breasts on the bones helped keep the meat juicy. To round out this rich centerpiece, we tossed cooked and cooled farro, fresh tomatoes, cucumbers, and mint with a zippy yogurt-lemon dressing. Mixing in some almonds added some nice crunch and favorable fat. We prefer the flavor and texture of whole farro; pearled farro can be used, but the texture may be softer. Do not use quick-cooking or presteamed farro (read the ingredient list on the package to determine this). The cooking time for farro can vary greatly among different brands, so we recommend beginning to check for doneness after 10 minutes.

- 1 cup whole farro
  Salt and pepper
- ¼ cup pomegranate molasses
- ½ teaspoon ground cinnamon
- 2 (12-ounce) bone-in split chicken breasts, skin removed, trimmed of all visible fat, and halved crosswise
- 3 tablespoons extra-virgin olive oil
- 2 tablespoons lemon juice
- 2 tablespoons 2 percent Greek yogurt
- 1 shallot, minced
- 1 English cucumber, halved lengthwise and cut into ¼-inch pieces
- 8 ounces cherry tomatoes, halved
- ¼ cup chopped fresh mint
- ¼ cup toasted sliced almonds

1. Bring 4 quarts water to boil in large pot. Add farro and 1 teaspoon salt and cook until grains are tender with slight chew, 15 to 30 minutes. Drain farro well. Transfer to platter and spread into even layer. Let cool completely, about 15 minutes.

2. Adjust oven rack to middle position and heat oven to 450 degrees. Set wire rack in aluminum foil–lined rimmed baking sheet and lightly spray with canola oil spray. Combine pomegranate molasses and cinnamon in small bowl; measure out and reserve 1 tablespoon glaze for serving.

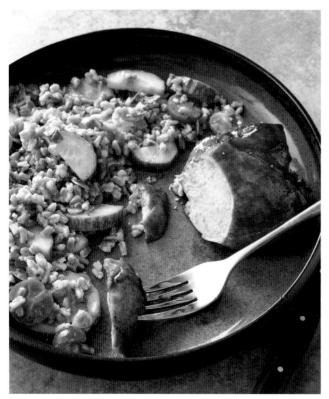

A glaze of spiced pomegranate molasses adds a new dimension to simple pan-roasted chicken.

3. Pound chicken breast pieces to uniform thickness as needed. Pat dry with paper towels and sprinkle with ¼ teaspoon salt and ⅛ teaspoon pepper. Transfer skinned side up to prepared rack and brush with 1½ tablespoons of glaze. Roast until chicken registers 160 degrees, 20 to 25 minutes, rotating sheet and brushing chicken with remaining glaze halfway through roasting.

4. Whisk oil, lemon juice, yogurt, shallot, ¼ teaspoon salt, and ¼ teaspoon pepper in large bowl until combined. Add farro, cucumber, tomatoes, mint, and almonds and gently toss to combine. Brush chicken with reserved glaze and serve with farro salad.

PER SERVING

Cal 480 • **Total Fat** 18g • **Sat Fat** 2.5g • **Chol** 70mg
Sodium 390mg • **Total Carbs** 54g • **Fiber** 6g • **Total Sugar** 13g
Added Sugar 0g • **Protein** 30g • **Total Carbohydrate Choices** 3.5

Braised Chicken Breasts with Chickpeas and Chermoula
SERVES 4

WHY THIS RECIPE WORKS Hearty and rustic, braised bone-in chicken breasts become juicy and tender as they simmer and lend their succulent flavor to the surrounding ingredients. We first browned skin-on breasts to develop lots of flavorful fond (we later discarded the skin in favor of a healthier dish). For this relatively quick-cooking braise, flavors needed to develop quickly. We added a very aromatic vegetable to the mix: Fennel, cooked until softened, worked perfectly, as its lively, licorice-like flavor added a soft but sturdy balance. Although beginning to take shape nicely, our dish lacked the hearty, starchy component that would make it a complete meal. Chickpeas were a natural fit; as they braised, they picked up great flavor from both the chicken and fennel. To pack even more flavor into our dish, we added homemade chermoula. This bold Moroccan green sauce worked overtime, seasoning the chickpeas and fennel and also serving as a bright, potent topping to drizzle over the juicy chicken. For a punch of freshness, we also stirred fennel fronds into the chickpea and fennel mixture. If you can't find fennel bulbs with their fronds intact, you can omit the fronds, or substitute minced parsley.

1½ cups fresh cilantro leaves
  6 tablespoons extra-virgin olive oil
  3 tablespoons lemon juice, plus lemon wedges for serving
  4 garlic cloves, minced
  1 teaspoon ground cumin
  1 teaspoon paprika
¼ teaspoon cayenne pepper
   Salt and pepper
  2 (12-ounce) bone-in split chicken breasts, trimmed of all visible fat and halved crosswise
  2 fennel bulbs, 2 tablespoons fronds minced, stalks discarded, bulbs halved, cored, and sliced thin
¾ cup unsalted chicken broth
  2 (15-ounce) cans no-salt-added chickpeas, rinsed

1. Process cilantro, ¼ cup oil, lemon juice, garlic, cumin, paprika, cayenne, and ¼ teaspoon salt in food processor until finely ground, about 1 minute, scraping down sides of bowl as needed. Transfer chermoula to bowl and set aside for serving.

2. Pound chicken breast pieces to uniform thickness as needed, pat dry with paper towels, and season with ¼ teaspoon salt and ¼ teaspoon pepper.

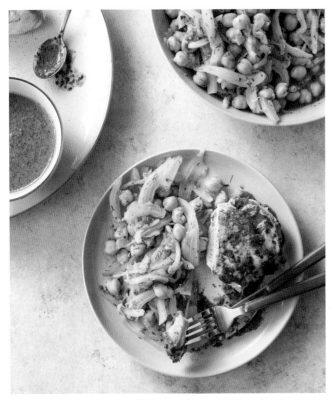

A fresh chermoula sauce of cilantro, lemon, and garlic gives hearty braised chicken a big punch of flavor.

3. Heat 1 tablespoon oil in Dutch oven over medium-high heat until just smoking. Cook breast pieces skin side down in pot until well browned, 4 to 6 minutes; transfer to plate.

4. Heat remaining 1 tablespoon oil in now-empty pot over medium heat until shimmering. Add fennel and cook until softened, about 5 minutes. Stir in broth, scraping up any browned bits. Stir in chickpeas and bring to simmer. Nestle chicken pieces into pot along with any accumulated juices. Reduce heat to medium-low, cover, and cook until chicken registers 160 degrees, 15 to 20 minutes.

5. Transfer chicken to plate and discard skin. Stir fennel fronds and 1 tablespoon chermoula into chickpea mixture. Top individual portions of chicken and chickpea mixture evenly with remaining chermoula. Serve with lemon wedges.

PER SERVING

Cal 550 • **Total Fat** 26g • **Sat Fat** 4g • **Chol** 100mg
Sodium 480mg • **Total Carbs** 35g • **Fiber** 10g • **Total Sugar** 6g
Added Sugar 0g • **Protein** 41g • **Total Carbohydrate Choices** 2

Cumin-Crusted Chicken Thighs with Cauliflower Couscous
SERVES 4

WHY THIS RECIPE WORKS Cauliflower is a versatile choice to replace pasta or another starchy side dish and a great way to increase the vegetable content of a meal. We used it to make a "couscous"-style side to accompany cumin-crusted boneless chicken thighs that cooked quickly and stayed moist. We pulsed the cauliflower in the food processor to a crumbly consistency before lightly sautéing it. We flavored our "couscous" with paprika and cumin and cooked it over medium-high heat to allow the edges to get crisp. After our cauliflower was done cooking, we stirred in pomegranate seeds, lime zest, and mint, which gave our dish a boost of fiber and color. Serving the finished dish with lime wedges provided a final bright, citrusy punch of flavor.

8 (3-ounce) boneless, skinless chicken thighs, trimmed of all visible fat
2 teaspoons cumin seeds
   Salt and pepper
2 tablespoons canola oil
1 head cauliflower (2 pounds), cored and cut into ½-inch pieces
1 teaspoon paprika
½ cup pomegranate seeds
½ cup chopped fresh mint
1½ teaspoons grated lime zest, plus lime wedges for serving

1. Pat chicken thighs dry with paper towels and sprinkle with 1 teaspoon cumin seeds, ¼ teaspoon salt, and ¼ teaspoon pepper. Heat 1 tablespoon oil in 12-inch nonstick skillet over medium-high heat until just smoking. Cook thighs, turning as needed, until well browned and register 175 degrees, about 8 minutes. Transfer chicken to plate, tent with aluminum foil, and let rest while preparing cauliflower.

2. Working in 2 batches, pulse cauliflower in food processor to ¼- to ⅛-inch pieces, about 6 pulses. Heat remaining 1 tablespoon oil in now-empty skillet over medium-high heat until shimmering. Add cauliflower, paprika, ⅛ teaspoon salt, ¼ teaspoon pepper, and remaining 1 teaspoon cumin seeds and cook, stirring occasionally, until just tender, about 7 minutes. Off heat, stir in pomegranate seeds, chopped mint, and lime zest. Serve chicken with couscous and lime wedges.

PER SERVING

Cal 320 • **Total Fat** 15g • **Sat Fat** 2.5g • **Chol** 160mg
Sodium 410mg • **Total Carbs** 10g • **Fiber** 4g • **Total Sugars** 5g
Added Sugars 0g • **Protein** 36g • **Total Carbohydrate Choices** >0.5

Poultry Safety and Handling

It's important to follow some basic safety procedures when storing, handling, and cooking chicken, turkey, and other poultry.

Refrigerating Keep poultry refrigerated until just before cooking. Bacteria thrive at temperatures between 40 and 140 degrees. This means leftovers should also be promptly refrigerated.

Freezing and Thawing Poultry can be frozen in its original packaging or after repackaging. If you are freezing it for longer than two months, rewrap (or wrap over the packaging) with aluminum foil or plastic wrap, or place it inside a zipper-lock bag. You can keep poultry frozen for several months, but after two months the texture and flavor will suffer. Don't thaw frozen poultry on the counter; this puts it at risk of growing bacteria. Thaw it in its packaging in the refrigerator (in a container to catch its juices), or in the sink under cold running water. Count on one day of defrosting in the refrigerator for every 4 pounds of bird.

Handling Raw Poultry When handling raw poultry, make sure to wash hands, knives, cutting boards, and counters (and anything else that has come into contact with the raw bird, its juices, or your hands) with hot, soapy water. Be careful not to let the poultry, its juices, or your unwashed hands touch foods that will be eaten raw. When seasoning raw poultry, touching the saltshaker or pepper mill can lead to cross-contamination. To avoid this, set aside the necessary salt and pepper before handling the poultry.

Rinsing The U.S. Department of Agriculture advises against washing poultry. Rinsing poultry will not remove or kill much bacteria, and the splashing of water around the sink can spread the bacteria found in raw poultry.

Cooking and Leftovers Poultry should be cooked to an internal temperature of 160 degrees to ensure that any bacteria have been killed (however, we prefer the flavor and texture of thigh meat cooked to 175 degrees). Leftover cooked poultry should be refrigerated and consumed within three days.

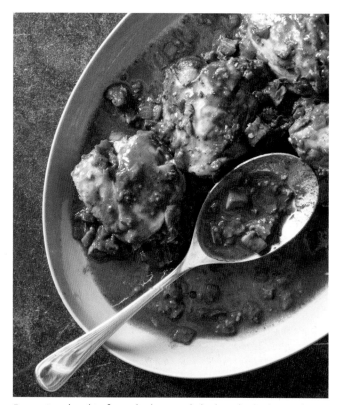

Removing the skin from the browned chicken thighs keeps the sauce from becoming greasy.

Braised Chicken Thighs with Mushrooms and Tomatoes
SERVES 4

WHY THIS RECIPE WORKS Classic chicken *cacciatore*, an Italian stew that includes earthy mushrooms, tomatoes, and red wine, should boast moist meat and a silken, robust sauce. Too often, though, the chicken is dry and the sauce greasy and unbalanced. Using chicken thighs and removing the skin after rendering the fat solved the problems of dry meat, soggy skin, and greasy sauce in our Italian-inspired braise. Cooking the chicken in a combination of red wine, chicken broth, and diced tomatoes, plus seasoning with fresh thyme, yielded moist, well-seasoned chicken. Portobello mushrooms gave the dish a meatier flavor, and fresh sage, to finish, highlighted our braise's woodsy notes. The Parmesan cheese rind is optional, but we highly recommend it for the rich, savory flavor it adds to the dish.

4 (5-ounce) bone-in chicken thighs, trimmed of all visible fat
   Salt and pepper
1 tablespoon extra-virgin olive oil
1 onion, chopped
6 ounces portobello mushroom caps, cut into ¾-inch pieces
1½ tablespoons all-purpose flour
4 garlic cloves, minced
2 teaspoons minced fresh thyme or ½ teaspoon dried
1½ cups dry red wine
½ cup unsalted chicken broth
1 (14.5-ounce) can no-salt-added diced tomatoes, drained
1 Parmesan cheese rind (optional)
2 teaspoons minced fresh sage

1. Adjust oven rack to middle position and heat oven to 300 degrees. Pat chicken thighs dry with paper towels and season with ¼ teaspoon salt and ¼ teaspoon pepper. Heat oil in Dutch oven over medium-high heat until just smoking. Brown thighs, 5 to 6 minutes per side; transfer to plate and discard skin.

2. Pour off all but 1 tablespoon fat from pot. Add onion, mushrooms, and ⅛ teaspoon salt and cook over medium heat until softened and lightly browned, 6 to 8 minutes. Stir in flour, garlic, and thyme and cook until fragrant, about 1 minute. Slowly whisk in wine, scraping up any browned bits and smoothing out any lumps.

3. Stir in broth, tomatoes, cheese rind, if using, and pinch salt and bring to simmer. Nestle thighs into pot and add any accumulated juices, cover, and transfer to oven. Cook until chicken registers 195 degrees, 35 to 40 minutes.

4. Remove pot from oven and transfer chicken to plate. Discard cheese rind, if using. Stir sage into sauce and season with pepper to taste. Spoon sauce evenly over each portion of chicken before serving.

PER SERVING

Cal 330 • **Total Fat** 10g • **Sat Fat** 2g • **Chol** 135mg
Sodium 420mg • **Total Carbs** 13g • **Fiber** 3g • **Total Sugar** 5g
Added Sugar 0g • **Protein** 31g • **Total Carbohydrate Choices** 1

REMOVING CHICKEN SKIN

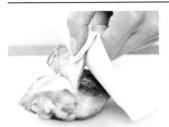

Chicken skin is often slippery, making it a challenge to remove by hand, even when the chicken has been browned. To simplify the task, use a paper towel to provide extra grip while pulling.

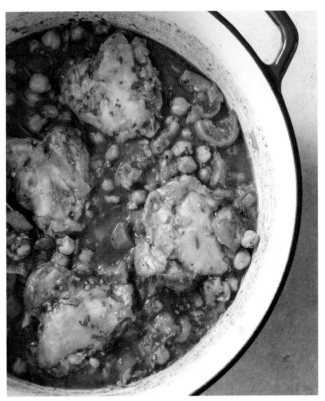

We flavor our chicken tagine with a warm mix of spices but temper their heat with dried apricots.

Chicken Tagine with Chickpeas and Apricots
SERVES 4

WHY THIS RECIPE WORKS Tagines are a North African specialty: exotically spiced, assertively flavored stews slow-cooked in earthenware vessels of the same name. They can include all manner of meats, vegetables, and fruit. Traditional recipes usually require a time-consuming cooking method, the special pot (the tagine), and hard-to-find ingredients; we wanted to make tagine more accessible. We found that braising in a Dutch oven was a serviceable substitute for stewing for hours in a tagine. To keep things easy we turned to meaty, bone-in chicken thighs and removed the skin after browning them. Chickpeas, carrots, onion, and garlic rounded out the stew. We created a spice blend for our tagine that was short on ingredients but created big flavor without adding any salt. Cumin and ginger lent depth, cinnamon brought warmth that tempered the cayenne's heat, and citrusy coriander boosted the stew's lemon flavor (as did a couple of broad ribbons of lemon zest); paprika colored the broth a deep, attractive red and lent a pleasant sweetness, as did the dried apricots.

3 (2-inch) strips lemon zest plus 3 tablespoons juice
5 garlic cloves, minced
4 (5-ounce) bone-in chicken thighs, trimmed of all visible fat
  Salt and pepper
1 tablespoon extra-virgin olive oil
1 large onion, halved and sliced ¼ inch thick
1¼ teaspoons paprika
½ teaspoon ground cumin
¼ teaspoon cayenne pepper
¼ teaspoon ground ginger
¼ teaspoon ground coriander
¼ teaspoon ground cinnamon
2 cups unsalted chicken broth
2 carrots, peeled, halved lengthwise, and sliced ½ inch thick
1 (15-ounce) can no-salt-added chickpeas, rinsed
½ cup dried apricots, halved
2 tablespoons chopped fresh cilantro

1. Adjust oven rack to middle position and heat oven to 300 degrees. Mince 1 strip lemon zest and combine with 1 teaspoon garlic in bowl; set aside.

2. Pat chicken thighs dry with paper towels and season with ¼ teaspoon salt and ¼ teaspoon pepper. Heat oil in Dutch oven over medium-high heat until just smoking. Brown thighs, 5 to 6 minutes per side; transfer to plate and discard skin.

3. Pour off all but 1 tablespoon fat from pot. Add onion, ¼ teaspoon salt, and remaining lemon zest strips and cook over medium heat until softened, about 5 minutes. Stir in paprika, cumin, cayenne, ginger, coriander, cinnamon, and remaining garlic and cook until fragrant, about 1 minute. Stir in broth, scraping up any browned bits.

4. Stir in carrots and chickpeas and bring to simmer. Nestle thighs into pot and add any accumulated juices, cover, and transfer to oven. Cook until chicken registers 195 degrees, 35 to 40 minutes.

5. Remove pot from oven. Transfer chicken to plate, tent with aluminum foil, and let rest while finishing sauce. Discard lemon zest. Stir in apricots, return sauce to simmer over medium heat, and cook until heated through, about 5 minutes. Stir in cilantro, lemon juice, and garlic–lemon zest mixture and season with pepper to taste.

6. Off heat, return chicken to pot along with any accumulated juices and let sit until heated through, about 2 minutes. Serve.

PER SERVING
Cal 290 • **Total Fat** 8g • **Sat Fat** 1.5g • **Chol** 80mg
Sodium 480mg • **Total Carbs** 31g • **Fiber** 7g • **Total Sugar** 14g
Added Sugar 0g • **Protein** 24g • **Total Carbohydrate Choices** 2

Latin-Style Chicken and Brown Rice
SERVES 4

WHY THIS RECIPE WORKS When done right, *arroz con pollo* (literally, "rice with chicken") is satisfying Latino comfort food—tender chicken nestled in rice rich with peppers, onions, and herbs. But the traditional method for making it takes all day; we wanted to turn this one-dish dinner into a fast but flavorful weeknight meal and keep it healthy at the same time. Using just boneless, skinless chicken thighs ensured that all the chicken would cook through at the same rate. To ensure the chicken was flavorful, we tossed it with a potent marinade of garlic and cider vinegar. The base for this dish was a mixture of sautéed chopped onion and green pepper to which we added broth and diced tomatoes. Switching out white rice for brown upped the fiber content. Once the chicken was perfectly cooked and the rice had absorbed most of the liquid, we simply shredded the chicken, let the rice steam for another 10 minutes, and then mixed in the pungent ingredients that are the hallmark of this dish: roasted red peppers, green olives, capers, and cilantro.

8 garlic cloves, minced
1 tablespoon cider vinegar
2 teaspoons minced fresh oregano or ½ teaspoon dried
  Pepper
1 pound boneless, skinless chicken thighs, trimmed of all visible fat
1 tablespoon canola oil
1 onion, chopped fine
1 green bell pepper, stemmed, seeded, and chopped
1 cup long-grain brown rice, rinsed
⅛ teaspoon red pepper flakes
¾ cup unsalted chicken broth
1 (14.5-ounce) can no-salt added diced tomatoes
½ cup jarred roasted red peppers, rinsed, patted dry, and sliced thin
½ cup pitted large brine-cured green olives, chopped
¼ cup minced fresh cilantro
2 tablespoons capers, rinsed
  Lemon wedges

1. Adjust oven rack to middle position and heat oven to 300 degrees. Combine half of garlic, vinegar, oregano, and ¼ teaspoon pepper in large bowl. Add chicken and toss to coat.

2. Heat oil in Dutch oven over medium heat until shimmering. Add onion and bell pepper and cook until softened, about 5 minutes. Stir in rice, pepper flakes, and remaining garlic and cook until fragrant, about 30 seconds. Stir in broth and tomatoes and their juice, scraping up any browned bits, and bring to simmer.

3. Nestle chicken on top of rice, cover, and transfer pot to oven. Cook until rice is tender and liquid is almost fully absorbed, 50 to 65 minutes.

4. Transfer chicken to cutting board, let cool slightly, then shred into bite-size pieces using 2 forks. Meanwhile, cover pot and let rice steam for 10 minutes.

5. Add chicken, red peppers, olives, cilantro, and capers to pot and gently fluff rice with fork to combine. Season with pepper to taste. Serve with lemon wedges.

PER SERVING

Cal 410 • **Total Fat** 12g • **Sat Fat** 1g • **Chol** 90mg
Sodium 570mg • **Total Carbs** 53g • **Fiber** 7g • **Total Sugar** 8g
Added Sugar 0g • **Protein** 29g • **Total Carbohydrate Choices** 3.5

Grilled Chicken Kebabs with Tomato-Feta Salad
SERVES 4

WHY THIS RECIPE WORKS Grilled chicken kebabs are a healthy option, but they often dry out on the grill. For this recipe, we first created a zesty vinaigrette that could pull double duty as the base for the marinade for the chicken and as the dressing for our simple tomato-feta salad. While the tomato salad sat in the fragrant dressing, we turned to the chicken—just ¼ cup of yogurt added to the vinaigrette made for a luxurious coating and ensured the chicken stayed moist on the grill. You will need four 12-inch metal skewers for this recipe.

- ¼ cup extra-virgin olive oil
- 1 teaspoon grated lemon zest plus 3 tablespoons juice
- 3 garlic cloves, minced
- 1 tablespoon minced fresh oregano
  Salt and pepper
- 1 pound cherry tomatoes, halved
- 3 ounces feta cheese, crumbled (¾ cup)
- ¼ cup thinly sliced red onion
- ¼ cup plain low-fat yogurt
- 1½ pounds boneless, skinless chicken breasts, trimmed of all visible fat and cut into 1-inch pieces

1. Whisk oil, lemon zest and juice, garlic, oregano, ¼ teaspoon salt, and ½ teaspoon pepper together in medium bowl. Reserve half of oil mixture in separate medium bowl. Add tomatoes, feta, and onion to remaining oil mixture and toss to coat. Season with pepper to taste and set salad aside for serving.

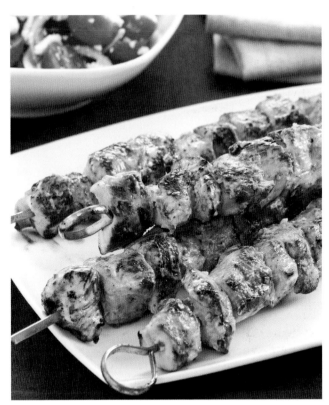

The yogurt in the dressing helps to coat the chicken and keep it moist on the grill.

2. Whisk yogurt into reserved oil mixture. Set aside half of yogurt dressing for serving. Add chicken to remaining yogurt dressing and toss to coat. Thread chicken onto four 12-inch metal skewers.

3A. FOR A CHARCOAL GRILL Open bottom vent completely. Light large chimney starter filled with charcoal briquettes (6 quarts). When top coals are partially covered with ash, pour evenly over grill. Set cooking grate in place, cover, and open lid vent completely. Heat grill until hot, about 5 minutes.

3B. FOR A GAS GRILL Turn all burners to high, cover, and heat grill until hot, about 15 minutes. Leave all burners on high.

4. Place skewers on grill and cook, turning occasionally, until chicken is well browned and registers 160 degrees, about 10 minutes. Using tongs, slide chicken off skewers onto serving platter. Serve chicken with salad and reserved dressing.

PER SERVING

Cal 400 • **Total Fat** 21g • **Sat Fat** 6g • **Chol** 145mg
Sodium 410mg • **Total Carbs** 9g • **Fiber** 2g • **Total Sugar** 6g
Added Sugar 0g • **Protein** 43g • **Total Carbohydrate Choices** 0.5

All About Spices

Just one or two spices can elevate an everyday dish to the next level. But spices can go rancid or stale, and often home cooks reach for old bottles of spices with little flavor. Here are a few tips to help you get the most from your spice rack.

Buying Spices

Grinding releases the compounds that give a spice its flavor and aroma, so it's best to buy spices whole and grind them before using; the longer a spice sits, the more its flavor fades. That said, there's no denying the convenience of preground spices. Try to buy preground spices in small quantities, from places likely to have high turnover.

Storing Spices Properly

Don't store spices and herbs on the counter close to the stove; heat, light, and moisture shorten their shelf life. Keep them in a cool, dark, dry place in well-sealed containers. To check whole spices for freshness, grind or finely grate a small amount and take a whiff. If the spice releases a lively aroma, it's still good to go. It's helpful to label each spice with the date opened; whole spices are generally good for two years and ground spices for one year.

Spice Rack Essentials

From arrowroot to mountain pepper to sumac to za'atar, there are hundreds of spices out there to choose from, but in the test kitchen there are only a few we believe are a must in every pantry. We have found we go through chili powder, cinnamon, cayenne, paprika, and peppercorns fairly quickly; all others we recommend buying on a need-to-use basis.

Blooming Spices Builds Flavor

We often like to bloom spices, a technique that removes any raw flavor or dustiness from spices and intensifies their flavor. To bloom spices, cook them briefly on the stovetop or in the microwave in a little oil or butter. As they dissolve, their essential oils are released from a solid state into solution form, where they mix and interact, producing a more complex flavor. Be careful to avoid burning them.

Getting a Good Grind

Freshly ground spices have superior aroma and vibrancy, and because whole spices have a longer shelf life than preground, grinding your own will help you get more out of the spices you buy. We recommend buying a designated blade-type coffee grinder for grinding spices.

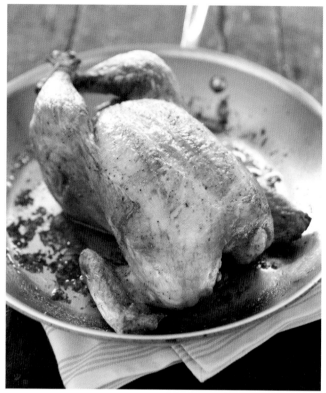

Our simplified roasting method uses a preheated skillet to jump-start the longer-cooking dark meat of a whole chicken.

Weeknight Skillet Roast Chicken
SERVES 4

WHY THIS RECIPE WORKS This is a recipe everyone should memorize. Given how popular and healthy roast chicken is, it's good to have a back-pocket recipe for busy nights that reliably delivers succulent meat with very little fuss or prep needed. Add a healthy side dish and you're done. And if you just need tender moist chicken to round out a salad or take to work, this recipe is your ticket. After systematically testing the various components and steps of typical recipes, we found we could just tie the legs together and tuck the wings underneath. We also discovered we could skip both the V-rack and flipping the chicken, which many recipes require, by using a preheated skillet and placing the chicken breast side up; this method gave the thighs a jump start on cooking, ensuring that the breast and thigh meat finish cooking at the same time. Starting the chicken in a 450-degree oven and then turning the oven off while the chicken finished cooking slowed the evaporation of juices, which gave moist, tender meat.

1 (4-pound) whole chicken, giblets discarded

1 tablespoon canola oil

½ teaspoon kosher salt

½ teaspoon pepper

  Lemon wedges

1. Adjust oven rack to middle position, place 12-inch oven-safe skillet on rack, and heat oven to 450 degrees. Pat chicken dry with paper towels. Rub entire surface with oil and sprinkle with salt and pepper. Tie legs together with twine and tuck wing tips behind back.

2. Transfer chicken breast side up to hot skillet in oven. Roast chicken until breast registers 120 degrees and thighs register 135 degrees, 25 to 35 minutes. Turn oven off and leave chicken in oven until breast registers 160 degrees and thighs register 175 degrees, 25 to 35 minutes.

3. Transfer chicken to carving board and let rest for 20 minutes. Carve chicken, discard skin, and serve with lemon wedges.

PER SERVING (½ BREAST PLUS 1 THIGH OR 1 DRUMSTICK)
Cal 240 • **Total Fat** 6g • **Sat Fat** 1.5g • **Chol** 160mg
Sodium 280mg • **Total Carbs** 0g • **Fiber** 0g • **Total Sugar** 0g
Added Sugar 0g • **Protein** 42g • **Total Carbohydrate Choices** 0

Asian Chicken Lettuce Wraps
SERVES 4

WHY THIS RECIPE WORKS Lettuce wraps are the perfect low-carb vehicle for delicious fillings. We wanted a light but flavor-packed filling and knew an Asian-inspired flavor profile was the way to go. Chicken lettuce wraps are most often made with ground or chopped chicken thighs. To lighten up our wraps, we turned to a combo of nutty, fiber-rich brown rice and store-bought lean ground chicken. Easy to make, we seasoned the chicken filling with minced jalapeño, fish sauce, and lime zest and juice. The bold flavors and simple ingredient list made this dish an easy weeknight dinner. Be sure to use ground chicken, not ground chicken breast (also labeled 99 percent fat free) in this recipe. To make this dish spicier, add the seeds from the chile.

1 cup short-grain brown rice, rinsed

1½ cups water

1 pound ground chicken

1 tablespoon canola oil

1 Thai or jalapeño chile, stemmed, seeded, and minced

2 teaspoons grated lime zest plus 1 tablespoon juice

2 tablespoons fish sauce

1 teaspoon cornstarch

¼ cup chopped fresh basil

3 scallions, sliced thin

¼ cup unsalted dry roasted peanuts, chopped

12 Bibb or Boston lettuce leaves

CARVING A WHOLE CHICKEN

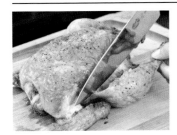

1. Cut chicken where leg meets breast.

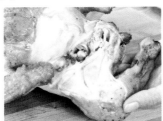

2. Pull leg quarter away from carcass. Separate joint by gently pressing leg out to side and pushing up on joint. Cut through joint to remove leg quarter.

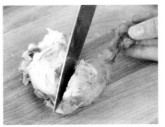

3. Cut through joint that connects drumstick to thigh. Repeat steps 1 through 3 on chicken's other side.

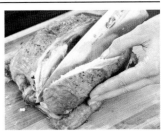

4. Cut down along side of breastbone, pulling breast meat away from breastbone as you cut. Remove wing from breast by cutting through wing joint. Discard skin and slice breast crosswise into slices. Repeat with other side.

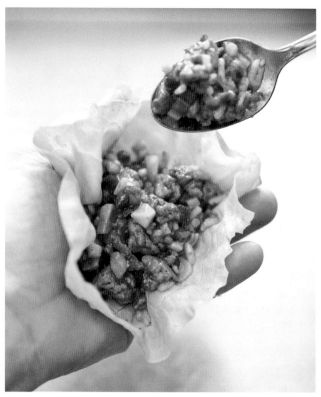

The superflavorful filling for these Asian lettuce wraps starts with lean ground chicken.

1. Bring rice and water to simmer in medium saucepan. Reduce heat to low, cover, and cook until rice is tender and water is absorbed, 45 to 50 minutes. Off heat, lay clean dish towel underneath lid and let rice sit for 10 minutes.

2. Mash chicken in bowl with back of wooden spoon until smooth and no strand-like pieces of meat remain. Heat oil in 12-inch nonstick skillet over medium heat until shimmering. Add ground chicken, chile, and lime zest and cook, breaking up meat with spoon, until no longer pink, about 5 minutes.

3. Whisk lime juice, fish sauce, and cornstarch together, then add to skillet and cook, stirring constantly, until sauce has thickened, about 45 seconds. Off heat, stir in basil, scallions, and peanuts. Gently fluff rice with fork. Divide chicken filling and rice evenly among lettuce leaves and serve.

PER 3-WRAP SERVING

Cal 440 • **Total Fat** 18g • **Sat Fat** 3.5g • **Chol** 75mg
Sodium 420mg • **Total Carbs** 44g • **Fiber** 4g • **Total Sugar** 1g
Added Sugar 0g • **Protein** 26g • **Total Carbohydrate Choices** 3

Stovetop Chicken Fajitas
SERVES 4

WHY THIS RECIPE WORKS This ingenious recipe can be made in a flash and delivers fajitas packed with chicken infused with pleasing orange undertones and the mild heat of chipotle chiles. Since sautéed red onion and bell pepper are a must when making fajitas, we started there and then set them aside until assembly time. Then we focused on boneless, skinless chicken. We poured some orange juice into our skillet and then added a hefty dose of minced cilantro, Worcestershire sauce, minced garlic, and chipotle. We slipped the chicken into this fragrant mixture and let it poach until perfectly tender, which took just 15 minutes. After we removed and shredded the chicken, we didn't want to waste a drop of the flavorful liquid. So we simmered it down until thickened, then stirred in mustard, more cilantro, chopped tomato, and sliced scallions. When the chicken had heated through in this mixture, our bright filling was complete and ready to stuff into warm whole-wheat tortillas.

- 1 tablespoon canola oil
- 2 red bell peppers, stemmed, seeded, and sliced thin
- 1 red onion, halved and sliced thin
- ½ cup orange juice
- ¾ cup minced fresh cilantro
- 1 tablespoon Worcestershire sauce
- 4 garlic cloves, minced
- 2 teaspoons minced canned chipotle chile in adobo sauce
  Salt and pepper
- 1½ pounds boneless, skinless chicken breasts, trimmed of all visible fat
- 1 teaspoon yellow mustard
- 1 tomato, cored, seeded, and chopped
- 3 scallions, sliced thin
- 8 (6-inch) 100 percent whole-wheat flour tortillas, warmed
  Lime wedges

1. Heat oil in 12-inch skillet over medium-high heat until just smoking. Add bell peppers and onion and cook until softened and well-browned, 5 to 7 minutes. Transfer to bowl and cover to keep warm.

2. Combine orange juice, ½ cup cilantro, Worcestershire, garlic, chipotle, ¼ teaspoon salt, and ⅛ teaspoon pepper in now-empty skillet and bring to simmer. Add chicken and bring to simmer. Reduce heat to medium-low, cover, and cook until chicken registers 160 degrees, 10 to 15 minutes, flipping chicken halfway through cooking.

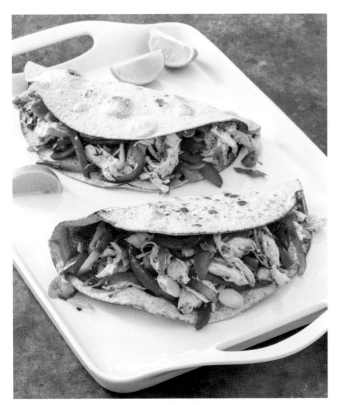

We use orange juice as the poaching liquid to produce tender, well-seasoned chicken for fajitas.

3. Transfer chicken to cutting board, let cool slightly, then shred into bite-size pieces using 2 forks.

4. Meanwhile, continue to simmer sauce over medium heat until slightly thickened and reduced to ¼ cup, about 5 minutes. Off heat, stir in mustard, tomato, scallions, remaining ¼ cup cilantro, and shredded chicken and let sit until heated through, about 2 minutes. Season with pepper to taste. Divide chicken filling and vegetable mixture evenly among tortillas and serve with lime wedges.

PER 2-FAJITA SERVING

Cal 520 • **Total Fat** 10g • **Sat Fat** 1.5g • **Chol** 125mg
Sodium 550mg • **Total Carbs** 57g • **Fiber** 9g • **Total Sugar** 5g
Added Sugar 0g • **Protein** 48g • **Total Carbohydrate Choices** 4

Know Your Labels

Many claims cited on poultry packaging have no government regulation, while those that do are often poorly enforced. Here's what you need to know.

Pay Attention to Processing

Processing is the major player in chicken's texture and flavor. We found that brands labeled "water-chilled" (soaked in a water bath in which they absorb up to 14 percent of their weight in water, which you pay for since chicken is sold by the pound) or "enhanced" (injected with broth and flavoring) are unnaturally spongy and are best avoided. Labeling laws say water gain must be shown on the product label, so these should be easily identifiable. When buying whole chickens or chicken parts, look for those that are labeled "air-chilled." Without the excess water weight, these brands are less spongy in texture and have more flavor.

Buyer Beware

USDA Organic is considered the gold standard seal for organic labeling. Poultry must eat organic feed that doesn't contain animal byproducts, be raised without antibiotics, and have access to the outdoors (how much, however, isn't regulated).

American Humane Certified is a program that verifies the use of standards that promote animal health and reduce stress, but these practices are widespread industry norms.

Raised Without Antibiotics and other claims regarding antibiotic use are important; too bad they're not strictly enforced. (The only rigorous enforcement is when the claim is subject to the USDA Organic seal.) Loopholes seem rife, like injecting the eggs—not the chickens—with antibiotics or feeding them feather meal laced with residual antibiotics from treated birds.

Natural and **All Natural** are ubiquitous on food labels. The USDA has defined the term just for fresh meat, stipulating only that no synthetic substances have been added to the cut. Producers may thus raise their chickens under the most unnatural circumstances on the most unnatural diets, inject birds with broth during processing, and still put the claim on their packaging.

Hormone-Free is empty reassurance, since the USDA does not allow the use of hormones or steroids in poultry production.

Vegetarian Fed and **Vegetarian Diet** sound healthy, but these terms aren't regulated by the government, so you're relying on the producer's notion of the claim.

Chicken Enchiladas
SERVES 6

WHY THIS RECIPE WORKS The things that make this Mexican dish so irresistible are the same things that make it so bad for you: the generous layer of melted cheese, greasy chicken, and heavy, sodium-laden sauce. For our take on this indulgent classic, we opted for boneless chicken breasts, which worked well when simmered gently in a potently flavored sauce; the meat was tender and infused with deep flavor. Instead of sprinkling all the cheese on top of the enchiladas, we mixed some in with the chicken and sauce for ultra-cheesy bites throughout. Canned chiles and minced cilantro added tangy, peppery notes and freshness. Using chipotle chile powder added layers of smoky, spicy flavor. Whole corn tortillas easily add more fiber to the casserole. When forming our enchiladas, simply rolling the filling in cold tortillas didn't cut it—the enchiladas broke and tore. Heating the tortillas in the microwave helped to make them pliable.

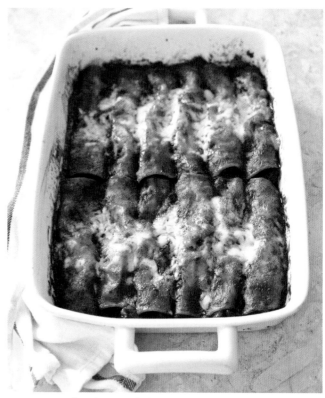

For corn tortillas that are pliable enough to easily roll and fill, we microwave them briefly.

1 tablespoon canola oil
1 onion, chopped fine
½ teaspoon salt
3 garlic cloves, minced
1 tablespoon chipotle chile powder
2 teaspoons ground cumin
1 (15-ounce) can no-salt-added tomato sauce
1¼ cups water
1 pound boneless, skinless chicken breasts, trimmed of all visible fat
4 ounces cheddar cheese, shredded (1 cup)
1 (4-ounce) can chopped green chiles, drained and chopped fine
½ cup minced fresh cilantro, plus ¼ cup leaves
12 (6-inch) corn tortillas
   Canola oil spray
¾ cup low-fat sour cream
   Lime wedges

1. Adjust oven rack to middle position and heat oven to 350 degrees. Heat oil in large saucepan over medium heat until shimmering. Add onion and salt and cook until softened, 5 to 7 minutes. Stir in garlic, chile powder, and cumin and cook until fragrant, about 30 seconds. Stir in tomato sauce and water, bring to simmer, and cook until slightly thickened, about 5 minutes. Add chicken and bring to simmer. Reduce heat to medium-low, cover, and cook until chicken registers 160 degrees, 10 to 15 minutes.

2. Transfer chicken to cutting board, let cool slightly, then shred into bite-size pieces using 2 forks. Strain sauce through fine-mesh strainer into bowl, pressing on solids to extract as much liquid as possible. Transfer solids to large bowl and stir in chicken, ½ cup strained sauce, ½ cup cheddar, chiles, and minced cilantro.

3. Wrap tortillas in clean dish towel and microwave until pliable, 30 to 90 seconds. Top each tortilla with ⅓ cup chicken mixture, roll tightly, and lay seam side down in 13 by 9-inch baking dish (2 columns of 6 tortillas will fit neatly across width of dish).

4. Lightly spray tops of enchiladas with oil spray. Pour remaining sauce over enchiladas and sprinkle remaining ½ cup cheddar evenly over top. Cover dish with aluminum foil and bake until enchiladas are hot throughout, about 25 minutes. Remove foil and continue to bake until cheese browns slightly, about 5 minutes.

5. Let enchiladas rest for 5 minutes. Sprinkle with cilantro leaves and serve with sour cream and lime wedges.

PER 2-ENCHILADA SERVING
Cal 360 • **Total Fat** 15g • **Sat Fat** 5g • **Chol** 80mg
Sodium 480mg • **Total Carbs** 32g • **Fiber** 6g • **Total Sugar** 6g
Added Sugar 0g • **Protein** 28g • **Total Carbohydrate Choices** 2

Chicken Pot Pie
SERVES 8

WHY THIS RECIPE WORKS With its buttery, flaky crust and tender chicken and vegetables coated in a velvety sauce, what's not to love about chicken pot pie? To make this family-friendly classic a little healthier, we cut back on the butter in both the crust and the filling. We started with the sauce, which relies on a butter-flour roux for its thickening power and richness. Fortunately, we found that simply toasting the flour let us ditch the butter; this easy step added deep flavor and also allowed us to add the flour to the stew without having it clump. Adding a bit of soy sauce to the filling helped ramp up its flavor even further. Moving on to the topping, we knew pie dough was out. We found that one sheet of puff pastry provided the perfect flaky, buttery topping without ratcheting up the saturated fat count significantly. To thaw frozen puff pastry, allow it to sit either in the refrigerator for 24 hours or on the counter for 30 minutes to 1 hour.

- 1 (9½ by 9-inch) sheet puff pastry, thawed
- ½ cup all-purpose flour
- 1 tablespoon canola oil
- 1 onion, chopped fine
- 1 celery rib, minced
    Salt and pepper
- 3½ cups unsalted chicken broth
- 1 tablespoon low-sodium soy sauce
- 2 pounds boneless, skinless chicken breasts, trimmed of all visible fat
- 3 carrots, peeled, halved lengthwise, and sliced ¼ inch thick
- 1 cup 1 percent low-fat milk
- ¾ cup frozen peas
- 2 tablespoons minced fresh parsley
- 2 teaspoons lemon juice

1. Adjust oven rack to middle position and heat oven to 425 degrees. Roll puff pastry into 13 by 9-inch rectangle on lightly floured counter and transfer to parchment paper–lined rimmed baking sheet. Using tip of paring knife, lightly score pastry in half lengthwise, then into quarters widthwise to create 8 segments, making sure not to cut through pastry completely. Bake pastry until puffed and lightly browned, about 8 minutes; let cool on sheet.

2. Toast flour in 12-inch nonstick skillet over medium-high heat, stirring often, until fragrant and lightly golden, about 5 minutes; transfer to medium bowl and let cool.

3. Meanwhile, heat oil in Dutch oven over medium heat until shimmering. Add onion, celery, and ½ teaspoon salt and cook until softened and lightly browned, 5 to 7 minutes. Stir in broth

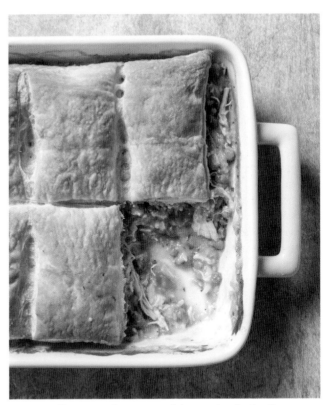

Frozen puff pastry makes an easy flaky topping for family-pleasing chicken pot pie.

and soy sauce, scraping up any browned bits. Add chicken and carrots and bring to simmer. Reduce heat to medium-low, cover, and cook until chicken registers 160 degrees, 10 to 15 minutes. Transfer chicken to carving board, let cool slightly, then shred into bite-size pieces using 2 forks.

4. Whisk milk into toasted flour until smooth, then whisk into cooking liquid in Dutch oven. Bring to simmer and cook, whisking constantly, until sauce thickens, about 2 minutes. Off heat, stir in chicken, peas, parsley, and lemon juice. Season with pepper to taste.

5. Transfer mixture to 13 by 9-inch baking dish. Place baked pastry on top and cut four 1-inch steam vents along center. Bake until pastry is deep golden and sauce is bubbling around edges, about 15 minutes. Let cool for 10 minutes before serving.

PER SERVING

Cal 350 • **Total Fat** 13g • **Sat Fat** 4.5g • **Chol** 85mg
Sodium 460mg • **Total Carbs** 25g • **Fiber** 3g • **Total Sugar** 6g
Added Sugar 0g • **Protein** 33g • **Total Carbohydrate Choices** 1.5

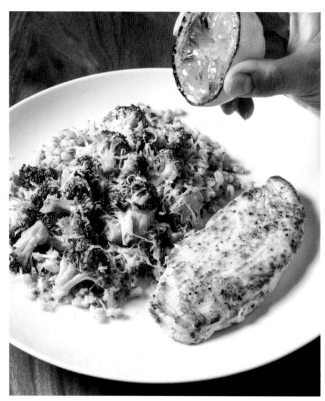
We infuse turkey cutlets with lots of lemony flavor by first caramelizing lemon halves in the cooking oil.

Turkey Cutlets with Barley and Broccoli
SERVES 4

WHY THIS RECIPE WORKS To update the traditional chicken-and-rice formula, we wanted to pair quick-cooking turkey cutlets with rustic, fiber-packed barley and nutritious broccoli. Since the cutlets cook so quickly, we prepared the barley first, simmering it with softened onion and garlic. To give the turkey and barley bright flavor, we employed a simple trick: We caramelized lemon halves in the cooking oil, infusing it (and thus the cutlets) with flavor. We seared the broccoli over high heat to get some tasty browning and then steamed it so that it cooked evenly. A light dusting of Parmesan added a savory richness, tying the dish together. Do not substitute hulled, hull-less, quick-cooking, or presteamed barley for the pearled barley in this recipe. The cooking time for pearled barley will vary from brand to brand (our preferred brand, Bob's Red Mill, is one of the longer cooking brands), so start checking barley for doneness after about 20 minutes.

¼ cup extra-virgin olive oil
1 onion, chopped fine
1 cup pearled barley, rinsed
3 garlic cloves, minced
2 cups unsalted chicken broth
¼ cup minced fresh parsley
  Salt and pepper
4 (4-ounce) turkey cutlets, ¼ inch thick, trimmed of all visible fat
1 lemon, zested to yield ½ teaspoon, halved and seeded
1 pound broccoli florets, cut into 1-inch pieces
⅛ teaspoon red pepper flakes
2 tablespoons grated Parmesan cheese

1. Heat 1 tablespoon oil in large saucepan over medium heat until shimmering. Add onion and cook until softened, about 5 minutes. Stir in barley and garlic and cook, stirring often, until lightly golden and fragrant, about 3 minutes.

2. Stir in broth and bring to simmer. Reduce heat to low, cover, and cook until barley is tender and broth is absorbed, 20 to 40 minutes. Add parsley, 1 tablespoon oil, and ⅛ teaspoon salt and gently fluff with fork to combine; cover to keep warm.

3. Meanwhile, pat cutlets dry with paper towels and sprinkle with ¼ teaspoon salt and ⅛ teaspoon pepper. Heat 1 teaspoon oil in 12-inch nonstick skillet over medium-high heat until shimmering. Cook lemon halves cut side down until browned, about 2 minutes; set aside. Heat 2 teaspoons oil in now-empty skillet until shimmering. Cook cutlets until well browned and tender, about 2 minutes per side. Transfer to plate and tent with aluminum foil.

4. Heat remaining 1 tablespoon oil in now-empty skillet over medium-high heat until just smoking. Add broccoli and cook, without stirring, until beginning to brown, about 2 minutes. Add 3 tablespoons water, cover, and cook until broccoli is bright green but still crisp, about 2 minutes. Uncover and continue to cook until water has evaporated and broccoli is crisp-tender, about 2 minutes. Off heat, add lemon zest, pepper flakes, ⅛ teaspoon salt, and ⅛ teaspoon pepper and toss to combine. Squeeze lemon halves over barley and cutlets. Serve with broccoli, sprinkling individual portions with Parmesan.

PER SERVING
Cal 500 • **Total Fat** 17g • **Sat Fat** 2.5g • **Chol** 45mg
Sodium 480mg • **Total Carbs** 49g • **Fiber** 12g • **Total Sugar** 4g
Added Sugar 0g • **Protein** 40g • **Total Carbohydrate Choices** 3

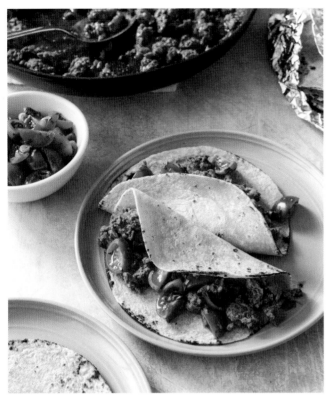

We ditch the usual fatty ground beef in favor of leaner turkey for a healthier taco filling.

Turkey Tacos
SERVES 4

WHY THIS RECIPE WORKS So maybe they're not authentic Mexican food, but ground meat tacos boast a comfort-food appeal that's undeniable. Ditching the ground beef in favor of ground turkey helped us slash the saturated fat in our healthier version of this popular dish, but its lean flavor needed a boost. To pump it up, we made a thick, zesty sauce using chicken broth, tomato sauce, and cider vinegar. Chili powder, garlic, and oregano provided the aromatic notes. Crunchy whole-grain corn tortillas were a given; soft tacos didn't do nearly as good a job securing the rich, hearty filling. Be sure to use ground turkey, not ground turkey breast (also labeled 99 percent fat-free), in this recipe.

SALSA
1 cup cherry tomatoes, quartered
2 scallions, sliced thin
1 tablespoon minced fresh cilantro
1½ teaspoons lime juice

TACOS
1 tablespoon canola oil
1 onion, chopped fine
3 garlic cloves, minced
2 tablespoons chili powder
1 teaspoon dried oregano
1 pound ground turkey
½ cup canned no-salt-added tomato sauce
½ cup unsalted chicken broth
2 teaspoons cider vinegar
Pepper
8 (6-inch) corn tortillas, warmed

1. FOR THE SALSA Combine all ingredients in bowl; set aside for serving.

2. FOR THE TACOS Heat oil in 12-inch nonstick skillet over medium-high heat until shimmering. Add onion and cook until softened, about 5 minutes. Stir in garlic, chili powder, and oregano and cook until fragrant, about 30 seconds. Add ground turkey and cook, breaking up meat with wooden spoon, until almost cooked through but still slightly pink, about 2 minutes.

2. Stir in tomato sauce, broth, and vinegar. Bring to simmer and cook until thickened, about 4 minutes. Season with pepper to taste. Divide filling evenly among tortillas and serve with salsa.

PER SERVING
Cal 320 • **Total Fat** 12g • **Sat Fat** 3.5g • **Chol** 45mg
Sodium 360mg • **Total Carbs** 26g • **Fiber** 7g • **Total Sugar** 5g
Added Sugar 0g • **Protein** 32g • **Total Carbohydrate Choices** 2

NOTES FROM THE TEST KITCHEN

Getting to Know: Ground Turkey

We prefer turkey that is ground from both white and dark meat. Typically labeled 93 percent fat-free, this ground turkey is moist and flavorful. By contrast, 99 percent fat-free ground turkey, which is all breast meat, is dry and chalky. When shopping for ground turkey, purchase just the amount you need from your supermarket butcher. Or, look for packaged ground turkey. But unlike packaged ground beef, packaged ground turkey is sold in uniform-size packaging, but the contents can vary in weight. Even among packages of the same brand, the amount of turkey can vary, from 1 pound to 1.3 pounds and so on. Our advice? Be sure to freeze the rest for another use. Otherwise, your tacos might not taste as saucy or your burgers might not be as moist.

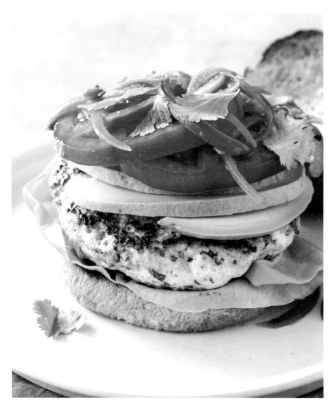

Mild, creamy ricotta cheese is the secret to moist and juicy turkey burgers.

Turkey Burgers
SERVES 4

WHY THIS RECIPE WORKS A burger is the quintessential comfort food, but it's not too surprising to learn that a classic beef burger is packed with saturated fat and salt. To satisfy a juicy burger craving, many of us have turned to lower-fat ground turkey, only to be disappointed with a dry, tasteless, and pale patty. We found that burgers made with a mixture of dark and white turkey meat (labeled 93 percent lean) had a decent meaty flavor and were relatively juicy. To add some moisture to the burgers, we mixed in a special ingredient: ricotta. This imparted a juicy, chewy texture, and its mild flavor allowed the turkey to stand out. Dijon and Worcestershire sauce amped up the savoriness of the burger. Tasters were divided on the necessity of a bun: The traditionalists insisted that a burger isn't a burger without a bun, while some felt that such a tasty burger just needed a few toppings to make it complete. Avocado brought some richness that was cut through by spicy vinegared onions. Be sure to use ground turkey, not ground turkey breast (also labeled 99 percent fat-free), in this recipe.

½ cup red wine vinegar
½ teaspoon red pepper flakes
1 small red onion, halved and sliced thin
1 pound ground turkey
3 ounces (⅓ cup) whole-milk ricotta cheese
¼ cup minced fresh cilantro, plus ¼ cup leaves
2 teaspoons Worcestershire sauce
2 teaspoons Dijon mustard
¼ teaspoon salt
¼ teaspoon pepper
1 tablespoon canola oil
4 100 percent whole-wheat hamburger buns, lightly toasted (optional)
1 avocado, halved, pitted, and sliced ¼ inch thick
1 head Bibb lettuce (8 ounces), leaves separated
1 tomato, cored and sliced ¼ inch thick

1. Microwave vinegar and pepper flakes in medium bowl until steaming, about 2 minutes. Stir in onion and let sit until ready to serve.

2. Break turkey into small pieces in large bowl, then add ricotta, minced cilantro, Worcestershire, mustard, salt, and pepper. Using your hands, lightly knead mixture until combined. Pat turkey mixture into four ¾-inch-thick patties, about 4 inches in diameter.

3. Heat oil in 12-inch nonstick skillet over medium heat until shimmering. Gently place patties in skillet, reshaping them as needed, and cook until browned and register 160 degrees, 5 to 7 minutes per side. Serve burgers on buns, if using, and top with avocado, lettuce, tomato, cilantro leaves, and onions.

PER SERVING WITH BUN

Cal 420 • **Total Fat** 17g • **Sat Fat** 5g • **Chol** 55mg
Sodium 530mg • **Total Carbs** 31g • **Fiber** 8g • **Total Sugar** 5g
Added Sugar 0g • **Protein** 33g • **Total Carbohydrate Choices** 2

PER SERVING WITHOUT BUN

Cal 290 • **Total Fat** 15g • **Sat Fat** 5g • **Chol** 55mg
Sodium 340mg • **Total Carbs** 9g • **Fiber** 7g • **Total Sugar** 3g
Added Sugar 0g • **Protein** 33g • **Total Carbohydrate Choices** 0.5

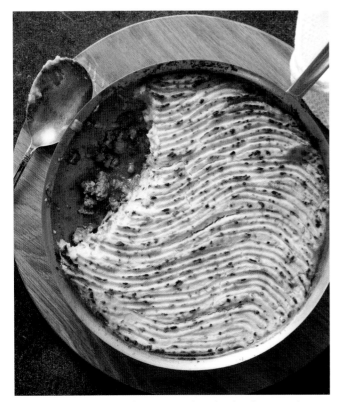

We skip the potatoes and top our turkey shepherd's pie with a creamy and fiber-rich cauliflower puree.

Turkey Shepherd's Pie
SERVES 6

WHY THIS RECIPE WORKS We wanted to refashion shepherd's pie into a high-nutrient dinner while keeping its hearty comforts. Substituting ground turkey for beef or lamb was a promising start. It's typical to brown the ground meat to add to the meatiness of the dish; however, doing so made it dry and tough. Instead, we seared mushrooms and onions as the base for a rich gravy, and enriched the gravy with Worcestershire sauce (for umami flavor) and carrots (for a touch of natural sweetness). Then we tossed the turkey with a little water, salt and pepper, and baking soda; the baking soda kept the meat moist and succulent as the turkey simmered in the gravy. For a nutrient-dense and carbohydrate-light topping, swapping out mashed russet potatoes for mild, fiber-rich cauliflower was an easy choice. We cooked a head of chopped florets until soft and pureed them until velvety smooth. Then we gently bound the mixture with an egg and stirred in chives for

flavor. Be sure to use ground turkey, not ground turkey breast (also labeled 99 percent fat-free), in this recipe. You will need a 10-inch broiler-safe skillet.

> 3 tablespoons extra-virgin olive oil
> 1 large head cauliflower (3 pounds), cored and cut into ½-inch pieces
> ½ cup plus 2 tablespoons water
>   Salt and pepper
> 1 large egg, lightly beaten
> 3 tablespoons minced fresh chives
> 1 pound ground turkey
> ¼ teaspoon baking soda
> 8 ounces cremini mushrooms, trimmed and chopped
> 1 onion, chopped
> 1 tablespoon no-salt-added tomato paste
> 2 garlic cloves, minced
> ¾ cup unsalted chicken broth
> 2 carrots, peeled and chopped
> 2 sprigs fresh thyme
> 1 tablespoon Worcestershire sauce
> 1 tablespoon cornstarch

1. Heat 2 tablespoons oil in Dutch oven over medium-low heat until shimmering. Add cauliflower and cook, stirring occasionally, until softened and beginning to brown, 10 to 12 minutes. Stir in ½ cup water and ½ teaspoon salt, cover, and cook until cauliflower falls apart easily when poked with fork, about 10 minutes.

2. Transfer cauliflower and any remaining liquid to food processor and let cool for 5 minutes. Process until smooth, about 45 seconds, scraping down sides of bowl as needed. Transfer to large bowl and stir in egg and chives; set aside.

3. Meanwhile, toss turkey, 1 tablespoon water, baking soda, ¼ teaspoon salt, and ¼ teaspoon pepper in bowl until thoroughly combined. Set aside for 20 minutes.

4. Heat remaining 1 tablespoon oil in broiler-safe 10-inch skillet over medium heat until shimmering. Add mushrooms and onion and cook until liquid has evaporated and fond begins to form on bottom of skillet, 10 to 12 minutes. Stir in tomato paste and garlic and cook until bottom of skillet is dark brown, about 2 minutes.

5. Stir in broth, scraping up any browned bits. Stir in carrots, thyme sprigs, and Worcestershire, bring to simmer, and reduce heat to medium-low. Pinch off turkey in ½-inch pieces, add to skillet, and bring to gentle simmer. Cover and cook until turkey is cooked through, 8 to 10 minutes, stirring and breaking up meat into small pieces halfway through cooking.

6. Whisk cornstarch and remaining 1 tablespoon water together, then stir mixture into filling and continue to simmer until thickened, about 1 minute. Discard thyme sprigs and season with pepper to taste.

7. Adjust oven rack 5 inches from broiler element and heat broiler. Transfer cauliflower mixture to 1-gallon zipper-lock bag. Using scissors, snip 1 inch off filled corner. Squeezing bag, pipe mixture in even layer over filling, making sure to cover entire surface. Smooth mixture with back of spoon, then use tines of fork to make ridges over surface. Place skillet on aluminum foil–lined rimmed baking sheet and broil until topping is golden brown and crusty and filling is bubbly, 10 to 15 minutes. Let cool for 10 minutes before serving.

PER SERVING

Cal 220 • **Total Fat** 9g • **Sat Fat** 2.5g • **Chol** 60mg
Sodium 490mg • **Total Carbs** 13g • **Fiber** 3g • **Total Sugar** 5g
Added Sugar 0g • **Protein** 23g • **Total Carbohydrate Choices** 1

TOPPING SHEPHERD'S PIE

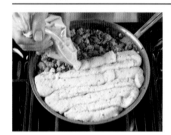

Transfer cauliflower mixture to 1-gallon zipper-lock bag and snip off 1 corner. Pipe mixture over filling, making sure to cover entire surface. Smooth with back of spoon, then make ridges with fork.

Easy Roast Turkey Breast
SERVES 12

WHY THIS RECIPE WORKS Bone-in turkey breasts are an underutilized cut, and a perfectly roasted breast is a great option for a smaller holiday gathering, especially if your guests prefer white meat. Other benefits: A breast requires less cooking time, which can free up your oven for other dishes, and it's much easier to carve than a whole bird. To start, we removed the backbone so the breast sat flat in the oven for even cooking and to make carving easier. Roasted right, the breast is flavorful and delivers lots of moist, tender meat. The trick, we found, was to use two different oven temperatures. Rather than trying to sear the cumbersome breast on the stovetop, we elevated it in a V-rack and started it out in a blazing hot oven to kick-start the browning process. Dropping the temperature to 325 degrees after 30 minutes allowed the meat

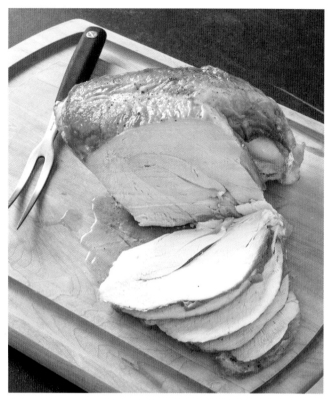

For moist, flavorful white meat, we start by soaking the turkey breast in a saltwater brine.

to gently finish cooking so it stayed moist and tender. Brining the turkey was the most efficient way to season the meat and allowed us to limit the amount of salt. If using a self-basting turkey (such as a frozen Butterball) or a kosher turkey, do not brine. Serve with any of the sauces on page 206.

1 (5-pound) bone-in turkey breast
¼ cup salt
1 teaspoon pepper

1. To remove backbone, use kitchen shears to cut through ribs following vertical line of fat where breast meets back, from tapered end of breast to wing joint. Using your hands, bend back away from breast to pop shoulder joint out of socket. With paring knife, cut through joint between bones to separate back from breast; discard backbone. Trim excess fat from breast. Dissolve salt in 4 quarts cold water in large container. Submerge turkey breast in brine, cover, and refrigerate for at least 3 hours or up to 6 hours.

2. Adjust oven rack to middle position and heat oven to 425 degrees. Set V-rack inside roasting pan and spray with vegetable oil spray. Remove turkey from brine, pat dry with paper towels, and sprinkle with pepper. Place turkey, skin side up, on prepared V-rack and add 1 cup water to pan. Roast turkey for 30 minutes.

3. Reduce oven temperature to 325 degrees and continue to roast until turkey registers 160 degrees, about 1 hour. Transfer turkey to carving board and let rest for 20 minutes. Carve turkey, discard skin, and serve.

PER SERVING

Cal 170 • **Total Fat** 2g • **Sat Fat** 0g • **Chol** 85mg
Sodium 310mg • **Total Carbs** 0g • **Fiber** 0g • **Total Sugar** 0g
Added Sugar 0g • **Protein** 35g • **Total Carbohydrate Choices** 0

REMOVING THE BACKBONE FROM A TURKEY BREAST

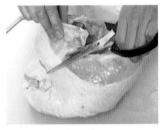

1. Using kitchen shears, cut through ribs following vertical line of fat where breast meets back, from tapered end of breast to wing joint.

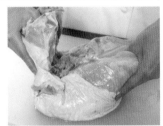

2. Using your hands, bend back away from breast to pop shoulder joint out of socket. Cut through joint to remove back.

Smoked Turkey Breast
SERVES 12

WHY THIS RECIPE WORKS For smoked turkey with plump, juicy white meat lightly perfumed with smoke, we chose a turkey breast, which cooked relatively quickly on the grill. Brining the turkey helped to flavor the meat and keep the lean white meat moist. Before grilling, we dried the skin and seasoned it with black pepper for a kick. Piercing the skin before grilling allowed some of the fat to drain away. Two cups of wood chips added enough smokiness without overwhelming the mild meat. After grilling the bird for an hour and a half, we had smoky, well-seasoned, juicy meat with golden, crisp skin. If you'd like to use wood chunks instead of wood chips when using a charcoal grill, substitute two medium wood chunks, soaked in water for 1 hour, for the wood chip packet. If using a self-basting turkey (such as a frozen Butterball) or a kosher turkey, do not brine.

1 (5-pound) bone-in turkey breast
¼ cup salt
1 teaspoon pepper
2 cups wood chips
1 (13 by 9-inch) disposable aluminum roasting pan (if using charcoal)

1. To remove backbone, use kitchen shears to cut through ribs following vertical line of fat where breast meets back, from tapered end of breast to wing joint. Using your hands, bend back away from breast to pop shoulder joint out of socket. With paring knife, cut through joint between bones to separate back from breast; discard backbone. Trim excess fat from breast. Dissolve salt in 4 quarts cold water in large container. Submerge turkey breast in brine, cover, and refrigerate for at least 3 hours or up to 6 hours.

2. Just before grilling, soak wood chips in water for 15 minutes, then drain. Using large piece of heavy-duty aluminum foil, wrap soaked chips in foil packet and cut several vent holes in top. Remove turkey from brine, pat dry with paper towels, and sprinkle with pepper. Poke skin all over with skewer.

3A. FOR A CHARCOAL GRILL Open bottom vent halfway and place disposable pan in center of grill. Light large chimney starter filled with charcoal briquettes (6 quarts). When top coals are partially covered with ash, pour into 2 even piles on either side of disposable pan. Place wood chip packet on coals. Set cooking grate in place, cover, and open lid vent halfway. Heat grill until hot and wood chips are smoking, about 5 minutes.

3B. FOR A GAS GRILL Remove cooking grate and place wood chip packet directly on primary burner. Set cooking grate in place, turn all burners to high, cover, and heat grill until hot and wood chips are smoking, about 15 minutes. Turn all burners to medium-low. (Adjust burners as needed to maintain grill temperature around 350 degrees.)

4. Clean and oil cooking grate. Place turkey breast, skin side up, in center of grill (over disposable pan if using charcoal). Cover (position lid vent over turkey if using charcoal) and cook until skin is well browned and breast registers 160 degrees, about 1½ hours.

5. Transfer turkey to carving board and let rest for 20 minutes. Carve turkey, discard skin, and serve.

PER SERVING

Cal 170 • **Total Fat** 2g • **Sat Fat** 0g • **Chol** 85mg
Sodium 310mg • **Total Carbs** 0g • **Fiber** 0g • **Total Sugar** 0g
Added Sugar 0g • **Protein** 35g • **Total Carbohydrate Choices** 0

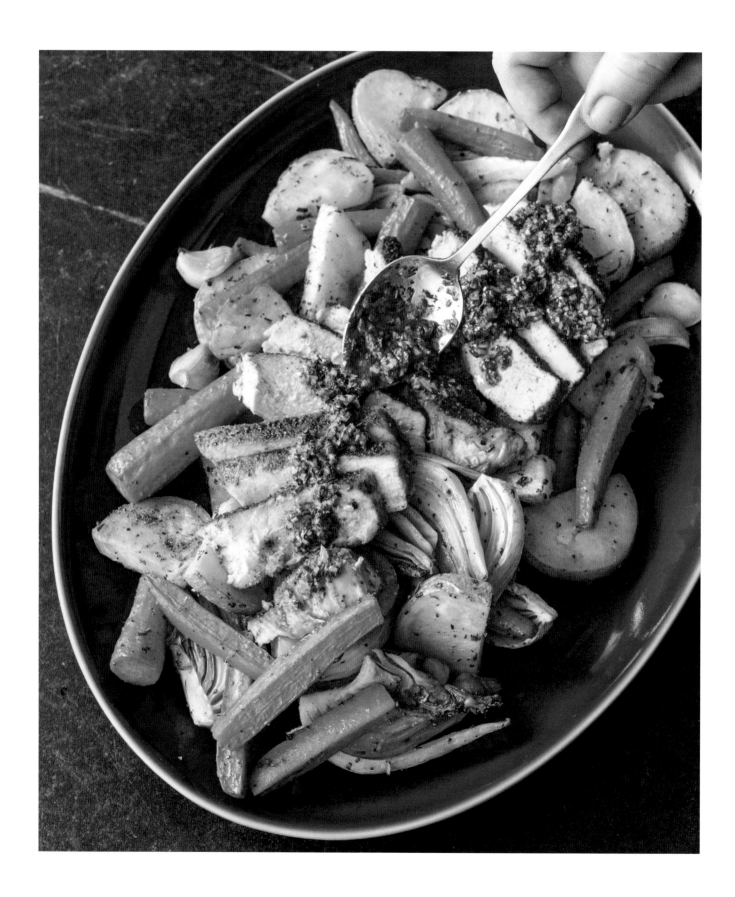

MEAT

Photo: One-Pan Roasted Pork Chops and Vegetables with Parsley Vinaigrette

A simple steak, or a poached (page 174) or pan-seared (page 175) chicken breast, is easy to prepare in a skillet and a great go-to option for a high-protein, carb-free main course. But sometimes you want to dress it up a little, so it's nice to have a variety of easy-to-execute pan sauces in your repertoire. Here are some of the test kitchen's favorites.

Porcini-Marsala Pan Sauce

MAKES ABOUT ½ CUP; ENOUGH FOR 4 SERVINGS

This recipe is meant to be started after you have seared steak or chicken in a skillet. Do not wash the skillet after searing—any remaining browned bits add important flavor to the sauce.

- ¾ cup unsalted chicken broth
- ¼ ounce dried porcini mushrooms, rinsed
- 1 shallot, minced
- ½ cup dry Marsala
- 2 tablespoons unsalted butter, cut into 2 pieces and chilled
- 1 tablespoon minced fresh parsley
  Pepper

1. Microwave ½ cup broth and mushrooms in covered bowl until steaming, about 1 minute. Let sit until softened, about 5 minutes. Drain mushrooms through fine-mesh strainer lined with coffee filter, reserving soaking liquid, and finely chop mushrooms.

2. Pour off all but 2 teaspoons fat from skillet. (Or, if necessary, add oil to equal 2 teaspoons.) Add shallot and ⅛ teaspoon salt and cook over medium heat until softened, 1 to 2 minutes. Off heat, stir in Marsala, scraping up any browned bits. Return skillet to medium heat and simmer until Marsala is reduced to glaze, about 3 minutes.

3. Stir in remaining ¼ cup broth, reserved soaking liquid, and mushrooms. Bring to simmer and cook until liquid is reduced to ⅓ cup, 4 to 6 minutes. Off heat, whisk in butter, 1 piece at a time, until combined, then whisk in parsley and any accumulated meat juices. Season with pepper to taste. Serve immediately.

PER 2-TABLESPOON SERVING

Cal 110 • **Total Fat** 6g • **Sat Fat** 3.5g • **Chol** 15mg
Sodium 220mg • **Total Carbs** 6g • **Fiber** 1g • **Total Sugar** 5g
Added Sugar 0g • **Protein** 2g • **Total Carbohydrate Choices** 0.5

Cognac and Mustard Pan Sauce

MAKES ABOUT ½ CUP; ENOUGH FOR 4 SERVINGS

This recipe is meant to be started after you have seared steak or chicken in a skillet. Do not wash the skillet after searing—any remaining browned bits add important flavor to the sauce.

- 1 shallot, minced
- ¼ cup cognac
- ¾ cup low-sodium beef broth
- 2 tablespoons unsalted butter, cut into 2 pieces and chilled
- 1 tablespoon whole-grain mustard
- 2 teaspoons minced fresh tarragon
- 1 teaspoon fresh lemon juice
  Pepper

1. Pour off all but 2 teaspoons fat from skillet. (Or, if necessary, add oil to equal 2 teaspoons.) Add shallot and cook over medium heat until softened, 1 to 2 minutes. Off heat, stir in cognac, scraping up any browned bits. Return skillet to medium heat and simmer until cognac is reduced to glaze, about 1 minute.

2. Stir in broth, bring to simmer, and cook until liquid is reduced to ½ cup, 10 to 12 minutes. Off heat, whisk in butter, 1 piece at a time, until combined, then whisk in mustard, tarragon, lemon juice, and any accumulated meat juices. Season with pepper to taste. Serve immediately.

PER 2-TABLESPOON SERVING

Cal 100 • **Total Fat** 6g • **Sat Fat** 3.5 • **Chol** 15mg
Sodium 180mg • **Total Carbs** 1g • **Fiber** 0g • **Total Sugar** 1g
Added Sugar 0g • **Protein** 1g • **Total Carbohydrate Choices** 0

Rustic Bell Pepper and Vinegar Pan Sauce

MAKES ABOUT 1½ CUPS; ENOUGH FOR 4 SERVINGS

This recipe is meant to be started after you have seared steak or chicken in a skillet. Do not wash the skillet after searing—any remaining browned bits add important flavor to the sauce.

- 1 red bell pepper, stemmed, seeded, and sliced thin
- 1 small red onion, halved and sliced thin
- 2 garlic cloves, minced
- 1 teaspoon minced fresh thyme or ¼ teaspoon dried
- 1 cup unsalted chicken broth
- 1 tablespoon balsamic vinegar
  Pepper

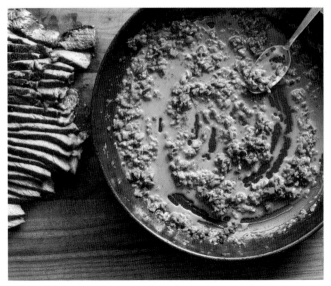

A flavorful pan sauce is a quick and easy way to enliven plain steak or chicken.

Pour off all but 2 teaspoons fat from skillet. (Or, if necessary, add oil to equal 2 teaspoons.) Add bell pepper and onion and cook over medium heat until softened, about 5 minutes. Stir in garlic and thyme and cook until fragrant, about 30 seconds. Stir in broth, scraping up any browned bits, and simmer until the sauce has thickened slightly, about 6 minutes. Stir in vinegar and any accumulated meat juices. Season with pepper to taste. Serve immediately.

PER 6-TABLESPOON SERVING

Cal 25 • Total Fat 0g • Sat Fat 0 • Chol 0mg
Sodium 35mg • Total Carbs 4g • Fiber 1g • Total Sugar 2g
Added Sugar 0g • Protein 2g • Total Carbohydrate Choices <0.5

Sun-Dried Tomato Relish

MAKES ABOUT ½ CUP; ENOUGH FOR 4 SERVINGS

This recipe is meant to be started after you have seared steak or chicken in a skillet. Do not wash the skillet after searing—any remaining browned bits add important flavor to the sauce.

    ½ cup unsalted chicken broth
      Pinch red pepper flakes
    ¼ cup oil-packed sun-dried tomatoes, rinsed, patted dry, and minced
    2 tablespoons extra-virgin olive oil
    1 tablespoon capers, rinsed and minced

    1 teaspoon lemon juice
    2 tablespoons minced fresh parsley
    1 tablespoon minced fresh mint
      Pepper

Pour off any fat from skillet. Add broth and pepper flakes, scraping up any browned bits, and cook over medium heat until liquid is reduced to 2 tablespoons, about 5 minutes. Stir in tomatoes, oil, capers, and lemon juice and bring to simmer. Off the heat, stir in parsley, mint, and any accumulated meat juices. Season with pepper to taste. Serve immediately.

PER 2-TABLESPOON SERVING

Cal 80 • Total Fat 8g • Sat Fat 1 • Chol 0mg
Sodium 85mg • Total Carbs 2g • Fiber 1g • Total Sugar 0g
Added Sugar 0g • Protein 1g • Total Carbohydrate Choices <0.5

Chimichurri

MAKES ABOUT ½ CUP; ENOUGH FOR 4 SERVINGS

    2 tablespoons hot tap water
    1 teaspoon dried oregano
      Salt and pepper
    ½ cup fresh parsley leaves
    ¼ cup fresh cilantro leaves
    3 garlic cloves, minced
    ¼ teaspoon red pepper flakes
    2 tablespoons red wine vinegar
    ¼ cup extra-virgin olive oil

    1. Combine hot water, oregano, and ¼ teaspoon salt in small bowl; let sit for 5 minutes to soften oregano.
    2. Pulse parsley, cilantro, garlic, and pepper flakes in food processor until coarsely chopped, about 10 pulses. Add water mixture and vinegar and pulse briefly to combine.
    3. Transfer mixture to medium bowl and slowly whisk in oil until incorporated. Cover and let sit at room temperature for at least 1 hour to allow flavors to meld. Season with pepper to taste. (Sauce can be refrigerated for up to 2 days. Bring to room temperature and whisk to recombine before serving.)

PER 2-TABLESPOON SERVING

Cal 130 • Total Fat 14g • Sat Fat 2 • Chol 0mg
Sodium 130mg • Total Carbs 1g • Fiber 0g • Total Sugar 0g
Added Sugar 0g • Protein 0g • Total Carbohydrate Choices <0.5

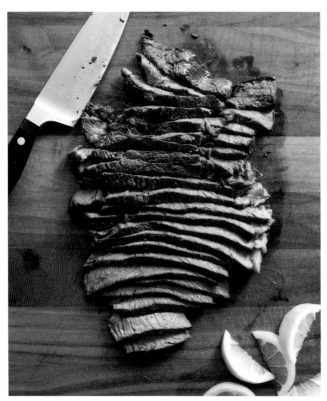

A very hot skillet and a few teaspoons of smoking oil are the secret to cooking a perfect steak indoors.

Pan-Seared Sirloin Steak
SERVES 4

WHY THIS RECIPE WORKS A well-caramelized exterior is essential to a great steak. We wanted a way to make a steak with a flavorful crust entirely on the stovetop. After cooking dozens of steaks, we found a few keys to success. The most important step is to get the pan really hot—if the pan isn't properly preheated, the interior of the steak will overcook before it develops a good crust, so make sure the oil is just smoking before adding the meat to the pan. Also, pat the steak dry before searing; any moisture on the exterior of the steak will prevent it from browning properly. Finally, use the right pan. A large traditional (not nonstick) skillet will ensure that the steak has enough room to sear and will encourage the development of browned bits, called fond, the secret to a flavorful pan sauce. We prefer this steak cooked to medium-rare, but if you prefer it more or less done, see our guidelines on page 209. You can serve the steak with one of the pan sauces on pages 206–7, if desired.

1 (1-pound) boneless beef top sirloin steak, 1 to 1½ inches thick, trimmed of all visible fat
¼ teaspoon salt
⅛ teaspoon pepper
2 teaspoons canola oil
Lemon wedges

1. Pat steak dry with paper towels and sprinkle with salt and pepper. Heat oil in 12-inch skillet over medium-high heat until just smoking. Brown steak well on first side, 3 to 5 minutes.

2. Flip steak and continue to cook until meat registers 120 to 125 degrees (for medium-rare), 5 to 10 minutes, reducing heat as needed to prevent scorching. Transfer steak to carving board, tent with aluminum foil, and let rest for 5 minutes. Slice steak thin and serve with lemon wedges.

PER SERVING
Cal 170 • **Total Fat** /g • **Sat Fat** 2g • **Chol** 70mg
Sodium 210mg • **Total Carbs** 0g • **Fiber** 0g • **Total Sugar** 0g
Added Sugar 0g • **Protein** 25g • **Total Carbohydrate Choices** 0

Skirt Steak with Pinto Bean Salad
SERVES 6

WHY THIS RECIPE WORKS Thin slices of skirt steak pair perfectly with a simple arugula and pinto bean salad. The dressing with chipotle chile and lime juice adds subtle spicy and smoky notes as well as a hit of brightness for a satisfying Southwestern flavor profile. We prefer these steaks cooked to medium-rare, but if you prefer them more or less done, see our guidelines on page 209. The steaks may overlap slightly in the skillet at first but will shrink as they cook. For a spicier dish, use the larger amount of chipotle.

2 (15-ounce) cans no-salt-added pinto beans, rinsed
¼ cup finely chopped red onion
¼ cup chopped fresh cilantro
3 tablespoons extra-virgin olive oil
2 tablespoons lime juice
1–2 teaspoons minced canned chipotle chile in adobo sauce
Salt and pepper
1 teaspoon paprika
1½ pounds skirt steak, trimmed of all visible fat and cut into thirds
5 ounces (5 cups) baby arugula
Lime wedges

1. Combine beans, onion, cilantro, 2 tablespoons oil, lime juice, chipotle, ¼ teaspoon salt, and ½ teaspoon pepper in bowl; set aside while preparing steak.

2. Combine paprika, ¼ teaspoon salt, and ¼ teaspoon pepper in bowl. Pat steaks dry with paper towels and sprinkle with paprika mixture. Heat remaining 1 tablespoon oil in 12-inch skillet over medium-high heat until just smoking. Cook steaks until well browned and meat registers 120 to 125 degrees (for medium-rare), about 2 minutes per side. Transfer steaks to carving board, tent with aluminum foil, and let rest for 5 minutes.

3. Add arugula to bean mixture and gently toss to combine. Season with pepper to taste. Slice steaks thin against grain and serve with bean salad and lime wedges.

PER SERVING

Cal 360 • Total Fat 21g • Sat Fat 6g • Chol 75mg
Sodium 280mg • Total Carbs 16g • Fiber 5g • Total Sugar 2g
Added Sugar 0g • Protein 28g • Total Carbohydrate Choices 1

One-Pan Roasted Steaks with Sweet Potatoes and Scallions

SERVES 6

WHY THIS RECIPE WORKS When we think steak dinner, some key characteristics spring to mind: tender, juicy meat, a flavorful browned crust, and robust sides like thick-cut potato wedges and a green vegetable. While we usually look to the grill or a ripping-hot skillet to turn out steaks with a strong crust, we saw potential in our sheet pan to easily prepare the whole meal in one go. Preheating the pan promised the sizzle we love. A pleasantly bitter coffee rub accentuated the meat's savoriness while chili powder added a touch of heat. We decided to use the preheating time to jump-start our side dish, so we sliced fiber-rich unpeeled sweet potatoes into wedges and let them soften in the pan as it heated up. Then we added the steaks, scattering some scallions over the potatoes to bring some greenery to the dish. To give our dish a final, flavorful flourish, we served our steaks with quick-pickled radishes. We prefer these steaks cooked to medium-rare, but if you prefer them more or less done, see our guidelines at right. The scallions should be left whole; trim off only the small roots.

6 radishes, trimmed and sliced thin
1 tablespoon lime juice, plus lime wedges for serving
  Salt and pepper
2 pounds sweet potatoes, unpeeled, cut lengthwise into 1-inch wedges
2 tablespoons extra-virgin olive oil

Taking the Temperature of Meat and Poultry

Since the temperature of beef and pork will continue to rise as the meat rests—an effect called carryover cooking—they should be removed from the oven, grill, or pan when they are 5 to 10 degrees below the desired serving temperature. Carryover cooking doesn't apply to poultry and fish (they lack the dense muscle structure of beef and pork and don't retain heat as well), so they should be cooked to the desired serving temperature. The following temperatures should be used to determine when to stop the cooking process.

FOR THIS INGREDIENT...	COOK TO THIS TEMPERATURE
Beef/Lamb	
Rare	115 to 120 degrees (120 to 125 degrees after resting)
Medium-Rare	120 to 125 degrees (125 to 130 degrees after resting)
Medium	130 to 135 degrees (135 to 140 degrees after resting)
Medium-Well	140 to 145 degrees (145 to 150 degrees after resting)
Well-Done	150 to 155 degrees (155 to 160 degrees after resting)
Pork	
Chops and Tenderloin	145 degrees (150 degrees after resting)
Loin Roasts	140 degrees (145 degrees after resting)
Chicken	
White Meat	160 degrees
Dark Meat	175 degrees

Thawing Steaks Quickly

We tested defrosting steaks on various surfaces to find the fastest method. After one hour, steaks left on wood and plastic cutting boards were still frozen solid; those on aluminum baking trays had thawed slightly more; and steaks left on heavy skillets were almost completely thawed. Why? Metal contains a lot of moving atoms, allowing it to transfer ambient heat much more quickly. To thaw steaks, place them, wrapped, in a skillet in a single layer. Flip the steaks every half hour until thawed.

- 2 teaspoons finely ground coffee
- 2 teaspoons chili powder
- 2 (12-ounce) boneless strip steaks, 1 to 1¼ inches thick, trimmed of all visible fat
- 16 scallions, trimmed

1. Adjust oven rack to lower-middle position and heat oven to 450 degrees. Combine radishes, lime juice, and ⅛ teaspoon salt in bowl; cover and refrigerate until ready to serve.

2. Toss potatoes with 1½ tablespoons oil, ¼ teaspoon salt, and ¼ teaspoon pepper in bowl. Arrange potatoes skin side down on half of rimmed baking sheet and roast until potatoes begin to soften, 25 to 30 minutes.

3. Meanwhile, combine coffee, chili powder, ¼ teaspoon salt, and ⅛ teaspoon pepper in bowl. Pat steaks dry with paper towels and sprinkle with coffee mixture. Toss scallions with remaining 1½ teaspoons oil, ⅛ teaspoon salt, and ¼ teaspoon pepper.

4. Lay scallions on top of potatoes. Arrange steaks on empty portion of sheet and roast until steaks register 120 to 125 degrees (for medium-rare) and potatoes are lightly browned and fully tender, 10 to 15 minutes, rotating sheet halfway through roasting.

5. Transfer steaks bottom side up to carving board as they finish cooking. Tent with aluminum foil and let rest for 5 minutes. Transfer vegetables to serving platter and tent with foil. Slice steaks thin and serve with vegetables, pickled radishes, and lime wedges.

PER SERVING
Cal 420 • **Total Fat** 21g • **Sat Fat** 7g • **Chol** 90mg
Sodium 480mg • **Total Carbs** 31g • **Fiber** 7g • **Total Sugar** 10g
Added Sugar 0g • **Protein** 26g • **Total Carbohydrate Choices** 2

NOTES FROM THE TEST KITCHEN

Letting Meat Rest

After cooking almost any piece of meat, it is crucial to allow the meat to rest. All steaks should rest for at least 5 minutes and all roasts should rest for at least 15 minutes. This is because the internal temperature of the meat will continue to rise anywhere from 5 to 10 degrees depending on the size of the cut of meat, an effect known as carryover cooking. During this time, as the protein molecules in the meat cool, they will reabsorb any accumulated meat juice and redistribute it throughout the meat. Plus, if you let your meat rest, it will be more tender and the juices will not run all over your plate or carving board when you slice into it.

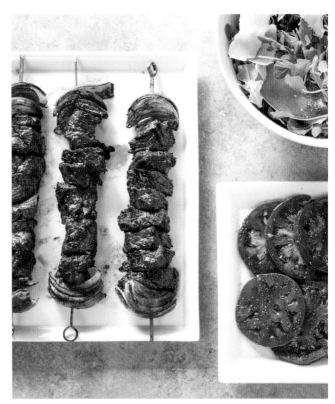

Our foolproof kebabs cook quickly on the grill and emerge beefy, tender, and full of flavor thanks to an easy marinade.

Grilled Balsamic Beef Skewers with Tomatoes and Salad
SERVES 8

WHY THIS RECIPE WORKS Richly marbled steak tips have great beefy flavor and tender texture. Grilling them on skewers and pairing them with a super simple salad plus a tomato side dish makes for a quick, fresh dinner. Sirloin steak tips, also known as flap meat, can be sold as whole steaks, cubes, and strips. To ensure uniform pieces, we prefer to buy whole steaks and cut them ourselves. We like the bright flavor of heirloom tomatoes here, but any ripe in-season tomatoes can be substituted. We prefer these steaks cooked to medium-rare, but if you like them more or less done, see our guidelines on page 209. You will need four 12-inch metal skewers for this recipe.

- ½ cup balsamic vinegar
- 7 tablespoons extra-virgin olive oil
- 2 tablespoons Dijon mustard
- 4 garlic cloves, minced
- ½ teaspoon red pepper flakes

Salt and pepper
2 pounds sirloin steak tips, trimmed of all visible fat
  and cut into 1-inch pieces
1 red onion, peeled and cut through root end into 8 wedges
2 tablespoons lemon juice
8 ounces (8 cups) arugula
1 ounce Parmesan cheese, shaved
2 large heirloom tomatoes, cored and sliced thin

1. Whisk vinegar, ¼ cup oil, mustard, garlic, pepper flakes, ½ teaspoon salt, and ½ teaspoon pepper together in large bowl. Transfer ½ cup vinegar mixture to small saucepan. Toss steak with remaining vinegar mixture and let marinate for 10 minutes.

2. Meanwhile, cook reserved ½ cup vinegar mixture over medium heat until slightly thickened, about 2 minutes; set aside basting sauce. Working with 1 skewer at a time, thread 1 onion wedge, followed by one-quarter of marinated steak, then 1 onion wedge onto each skewer.

3A. FOR A CHARCOAL GRILL Open bottom grill vent completely. Light large chimney starter filled with charcoal briquettes (6 quarts). When top coals are partially covered with ash, pour evenly over grill. Set cooking grate in place, cover, and open lid vent completely. Heat grill until hot, about 5 minutes.

3B. FOR A GAS GRILL Turn all burners to high, cover, and heat grill until hot, about 15 minutes. Leave all burners on high.

4. Clean and oil cooking grate. Place skewers on grill and cook (covered if using gas), turning and basting with sauce every 2 minutes, until well charred and meat registers 120 to 125 degrees (for medium-rare), 10 to 12 minutes. Transfer to plate, tent with aluminum foil, and let rest for 5 minutes.

5. Whisk lemon juice, ¼ teaspoon salt, and ⅛ teaspoon pepper, and 2 tablespoons oil in large bowl. Add arugula and gently toss to coat. Sprinkle salad with Parmesan. Arrange tomatoes on serving platter, then drizzle with remaining 1 tablespoon oil and season with pepper. Using tongs, slide steak and onions off skewers onto platter with tomatoes and season with pepper to taste. Serve with salad.

PER SERVING

Cal 340 • **Total Fat** 23g • **Sat Fat** 6g • **Chol** 80mg
Sodium 430mg • **Total Carbs** 6g • **Fiber** 1g • **Total Sugar** 4g
Added Sugar 0g • **Protein** 26g • **Total Carbohydrate Choices** 0.5

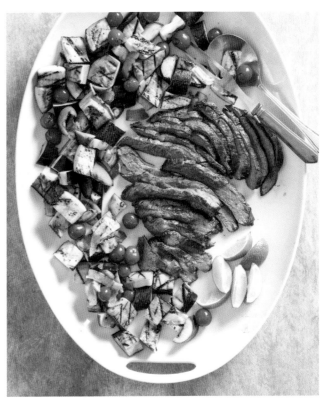

Flank steak is lean, tender, and quick-cooking as well as being a great source of protein and vitamins.

Grilled Flank Steak with Summer Vegetables

SERVES 6

WHY THIS RECIPE WORKS Rich and beefy flank steak is thin, flat, and quick-cooking, making it ideal for grilling. It is also relatively inexpensive, so you can serve it at a dinner party without breaking the bank. We chose fresh zucchini, eggplant, red onion, and cherry tomatoes for our vegetables, taking care to grill each element to perfection. We prefer this steak cooked to medium-rare, but if you prefer it more or less done, see our guidelines on page 209. You will need four 12-inch metal skewers for this recipe.

1 red onion, sliced into ½-inch-thick rounds
8 ounces cherry tomatoes
2 zucchini, sliced lengthwise into ¾-inch-thick planks
1 pound eggplant, sliced lengthwise into ¾-inch-thick planks
2 tablespoons extra-virgin olive oil
  Salt and pepper
1½ pounds flank steak, trimmed of all visible fat
  Lime wedges

1. Thread onion rounds from side to side onto two 12-inch metal skewers. Thread cherry tomatoes onto two 12-inch metal skewers. Brush onion rounds, tomatoes, zucchini, and eggplant with oil and sprinkle with ½ teaspoon pepper. Pat steak dry with paper towels and sprinkle with ¼ teaspoon salt and ⅛ teaspoon pepper.

2A. FOR A CHARCOAL GRILL Open bottom grill vent completely. Light large chimney starter filled with charcoal briquettes (6 quarts). When top coals are partially covered with ash, pour evenly over grill. Set cooking grate in place, cover, and open lid vent completely. Heat grill until hot, about 5 minutes.

2B. FOR A GAS GRILL Turn all burners to high, cover, and heat grill until hot, about 15 minutes. Leave all burners on high.

3. Clean and oil cooking grate. Place steak, onion and tomato skewers, zucchini, and eggplant on grill. Cook (covered if using gas), flipping steak and turning vegetables as needed, until steak is well browned and registers 120 to 125 degrees (for medium-rare) and vegetables are slightly charred and tender, 7 to 12 minutes. Transfer steak and vegetables to carving board as they finish grilling and tent with aluminum foil. Let steak rest for 10 minutes.

4. Meanwhile, using tongs, slide tomatoes and onions off skewers. Cut onion rounds, zucchini, and eggplant into 2- to 3-inch pieces. Arrange vegetables on serving platter and season with pepper to taste. Slice steak thin against grain on bias and arrange on platter with vegetables. Serve with lime wedges.

PER SERVING

Cal 270 • **Total Fat** 15g • **Sat Fat** 4.5g • **Chol** 75mg
Sodium 170mg • **Total Carbs** 10g • **Fiber** 3g • **Total Sugar** 6g
Added Sugar 0g • **Protein** 26g • **Total Carbohydrate Choices** 0.5

Beef en Cocotte with Mushrooms
SERVES 12

WHY THIS RECIPE WORKS The French method of cooking *en cocotte* (in a covered pot in a low oven), combines the best of braising and roasting. The low, slow heat allows the fibers to break down, rendering a tough piece of meat tender. We discovered that a top sirloin roast was the best option; not only was it very tender when done, it also had a concentrated beefy flavor. We started by searing the roast to create meaty fond, then cooked non-starchy onions, cremini mushrooms, and porcini mushrooms for an even more flavorful umami base. We then deglazed the pan with wine and cognac, and had, along with some tarragon, a decadent braising liquid—and the beginnings of a sumptuous sauce. We prefer this roast cooked to medium-rare, but if you prefer it more or less done, see our guidelines on page 209.

1 (3-pound) top sirloin roast, trimmed of all visible fat and tied at 1½-inch intervals
  Salt and pepper
4 teaspoons canola oil
8 ounces cremini mushrooms, trimmed and sliced thin
1 onion, halved and sliced thin
½ ounce dried porcini mushrooms, rinsed and minced
6 garlic cloves, lightly crushed and peeled
1 tablespoon no-salt-added tomato paste
¼ cup dry white wine
2 tablespoons cognac
2 sprigs fresh tarragon, plus 2 tablespoons minced
2 cups unsalted chicken broth

1. Adjust oven rack to lowest position and heat oven to 250 degrees. Pat roast dry with paper towels and sprinkle with ¾ teaspoon salt and ½ teaspoon pepper. Heat 2 teaspoons oil in Dutch oven over medium-high heat until just smoking. Brown beef on all sides, about 10 minutes; transfer to plate.

2. Add cremini mushrooms, onion, porcini mushrooms, and remaining 2 teaspoons oil to fat left in pot. Cover and cook until mushrooms release their moisture, about 5 minutes. Uncover and continue to cook, stirring often, until liquid has evaporated and vegetables are well browned, 5 to 7 minutes.

3. Stir in garlic and tomato paste and cook until fragrant, about 30 seconds. Stir in wine and cognac, scraping up any browned bits, and cook until nearly evaporated, about 1 minute. Add tarragon sprigs.

4. Nestle roast into pot along with any accumulated juices. Place large sheet of aluminum foil over pot and press to seal, then cover tightly with lid. Transfer pot to oven and cook until meat registers 120 to 125 degrees (for medium-rare), 45 to 75 minutes.

5. Transfer roast to carving board, tent with foil, and let rest for 20 minutes. Discard tarragon sprigs. Stir broth into cooking liquid and simmer over medium-high heat until thickened slightly, about 2 minutes. Off heat, stir in minced tarragon and season with pepper to taste; cover to keep warm.

6. Discard twine. Slice roast thin and transfer to serving platter. Spoon sauce over meat and serve.

PER SERVING

Cal 190 • **Total Fat** 6g • **Sat Fat** 1.5g • **Chol** 80mg
Sodium 240mg • **Total Carbs** 3g • **Fiber** 1g • **Total Sugar** 1g
Added Sugar 0g • **Protein** 28g • **Total Carbohydrate Choices** <0.5

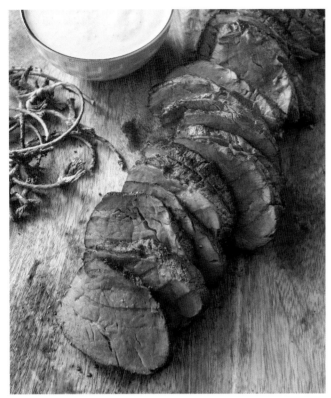

A beef tenderloin is a company-worthy roast that's also a great source of lean protein.

Roast Beef Tenderloin

SERVES 12

WHY THIS RECIPE WORKS When devising a no-fuss recipe for perfectly cooked roast beef tenderloin, we chose to work with Châteaubriand, the smaller center-cut roast. To flavor the meat, we salted it, covered it in plastic wrap, and let it rest on the counter for an hour. We reversed the usual cooking process, roasting the meat first and then searing it, to eliminate the ring of overdone meat just below the crust and to give the roast an appealing ruby coloring from edge to edge. Flavorful horseradish sauce is a classic accompaniment to roast tenderloin. Buy refrigerated prepared horseradish, not the shelf-stable kind, which contains preservatives and additives. We prefer this roast cooked to medium-rare, but if you prefer it more or less done, see our guidelines on page 209.

HORSERADISH SAUCE

½ cup mayonnaise

¼ cup sour cream

3 tablespoons prepared horseradish

2 tablespoons lemon juice

½ teaspoon garlic powder

Salt and pepper

BEEF TENDERLOIN

¾ teaspoon salt

1 (3-pound) center-cut beef tenderloin roast, trimmed of all visible fat and tied at 1½-inch intervals

½ teaspoon pepper

2 teaspoons canola oil

1. FOR THE HORSERADISH SAUCE Combine mayonnaise, sour cream, horseradish, lemon juice, garlic powder, ¼ teaspoon salt, and ⅛ teaspoon pepper in bowl. Adjust consistency with water as needed and season with pepper to taste. Cover and refrigerate until ready to serve. (Sauce can be refrigerated for up to 2 days.)

2. FOR THE BEEF TENDERLOIN Sprinkle salt evenly over roast, cover loosely with plastic wrap, and let sit at room temperature for 1 hour.

3. Adjust oven rack to middle position and heat oven to 300 degrees. Pat roast dry with paper towels. Sprinkle roast evenly with pepper and transfer to wire rack set in rimmed baking sheet. Roast until meat registers 120 to 125 degrees (for medium-rare), 40 to 55 minutes, flipping roast halfway through roasting.

4. Heat oil in 12-inch skillet over medium-high heat until just smoking. Brown roast on all sides, 4 to 8 minutes. Transfer roast to carving board, tent with aluminum foil, and let rest for 15 minutes. Discard twine and slice roast thin. Serve with sauce.

PER SERVING

Cal 250 • **Total Fat** 16g • **Sat Fat** 4g • **Chol** 80mg
Sodium 330mg • **Total Carbs** 1g • **Fiber** 0g • **Total Sugar** 1g
Added Sugar 0g • **Protein** 25g • **Total Carbohydrate Choices** <0.5

Pomegranate-Braised Beef Short Ribs with Prunes and Sesame

SERVES 8

WHY THIS RECIPE WORKS This braise takes its cue from a popular combination in Moroccan tagines: meltingly tender beef and chewy, tangy prunes. We found that using unsweetened pomegranate juice as the braising liquid gave our sauce the perfect touch of tartness to balance the meatiness of the beef. *Ras el hanout*, the complex Moroccan spice blend that traditionally features a host of warm spices, added a pleasing, piquant aroma. We chose short ribs for their intense, beefy flavor and first roasted them in the oven; this enabled us to render and discard some saturated fat. After braising the ribs in the pomegranate juice, we defatted the cooking liquid, then blended it with the vegetables and some of the prunes to create a velvety sauce. We added the remaining prune halves to the sauce and garnished the finished dish with toasted sesame seeds and cilantro. You can find ras el hanout in the spice aisle of most well-stocked supermarkets.

4 pounds bone-in English-style short ribs, trimmed
   Salt and pepper
4 cups unsweetened pomegranate juice
1 cup water
2 tablespoons extra-virgin olive oil
1 onion, chopped fine
1 carrot, peeled and chopped fine
¼ cup toasted sesame seeds
2 tablespoons ras el hanout
4 garlic cloves, minced
1 cup prunes, halved
1 tablespoon red wine vinegar
2 tablespoons chopped fresh cilantro

1. Adjust oven rack to lower-middle position and heat oven to 450 degrees. Pat short ribs dry with paper towels and sprinkle with ½ teaspoon salt and ¼ teaspoon pepper. Arrange ribs bone side down in single layer in large roasting pan and roast until meat begins to brown, about 45 minutes.

2. Discard any accumulated fat and juices in pan and continue to roast until meat is well browned, 15 to 20 minutes. Transfer ribs to bowl and tent loosely with aluminum foil; set aside. Stir pomegranate juice and water into pan, scraping up any browned bits; set aside.

3. Reduce oven temperature to 300 degrees. Heat oil in Dutch oven over medium heat until shimmering. Add onion, carrot, and ¼ teaspoon salt and cook until softened, about 5 minutes. Stir in 2 tablespoons sesame seeds, ras el hanout, and garlic and cook until fragrant, about 30 seconds.

4. Stir in pomegranate mixture from roasting pan and half of prunes and bring to simmer. Nestle short ribs bone side up into

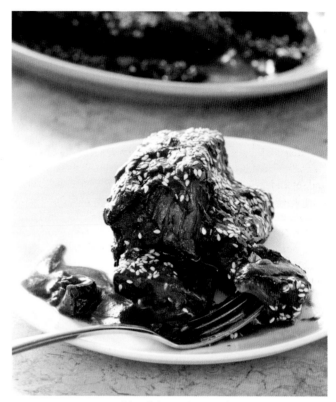

Our Moroccan-inspired beef short ribs use chopped prunes to enrich the velvety sauce.

pot and bring to simmer. Cover, transfer pot to oven, and cook until ribs are tender and fork slips easily in and out of meat, about 2½ hours.

5. Transfer short ribs to bowl, discard any loose bones, and tent with aluminum foil. Strain braising liquid through fine-mesh strainer into fat separator; transfer solids to blender. Let braising liquid settle for 5 minutes, then pour defatted liquid into blender with solids and process until smooth, about 1 minute.

6. Transfer sauce to now-empty pot and stir in vinegar and remaining prunes. Return short ribs and any accumulated juices to pot, bring to gentle simmer over medium heat, and cook, spooning sauce over ribs occasionally, until heated through, about 5 minutes. Season with pepper to taste. Transfer short ribs to serving platter, spoon 1 cup sauce over top, and sprinkle with cilantro and remaining 2 tablespoons sesame seeds. Serve, passing remaining sauce separately.

PER SERVING
Cal 360 • **Total Fat** 16g • **Sat Fat** 5g • **Chol** 55mg
Sodium 290mg • **Total Carbs** 37g • **Fiber** 3g • **Total Sugar** 27g
Added Sugar 0g • **Protein** 20g • **Total Carbohydrate Choices** 2.5

Orange-Sesame Beef and Vegetable Stir-Fry

SERVES 4

WHY THIS RECIPE WORKS Beef and broccoli is a classic combination for a stir-fry. Flank steak is the perfect choice for the beef as it is lean but has beefy flavor. For more nutritional punch and to up the vegetable quotient, we added two colorful red bell peppers. A simple and flavor-packed sauce with orange juice and neutral-tasting chicken broth as its base was easy to just whisk together and set aside while we prepared all the other ingredients. To avoid the grease trap that is so often a downfall of many stir-fries, we first steamed our vegetables until they were perfectly crisp and tender. Next we sautéed the thinly sliced beef and aromatics in heart-healthy canola oil before adding in the vegetables and sauce to heat through quickly. To make slicing the flank steak easier, put it in the freezer for 15 minutes.

SAUCE

½ cup unsalted chicken broth
½ cup orange juice
3 tablespoons low-sodium soy sauce
2 tablespoons toasted sesame oil
1½ tablespoons cornstarch

STIR-FRY

3 scallions, minced
3 garlic cloves, minced
1 tablespoon grated fresh ginger
1 tablespoon canola oil
⅛ teaspoon red pepper flakes
1 pound broccoli, florets cut into 1-inch pieces, stalks peeled and sliced thin
⅓ cup water
2 red bell peppers, stemmed, seeded, and cut into 2-inch-long matchsticks
12 ounces flank steak, trimmed of all visible fat, sliced thin against grain into 2-inch-long pieces
½ teaspoon toasted sesame oil
Pinch salt
1 tablespoon toasted sesame seeds

1. FOR THE SAUCE Whisk all ingredients together in bowl.

2. FOR THE STIR-FRY Combine scallions, garlic, ginger, 1 teaspoon canola oil, and pepper flakes in small bowl; set aside.

3. Cook broccoli and water in covered 12-inch nonstick skillet over high heat until water is boiling and broccoli is green and beginning to soften, about 2 minutes. Uncover, add bell peppers, and cook until water has evaporated and vegetables are crisp-tender, about 3 minutes; transfer to colander.

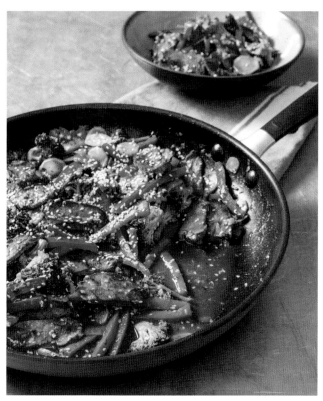

To boost the nutritional profile of our beef stir-fry, we use more vegetables than meat.

4. Heat 1 teaspoon canola oil in now-empty skillet over high heat until just smoking. Add half of beef in single layer and cook without stirring for 1 minute. Continue to cook, stirring occasionally, until spotty brown on both sides, about 1 minute; transfer to clean bowl. Repeat with remaining beef and 1 teaspoon canola oil; transfer to bowl.

5. Add scallion mixture to again-empty skillet and cook over high heat, mashing mixture into skillet, until fragrant, about 30 seconds. Stir in beef and cooked vegetables. Whisk sauce to recombine, then add to skillet and cook, stirring constantly, until sauce has thickened, about 30 seconds. Stir in sesame oil and salt, then sprinkle with sesame seeds. Serve immediately.

PER SERVING
Cal 320 • **Total Fat** 17g • **Sat Fat** 3.5g • **Chol** 55mg
Sodium 530mg • **Total Carbs** 18g • **Fiber** 4g • **Total Sugar** 7g
Added Sugar 0g • **Protein** 23g • **Total Carbohydrate Choices** 1

Getting to Know Beef

Compared to lean cuts of chicken and pork, lean cuts of beef pack more fat, calories, and cholesterol per ounce. But this doesn't mean you need to strip beef from your diet. Beef is a source of high-quality protein and can be healthy as long as you trim away all of the visible fat, are mindful of portion size, and eat it in moderation (up to 2 times per week). For example, if you don't trim your steak, you could be unknowingly adding up to 20 grams of fat and 180 calories to your meal; beef fat has 8 grams of saturated fat per ounce. Rather than cut the portion size down too much, we allot 4 ounces of beef (raw weight) per person, which is a satisfyingly ample amount for dinner.

PER 4 OUNCES	CAL	UNSAT FAT	SAT FAT
Boneless Top Sirloin, Trimmed of Visible Fat	149	5g	2g
Boneless Strip Loin, Trimmed of Visible Fat	156	6g	2g
Flank Steak, Trimmed of Visible Fat	160	6g	2g
Skirt Steak, Trimmed of Visible Fat	194	11g	4g
Blade Steak, Trimmed of Visible Fat	158	7g	3g
Steak Tips, Trimmed of Visible Fat	161	6g	2g
Beef Tenderloin, Trimmed of Visible Fat	174	7g	3g

CUTTING UP FLANK STEAK FOR STIR-FRY

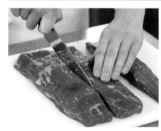

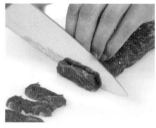

1. To make slicing flank steak easier, freeze it until firm, about 15 minutes. Slice meat lengthwise (with the grain) into 2-inch-wide strips.

2. Slice each 2-inch strip thin (against grain) into ¼-inch-thick slices.

Stir-Fried Beef with Bok Choy and Green Beans
SERVES 4

WHY THIS RECIPE WORKS Chinese restaurant stir-fries are beloved for their thin strips of meat in succulent sauce, but all too often the meat is chewy, the sauce is loaded with sodium, and the vegetables are few and far between. To boost the nutritional profile of this beef stir-fry, we first used more vegetables than meat: bok choy, green beans, and carrots provided color, crispness, and a little sweetness. Lean flank steak delivered plenty of protein, great beef flavor, and a moderate chew. Cornstarch worked double duty, preventing the meat from drying out and thickening the sauce. To make slicing the flank steak easier, put it in the freezer for 15 minutes.

SAUCE
- ¼ cup water
- 2 tablespoons dry sherry or Chinese rice wine
- 1 tablespoon low-sodium soy sauce
- 1½ teaspoons cornstarch
- 1 tablespoon oyster sauce
- 2 teaspoons rice vinegar
- 2 teaspoons coarsely ground pepper
- 1½ teaspoons toasted sesame oil

STIR-FRY
- 1 tablespoon dry sherry or Chinese rice wine
- 1 tablespoon low-sodium soy sauce
- 1½ teaspoons cornstarch
- 12 ounces flank steak, trimmed of all visible fat, sliced thin against grain into 2-inch-long pieces
- 2 tablespoons canola oil
- 3 garlic cloves, minced
- 1 tablespoon grated fresh ginger
- 1 pound bok choy, stalks and greens separated, stalks cut on bias into ¼-inch slices and greens cut into ½-inch strips
- 8 ounces green beans, trimmed and cut into 2-inch lengths
- 1 carrot, peeled and shredded

1. FOR THE SAUCE Whisk all ingredients together in bowl.

2. FOR THE STIR-FRY Whisk sherry, soy sauce, and cornstarch together in large bowl. Add beef to soy sauce mixture, tossing to coat, and set aside for 15 to 30 minutes. Combine 2 teaspoons oil, garlic, and ginger in separate bowl; set aside.

3. Heat 1 teaspoon oil in 12-inch nonstick skillet over high heat until just smoking. Add half of beef in single layer and cook without stirring for 1 minute. Continue to cook, stirring occasionally, until spotty brown on both sides, about 1 minute; transfer to clean bowl. Repeat with remaining beef and 1 teaspoon oil; transfer to bowl.

4. Heat remaining 2 teaspoons oil in now-empty skillet over high heat until just smoking. Add bok choy stalks and green beans and cook, stirring occasionally, until vegetables are spotty brown and crisp-tender, about 5 minutes. Push vegetables to sides of skillet. Add garlic mixture to center and cook, mashing mixture into skillet, until fragrant, 30 to 60 seconds. Stir mixture into vegetables. Stir in bok choy greens, carrot, and beef.

5. Whisk sauce to recombine, then add to skillet and cook, stirring constantly, until sauce has thickened, about 30 seconds. Serve immediately.

PER SERVING

Cal 270 • **Total Fat** 15g • **Sat Fat** 3g • **Chol** 60mg
Sodium 520mg • **Total Carbs** 12g • **Fiber** 3g • **Total Sugar** 4g
Added Sugar 0g • **Protein** 22g • **Total Carbohydrate Choices** 1

Steak Tacos with Jícama Slaw
SERVES 4

WHY THIS RECIPE WORKS To develop indoor steak tacos as tender, juicy, and rich-tasting as grilled, we chose flank steak and seared it to achieve the browned exterior and crisp, brittle edges characteristic of grilled meat. A paste of cilantro, scallions, garlic, and jalapeño gave our steak a flavor boost. And a bright jícama slaw with cilantro and lime was the perfect accompaniment for the rich meat. We prefer this steak cooked to medium-rare, but if you prefer it more or less done, see our guidelines on page 209. To make this dish spicier, include the seeds from the chile.

SLAW
    1 pound jícama, peeled and cut into 3-inch-long matchsticks
¼ cup thinly sliced red onion
    3 tablespoons chopped fresh cilantro
    1 tablespoon extra-virgin olive oil
    1 teaspoon grated lime zest plus 2 tablespoons juice
¼ teaspoon salt

TACOS
½ cup fresh cilantro leaves
    3 scallions, chopped
    3 garlic cloves, peeled
    1 jalapeño chile, stemmed, seeded, and chopped

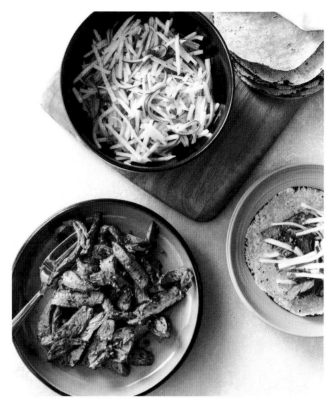

Delicately flavored and crunchy jícama makes a lively refreshing slaw to top spicy steak tacos.

½ teaspoon ground cumin
    2 tablespoons extra-virgin olive oil
    1 tablespoon lime juice
    1 (1-pound) flank steak, trimmed of all visible fat and cut lengthwise into 3 equal pieces
        Salt and pepper
12 (6-inch) corn tortillas, warmed

1. FOR THE SLAW Combine all ingredients in bowl. Cover and refrigerate until ready to serve.

2. FOR THE TACOS Pulse cilantro, scallions, garlic, jalapeño, cumin, and 4 teaspoons oil in food processor to paste, 10 to 12 pulses, scraping down sides of bowl as needed. Transfer 2 tablespoons herb paste to bowl, whisk in lime juice, and set aside for serving.

3. Using fork, poke each piece of steak 10 to 12 times on each side. Sprinkle steaks with ¼ teaspoon salt and place in 13 by 9-inch baking dish. Coat steaks thoroughly with remaining herb paste, cover dish, and refrigerate at least 30 minutes or up to 1 hour.

4. Scrape herb paste off steaks and pat dry with paper towels. Heat remaining 2 teaspoons oil in 12-inch nonstick skillet over medium-high heat until just smoking. Cook steaks until well browned and meat registers 120 to 125 degrees (for medium-rare), 5 to 7 minutes per side, adjusting heat as needed to prevent scorching. Transfer steaks to carving board and let rest for 5 minutes.

5. Slice steaks thin against grain on bias and transfer to large bowl. Toss steak with reserved herb mixture and season with pepper to taste. Divide steak evenly among tortillas and top with slaw. Serve.

PER SERVING

Cal 480 • **Total Fat** 19g • **Sat Fat** 4g • **Chol** 70mg
Sodium 370mg • **Total Carbs** 47g • **Fiber** 9g • **Total Sugar** 3g
Added Sugar 0g • **Protein** 29g • **Total Carbohydrate Choices** 3

Meatloaf with Mushroom Gravy
SERVES 6

WHY THIS RECIPE WORKS For an all-beef meatloaf that is tender and flavorful—not dry and grainy—we started with 93 percent lean ground beef rather than ground chuck or meatloaf mix. For moisture and some extra flavor, we swapped the usual dry bread crumbs for a single slice of whole-wheat bread. An untraditional ingredient, low-sodium soy sauce, also amped up the moisture and flavor of our meatloaf. Sautéed mushrooms, broken down in the food processor so they would blend in with the beef, added even more moisture and gave our meatloaf serious substance and heartiness. Baking the meatloaf elevated on a rimmed baking sheet instead of in a loaf pan eliminated the risk of it becoming soggy. A flavorful mushroom gravy made this meatloaf special, while still fitting into a diabetic-friendly diet.

3 tablespoons canola oil
1 onion, chopped fine
20 ounces cremini mushrooms, trimmed and sliced thin
3 garlic cloves, minced
1½ teaspoons minced fresh thyme
1 (1¼-ounce) slice 100 percent whole-wheat sandwich bread, torn into pieces
1 large egg
3 tablespoons minced fresh parsley
1 tablespoon low-sodium soy sauce
1 tablespoon Dijon mustard

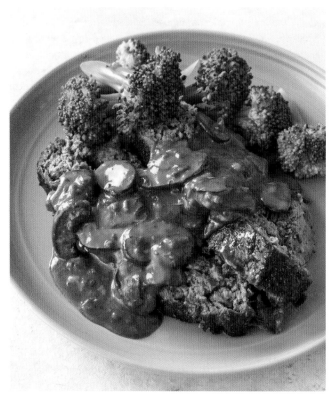

Fresh and dried mushrooms plus a little soy sauce add both moisture and flavor to our lean ground beef meatloaf and gravy.

Pepper
1½ pounds 93 percent lean ground beef
¼ ounce dried porcini mushrooms, rinsed and minced
2 tablespoons all-purpose flour
2 cups low-sodium beef broth
1 teaspoon Worcestershire sauce

1. Adjust oven rack to middle position and heat oven to 375 degrees. Set wire rack inside rimmed baking sheet and arrange 8 by 6-inch piece of aluminum foil in center of rack. Using skewer, poke holes in foil every ½-inch.

2. Heat 1 tablespoon oil in 12-inch nonstick skillet over medium heat until shimmering. Add onion and cook until softened, about 5 minutes. Stir in half of cremini mushrooms and cook until they have released their liquid and are lightly browned, about 10 minutes. Stir in garlic and 1 teaspoon thyme and cook until fragrant, about 30 seconds. Transfer to food processor and let cool for 5 minutes. Add bread and process until smooth, about 25 seconds, scraping down sides of bowl as needed.

3. Whisk egg, 2 tablespoons parsley, soy sauce, mustard, and ½ teaspoon pepper together in large bowl. Add mushroom mixture and beef and mix with hands until evenly combined. Using hands, shape mixture into 8 by 6-inch loaf on top of prepared foil. Bake until meatloaf registers 160 degrees, 50 to 60 minutes.

4. Meanwhile, heat remaining 2 tablespoons oil in now-empty skillet over medium-high heat until shimmering. Add porcini mushrooms and remaining cremini mushrooms and cook, stirring occasionally, until they have released their liquid and are deep golden brown, 6 to 8 minutes. Stir in remaining ½ teaspoon thyme and cook until fragrant, about 30 seconds. Add flour and cook, stirring frequently, until golden, about 2 minutes. Slowly whisk in broth and Worcestershire, scraping up any browned bits. Bring to simmer and cook, whisking occasionally, until thickened, 8 to 10 minutes. Cover gravy to keep warm.

5. Transfer meatloaf to cutting board, tent with foil, and let rest for 10 minutes. Stir remaining 1 tablespoon parsley into gravy and season with pepper to taste. Slice meatloaf and serve with gravy.

PER SERVING

Cal 310 • **Total Fat** 16g • **Sat Fat** 4g • **Chol** 100mg
Sodium 430mg • **Total Carbs** 12g • **Fiber** 2g • **Total Sugar** 3g
Added Sugar 0g • **Protein** 30g • **Total Carbohydrate Choices** 1

Stuffed Bell Peppers
SERVES 4

WHY THIS RECIPE WORKS Stuffed bell peppers can be problematic, with bland fillings and tough or mushy peppers, so we knew that creating an easy stuffed pepper recipe would require some tinkering. We started by boiling our peppers in water to soften the exteriors. This did two things: It parcooked the peppers to the perfect consistency so they needed less time in the oven, and we were then able to use the leftover boiling water to cook the rice until perfectly tender. For our filling, we built a flavorful base with carrots, onion, garlic, tomato paste, and chili powder. We added relatively lean beef to bulk up the protein, some tomatoes for freshness, and some cheese to bind everything together into a filling with a creamy texture. Fresh parsley and lemon juice added much welcome brightness to round out the filling. Since the filling was mostly hot, we stuffed the peppers, topped them with extra cheese, and put them in the oven until the cheese had melted and the filling was hot throughout. When shopping for the bell peppers, choose peppers of equal size and with broad bases that will allow them to stand upright in the pan. If the peppers don't stand upright, trim the bottoms slightly until they are level.

4 red bell peppers
Salt and pepper
½ cup long-grain brown rice
1 tablespoon extra-virgin olive oil
2 carrots, peeled and chopped fine
1 onion, chopped fine
6 garlic cloves, minced
2 teaspoons no-salt-added tomato paste
1 teaspoon chili powder
8 ounces 93 percent lean ground beef
2 tomatoes, cored, seeded, and chopped
¼ cup unsalted chicken broth
4 ounces extra-sharp cheddar cheese, shredded (1 cup)
2 tablespoons minced fresh parsley
1 tablespoon lemon juice

1. Bring 4 quarts water to boil in large pot. Trim ½ inch off top of each pepper, then remove seeds and core. Add 1 teaspoon salt to water, then submerge peppers and cook until they just begin to soften, about 5 minutes. Remove peppers from water, let drain, and place cut-side up on paper towel–lined plate to cool.

2. Return water to boil. Add rice and cook until tender, 25 to 30 minutes. Drain thoroughly and transfer to large bowl.

3. Adjust oven rack to middle position and heat oven to 350 degrees. Heat oil in 12-inch nonstick skillet over medium heat until shimmering. Add carrots, onion, and ⅛ teaspoon salt and cook until softened, about 5 minutes. Stir in garlic, tomato paste, and chili powder and cook until fragrant, about 30 seconds.

4. Add beef and cook, breaking up meat with wooden spoon, until no longer pink, about 5 minutes. Stir in tomatoes and chicken broth, scraping up any browned bits, and cook until tomatoes begin to break down, 1 to 2 minutes.

5. Stir beef mixture, ¾ cup cheddar, parsley, and lemon juice into rice and season with pepper to taste. Pat inside of peppers dry with paper towels, then place peppers in 8-inch square baking dish. Divide filling evenly among peppers and top with remaining ¼ cup cheddar. Bake until cheese is melted and filling is heated through, about 30 minutes. Serve.

PER SERVING

Cal 400 • **Total Fat** 18g • **Sat Fat** 7g • **Chol** 65mg
Sodium 410mg • **Total Carbs** 38g • **Fiber** 6g • **Total Sugar** 11g
Added Sugar 0g • **Protein** 24g • **Total Carbohydrate Choices** 2.5

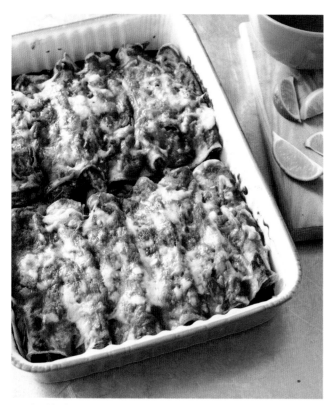

Tender blade steaks, along with a sprinkle of sharp cheddar cheese, give our beef enchiladas big flavor.

Beef Enchiladas

SERVES 6

WHY THIS RECIPE WORKS Traditional beef enchiladas, with silky, slow-cooked meat and a blanket of hearty chile sauce, are the ultimate in Mexican comfort food. But as with many comfort-food favorites, from-scratch enchiladas aren't exactly easy to make, nor are they high on the list of healthy dinner options. We wanted to simplify the enchilada-making process but still maintain some of the authentic flavor—all while keeping them a diabetic-friendly option. Since we were after simplicity and convenience, we turned to canned tomato sauce. We infused it with aromatics, chili powder, and spices for an easy yet deeply flavored sauce that wasn't overly acidic. Many enchilada fillings rely on beef chuck for intense beefy flavor, but this hefty cut from the shoulder requires a lengthy braise of 4 to 5 hours. Instead, we browned and simmered top blade steaks (smaller and conveniently inexpensive cuts also from the shoulder) in our sauce. This gave us a rich, meaty filling in half the time. For piquancy, freshness, and a salty finish, we added pickled jalapeños, cilantro, and a bit of *queso fresco* to the mix. We filled and rolled tortillas, then topped them with our

flavorful sauce and a light sprinkling of sharp cheddar cheese for just the right amount of gooey appeal that didn't leave us feeling weighed down. For a spicier dish, use the larger amount of pickled jalapeño chiles.

1½ pounds beef blade steaks, trimmed of all visible fat
   Pepper
   2 tablespoons canola oil
   2 onions, chopped fine
   ¼ cup chili powder
   5 garlic cloves, minced
   1 tablespoon ground coriander
   1 tablespoon ground cumin
   2 (15-ounce) cans no-salt-added tomato sauce
1½ cups water
   4 ounces queso fresco, crumbled (1 cup)
   ⅓ cup chopped fresh cilantro
2–4 tablespoons chopped jarred jalapeños
  12 (6-inch) corn tortillas
   2 ounces sharp cheddar cheese, shredded (½ cup)
   Lime wedges

1. Pat steaks dry with paper towels and sprinkle with ¼ teaspoon pepper. Heat oil in Dutch oven over medium-high heat until just smoking. Brown steaks, 2 to 3 minutes per side; transfer to plate.

2. Add onions to fat left in pot and cook over medium heat until softened, 6 to 8 minutes. Stir in chili powder, garlic, coriander, and cumin and cook until fragrant, about 1 minute. Stir in tomato sauce and water, scraping up any browned bits, and bring to simmer. Nestle steaks into pot along with any accumulated juices. Reduce heat to medium-low, cover, and cook, stirring occasionally, until steaks are tender and knife slips easily in and out of meat, about 1½ hours.

3. Adjust oven rack to middle position and heat oven to 350 degrees. Transfer steaks to cutting board, let cool slightly, then shred into bite-size pieces using 2 forks; discard gristle.

4. Strain sauce through fine-mesh strainer into 4-cup liquid measuring cup, pressing on solids to extract as much sauce as possible; discard solids. (You should have 2 cups sauce; add water as needed to equal 2 cups.) Combine beef, ½ cup sauce, queso fresco, cilantro, and jalapeños in bowl and season with pepper to taste.

5. Spread ¾ cup sauce in bottom of 13 by 9-inch baking dish. Wrap tortillas in clean kitchen towel and microwave until pliable, 30 to 90 seconds. Top each tortilla with ¼ cup beef mixture, roll tightly, and lay seam side down in dish (2 columns of 6 tortillas will fit neatly across width of dish).

6. Spread ¼ cup sauce evenly over enchiladas. Sprinkle with cheddar, cover with aluminum foil, and bake until hot throughout, about 25 minutes. Remove foil and continue to bake until cheese browns slightly, 5 to 10 minutes.

7. Let enchiladas rest for 5 minutes. Microwave remaining sauce until warm, about 30 seconds. Serve enchiladas, passing sauce and lime wedges separately.

Stuffed Pork Chops
SERVES 6

WHY THIS RECIPE WORKS Making stuffed pork chops starts with choosing the right cut of pork: lean and convenient boneless chops. For the stuffing, we hit up our crisper drawer; sautéed spinach and fennel made for a fresher and healthier alternative to the usual sausage and bread-crumb combo. Goat cheese gave the filling some richness and helped bind the elements, while lemon zest contributed brightness. A spice rub of coriander, cumin, and crushed fennel seeds on the outside of the chops added more layers of flavor and echoed the anise-like notes of the sautéed fennel. To cook our chops, we "seared" them on a preheated sheet pan; a spritz of vegetable oil spray ensured they emerged from the oven nicely golden. Cooking 3 whole chops and serving a half chop per person cut into ½-inch-thick slices made for a stunning presentation and appropriate portion size.

1 tablespoon extra-virgin olive oil
½ small fennel bulb, stalks discarded, cored, and chopped fine
1 shallot, minced
  Salt and pepper
2 garlic cloves, minced
2 tablespoons dry white wine
6 ounces (6 cups) baby spinach
1½ ounces goat cheese, crumbled (⅓ cup)
¼ teaspoon grated lemon zest
3 (8-ounce) boneless pork chops, about 1 inch thick, trimmed of all visible fat
1 teaspoon fennel seeds, toasted and crushed

1 teaspoon ground coriander
½ teaspoon ground cumin
  Vegetable oil spray

1. Adjust oven rack to upper-middle position, place rimmed baking sheet on rack, and heat oven to 475 degrees. Heat oil in 12-inch nonstick skillet over medium heat until shimmering. Add fennel, shallot, and ⅛ teaspoon salt and cook until softened and lightly browned, 5 to 7 minutes. Stir in garlic and cook until fragrant, about 30 seconds. Stir in wine, scraping up any browned bits, and cook until evaporated. Stir in spinach and cook until wilted, about 2 minutes. Transfer to bowl, let cool for 5 minutes, then stir in goat cheese and lemon zest. Season with pepper to taste.

2. Working with 1 chop at a time, use paring knife to cut 1-inch opening in side of chop. Through opening, continue to cut large pocket inside center of chop for filling; use fingers to help enlarge pocket if necessary. Repeat with remaining chops.

3. Pat chops dry with paper towels. Using spoon and your fingers, gently stuff chops with spinach filling. Combine fennel seeds, coriander, cumin, ¼ teaspoon salt, and ½ teaspoon pepper in bowl, then rub spice mixture evenly over chops. Spray both sides of chops with oil spray. Lay chops on preheated sheet and roast until pork registers 145 degrees, 10 to 14 minutes, flipping chops halfway through roasting. Transfer chops to carving board, tent with aluminum foil, and let rest for 5 minutes. Slice chops ½ inch thick and serve.

STUFFING PORK CHOPS

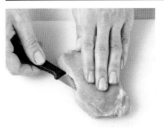 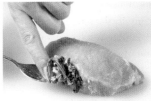

1. Insert small sharp knife through side of chop until tip almost reaches opposite edge. Swing knife through meat, creating large pocket.

2. Use your finger to widen pocket almost to edge of chop. Spoon small amount of filling into chop.

Pork Chops with Braised Cabbage
SERVES 4

WHY THIS RECIPE WORKS Pork chops and cabbage are a classic combination, but the pork often winds up dry, and the cabbage bland and mushy. We wanted a simple, one-pot version that turned out perfectly cooked chops and cabbage. We started by browning the chops to develop fond in the pot. After transferring the chops to a plate, we softened carrots and onion in the pot along with some aromatics before adding a hefty amount of cabbage and our cooking liquid (broth and white wine). We then returned the chops to the pot so they could finish cooking. Once the pork was cooked through, we transferred the chops to a carving board to rest while the cabbage finished cooking and the liquid evaporated. Sour cream, mustard, and vinegar gave the cabbage an extra pop of brightness (plus a bit of creaminess) before serving.

2 (10-ounce) bone-in center-cut pork chops, 1 inch thick, trimmed of all visible fat
 Salt and pepper
2 teaspoons canola oil
2 carrots, peeled and chopped
1 onion, halved and sliced thin
2 garlic cloves, minced
1 teaspoon minced fresh thyme or ¼ teaspoon dried
¼ teaspoon cumin seeds, toasted
½ head green cabbage (about 1 pound), cored and sliced thin
½ cup unsalted chicken broth
¼ cup dry white wine
⅓ cup low-fat sour cream
1 tablespoon whole-grain mustard
1 teaspoon cider vinegar

1. Pat chops dry with paper towels and sprinkle with ¼ teaspoon salt and ⅛ teaspoon pepper. Heat oil in Dutch oven over medium-high heat until just smoking. Brown chops well on first side, about 3 minutes; transfer to plate.

2. Add carrots and onion to fat left in pot and cook over medium heat until softened, 6 to 8 minutes. Stir in garlic, thyme, and cumin and cook until fragrant, about 30 seconds.

3. Stir in cabbage, broth, wine, and ⅛ teaspoon salt, bring to simmer, and cook until cabbage begins to soften, about 10 minutes. Nestle chops browned side up into pot and continue to cook until cabbage is wilted and pork registers 145 degrees, 5 to 10 minutes.

4. Transfer chops to carving board, tent with aluminum foil, and let rest while finishing cabbage. Continue to cook cabbage over medium heat until liquid has completely evaporated, 2 to 4 minutes.

5. Combine sour cream and mustard in bowl and season with pepper to taste. Off heat, stir vinegar and 2 tablespoons sour cream-mustard mixture into cabbage and season with pepper to taste. Carve chops from bones and slice ½ inch thick. Serve with cabbage, passing remaining sour cream mixture separately.

PER SERVING
Cal 320 • **Total Fat** 11g • **Sat Fat** 3g • **Chol** 85mg
Sodium 480mg • **Total Carbs** 16g • **Fiber** 5g • **Total Sugar** 10g
Added Sugar 0g • **Protein** 35g • **Total Carbohydrate Choices** 1

One-Pan Roasted Pork Chops and Vegetables with Parsley Vinaigrette
SERVES 4

WHY THIS RECIPE WORKS Thick-cut bone-in pork chops deliver the succulence of a larger roast but cook in just 10 to 15 minutes, making them perfect weeknight treats. They stand up to high heat and bold flavors, so it was natural to pair them with roasted root vegetables and to season everything well for a memorably flavor-packed one-pan meal. We partially roasted the vegetables—a rustic mix of thick-sliced Yukon Gold potatoes, carrot sticks, and fennel wedges—to give them a good head start. To add base notes of flavor, we first tossed them with minced fresh rosemary and peeled whole garlic cloves, which turn deliciously creamy when roasted. Once the vegetables had softened and taken on some color, we added our pork chops, which we'd seasoned with a bold rub of pepper, salt, paprika, and coriander for a deeply flavored crust. We whisked up a simple parsley vinaigrette to drizzle over the pork, ensuring our meal would end on a high note.

1 pound Yukon Gold potatoes, unpeeled, halved lengthwise and sliced ½ inch thick
1 pound carrots, peeled and cut into 3-inch lengths, thick ends quartered lengthwise
1 fennel bulb, stalks discarded, bulb halved, cored, and cut into ½-inch-thick wedges
10 garlic cloves, peeled
3 tablespoons plus 1 teaspoon extra-virgin olive oil
2 teaspoons minced fresh rosemary or ¾ teaspoon dried

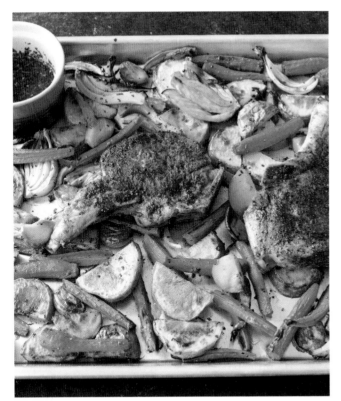

Roasting boldly seasoned thick-cut pork chops on top of plenty of root vegetables provides an easy-prep weeknight meal.

Salt and pepper
1 teaspoon paprika
1 teaspoon ground coriander
2 (10-ounce) bone-in center-cut pork chops, 1 inch thick, trimmed of all visible fat
4 teaspoons red wine vinegar
2 tablespoons minced fresh parsley
1 small shallot, minced

1. Adjust oven rack to upper-middle position and heat oven to 450 degrees. Toss potatoes, carrots, fennel, garlic, 1 tablespoon oil, rosemary, ¼ teaspoons salt, and ¼ teaspoon pepper together in bowl. Spread vegetables into single layer on rimmed baking sheet. Roast until beginning to soften, about 25 minutes.

2. Combine 1 teaspoon oil, paprika, coriander, ¼ teaspoon salt, and 1 teaspoon pepper in bowl. Pat pork dry with paper towels, then rub with spice mixture. Lay chops on top of vegetables and continue to roast until pork register 145 degrees and vegetables are tender, 10 to 15 minutes, rotating sheet halfway through roasting.

3. Remove sheet from oven, tent with aluminum foil, and let rest for 5 minutes. Whisk remaining 2 tablespoons oil, vinegar, parsley, shallot, ¼ teaspoon salt, and ¼ teaspoon pepper together in bowl. Transfer chops to carving board, carve meat from bone, and slice ½ inch thick. Drizzle vinaigrette over pork before serving with vegetables.

PER SERVING

Cal 480 • **Total Fat** 19g • **Sat Fat** 4g • **Chol** 80mg
Sodium 640mg • **Total Carbs** 39g • **Fiber** 7g • **Total Sugar** 8g
Added Sugar 0g • **Protein** 36g • **Total Carbohydrate Choices** 2.5

Spice-Rubbed Pork Tenderloin with Fennel, Tomatoes, Artichokes, and Olives
SERVES 4

WHY THIS RECIPE WORKS When done right, nothing can match the fine-grained, buttery-smooth texture of pork tenderloin. Since it has a tendency to be bland, it benefits from bold seasoning. We wondered if a dry rub might allow us to skip the step of browning, adding both flavor and color to our tenderloin without the extra work. We were looking for a distinct flavor profile and reasoned that herbes de Provence would easily give a distinctly Mediterranean flavor to our pork. A little of this spice goes a long way; a mere 1 teaspoon was sufficient to flavor and coat a tenderloin without overwhelming the pork. For a vegetable that would complement both the rub and the pork, we thought of sweet, mild fennel and supplemented it with artichokes, kalamata olives, and cherry tomatoes. After jump-starting the fennel in the microwave, we cooked the tenderloin on top of the vegetables on a baking sheet. In less than an hour, we were transported to Provence with a weeknight dinner that was low on fuss but high on flavor.

TRIMMING PORK SILVERSKIN

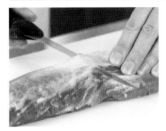

Silverskin is a swath of connective tissue located between the meat and the fat that covers its surface. To remove silverskin, simply slip a knife under it, angle slightly upward, and use a gentle back-and-forth motion to cut it away.

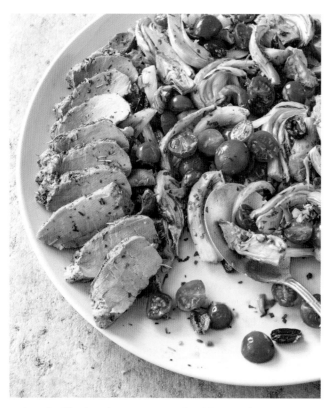

A dry rub of herbes de Provence easily adds great flavor and color to roasted pork tenderloin.

2 large fennel bulbs, stalks discarded, bulbs halved, cored, and sliced ½ inch thick

12 ounces frozen artichoke hearts, thawed and patted dry

½ cup pitted kalamata olives, halved

3 tablespoons extra-virgin olive oil

1 teaspoon herbes de Provence
   Salt and pepper

1 (1-pound) pork tenderloin, trimmed of all visible fat

1 pound cherry tomatoes, halved

1 tablespoon grated lemon zest

2 tablespoons minced fresh parsley

1. Adjust oven rack to lower-middle position and heat oven to 450 degrees. Microwave fennel and 2 tablespoons water in covered bowl until softened, about 5 minutes. Drain fennel well, then toss with artichoke hearts, olives, and 2 tablespoons oil.

2. Combine herbes de Provence, ¼ teaspoon salt, and ¼ teaspoon pepper in bowl. Pat tenderloin dry with paper towels, then rub with remaining 1 tablespoon oil and sprinkle with herb mixture. Spread vegetables into even layer on rimmed baking sheet, then lay tenderloin on top. Roast until pork registers 145 degrees, 25 to 30 minutes, rotating sheet halfway through roasting.

3. Remove sheet from oven. Transfer tenderloin to carving board, tent with aluminum foil, and let rest while vegetables finish cooking. Stir tomatoes and lemon zest into vegetables and continue to roast until fennel is tender and tomatoes have softened, about 10 minutes. Stir in parsley and season with pepper to taste. Slice pork ½ inch thick and serve with vegetables.

PER SERVING

Cal 330 • **Total Fat** 15g • **Sat Fat** 2.5g • **Chol** 75mg
Sodium 400mg • **Total Carbs** 22g • **Fiber** 11g • **Total Sugar** 8g
Added Sugar 0g • **Protein** 28g • **Total Carbohydrate Choices** 1.5

One-Pan Roasted Pork Tenderloin with Green Beans and Potatoes
SERVES 4

WHY THIS RECIPE WORKS To create a satisfying one-pan meal of roasted pork and vegetables, we seasoned green beans and tossed them with flavorful aromatics—scallions, garlic, and lemon zest—and arranged them down the middle of a baking sheet, perching a tenderloin atop the beans to protect the lean meat from drying out while the vegetables roasted. As a complement, we chose quick-cooking fingerling potatoes. We simply halved them, tossed them with more of the aromatics, and arranged them cut sides down on the sheet for some tasty browning. Brushing a small amount of hoisin sauce over the lean cut of meat and roasting it for only 25 minutes produced perfectly cooked pork with balanced richness and beautiful browning. While the tenderloin rested, we gave the vegetables a little extra time in the oven to pick up some color.

1 pound green beans, trimmed

2 tablespoons extra-virgin olive oil

2 scallions, sliced thin

2 garlic cloves, minced

½ teaspoon grated lemon zest, plus lemon wedges
   for serving
   Salt and pepper

1 pound fingerling potatoes, unpeeled, halved lengthwise

1 tablespoon hoisin sauce

1 teaspoon water

1 (1-pound) pork tenderloin, trimmed of all visible fat

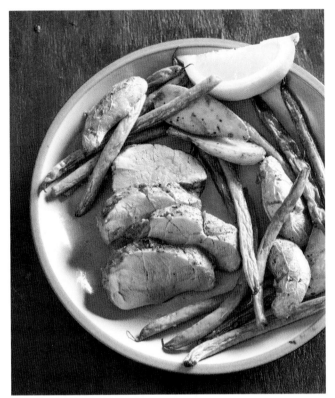

Pork tenderloin and fingerling potatoes cook relatively quickly and deliver a satisfying one-pan meal in about an hour.

1. Adjust oven rack to lower-middle position and heat oven to 450 degrees. Toss green beans with 1 tablespoon oil, half of scallions, half of garlic, lemon zest, ⅛ teaspoon salt, and ¼ teaspoon pepper in bowl. Arrange green beans crosswise down center of rimmed baking sheet, leaving room on both sides for potatoes. Toss potatoes with remaining 1 tablespoon oil, remaining scallions, remaining garlic, ¼ teaspoon salt, and ¼ teaspoon pepper in now-empty bowl. Place potatoes cut sides down on either side of green beans.

2. Whisk hoisin and water together in bowl. Pat tenderloin dry with paper towels, brush with hoisin mixture, and sprinkle with ¼ teaspoon salt and ⅛ teaspoon pepper. Lay tenderloin on top of green beans and roast until pork registers 145 degrees, 20 to 25 minutes, rotating sheet halfway through cooking.

3. Remove sheet from oven. Transfer tenderloin to carving board, tent with aluminum foil, and let rest while vegetables finish cooking. Gently stir vegetables on sheet to combine and continue to roast until tender and golden, 5 to 10 minutes. Slice pork ½ inch thick and serve with vegetables and lemon wedges.

PER SERVING

Cal 320 • **Total Fat** 10g • **Sat Fat** 2g • **Chol** 75mg
Sodium 500mg • **Total Carbs** 30g • **Fiber** 6g • **Total Sugar** 5g
Added Sugar 0g • **Protein** 28g • **Total Carbohydrate Choices** 2

Garlic Pork Roast
SERVES 8

WHY THIS RECIPE WORKS To make our garlic pork roast as garlicky as possible, we started with an impressive 18 cloves. We also wanted to take advantage of garlic's versatility, as it boasts different qualities when raw versus cooked, so we incorporated the garlic into our roast in three different ways. First, we used several raw cloves to make a marinade for the pork loin. We then toasted whole cloves and mashed them into a paste that we spread throughout the inside of the pork before rolling it up for roasting. Finally, we microwaved butter with more toasted garlic cloves to get a flavorful butter sauce that we brushed on the pork after it came out of the oven, just before serving. We found that leaving a ⅛-inch-thick layer of fat on top of the roast is ideal; if your roast has a thicker fat cap, trim it to be ⅛ inch thick.

1 (2-pound) boneless center-cut pork loin roast, fat trimmed to ⅛ inch
18 garlic cloves (10 peeled and smashed, 8 unpeeled)
4 teaspoons extra-virgin olive oil
   Salt and pepper
1½ teaspoons minced fresh thyme
¼ teaspoon red pepper flakes
1 tablespoon unsalted butter

1. Slice roast open down middle, from end to end, about two-thirds through pork. Gently press roast open. Carefully slice into sides of roast, being careful not to cut through, and press pork flat. Combine crushed garlic, 1 teaspoon oil, ½ teaspoon salt, and ¼ teaspoon pepper in bowl, then spread mixture evenly over roast. Wrap roast tightly with plastic wrap and refrigerate for at least 1 hour or up to 24 hours.

2. Toast unpeeled garlic cloves in 12-inch skillet over medium heat until fragrant and color deepens slightly, about 8 minutes; set aside. When cool enough to handle, peel garlic. Mince 6 cloves, transfer to bowl, and add 1 teaspoon oil, thyme, pepper flakes, and ¼ teaspoon pepper. Mash mixture to paste with back of fork.

3. Adjust oven rack to lower-middle position and heat oven to 325 degrees. Set wire rack inside aluminum foil–lined rimmed baking sheet. Pat roast dry with paper towels. Spread garlic paste inside surface of pork, leaving ½-inch border on all sides. Wrap sides of pork around garlic paste, then tie at 1½-inch intervals with kitchen twine. Sprinkle with ¼ teaspoon pepper.

4. Heat remaining 2 teaspoons oil in 12-inch skillet over medium-high heat until just smoking. Brown roast on all sides, 6 to 10 minutes. Transfer to prepared rack in baking sheet and roast until pork registers 140 degrees, 50 to 60 minutes.

5. Mince remaining 2 toasted garlic cloves and place in bowl. Add butter and microwave until garlic is golden and butter is melted, about 1 minute, stirring halfway through microwaving. Transfer roast to carving board and brush with garlic butter. Tent with foil and let rest for 15 minutes. Discard twine and slice roast ½ inch thick. Serve.

PER SERVING

Cal 190 • **Total Fat** 8g • **Sat Fat** 2.5g • **Chol** 75mg
Sodium 200mg • **Total Carbs** 2g • **Fiber** 0g • **Total Sugar** 0g
Added Sugar 0g • **Protein** 26g • **Total Carbohydrate Choices** <0.5

NOTES FROM THE TEST KITCHEN

Natural Versus Enhanced Pork

Because modern pork is so lean and therefore somewhat bland and prone to dryness if overcooked, many producers now inject their fresh pork products with a sodium solution. So-called enhanced pork is now the only option at many supermarkets, especially when buying lean cuts like the tenderloin. (You can determine the difference by reading the label; if the pork has been enhanced it will have an ingredient list.) Enhanced pork is injected with a solution of water, salt, sodium phosphates, sodium lactate, potassium lactate, sodium diacetate, and varying flavor agents, generally adding 7 to 15 percent extra weight. While enhanced pork does cook up juicier (it has been pumped full of water!), we find the texture almost spongy, and the flavor is often unpleasantly salty. We prefer the genuine pork flavor of natural pork and rely on brining to keep it juicy. Also, enhanced pork loses six times the moisture that natural pork loses when frozen and thawed—yet another reason to avoid enhanced pork.

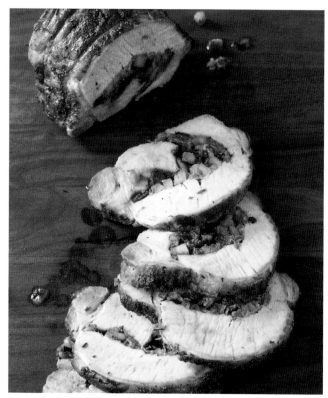

Just a few strategic cuts with a sharp knife and a pork loin roast is ready for a flavorful apple and fig stuffing.

Easy Stuffed Pork Loin with Figs and Balsamic Vinegar
SERVES 8

WHY THIS RECIPE WORKS Roast stuffed pork loin is an impressive centerpiece to a holiday meal. We worked to prevent some of the usual problems: meat that turns out tough and dry; stuffing with a dull flavor; and a roast that looks sloppy, with stuffing oozing out. For a flavorful stuffing, we created a sweet and tangy apple, shallot, and fig mixture. Precooking the stuffing ensured that the meat didn't have to roast until it was overcooked and dry. We found that leaving a ⅛-inch-thick layer of fat on top of the roast is ideal; if your roast has a thicker fat cap, trim it to be ⅛ inch thick.

1 tablespoon unsalted butter

1 Granny Smith apple, peeled, cored, and cut into ¼-inch pieces

2 shallots, halved and sliced thin

1 tablespoon minced fresh thyme

Pinch red pepper flakes

½ cup unsalted chicken broth

¼ cup dried figs, stemmed and chopped coarse

1 tablespoon balsamic vinegar

Salt and pepper

1 (2-pound) boneless center-cut pork loin roast, fat trimmed to ⅛ inch

1 teaspoon minced fresh rosemary or ¼ teaspoon dried

1 teaspoon ground coriander

1. Adjust oven rack to lower-middle position and heat oven to 375 degrees. Set wire rack inside aluminum foil–lined rimmed baking sheet.

2. Melt butter in 12-inch skillet over medium heat. Add apple and shallots and cook until softened and lightly browned, 10 to 12 minutes. Stir in 1 teaspoon thyme and pepper flakes and cook until fragrant, about 30 seconds. Stir in broth, figs, vinegar, and ¼ teaspoon salt, scraping up any browned bits, and cook until liquid has almost completely evaporated, 1 to 2 minutes; transfer to bowl and let cool slightly.

3. Slice roast open down middle, from end to end, about two-thirds through pork. Gently press roast open. Carefully slice into sides of roast, being careful not to cut through, and press pork flat. Sprinkle inside of roast with ¼ teaspoon salt and ⅛ teaspoon pepper, then spread stuffing evenly down center leaving ½-inch border on all sides. Wrap sides of pork around filling, then tie at 1½-inch intervals with kitchen twine.

4. Combine remaining 2 teaspoons thyme, rosemary, coriander, ¼ teaspoon salt, and ⅛ teaspoon pepper in bowl. Pat roast dry with paper towels and sprinkle with spice mixture. Place roast on prepared rack in baking sheet and roast until pork registers 140 degrees, 50 to 70 minutes.

5. Transfer roast to carving board, tent with aluminum foil, and let rest for 15 minutes. Discard twine and slice roast ½ inch thick. Serve.

PER SERVING

Cal 190 • **Total Fat** 6g • **Sat Fat** 5g • **Chol** 75mg
Sodium 280mg • **Total Carbs** 7g • **Fiber** 1g • **Total Sugar** 5g
Added Sugar 0g • **Protein** 26g • **Total Carbohydrate Choices** 0.5

PREPARING A STUFFED PORK LOIN

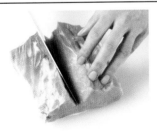 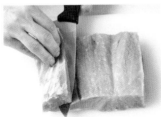 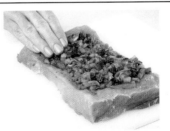 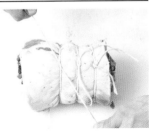

1. Slice pork open down middle, from end to end, about two-thirds through meat.

2. Gently press pork loin open. Carefully slice into sides of roast, being careful not to cut through, and press pork flat.

3. Season inside of pork, then mound filling evenly down center of roast.

4. Wrap sides of pork around filling, then tie roast closed with butcher's twine at 1½-inch intervals. Don't tie roast too tight or you may squeeze out filling.

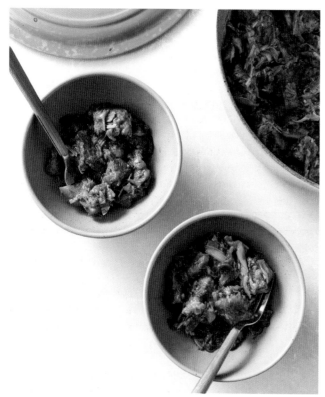

Leeks are a great source of fiber and antioxidants—this pork dish contains a full two pounds of them.

Greek-Style Braised Pork with Leeks
SERVES 6

WHY THIS RECIPE WORKS Pork braised with an abundant amount of leeks in white wine is a classic Greek dish. For our version, we browned the pork to add deep flavor. Because leeks are milder than onions, we used a full 2 pounds to ensure that we got a ton of flavor. After sautéing the leeks in the fat left from searing the pork, we built our aromatic base by cooking diced tomatoes and garlic. We then combined everything with white wine, chicken broth, and a bay leaf and put it all in the oven to cook low and slow until the pork was meltingly tender and the leeks were soft. A sprinkle of fresh oregano added pleasant earthy and minty notes. Pork butt roast is often labeled "Boston butt" in the supermarket.

1½ pounds boneless pork butt roast, trimmed of all visible fat and cut into 1-inch pieces
    Salt and pepper
2 tablespoons extra-virgin olive oil
2 pounds leeks, white and light green parts only, halved lengthwise, sliced 1 inch thick, and washed thoroughly
2 garlic cloves, minced
½ teaspoon grated lemon zest
1 (14.5-ounce) can no-salt-added diced tomatoes
1 cup dry white wine
½ cup unsalted chicken broth
1 bay leaf
2 teaspoons chopped fresh oregano

1. Adjust oven rack to lower-middle position and heat oven to 325 degrees. Pat pork dry with paper towels and sprinkle with ½ teaspoon salt and ¼ teaspoon pepper. Heat 1 tablespoon oil in Dutch oven over medium-high heat until just smoking. Brown pork on all sides, about 8 minutes; transfer to bowl.

2. Add remaining 1 tablespoon oil, leeks, ¼ teaspoon salt, and ½ teaspoon pepper to fat left in pot and cook over medium heat until softened and lightly browned, 5 to 7 minutes. Stir in garlic and lemon zest and cook until fragrant, about 30 seconds. Stir in tomatoes and their juice, scraping up any browned bits, and cook until tomato liquid is nearly evaporated, 10 to 12 minutes.

3. Stir in wine, broth, bay leaf, and pork along with any accumulated juices and bring to simmer. Cover, transfer pot to oven, and cook until pork is tender, 1 to 1½ hours. Discard bay leaf. Stir in oregano and season with pepper to taste. Serve.

PER SERVING
Cal 300 • **Total Fat** 13g • **Sat Fat** 3.5g • **Chol** 75mg
Sodium 310mg • **Total Carbs** 14g • **Fiber** 2g • **Total Sugar** 5g
Added Sugar 0g • **Protein** 24g • **Total Carbohydrate Choices** 1

Grilled Spiced Pork Skewers with Onion and Caper Relish
SERVES 6

WHY THIS RECIPE WORKS For grilled pork skewers that were moist and flavorful, we turned to boneless country-style ribs, which are quick-cooking and tender, yet have enough fat to keep them from drying out. The flavorful North African–inspired seasonings of garlic, lemon, coriander, cumin, nutmeg, and cinnamon did double duty, first in a marinade and later in a basting sauce. As a base for the relish, we grilled onions alongside the pork. We mixed the grilled onions with a zesty combination of olives, capers, balsamic vinegar, and parsley for a bright, potent sauce that perfectly complemented the skewers. You will need six 12-inch metal skewers for this recipe.

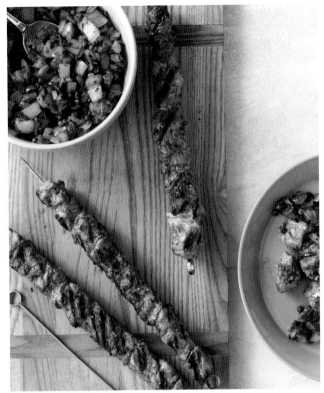

For flavorful and juicy pork kebabs, we use boneless country-style ribs and marinate them in warm spices.

6 tablespoons extra-virgin olive oil

5 garlic cloves, minced

1 tablespoon grated lemon zest

1 tablespoon ground coriander

2 teaspoons ground cumin

½ teaspoon ground nutmeg

½ teaspoon ground cinnamon

Salt and pepper

1½ pounds boneless country-style pork ribs, trimmed of all visible fat and cut into 1-inch pieces

2 onions, sliced into ½-inch-thick rounds

½ cup pitted kalamata olives, chopped

¼ cup capers, rinsed

3 tablespoons balsamic vinegar

2 tablespoons minced fresh parsley

1. Whisk ¼ cup oil, garlic, lemon zest, coriander, cumin, nutmeg, cinnamon, ¼ teaspoon salt, and ½ teaspoon pepper together in medium bowl. Measure out and reserve 2 tablespoons

marinade. Combine remaining marinade and pork in 1-gallon zipper-lock bag and toss to coat. Press out as much air as possible and seal bag. Refrigerate for at least 1 hour or up to 2 hours, flipping bag every 30 minutes.

2. Remove pork from bag and pat dry with paper towels. Thread pork tightly onto four 12-inch metal skewers. Thread onion rounds from side to side onto two 12-inch metal skewers and brush with 1 tablespoon oil.

3A. FOR A CHARCOAL GRILL Open bottom vent completely. Light large chimney starter three-quarters filled with charcoal briquettes (4½ quarts). When top coals are partially covered with ash, pour evenly over grill. Set cooking grate in place, cover, and open lid vent completely. Heat grill until hot, about 5 minutes.

3B. FOR A GAS GRILL Turn all burners to high, cover, and heat grill until hot, about 15 minutes. Turn all burners to medium-high.

4. Clean and oil cooking grate. Place pork and onion skewers on grill and cook (covered if using gas), turning skewers every 2 minutes and basting pork with reserved marinade, until pork is browned and registers 145 degrees and onions are slightly charred and tender, 10 to 15 minutes. Transfer pork and onions to cutting board as they finish grilling and tent with aluminum foil. Let pork rest while preparing relish.

5. Coarsely chop onions and combine with remaining 1 tablespoon oil, olives, capers, vinegar, and parsley. Season with pepper to taste. Using tongs, slide pork off skewers onto serving platter. Serve with relish.

PER SERVING

Cal 330 • **Total Fat** 21g • **Sat Fat** 4.5g • **Chol** 85mg
Sodium 350mg • **Total Carbs** 7g • **Fiber** 2g • **Total Sugar** 3g
Added Sugar 0g • **Protein** 25g • **Total Carbohydrate Choices** 0.5

NOTES FROM THE TEST KITCHEN

Buying Country-Style Pork Ribs

Country-style ribs aren't actually ribs at all. They're well-marbled pork chops cut from the upper side of the rib cage, from the fatty blade end of the loin. Because they contain a good amount of intramuscular fat, they are a favorite to make into kebabs, particularly when we want only a small amount of juicy, tender pork. At the meat counter, these "ribs" can have widely varying proportions of light and dark meat, so be sure to choose those with a greater amount of dark.

Spicy Mexican Shredded Pork Tostadas
SERVES 6

WHY THIS RECIPE WORKS Simmered for hours with aromatics and spices and then shredded and browned in oil until crisp, pork *tinga* is comfort food with a distinctly south-of-the-border feel. Served atop a crunchy whole-grain corn tostada with fresh garnishes, it's rich and flavorful and offers a variety of appealing textures. We looked to slim down this heavyweight dish, since much of its fat comes from the well-marbled pork butt traditionally called for. Switching to pork tenderloin was a nonstarter: The leaner cut couldn't withstand the lengthy cooking time needed to develop the intense, deep flavor. Instead, we scaled back the amount of pork butt and supplemented it with hearty, fiber-rich pinto beans for an equally satisfying dish. Pork butt roast is often labeled "Boston butt" in the supermarket.

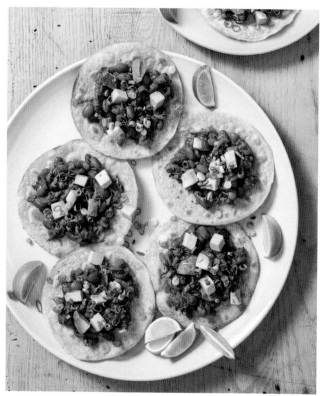

Cutting back on the amount of pork and adding pinto beans makes a healthier topping for crisp corn tostadas.

1 pound boneless pork butt roast, trimmed of all visible fat and cut into 1-inch pieces
2 onions, 1 quartered and 1 chopped fine
5 garlic cloves (3 peeled and smashed, 2 minced)
4 sprigs fresh thyme
2 bay leaves
12 (6-inch) corn tortillas
  Vegetable oil spray
2 teaspoons canola oil
½ teaspoon dried oregano
1 (15-ounce) can no-salt-added tomato sauce
1 (15-ounce) can no-salt-added pinto beans, rinsed
1 tablespoon minced canned chipotle chile in adobo sauce
  Salt and pepper
3 avocados, halved, pitted, and cut into ½-inch pieces
3 scallions, sliced thin
  Lime wedges

1. Bring 4 cups water, pork, quartered onion, smashed garlic, thyme sprigs, and bay leaves to simmer in large saucepan over medium-high heat, skimming off any foam that rises to surface. Reduce heat to medium-low, partially cover, and cook until meat is tender, 1¼ to 1½ hours.

2. Meanwhile, adjust oven racks to upper-middle and lower-middle positions and heat oven to 450 degrees. Spread tortillas over 2 rimmed baking sheets, spray both sides with oil spray, and bake until brown and crisp, 8 to 10 minutes, switching and rotating sheets halfway through baking.

3. Drain pork, reserving 1 cup of cooking liquid. Discard onion, garlic, thyme sprigs, and bay leaves. Return pork to saucepan and, using potato masher, mash until pork is shredded into rough ½-inch pieces.

4. Heat oil in 12-inch nonstick skillet over medium-high heat until just smoking. Add pork and chopped onion and cook until pork is well-browned and crisp, 5 to 7 minutes. Stir in minced garlic and oregano and cook until fragrant, about 30 seconds. Stir in reserved cooking liquid, tomato sauce, beans, chipotle, and ½ teaspoon salt. Bring to simmer and cook until almost all liquid has evaporated, 5 to 7 minutes. Season with pepper to taste. Spoon pork mixture evenly onto tostadas, top with avocados, and sprinkle with scallions. Serve with lime wedges.

PER SERVING

Cal 460 • **Total Fat** 24g • **Sat Fat** 4g • **Chol** 50mg
Sodium 280mg • **Total Carbs** 42g • **Fiber** 12g • **Total Sugar** 4g
Added Sugar 0g • **Protein** 22g • **Total Carbohydrate Choices** 3

Mexican Pork and Rice
SERVES 6

WHY THIS RECIPE WORKS Spiced with chipotle chiles and bathed in a tomatoey sauce, pork with Mexican flavors is a rich stew-like dish. Rather than spooning braised pork and sauce onto tortillas or tostadas, we used brown rice to absorb the sauce's flavors in this simple one-pot meal. The challenge lay in maintaining the dish's bold essence while achieving perfectly tender pork and well-cooked rice, all in the same pot. Early attempts were lackluster in flavor, so we cut the pork into cubes and browned each side to develop a golden-brown crust. The technique worked, imparting a meaty richness to the rice as it simmered away. We built upon our rich fond by adding onions, garlic, herbs, and chipotle chile in adobo sauce. The chipotles lent a subtle heat, as well as smokiness and depth. To provide a more substantial, meaty bite with the rice, we added pinto beans, which perfectly complemented our flavor profile. Finally, we finished our dish with a sprinkling of healthy peas and fresh chopped scallions and cilantro, along with a splash of lime juice. Pork butt roast is often labeled Boston Butt in the supermarket. You will need a Dutch oven with a tight-fitting lid for this recipe.

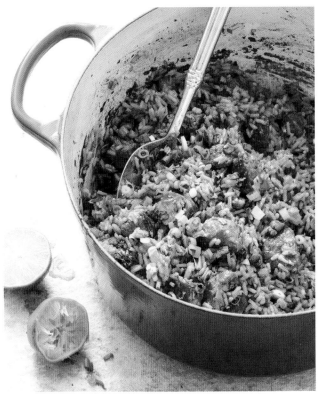

Brown rice, pinto beans, and frozen peas easily add fiber to this flavorful one-pot Mexican pork dinner.

1 tablespoon extra-virgin olive oil
2 onions, chopped fine
Salt and pepper
5 garlic cloves, minced
1 tablespoon minced canned chipotle chile in adobo sauce
2 teaspoons minced fresh oregano or ½ teaspoon dried
1 teaspoon minced fresh thyme or ¼ teaspoon dried
2 cups unsalted chicken broth
1 (8-ounce) can no-salt-added tomato sauce
1½ pounds boneless pork butt roast, trimmed of all visible fat and cut into 1-inch pieces
1 cup long-grain brown rice, rinsed
2 (15-ounce) cans no-salt-added pinto beans, rinsed
1 cup frozen peas
½ cup minced fresh cilantro
3 scallions, sliced thin
1 tablespoon lime juice, plus lime wedges for serving

1. Adjust oven rack to lower-middle position and heat oven to 300 degrees. Heat oil in Dutch oven over medium heat until shimmering. Add onions and ½ teaspoon salt and cook until softened, about 5 minutes. Stir in garlic, chipotle, oregano, and thyme and cook until fragrant, about 30 seconds. Stir in broth and tomato sauce, scraping up any browned bits, and bring to simmer. Stir in pork, cover, and transfer pot to oven. Cook until pork is tender, 1¼ to 1½ hours.

2. Remove pot from oven and increase oven temperature to 350 degrees. Stir in rice and beans, cover, and return pot to oven. Cook until rice is tender and all liquid has been absorbed, 40 to 50 minutes, gently stirring rice from bottom of pot to top halfway through cooking.

3. Remove pot from oven. Sprinkle peas over rice mixture, cover, and let sit until heated through, about 5 minutes. Add ¼ cup cilantro, scallions, and lime juice and gently fluff with fork to combine. Season with pepper to taste. Sprinkle with remaining ¼ cup cilantro and serve with lime wedges.

PER SERVING

Cal 440 • **Total Fat** 12g • **Sat Fat** 3.5g • **Chol** 75mg
Sodium 360mg • **Total Carbs** 50g • **Fiber** 9g • **Total Sugar** 8g
Added Sugar 0g • **Protein** 33g • **Total Carbohydrate Choices** 3

Braised Lamb with Tomatoes and Red Wine

SERVES 6

WHY THIS RECIPE WORKS When buying lamb, many people turn to the tried-and-true—and expensive—rib or loin chop. The tougher cut, boneless lamb leg, often doesn't get a second look. The leg's assertive flavor and somewhat chewy texture are particularly well suited to braising; we wanted a recipe for braised lamb leg that would yield tender meat and a rich, flavorful sauce. After browning the lamb to create flavorful fond, we sautéed onion and garlic, then deglazed the pan with wine. Tomatoes balanced out the acidity of the wine and cinnamon added warmth. We then returned the lamb to the pot and braised it until it was meltingly tender. As the lamb braised, the tomatoes broke down and created a luscious sauce. After trimming the lamb, you should have about 1½ pounds of meat.

> 2 pounds boneless lamb leg, trimmed of all visible fat and cut into 1-inch pieces
> Salt and pepper
> 2 tablespoons extra-virgin olive oil
> 1 onion, chopped fine
> 3 garlic cloves, minced
> ¼ teaspoon ground cinnamon
> ½ cup dry red wine
> 1 (28-ounce) can no-salt-added whole peeled tomatoes, drained and chopped
> 2 tablespoons minced fresh parsley

1. Adjust oven rack to lower-middle position and heat oven to 300 degrees. Pat lamb dry with paper towels and sprinkle with ½ teaspoon salt and ¼ teaspoon pepper. Heat 1 tablespoon oil in Dutch oven over medium-high heat until just smoking. Brown lamb on all sides, 8 to 10 minutes; transfer to bowl.

2. Add remaining 1 tablespoon oil and onions to fat left in pot and cook over medium heat until onions are softened, about 5 minutes. Stir in garlic and cinnamon and cook until fragrant, about 30 seconds. Stir in wine, scraping up any browned bits, and cook until reduced by half, about 1 minute.

3. Stir in tomatoes and lamb along with any accumulated juices and bring to simmer. Cover, transfer pot to oven, and cook until meat is tender, 1¼ to 1½ hours. Stir in parsley and season with pepper to taste. Serve.

PER SERVING

Cal 260 • **Total Fat** 12g • **Sat Fat** 3.5g • **Chol** 85mg
Sodium 380mg • **Total Carbs** 6g • **Fiber** 1g • **Total Sugar** 3g
Added Sugar 0g • **Protein** 29g • **Total Carbohydrate Choices** 0.5

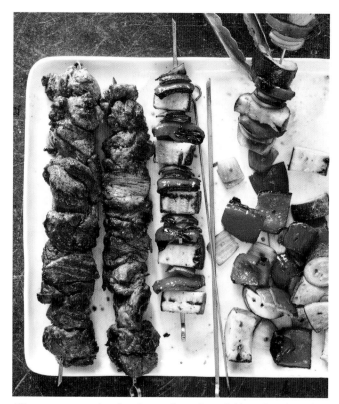

We cut our own chunks of meat from flavorful boneless leg of lamb and marinate them for just an hour before grilling.

Grilled Lamb Shish Kebabs

SERVES 6

WHY THIS RECIPE WORKS Shish kebab has its challenges, from overcooked meat to bland flavors; we wanted a foolproof method that would give us flavorful and perfectly cooked vegetables and meat. We opted to use a boneless leg of lamb: It's inexpensive, has bold lamb flavor, and cooks up tender in just minutes. We found three vegetables that worked well: bell peppers, red onions, and zucchini. They have similar textures and cook through at about the same rate when cut appropriately. Just 1 hour of marinating was enough to give the kebabs good flavor. Reserving some of the marinade allowed us to flavor our vegetables while they cooked. You will need six 12-inch metal skewers for this recipe. After trimming the lamb, you should have about 1½ pounds of meat. If you have long, thin pieces of meat, roll or fold them into approximate 2-inch cubes before skewering. We prefer the lamb cooked to medium-rare, but if you prefer it more or less done, see our guidelines on page 209.

MARINADE

- 6 tablespoons extra-virgin olive oil
- 7 large fresh mint leaves
- 2 teaspoons chopped fresh rosemary
- 2 garlic cloves, peeled
- ½ teaspoon salt
- ½ teaspoon grated lemon zest plus 2 tablespoons juice
- ¼ teaspoon pepper

LAMB AND VEGETABLES

- 2 pounds boneless leg of lamb, trimmed of all visible fat and cut into 2-inch pieces
- 2 zucchini or yellow summer squash, halved lengthwise and sliced 1 inch thick
- 2 red or green bell peppers, stemmed, seeded, and cut into 1½-inch pieces
- 2 red onions, cut into 1-inch pieces, 3 layers thick

1. FOR THE MARINADE Process all ingredients in food processor until smooth, about 1 minute, scraping down sides of bowl as needed. Transfer 3 tablespoons marinade to large bowl and set aside.

2. FOR THE LAMB AND VEGETABLES Place remaining marinade and lamb in 1-gallon zipper-lock bag and toss to coat. Press out as much air as possible and seal bag. Refrigerate for at least 1 hour or up to 2 hours, flipping bag every 30 minutes.

3. Add zucchini, bell peppers, and onions to bowl with reserved marinade and toss to coat. Cover and let sit at room temperature for at least 30 minutes.

4. Remove lamb from bag and pat dry with paper towels. Thread lamb tightly onto two 12-inch metal skewers. In alternating pattern of zucchini, bell pepper, and onion, thread vegetables onto four 12-inch metal skewers.

5A. FOR A CHARCOAL GRILL Open bottom vent completely. Light large chimney starter mounded with charcoal briquettes (7 quarts). When top coals are partially covered with ash, pour evenly over center of grill, leaving 2-inch gap between grill wall and charcoal. Set cooking grate in place, cover, and open lid vent completely. Heat grill until hot, about 5 minutes.

5B. FOR A GAS GRILL Turn all burners to high, cover, and heat grill until hot, about 15 minutes. Leave primary burner on high and turn other burner(s) to medium-low.

6. Clean and oil cooking grate. Place lamb skewers on grill (directly over coals if using charcoal or over hotter side of grill if using gas). Place vegetable skewers on grill (near edge of coals but still over coals if using charcoal or on cooler side of grill if using gas). Cook (covered if using gas), turning skewers every

3 to 4 minutes, until lamb is well browned and registers 120 to 125 degrees (for medium-rare), 10 to 15 minutes. Transfer lamb skewers to serving platter, tent loosely with aluminum foil, and let rest while finishing vegetables.

7. Continue to cook vegetable skewers until tender and lightly charred, 5 to 7 minutes; transfer to platter. Using tongs, slide lamb and vegetables off skewers onto serving platter. Serve.

PER SERVING

Cal 300 • **Total Fat** 17g • **Sat Fat** 4g • **Chol** 85mg
Sodium 270mg • **Total Carbs** 9g • **Fiber** 2g • **Total Sugar** 5g
Added Sugar 0g • **Protein** 29g • **Total Carbohydrate Choices** 0.5

Roast Butterflied Leg of Lamb with Coriander, Cumin, and Mustard Seeds
SERVES 12

WHY THIS RECIPE WORKS There is no better centerpiece for a special occasion than an aromatic roasted leg of lamb. Here we swapped in a butterflied leg of lamb for the usual bone-in or boned, rolled, and tied leg options, which kept things easy and allowed more thorough seasoning, created a great ratio of crust to meat, and meant faster, more even cooking. By first roasting the lamb in a 250-degree oven, we were able to keep the meat juicy, and a final blast under the broiler was all it took to crisp and brown the exterior. We ditched the usual spice rub (which had a tendency to scorch under the broiler) in favor of a slow-cooked spice-infused oil that seasoned the lamb during cooking. We prefer the lamb cooked to medium-rare, but if you prefer it more or less done, see our guidelines on page 209.

- 1 (2½-pound) boneless half leg of lamb
- 1½ teaspoons kosher salt
- ⅓ cup extra-virgin olive oil
- 3 shallots, sliced thin
- 4 garlic cloves, peeled and smashed
- 1 (1-inch) piece ginger, peeled, sliced into ½-inch-thick rounds, and smashed
- 1 tablespoon coriander seeds
- 1 tablespoon cumin seeds
- 1 tablespoon mustard seeds
- 3 bay leaves
- 2 (2-inch) strips lemon zest

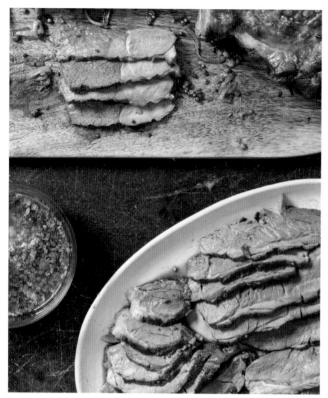

We pound a butterflied leg of lamb to an even thickness then roast it directly on top of a fragrant mix of aromatics and spices.

1. Place lamb on cutting board with fat cap facing down. Using sharp knife, trim any pockets of fat and connective tissue from underside of lamb. Flip lamb over, trim fat cap to ⅛ inch, and pound roast to even 1-inch thickness. Cut slits, spaced ½ inch apart, in fat cap in crosshatch pattern, being careful to cut down to but not into meat. Rub salt over entire roast and into slits. Let sit, uncovered, at room temperature for 1 hour.

2. Meanwhile, adjust oven rack to lower-middle position and second rack 4 to 5 inches from broiler element and heat oven to 250 degrees. Stir together oil, shallots, garlic, ginger, coriander seeds, cumin seeds, mustard seeds, bay leaves, and lemon zest in rimmed baking sheet and bake on lower rack until spices are softened and fragrant and shallots and garlic turn golden, about 1 hour. Remove sheet from oven and discard bay leaves.

3. Pat lamb dry with paper towels and transfer fat side up to sheet (directly on top of spices). Roast on lower rack until lamb registers 120 degrees, 20 to 25 minutes. Remove sheet from oven and heat broiler. Broil lamb on upper rack until surface is well browned and charred in spots and lamb registers 120 to 125 degrees (for medium-rare), 3 to 8 minutes.

4. Remove sheet from oven and transfer lamb to carving board (some spices will cling to bottom of roast). Tent loosely with aluminum foil and let rest for 20 minutes.

5. Slice lamb with grain into 2 equal pieces. Turn each piece and slice against grain into ¼-inch-thick slices. Serve.

PER SERVING

Cal 150 • **Total Fat** 7g • **Sat Fat** 2.5g • **Chol** 60mg
Sodium 220mg • **Total Carbs** 0g • **Fiber** 0g • **Total Sugar** 0g
Added Sugar 0g • **Protein** 19g • **Total Carbohydrate Choices** 0

VARIATIONS
Roast Butterflied Leg of Lamb with Coriander, Rosemary, and Red Pepper
Omit cumin and mustard seeds. Toss 6 sprigs fresh rosemary and ½ teaspoon red pepper flakes with oil mixture in step 2.

PER SERVING

Cal 150 • **Total Fat** 7g • **Sat Fat** 2.5g • **Chol** 60mg
Sodium 220mg • **Total Carbs** 0g • **Fiber** 0g • **Total Sugar** 0g
Added Sugar 0g • **Protein** 19g • **Total Carbohydrate Choices** 0

Roast Butterflied Leg of Lamb with Coriander, Fennel, and Black Pepper
Substitute fennel seeds for cumin seeds and black peppercorns for mustard seeds.

PER SERVING

Cal 150 • **Total Fat** 7g • **Sat Fat** 2.5g • **Chol** 60mg
Sodium 220mg • **Total Carbs** 0g • **Fiber** 0g • **Total Sugar** 0g
Added Sugar 0g • **Protein** 19g • **Total Carbohydrate Choices** 0

Harissa-Rubbed Roast Boneless Leg of Lamb with Warm Cauliflower Salad
SERVES 12

WHY THIS RECIPE WORKS The robust, fragrant flavor profile of North African cuisine is a perfect pairing with rich, meaty lamb. We again took advantage of the broad surface area of a boneless leg of lamb by rubbing it with Tunisian-inspired harissa paste. We bloomed paprika, coriander, Aleppo pepper, cumin, caraway, and garlic in oil in the microwave and applied our quick homemade harissa to the inside of the leg before rolling it up and tying it to make a compact roast. We seared the exterior of the meat on all sides to build up some browning before moving the lamb to the oven, where it finished roasting to a juicy medium-rare. We also applied more of the harissa to the outside of the roast in between the two cooking steps. Then, to keep the flavorful fat and fond from going to waste, we prepared a quick vegetable side while the roast rested by tossing cauliflower florets with the pan drippings and roasting them until tender and browned. Combining the warm cauliflower with shredded carrots, sweet raisins, cilantro, and toasted almonds produced a side that paired perfectly with the fragrant, richly spiced lamb. If you can't find Aleppo pepper, you can substitute ¾ teaspoon paprika plus ¾ teaspoon finely chopped red pepper flakes. We prefer the lamb cooked to medium-rare, but if you prefer it more or less done, see our guidelines on page 209.

½ cup extra-virgin olive oil
6 garlic cloves, minced
2 tablespoons paprika
1 tablespoon ground coriander
1 tablespoon ground dried Aleppo pepper
1 teaspoon ground cumin
¾ teaspoon caraway seeds
   Salt and pepper
1 (2½-pound) boneless half leg of lamb
1 head cauliflower (2 pounds), cored and cut into 1-inch florets
½ red onion, sliced ¼ inch thick
1 cup shredded carrots
½ cup raisins
¼ cup fresh cilantro leaves
2 tablespoons sliced almonds, toasted
1 tablespoon lemon juice, plus extra for seasoning

1. Combine 6 tablespoons oil, garlic, paprika, coriander, Aleppo pepper, cumin, caraway seeds, and ¾ teaspoon salt in bowl and microwave until bubbling and very fragrant, about 1 minute, stirring halfway through microwaving. Let cool to room temperature.

2. Adjust oven rack to lower-middle position and heat oven to 375 degrees. Set V-rack in large roasting pan and spray with vegetable oil spray. Place lamb on cutting board with fat cap facing up. Using sharp knife, trim fat cap to ⅛ inch. Flip lamb over and trim any pockets of fat and connective tissue from underside of lamb (side that was closest to bone). Pound roast to even 1-inch thickness, then rub with 2 tablespoons spice paste. Roll roast tightly into cylinder, tie at 1½-inch intervals with kitchen twine, then rub exterior with 1 tablespoon oil.

3. Heat remaining 1 tablespoon oil in 12-inch skillet over medium-high heat until just smoking. Brown lamb on all sides, about 8 minutes. Brush lamb all over with remaining spice paste

and place fat side down in prepared V-rack. Roast until lamb registers 120 to 125 degrees (for medium-rare), about 1 hour, flipping lamb halfway through roasting. Transfer lamb to carving board, tent with aluminum foil, and let rest while making salad.

4. Increase oven temperature to 475 degrees. Pour off all but 3 tablespoons fat from pan; discard any charred drippings. Add cauliflower, ½ teaspoon salt, and ½ teaspoon pepper to fat left in pan and toss to coat. Cover with foil and roast until cauliflower is softened, about 5 minutes.

5. Remove foil and spread onion evenly over cauliflower. Roast until vegetables are tender and cauliflower is golden brown, 10 to 15 minutes, stirring halfway through roasting. Transfer vegetable mixture to serving bowl, add carrots, raisins, cilantro, almonds, and lemon juice and toss to combine. Season with pepper and lemon juice to taste. Slice lamb ½ inch thick and serve with salad.

PER SERVING
Cal 260 • **Total Fat** 15g • **Sat Fat** 3.5g • **Chol** 60mg
Sodium 340mg • **Total Carbs** 10g • **Fiber** 2g • **Total Sugar** 6g
Added Sugar 0g • **Protein** 21g • **Total Carbohydrate Choices** 0.5

PREPARING BONELESS LEG OF LAMB

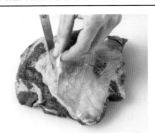

1. Place lamb on cutting board with fat cap facing up. Using sharp knife, trim fat cap to ⅛ inch.

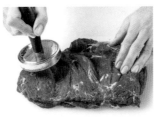

2. Flip lamb over and trim any pockets of fat and connective tissue from underside of lamb. Pound roast to even 1-inch thickness.

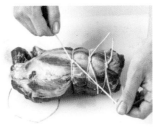

3. Rub with 2 tablespoons spice paste. Roll roast tightly into cylinder, tie at 1½-inch intervals with kitchen twine, then rub exterior with 1 tablespoon oil.

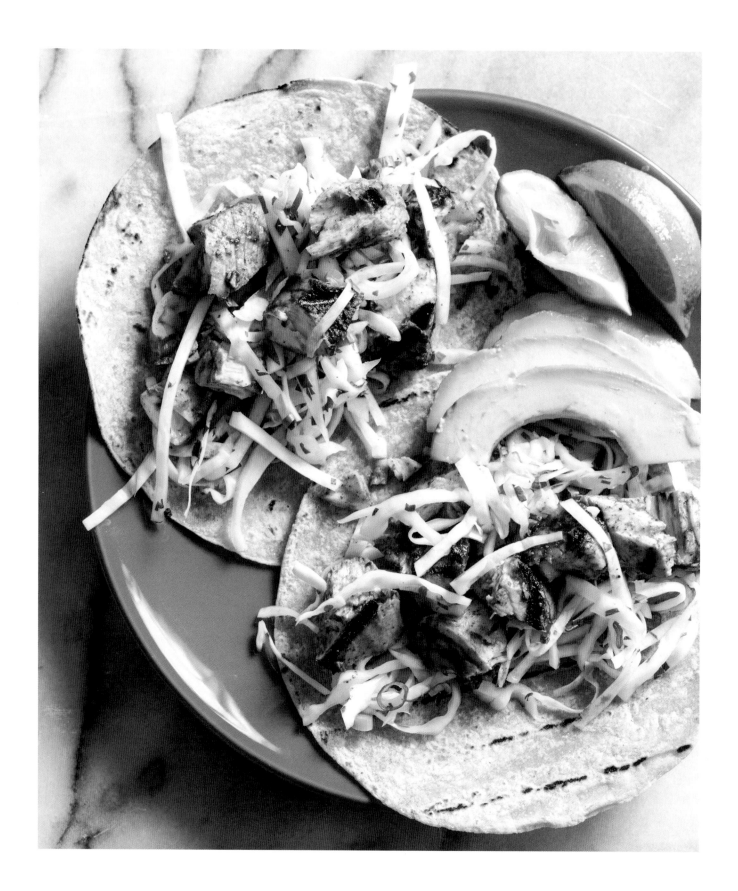

SEAFOOD

Photo: Grilled Fish Tacos

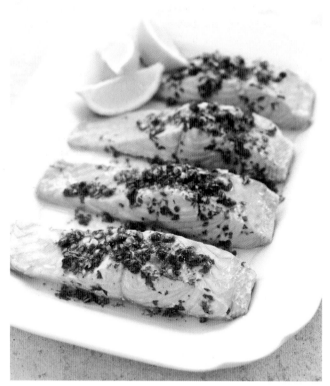

We poach salmon on a bed of lemons and herbs, then make a vibrant vinaigrette with the cooking liquid.

Poached Salmon with Herb and Caper Vinaigrette
SERVES 4

WHY THIS RECIPE WORKS It's no wonder salmon is so popular: Its flesh is rich-tasting thanks to high levels of heart-healthy omega-3 fatty acids. A great way to ensure moist, tender salmon is to poach it. And a vinaigrette packed with fresh herbs offers surprising nutritional value. Poaching the salmon in just enough liquid to come half an inch up its sides meant we didn't need much to boost the flavor of the liquid. However, the portion of the salmon that wasn't submerged needed to be steamed to cook through properly, and the low poaching cooking temperature didn't create enough steam. Cutting the water with some wine lowered the boiling point; the alcohol helped to produce more vapor even at the lower temperature. To keep the bottoms of the fillets from overcooking, we placed them on top of lemon slices. After poaching, we reduced the poaching liquid and added some olive oil and capers for an easy vinaigrette-style sauce. If using wild salmon, which contains less fat than farmed salmon, cook the fillets until they register 120 degrees (for medium-rare). For information on salmon, see page 245.

1 lemon, sliced into ¼-inch-thick rounds, plus lemon wedges for serving
2 tablespoons minced fresh parsley, stems reserved
2 tablespoons minced fresh tarragon, stems reserved
2 shallots, minced
½ cup dry white wine
½ cup water
1 (1½-pound) skinless salmon fillet, 1 inch thick
  Salt and pepper
2 tablespoons capers, rinsed and minced
1 tablespoon extra-virgin olive oil

1. Arrange lemon slices in single layer over bottom of 12-inch skillet. Scatter parsley stems, tarragon stems, and half of shallots over lemon slices then add wine and water.

2. Cut salmon crosswise into 4 fillets. Pat dry with paper towels and season with ¼ teaspoon salt and ⅛ teaspoon pepper. Lay salmon fillets, skinned-side down, on top of lemons and herb sprigs. Set pan over high heat and bring to simmer. Reduce heat to low, cover, and cook until centers are still translucent when checked with tip of paring knife and register 125 degrees (for medium-rare), 10 to 12 minutes.

3. Transfer salmon, herb sprigs, and lemon slices to paper towel–lined plate, cover with aluminum foil, and let drain while finishing sauce.

4. Return cooking liquid to medium-high heat and simmer until reduced to 1 tablespoon, 3 to 5 minutes. Combine remaining shallots, minced parsley, minced tarragon, capers, and oil in bowl. Strain reduced cooking liquid through fine-mesh strainer into bowl, whisk to combine, and season with pepper to taste.

5. Gently transfer drained salmon to individual serving plates, discarding lemon slices and herb stems. Spoon vinaigrette evenly over tops and serve.

PER SERVING

Cal 420 • **Total Fat** 26g • **Sat Fat** 6g • **Chol** 95mg
Sodium 350mg • **Total Carbs** 4g • **Fiber** 1g • **Total Sugar** 1g
Added Sugar 0g • **Protein** 35g • **Total Carbohydrate Choices** <0.5

VARIATION
Poached Salmon with Herb-Dijon Vinaigrette
Substitute 2 tablespoons minced fresh dill, stems reserved, for tarragon and add 1 tablespoon Dijon mustard to shallot-herb mixture in step 4. Omit capers.

PER SERVING

Cal 430 • **Total Fat** 26g • **Sat Fat** 6g • **Chol** 95mg
Sodium 340mg • **Total Carbs** 4g • **Fiber** 1g • **Total Sugar** 1g
Added Sugar 0g • **Protein** 35g • **Total Carbohydrate Choices** <0.5

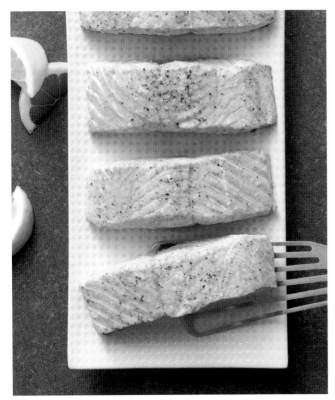

The key to moist oven-roasted salmon is threefold: a preheated roasting pan, a hot oven at first, then a lower oven to finish.

Oven-Roasted Salmon
SERVES 4

WHY THIS RECIPE WORKS Perfectly roasted salmon is a blank canvas for many healthy relishes and sauces, but you need a method for ensuring fish that cooks up tender, not dry. Our hybrid roasting method solves this common problem by heating the oven to 500 degrees before dropping the temperature to 275. The initial blast of heat firms the exterior and renders some fat while the fish gently cooks. We also place the baking sheet in the oven as it preheats, which jump-starts the cooking of the salmon. To ensure uniform pieces of fish that cooked at the same rate, we found it best to buy a whole center-cut fillet and cut it into four pieces ourselves. If using wild salmon, which contains less fat than farmed salmon, cook the fillets until they register 120 degrees (for medium-rare). For information on salmon, see page 245. Serve with one of the sauces on pages 242–243, if desired.

1 (1½-pound) skin-on salmon fillet, 1 inch thick
1 teaspoon extra-virgin olive oil
¼ teaspoon salt
⅛ teaspoon pepper

1. Adjust oven rack to lowest position, place aluminum foil–lined rimmed baking sheet on rack, and heat oven to 500 degrees. Cut salmon crosswise into 4 fillets, then make 4 or 5 shallow slashes about an inch apart along skin side of each piece, being careful not to cut into flesh. Pat fillets dry with paper towels, rub with oil, and sprinkle with salt and pepper.

2. Once oven reaches 500 degrees, reduce oven temperature to 275 degrees. Remove sheet from oven and carefully place salmon, skin-side down, on hot sheet. Roast until centers are still translucent when checked with tip of paring knife and register 125 degrees (for medium-rare), 8 to 12 minutes.

3. Slide spatula along underside of fillets and transfer to individual serving plates or serving platter, leaving skin behind; discard skin. Serve.

PER SERVING
Cal 360 • **Total Fat** 24g • **Sat Fat** 5g • **Chol** 95mg
Sodium 250mg • **Total Carbs** 0g • **Fiber** 0g • **Total Sugar** 0g
Added Sugar 0g • **Protein** 35g • **Total Carbohydrate Choices** 0

SCORING SALMON FILLETS

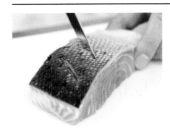

Salmon skin needs to be scored to keep it from buckling. Using a sharp or serrated knife, cut four or five shallow slashes, about an inch apart, through the skin of each piece of salmon, being careful not to cut into the fish.

Sesame Salmon with Napa Cabbage Slaw
SERVES 4

WHY THIS RECIPE WORKS For a simple, fresh supper, we paired seared salmon—coated in a sprinkling of sesame seeds—with a vibrant, fiber-rich slaw. Napa cabbage and grapefruit pieces were the base of our slaw and provided a light contrast to the rich fish. Shredded carrots added more texture, and thinly sliced jalapeño added just enough heat. We kept our slaw dressing simple: Rice vinegar, sesame oil, and just a bit of salt and pepper enhanced the flavor of the vegetables and complemented the sesame seeds on the salmon. To ensure uniform pieces of fish that cooked at the same rate, we found it best to buy a whole center-cut fillet and cut it into four pieces ourselves. For information on salmon, see page 245. Shred the carrots on the large holes of a box grater.

3 tablespoons unseasoned rice vinegar
1 tablespoon canola oil
2 teaspoons toasted sesame oil
  Salt and pepper
1 red grapefruit
½ head napa cabbage, cored and sliced thin (5½ cups)
3 carrots, peeled and shredded
3 scallions, sliced thin
1 jalapeño chile, stemmed, seeded, and sliced thin
1 (1½-pound) skin-on salmon fillet, 1 inch thick
1 teaspoon sesame seeds

1. Whisk vinegar, canola oil, sesame oil, ⅛ teaspoon salt, and ⅛ teaspoon pepper together in large bowl. Cut away peel and pith from grapefruit. Quarter grapefruit, then slice crosswise into ¼-inch-thick pieces. Add grapefruit pieces, cabbage, carrots, scallions, and jalapeño to dressing in bowl and toss to combine. Set aside.

2. Cut salmon crosswise into 4 fillets. Pat dry with paper towels and sprinkle with ¼ teaspoon salt and ⅛ teaspoon pepper. Sprinkle flesh sides of fillets evenly with sesame seeds.

3. Arrange salmon skin side down in 12-inch nonstick skillet. Place skillet over medium-high heat and cook until fat from skin renders, about 7 minutes. Flip salmon and continue to cook until centers are still translucent when checked with tip of paring knife and register 125 degrees (for medium-rare), about 7 minutes. Remove skin from salmon and serve with slaw.

PER SERVING

Cal 490 • **Total Fat** 29g • **Sat Fat** 6g • **Chol** 95mg
Sodium 410mg • **Total Carbs** 18g • **Fiber** 7g • **Total Sugar** 10g
Added Sugar 0g • **Protein** 38g • **Total Carbohydrate Choices** 1

Pomegranate Roasted Salmon with Lentils and Chard
SERVES 4

WHY THIS RECIPE WORKS Here we amplified the benefits of salmon by pairing it with high-fiber lentils, nutritious Swiss chard, and pomegranate molasses and seeds, a rich source of B vitamins. While chard stems are often discarded, they have great flavor, so we softened then simmered them with our lentils, stirring in the leaves near the end. For the salmon, we wanted sweetness without a sugary glaze, so we painted it with pomegranate molasses. Fresh pomegranate seeds tied the dish together. To ensure uniform pieces of fish that cooked at the same rate, we found it best to buy a whole center-cut fillet and cut it into four pieces ourselves.

If using wild salmon, which contains less fat than farmed salmon, cook the fillets until they register 120 degrees (for medium-rare). For information on salmon, see page 245. *Lentilles du Puy*, also called French green lentils, are our first choice, but brown, black, or regular green lentils will work (cooking times will vary).

1 tablespoon plus 1 teaspoon extra-virgin olive oil
12 ounces Swiss chard, stemmed, ½ cup stems chopped fine, leaves cut into 2-inch pieces
1 small onion, chopped fine
2 garlic cloves, minced
4 sprigs fresh thyme
  Salt and pepper
1½ cups unsalted chicken broth
¾ cup lentilles du Puy, picked over and rinsed
1 (1½-pound) skin-on salmon fillet, 1 inch thick
2 tablespoons pomegranate molasses
½ cup pomegranate seeds

1. Heat 1 tablespoon oil in large saucepan over medium-high heat until shimmering. Add chard stems, onion, garlic, thyme, and ⅛ teaspoon salt and cook, stirring frequently, until softened, about 5 minutes. Stir in broth and lentils and bring to boil. Reduce heat to low, cover, and simmer, stirring occasionally, until lentils are mostly tender but still intact, 45 to 55 minutes.

2. Adjust oven rack to lowest position, place aluminum foil–lined rimmed baking sheet on rack, and heat oven to 500 degrees. Uncover lentils and stir in chard leaves. Increase heat to medium-low and continue to cook until chard leaves are tender and lentils are completely tender, about 4 minutes. Off heat, discard thyme sprigs and season with pepper to taste; cover to keep warm.

3. Cut salmon crosswise into 4 fillets. Pat dry with paper towels. Brush with remaining 1 teaspoon oil, then brush with 1 tablespoon pomegranate molasses and sprinkle with ¼ teaspoon salt and ⅛ teaspoon pepper. Once oven reaches 500 degrees, reduce oven temperature to 275 degrees. Remove sheet from oven and carefully place salmon skin-side down on hot sheet. Roast until centers are still translucent when checked with tip of paring knife and register 125 degrees (for medium-rare), 4 to 6 minutes.

4. Brush salmon with remaining 1 tablespoon pomegranate molasses. Slide spatula under fillets and transfer to individual serving plates or serving platter, leaving skin behind; discard skin. Stir pomegranate seeds into lentil mixture and serve with salmon.

PER SERVING

Cal 580 • **Total Fat** 29g • **Sat Fat** 6g • **Chol** 95mg
Sodium 540mg • **Total Carbs** 35g • **Fiber** 8g • **Total Sugar** 9g
Added Sugar 0g • **Protein** 46g • **Total Carbohydrate Choices** 2

Black Rice Bowls with Salmon
SERVES 4

WHY THIS RECIPE WORKS Black rice, an ancient grain that was once reserved for the emperors of China, contains more protein, fiber, and iron than any other rice variety. We decided to use it in a Japanese-style rice bowl with healthful salmon as the star. To ensure well-seasoned grains with a bit of chew, we boiled the rice like pasta, and then drizzled it with a mix of rice vinegar, mirin, miso, and ginger. We roasted salmon fillets until medium-rare and then arranged them atop the rice before garnishing our bowls with radishes, avocado, cucumber, and scallions. To ensure uniform pieces of salmon that cooked at the same rate, we found it best to buy a whole center-cut fillet and cut it into four pieces ourselves. If using wild salmon, which contains less fat than farmed salmon, cook the fillets until they register 120 degrees (for medium-rare). For information on salmon, see page 245.

¾ cup black rice
   Salt and pepper
¼ cup unseasoned rice vinegar
¼ cup mirin
1 tablespoon white miso
1 teaspoon grated fresh ginger
½ teaspoon grated lime zest plus 2 tablespoons juice
1 (1½-pound) skin-on salmon fillet, 1 inch thick
1 teaspoon extra-virgin olive oil
4 radishes, trimmed, halved, and sliced thin
1 cucumber, halved lengthwise, seeded, and sliced thin
½ avocado, sliced thin
2 scallions, sliced thin

1. Bring 2 quarts water to boil in large saucepan over medium-high heat. Add rice and ½ teaspoon salt and cook until rice is tender, 20 to 25 minutes. Drain rice and transfer to large bowl.

2. Whisk vinegar, mirin, miso, ginger, lime zest and juice, ⅛ teaspoon salt, and ⅛ teaspoon pepper in small bowl until miso is fully incorporated. Measure out ¼ cup vinegar mixture and drizzle over rice. Let rice cool to room temperature, tossing occasionally, about 20 minutes. Set remaining dressing aside for serving.

3. While rice is cooking, adjust oven rack to lowest position, place aluminum foil–lined rimmed baking sheet on rack, and heat oven to 500 degrees. Cut salmon crosswise into 4 fillets. Pat salmon dry with paper towels, rub with oil, and sprinkle with ¼ teaspoon salt and ⅛ teaspoon pepper.

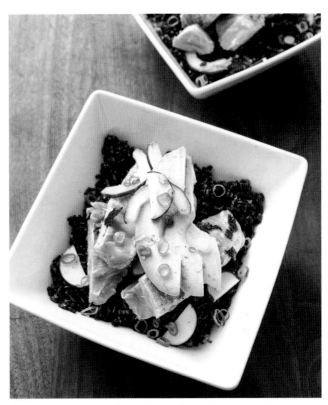

This easy Japanese-style bowl is packed with protein, fiber, and healthy fat thanks to roasted salmon, black rice, and avocado.

4. Once oven reaches 500 degrees, reduce oven temperature to 275 degrees. Remove sheet from oven and carefully place salmon skin-side down on hot sheet. Roast until centers are still translucent when checked with tip of paring knife and thickest part registers 125 degrees (for medium-rare), 4 to 6 minutes.

5. Flake salmon into large 3-inch pieces. Portion rice into 4 individual serving bowls and top with salmon, radishes, cucumber, and avocado. Sprinkle with scallions and drizzle with reserved dressing. Serve.

PER SERVING

Cal 580 • **Total Fat** 29g • **Sat Fat** 6 • **Chol** 95mg
Sodium 490mg • **Total Carbs** 37g • **Fiber** 5g • **Total Sugar** 7g
Added Sugar 0g • **Protein** 39g • **Total Carbohydrate Choices** 2.5

Homemade sauces are easy to make and a nice way to dress up a simply prepared piece of fish such as Oven-Roasted Salmon (page 239) and Sautéed Sole (page 247). These fresh relishes, mustard vinaigrette, and creamy sauces are really flavorful so a little goes a long way. Here are a few of the test kitchen's favorites to try.

Fresh Tomato Relish

MAKES 1 CUP

Be sure to use super-ripe tomatoes in this simple relish.

- 2 tomatoes, cored, seeded, and cut into ¼-inch pieces
- 1 small shallot, minced
- 1 small garlic clove, minced
- 2 tablespoons chopped fresh basil
- 1 tablespoon extra-virgin olive oil
- 1 teaspoon red wine vinegar
  Pepper

Combine all ingredients in bowl, let sit for 15 minutes, and season with pepper to taste.

PER ¼-CUP SERVING
Cal 45 • **Total Fat** 3.5g • **Sat Fat** 0.5g • **Chol** 0mg
Sodium 0mg • **Total Carbs** 3g • **Fiber** 1g • **Total Sugar** 2g
Added Sugar 0g • **Protein** 1g • **Total Carbohydrate Choices** <0.5

Grapefruit-Basil Relish

MAKES 1 CUP

The sweetness of this relish depends on the sweetness of the grapefruits.

- 2 red grapefruits
- 1 small shallot, minced
- 2 tablespoons chopped fresh basil
- 2 teaspoons lemon juice
- 2 teaspoons extra-virgin olive oil
  Pepper

Cut away peel and pith from grapefruits. Cut grapefruits into 8 wedges, then slice crosswise into ½-inch-thick pieces. Place grapefruit in strainer set over bowl and let drain for 15 minutes; measure out and reserve 1 tablespoon drained juice. Combine reserved juice, shallot, basil, lemon juice, and oil in bowl. Stir in grapefruit and let sit for 15 minutes. Season with pepper to taste. (Relish can be refrigerated for up to 2 days.)

PER ¼-CUP SERVING
Cal 80 • **Total Fat** 2.5g • **Sat Fat** 0g • **Chol** 0mg
Sodium 0mg • **Total Carbs** 17g • **Fiber** 6g • **Total Sugar** 10g
Added Sugar 0g • **Protein** 1g • **Total Carbohydrate Choices** 1

Mustard Vinaigrette with Lemon and Parsley

MAKES ½ CUP

- 3 tablespoons extra-virgin olive oil
- 2 tablespoons lemon juice
- 5 teaspoons whole-grain mustard
- 1 small shallot, minced
- 1 tablespoon water
- 2 teaspoons minced fresh parsley
  Pepper

Whisk oil, lemon juice, mustard, shallot, water, and parsley together in bowl and season with pepper to taste. Let sit for 10 minutes. (Vinaigrette can be refrigerated for up to 24 hours; whisk to recombine before serving.)

PER 2-TABLESPOON SERVING
Cal 110 • **Total Fat** 11g • **Sat Fat** 1.5g • **Chol** 0mg
Sodium 125mg • **Total Carbs** 1g • **Fiber** 0g • **Total Sugar** 0g
Added Sugar 0g • **Protein** 0g • **Total Carbohydrate Choices** <0.5

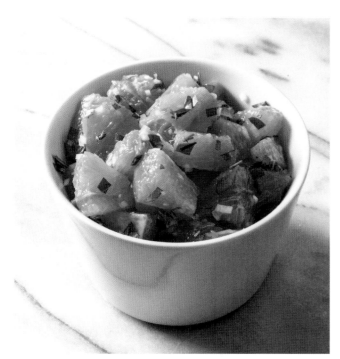

A bright and fresh relish makes a nice finishing touch for a simple piece of fish.

Tartar Sauce

MAKES ¹/₂ CUP

This briny sauce is the classic accompaniment for fish.

- ¼ cup mayonnaise
- 2 tablespoons low-fat sour cream
- 2 tablespoons finely chopped red onion
- 3 cornichons, minced, plus 2 teaspoons cornichon pickling juice
- 1 tablespoon capers, rinsed and minced
  Water
  Pepper

Combine mayonnaise, sour cream, onion, cornichons and juice, and capers in bowl. Add water as needed to thin sauce consistency and season with pepper to taste. Cover and refrigerate for 30 minutes before serving. (Sauce can be refrigerated for up to 24 hours.)

PER 2-TABLESPOON SERVING

Cal 100 • **Total Fat** 11g • **Sat Fat** 2g • **Chol** 5mg
Sodium 200mg • **Total Carbs** 2g • **Fiber** 0g • **Total Sugar** 2g
Added Sugar 0g • **Protein** 1g • **Total Carbohydrate Choices** <0.5

Creamy Dill Sauce

MAKES ¹/₂ CUP

This creamy sauce goes especially well with salmon.

- ¼ cup mayonnaise
- 2 tablespoons low-fat sour cream
- 1 small shallot, minced
- 1 tablespoon lemon juice
- 1 tablespoon minced fresh dill
  Water
  Pepper

Combine mayonnaise, sour cream, shallot, lemon juice, and dill in bowl. Add water as needed to thin sauce consistency and season with pepper to taste. Cover and refrigerate for 30 minutes before serving. (Sauce can be refrigerated for up to 24 hours.)

PER 2-TABLESPOON SERVING

Cal 100 • **Total Fat** 11g • **Sat Fat** 2g • **Chol** 5mg
Sodium 95mg • **Total Carbs** 1g • **Fiber** 0g • **Total Sugar** 1g
Added Sugar 0g • **Protein** 1g • **Total Carbohydrate Choices** <0.5

Creamy Chipotle Chile Sauce

MAKES ¹/₂ CUP

You can vary the spiciness of this sauce by adjusting the amount of chipotle.

- ¼ cup mayonnaise
- 2 tablespoons low-fat sour cream
- 1 tablespoon lime juice
- 2 teaspoons minced fresh cilantro
- 1 garlic clove, minced
- ½ teaspoon minced canned chipotle chile in adobo sauce
  Water
  Pepper

Combine mayonnaise, sour cream, lime juice, cilantro, garlic, and chipotle in bowl. Add water as needed to thin sauce consistency and season with pepper to taste. Cover and refrigerate for 30 minutes before serving. (Sauce can be refrigerated for up to 24 hours.)

PER 2-TABLESPOON SERVING

Cal 100 • **Total Fat** 11g • **Sat Fat** 2g • **Chol** 5mg
Sodium 95mg • **Total Carbs** 1g • **Fiber** 0g • **Total Sugar** 1g
Added Sugar 0g • **Protein** 1g • **Total Carbohydrate Choices** <0.5

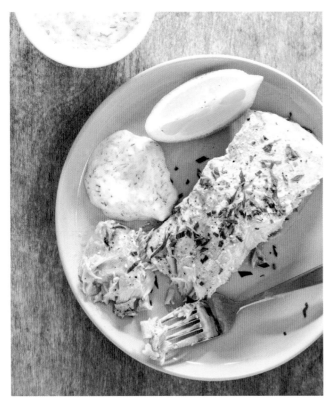

For a side of salmon that is moist and fuss-free, we use a simple oven-poaching method, no fish poacher required.

Oven-Poached Side of Salmon
SERVES 10

WHY THIS RECIPE WORKS An easy way to cook and serve a large piece of salmon is to poach it and then chill it. Our method eliminates the need for a large, unwieldy fish poacher. We simply wrap the seasoned fish in foil and place it directly on the oven rack, which offers more even cooking than using a baking sheet. Cooking the salmon low and slow yields the best results. If serving a big crowd, you can oven-poach two individually wrapped sides of salmon in the same oven (on the upper- and lower-middle racks) without altering the cooking time. If using wild salmon, which contains less fat than farmed salmon, cook the fillets until they register 120 degrees (for medium-rare). For information on salmon, see page 245. Serve with one of the sauces on pages 242–243, if desired.

  1 (4-pound) skin-on side of salmon, pinbones removed
  1 teaspoon salt
  ½ teaspoon pepper
  2 tablespoons cider vinegar

  6 sprigs plus 2 tablespoons minced fresh tarragon or dill
  2 lemons, sliced into ¼-inch-thick rounds, plus lemon wedges for serving

1. Adjust oven rack to middle position and heat oven to 250 degrees. Cut three sheets of heavy-duty aluminum foil to be 1 foot longer than side of salmon. Working with 2 pieces of foil, fold up 1 long side of each by 3 inches. Lay sheets side by side with folded sides touching, then fold edges together to create secure seam, and press seam flat. Center third sheet of foil over seam. Spray foil lightly with canola oil spray.

2. Pat salmon dry with paper towels and sprinkle with salt and pepper. Lay salmon, skin side down, in center of foil. Sprinkle with vinegar, then top with tarragon sprigs and lemon slices. Fold foil up over salmon to create seam on top and gently fold foil edges together to secure, leaving small air pocket at top.

3. Lay foil-wrapped fish directly on oven rack (without baking sheet) and cook until opaque throughout when checked with tip of paring knife and registers 135 to 140 degrees, 45 to 60 minutes.

4. Remove fish from oven, open foil, and let salmon cool for 30 minutes. Pour off any accumulated liquid. Reseal salmon in foil and refrigerate until cold, about 1 hour. (Poached salmon can be refrigerated for up to 2 days. Let salmon sit at room temperature for 30 minutes before serving.)

5. Unwrap salmon and brush away lemon slices, tarragon sprigs, and any solidified poaching liquid. Carefully transfer fish to serving platter, sprinkle with minced tarragon, and serve with lemon wedges.

PER SERVING

Cal 380 • **Total Fat** 25g • **Sat Fat** 6g • **Chol** 100mg
Sodium 340mg • **Total Carbs** 0g • **Fiber** 0g • **Total Sugar** 0g
Added Sugar 0g • **Protein** 37g • **Total Carbohydrate Choices** 0

Salmon Tacos with Super Slaw
SERVES 6

WHY THIS RECIPE WORKS California-style fish tacos generally feature deep-fried fish, a tangy cabbage slaw, and a creamy sauce. We wanted to boost the nutrition of each element for a supercharged take on tacos. Since we were forgoing the frying, we opted for salmon, which is richer than the more typically used cod or other white fish. A flavorful spice rub gave the fillets a nice crust. For a slaw that would stand up to the salmon, we wondered if we could incorporate nutrient-rich dark leafy greens, and collards proved just the ticket. When thinly sliced, they required no precooking. Combined with crunchy radishes, cooling jícama, red onion,

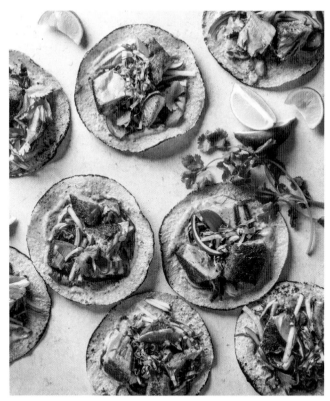

We turn tacos into a nutritional powerhouse by topping corn tortillas with a collard green–jícama slaw and chunks of salmon.

cilantro, and lime, they perfectly complemented the fish. To ensure uniform pieces of fish that cooked at the same rate, we found it best to buy a whole center-cut fillet and cut it into four pieces ourselves. If using wild salmon, which contains less fat than farmed salmon, cook the fillets until they register 120 degrees (for medium-rare). For information on salmon, see box at right. You can substitute 2 cups thinly sliced purple cabbage for the collards if desired.

¼ teaspoon grated lime zest plus 2 tablespoons juice, plus lime wedges for serving
 Salt and pepper
4 ounces collard greens, stemmed and sliced thin (2 cups)
4 ounces jícama, peeled and cut into 2-inch-long matchsticks
4 radishes, trimmed and cut into 1-inch-long matchsticks
½ small red onion, halved and sliced thin
¼ cup fresh cilantro leaves
1½ teaspoons chili powder
1 (1½-pound) skin-on salmon fillet, 1 inch thick
1 tablespoon canola oil
1 avocado, halved, pitted, and cut into ½-inch pieces
12 (6-inch) corn tortillas, warmed
 Hot sauce

1. Whisk lime zest and juice and ¼ teaspoon salt together in large bowl. Add collards, jícama, radishes, onion, and cilantro and toss to combine.

2. Combine chili powder, ¾ teaspoon salt, and ¼ teaspoon pepper in small bowl. Cut salmon crosswise into 4 fillets. Pat dry with paper towels and sprinkle evenly with spice mixture. Heat oil in 12-inch nonstick skillet over medium-high heat until shimmering. Cook salmon, skin side up, until well browned, 3 to 5 minutes. Gently flip salmon using 2 spatulas and continue to cook until salmon is still translucent when checked with tip of paring knife and registers 125 degrees (for medium-rare), 3 to 5 minutes. Transfer salmon to plate and let cool slightly, about 2 minutes. Using 2 forks, flake fish into 2-inch pieces, discarding skin.

3. Divide fish, collard slaw, and avocado evenly among tortillas, and drizzle with hot sauce to taste. Serve.

PER SERVING
Cal 440 • **Total Fat** 24g • **Sat Fat** 4.5g • **Chol** 60mg
Sodium 490mg • **Total Carbs** 29g • **Fiber** 6g • **Total Sugar** 1g
Added Sugar 0g • **Protein** 27g • **Total Carbohydrate Choices** 2

NOTES FROM THE TEST KITCHEN

Farmed and Wild Salmon Are Both Healthy

We love salmon because it's rich without being aggressively fishy. Salmon's rich flavor is due to how its fat is stored: Unlike the fat in white fish, which is mostly stored in the liver, the fat in salmon is spread throughout the flesh (much of it in the form of healthy omega-3 fatty acids). Wild salmon is praised for its optimal fat content (and flavor), but both wild and farm-raised salmon contain high levels of omega-3 fats. The farm-raised variety actually has higher absolute levels of omega-3s and higher total fat; also, the saturated fat content of farmed salmon may be higher than wild. Because wild salmon is leaner than farmed, it can be prone to overcooking, so we cook it to a slightly lower temperature.

SPECIES	WILD VS. FARMED	FAT (GRAMS PER 100G FLESH)	IDEAL INTERNAL TEMP. (F)
Atlantic	Farmed	13.42	125
King (Chinook)	Wild	11.73	120
Sockeye (Red)	Wild	7.28	120
Coho (Silver)	Wild	5.57	120
Chum	Wild	3.67	120

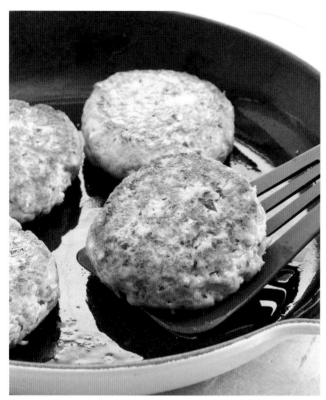

A mix of yogurt and mayonnaise plus just 1 slice of whole-wheat sandwich bread serve as the binder for our moist salmon cakes.

Salmon Cakes with Lemon-Herb Sauce

SERVES 4

WHY THIS RECIPE WORKS A good salmon cake delivers rich flavor and tender texture; the best veers away from flavor-muting binders at all costs. We used a food processor to coarsely chop salmon so it is not overly dense. A single slice of whole-wheat bread provided just enough binding without compromising flavor, and a combination of shallot, parsley, mustard, and capers complemented the salmon; a bit of yogurt ensured our patties would stay moist. We sautéed the patties rather than placing then inside the oven for better control over the heat, resulting in perfectly cooked cakes with great color. A quick lemon-parsley sauce built on a base of equal parts yogurt and mayonnaise added a touch of class. Be sure to use raw salmon here; do not substitute cooked or canned salmon. If using wild salmon, which contains less fat than farmed salmon, cook the cakes until they register 120 degrees (for medium-rare). For information on salmon, see page 245. Don't overprocess the salmon in step 2, or the cakes will have a pasty texture.

¼ cup low-fat plain yogurt
3 tablespoons minced fresh parsley
2 tablespoons mayonnaise
2 teaspoons lemon juice, plus lemon wedges for serving
1 scallion, minced
  Salt and pepper
1 shallot, minced
1 tablespoon Dijon mustard
2 teaspoons capers, rinsed and minced
1 (1¼-ounce) slice hearty 100 percent whole-wheat sandwich bread, crust removed, torn into 1-inch pieces
1 pound skinless salmon fillet, cut into 1-inch pieces
2 teaspoons extra-virgin olive oil

1. Combine 2 tablespoons yogurt, 1 tablespoon parsley, mayonnaise, lemon juice, scallion, and pinch pepper in small bowl. Cover and refrigerate until ready to serve. Whisk shallot, remaining 2 tablespoons yogurt, remaining 2 tablespoons parsley, mustard, capers, ⅛ teaspoon salt, and ⅛ teaspoon pepper together in large bowl.

2. Pulse bread in food processor to coarse crumbs, about 4 pulses, then transfer to bowl with shallot mixture. Working in 2 batches, pulse salmon in now-empty food processor until coarsely ground, about 4 pulses; transfer to bowl with bread crumbs and gently toss until well combined. Pat salmon mixture into four ¾-inch-thick cakes, about 4 inches in diameter.

3. Heat oil in 12-inch nonstick skillet over medium heat until shimmering. Gently add cakes to skillet and cook until browned and centers are still translucent when checked with tip of paring knife and register 125 degrees (for medium-rare), 3 to 5 minutes per side. Serve with sauce and lemon wedges.

PER SERVING

Cal 340 • **Total Fat** 23g • **Sat Fat** 4.5g • **Chol** 65mg
Sodium 350mg • **Total Carbs** 4g • **Fiber** 1g • **Total Sugar** 2g
Added Sugar 0g • **Protein** 25g • **Total Carbohydrate Choices** <0.5

SKINNING SALMON FILLETS

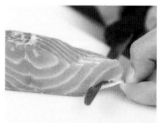

1. Using tip of boning knife (or sharp chef's knife), begin to cut skin away from fish at corner of fillet.

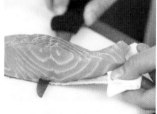

2. When enough skin is exposed, grasp skin firmly with piece of paper towel, hold taut, and carefully slice flesh off skin.

Lemony Steamed Spa Fish
SERVES 4

WHY THIS RECIPE WORKS This method for cooking sole fillets is the essence of simplicity and requires nothing more than a Dutch oven and a steamer basket. Since sole fillets are so thin and delicate, the trick here is to roll each fillet into a tiny bundle. To infuse them with a touch of lemony flavor, we lined the steamer basket with lemon rounds and then also covered the fish bundles with more rounds before steaming them. You can substitute flounder for the sole. Do not use fillets thinner than ¼ inch as they will overcook very quickly. Serve with one of the sauces on pages 242–243, if desired.

    2 lemons, sliced into ¼-inch-thick rounds,
      plus lemon wedges for serving
    4 (6-ounce) sole fillets, ¼ to ½ inch thick
    ¼ teaspoon salt
    ⅛ teaspoon pepper
    1 tablespoon minced fresh chives, tarragon,
      cilantro, basil, or parsley

1. Place steamer basket in Dutch oven and add water until it just touches bottom of basket. Line basket with half of lemon slices, cover pot, and bring water to boil over high heat. Meanwhile, pat sole dry with paper towels, sprinkle with salt and pepper, and roll each fillet into bundle.

2. Reduce heat to medium-low and bring water to simmer. Lay fish bundles in basket, seam-side down, and top with remaining lemon slices. Cover pot and steam until sole flakes apart when gently prodded with paring knife, 4 to 6 minutes.

3. Gently transfer fish bundles to individual serving plates (discarding lemon slices), sprinkle with herbs, and serve with lemon wedges.

PER SERVING
Cal 120 • **Total Fat** 3.5g • **Sat Fat** 1g • **Chol** 75mg
Sodium 280mg • **Total Carbs** 0g • **Fiber** 0g • **Total Sugar** 0g
Added Sugar 0g • **Protein** 21g • **Total Carbohydrate Choices** 0

ROLLING UP A THIN FILLET

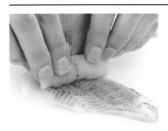

With the sole fillets skinned-side up, roll the fillets into tight bundles, starting at the tail end.

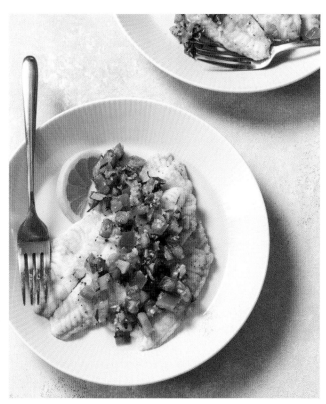

The less you fuss with delicate sole when cooking it the better — we simply flour it and give it a good sear in extra-virgin olive oil.

Sautéed Sole
SERVES 4

WHY THIS RECIPE WORKS Delicate sole tastes great when sautéed in flavorful, heart-healthy olive oil. First, though, we give it a light coating of flour, which protects the fish and creates just a bit of a browned crust during sautéing. You can substitute flounder for the sole. Fish fillets are sold in a range of sizes. Do not use fillets thinner than ¼ inch, as they will overcook very quickly. Serve with one of the sauces on pages 242–243, if desired.

    ½ cup all-purpose flour
    8 (2-ounce) skinless sole fillets, ¼ to ½ inch thick
    ¼ teaspoon salt
    ⅛ teaspoon pepper
    ¼ cup extra-virgin olive oil
      Lemon wedges

1. Place flour in shallow dish. Pat sole dry with paper towels and sprinkle with salt and pepper. Working with 1 fillet at a time, dredge in flour to coat, shaking off any excess.

2. Heat 2 tablespoons oil in 12-inch nonstick skillet over medium-high heat until shimmering. Place half of sole in skillet and cook until lightly browned on first side, 2 to 3 minutes. Gently flip sole using 2 spatulas and continue to cook until sole flakes apart when gently prodded with paring knife, 30 to 60 seconds.

3. Transfer sole to serving platter and tent loosely with aluminum foil. Wipe skillet clean with paper towels and repeat with remaining 2 tablespoons oil and fillets. Serve with lemon wedges.

PER SERVING

Cal 220 • **Total Fat** 16g • **Sat Fat** 2.5g • **Chol** 50mg
Sodium 240mg • **Total Carbs** 3g • **Fiber** 0g • **Total Sugar** 0g
Added Sugar 0g • **Protein** 14g • **Total Carbohydrate Choices** <0.5

Cod in Coconut Broth with Lemon Grass and Ginger
SERVES 4

WHY THIS RECIPE WORKS We liked the idea of bathing lean, mineral-rich cod in a flavorful liquid with lots of aromatics. A Thai-style approach drew upon the flavors of coconut soup to build a lush broth seasoned with lemon grass, ginger, and garlic. Poaching the cod in this broth ensured the flavors infused the fish and allowed it to cook gently and evenly. Mild leeks and sweet carrots complemented the delicate cod, a little coconut milk added richness, and a bit of fish sauce added a savory note. A garnish of peanuts, cilantro, and a serrano chile added welcome color, aroma, and crunch. Best of all, this dish came together quickly and in just one pan, making it an elegant but weeknight-friendly meal. You can substitute halibut, haddock, red snapper, or sea bass for the cod. If you can't find a serrano chile, substitute a red Fresno chile.

1 tablespoon canola oil
1 leek, white and light green parts only, halved lengthwise, sliced thin, and washed thoroughly
4 garlic cloves, minced
1 tablespoon grated fresh ginger
1 cup water
2 carrots, peeled and cut into 2-inch-long matchsticks
1 (10-inch) stalk lemon grass, trimmed to bottom 6 inches and bruised with back of knife
4 (6-ounce) skinless cod fillets, 1 to 1½ inches thick
Salt and pepper

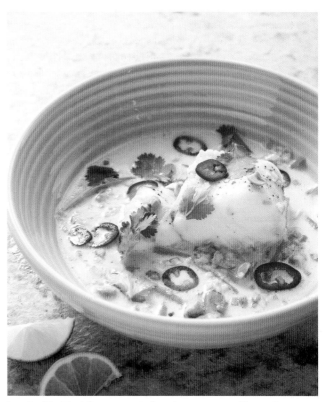

Inspired by Thai flavors, we infused a coconut milk poaching medium with them for a healthy way to cook cod.

⅓ cup canned light coconut milk
1 tablespoon lime juice, plus lime wedges for serving
1 teaspoon fish sauce
2 tablespoons chopped dry-roasted peanuts
2 tablespoons fresh cilantro leaves
1 serrano chile, stemmed and sliced thin

1. Heat oil in 12-inch nonstick skillet over medium heat until shimmering. Add leek and cook, stirring occasionally, until lightly browned, 4 to 6 minutes. Stir in garlic and ginger and cook until fragrant, about 30 seconds.

2. Stir in water, carrots, and lemon grass and bring to simmer. Pat cod dry with paper towels and sprinkle with ⅛ teaspoon salt and ⅛ teaspoon pepper. Nestle fish into skillet and bring to simmer. Reduce heat to low, cover, and cook until cod flakes apart when gently prodded with paring knife and registers 140 degrees, 8 to 12 minutes.

3. Carefully transfer fish to individual shallow serving bowls. Discard lemon grass. Using slotted spoon, divide leeks and carrots evenly among bowls. Off heat, whisk coconut milk, lime juice, and fish sauce into broth and season with pepper to taste. Ladle broth over fish. Sprinkle with peanuts, cilantro, and chile. Serve with lime wedges.

PER SERVING

Cal 250 • Total Fat 8g • Sat Fat 2g • Chol 75mg
Sodium 290mg • Total Carbs 10g • Fiber 2g • Total Sugar 3g
Added Sugar 0g • Protein 33g • Total Carbohydrate Choices 0.5

Baked Cod Provençal
SERVES 4

WHY THIS RECIPE WORKS Taking inspiration from the summer markets in the south of France, we put together this simple recipe pairing meaty cod with lots of aromatics, fresh herbs, and antioxidant-rich cherry tomatoes. First we created a flavorful base on which to bake our cod: quartered cherry tomatoes, minced shallots and garlic, capers, and fresh thyme—all combined with olive oil and a little white wine. To keep our cod moist as it cooked, we rubbed it with olive oil, lemon zest, and salt and pepper. As the fish cooked, the tomatoes released their juices and softened perfectly, then mingled with all the aromatics. A sprinkling of fresh basil just before serving gave this dish a hit of bright flavor. We like to spoon the tomato mixture over the cod when serving. You can substitute halibut, haddock, red snapper, or sea bass for the cod.

2 tablespoons extra-virgin olive oil
1½ pounds cherry tomatoes, quartered
2 shallots, minced
¼ cup dry white wine
2 tablespoons capers, rinsed
2 garlic cloves, minced
1 teaspoon minced fresh thyme or ¼ teaspoon dried
  Salt and pepper
½ teaspoon grated lemon zest, plus lemon wedges
  for serving
4 (6-ounce) skinless cod fillets, 1 to 1½ inches thick
2 tablespoons chopped fresh basil

1. Adjust oven rack to middle position and heat oven to 400 degrees. Combine 2 teaspoons oil, tomatoes, shallots, wine, capers, garlic, thyme, ⅛ teaspoon salt, and ¼ teaspoon pepper in 13 by 9-inch baking dish, stirring to combine.

2. Combine remaining 4 teaspoons oil, lemon zest, ⅛ teaspoon salt, and ¼ teaspoon pepper in bowl. Pat cod dry with paper towels then rub with oil mixture. Nestle, skinned side down, into tomato mixture.

3. Bake until cod flakes apart when gently prodded with paring knife and registers 140 degrees, 20 to 25 minutes. Sprinkle with basil and serve with lemon wedges.

PER SERVING

Cal 260 • Total Fat 9g • Sat Fat 1.5g • Chol 75mg
Sodium 350mg • Total Carbs 11g • Fiber 3g • Total Sugar 6g
Added Sugar 0g • Protein 32g • Total Carbohydrate Choices 1

Lemon-Herb Cod Fillets with Garlic Potatoes
SERVES 4

WHY THIS RECIPE WORKS The magical thing about this recipe is that it is an ingenious way to cook and present cod and potatoes without resorting to tons of butter—in fact, without any butter. We simply relied on the cooking method and heart-healthy extra-virgin olive oil. We decided to cut our potatoes into thin rounds, parcook them in the microwave with garlic and olive oil, then bake the fish and the potatoes together. The fillets were nestled on top of the potatoes in a casserole dish. Lemon slices placed atop the cod basted it as it baked, and sprigs of thyme added subtle seasoning to the fish. In the oven, the potatoes got nicely crisped and infused with flavor while the fish cooked through gently and evenly. Best of all, the side dish and entrée were ready at the same time. You can substitute halibut, haddock, red snapper, or sea bass for the cod.

1½ pounds russet potatoes, unpeeled, sliced into
  ¼-inch-thick rounds
¼ cup extra-virgin olive oil
3 garlic cloves, minced
  Salt and pepper
4 (6-ounce) skinless cod fillets, 1 to 1½ inches thick
4 sprigs fresh thyme
1 lemon, sliced into ¼-inch-thick rounds

1. Adjust oven rack to lower-middle position and heat oven to 425 degrees. Toss potatoes, 2 tablespoons oil, garlic, ⅛ teaspoon salt, and ¼ teaspoon pepper together in bowl. Microwave, uncovered, until potatoes are just tender, 12 to 14 minutes, stirring halfway through microwaving.

2. Transfer potatoes to 13 by 9-inch baking dish and press gently into even layer. Pat cod dry with paper towels, rub with remaining 2 tablespoons oil, and sprinkle with ¼ teaspoon salt and ⅛ teaspoon pepper. Arrange skinned side down on top of potatoes, then place thyme sprigs and lemon slices on top. Bake until cod flakes apart when gently prodded with paring knife and registers 140 degrees, 15 to 18 minutes. Slide spatula underneath potatoes and cod and carefully transfer to individual serving plates. Serve.

PER SERVING

Cal 400 • **Total Fat** 15g • **Sat Fat** 2g • **Chol** 75mg
Sodium 280mg • **Total Carbs** 32g • **Fiber** 2g • **Total Sugar** 1g
Added Sugar 0g • **Protein** 34g • **Total Carbohydrate Choices** 2

ASSEMBLING COD AND POTATOES

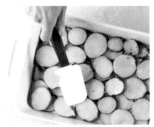

1. Transfer microwaved potatoes to 13 by 9-inch baking dish and press gently into even layer.

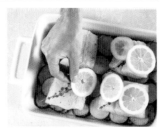

2. Arrange cod skinned side down on top of potatoes, drizzle with oil, then top with thyme sprigs and lemon slices.

Nut-Crusted Cod Fillets
SERVES 4

WHY THIS RECIPE WORKS Breaded and fried fish is undeniably delicious when done right, but we wanted a more nutritious path to moist, delicate fish with a crunchy coating, not to mention avoiding the hassle of deep-frying. Baking instead of frying was an obvious starting point, but we also wanted to rework the coating. We replaced half the bread crumbs with ground pistachios, which offered more nutrients as well as richness and fragrance. We skipped traditional bread crumbs, which are prone to sogginess, and opted for whole-wheat panko. Toasting the two components together with aromatics brought out their flavors and ensured the topping would remain extra crisp. To help the coating adhere to the fillets, we brushed the vitamin B–rich fish with a mixture of yogurt, egg yolk, and lemon zest before pressing on the crumbs.

Because our crust was so flavorful, we only needed to coat the tops of the fillets, making them easy to bake without crumbs falling off the sides or getting soggy underneath. Baking the fillets on a wire rack set in a baking sheet ensured even cooking. You can substitute halibut, haddock, red snapper, or sea bass for the cod. Any nut will work for the topping, but we particularly liked pistachios and hazelnuts.

½ cup shelled unsalted pistachios
2 tablespoons canola oil
1 large shallot, minced
  Salt and pepper
1 garlic clove, minced
1 teaspoon minced fresh thyme or ¼ teaspoon dried
½ cup 100 percent whole-wheat panko bread crumbs
2 tablespoons minced fresh parsley
1 tablespoon plain low-fat yogurt
1 large egg yolk
½ teaspoon grated lemon zest, plus lemon wedges
  for serving
4 (6-ounce) skinless cod fillets, 1 to 1½ inches thick

1. Adjust oven rack to middle position and heat oven to 300 degrees. Set wire rack in rimmed baking sheet and spray lightly with canola oil spray. Process pistachios in food processor until finely chopped, 20 to 30 seconds. Heat oil in 12-inch nonstick skillet over medium heat until shimmering. Add shallot and ⅛ teaspoon salt and cook until softened, about 3 minutes. Stir in garlic and thyme and cook until fragrant, about 30 seconds. Reduce heat to medium-low and add pistachios, panko, and ¼ teaspoon pepper. Cook, stirring frequently, until well browned and crisp, about 8 minutes. Transfer nut mixture to shallow dish and let cool for 10 minutes. Stir in parsley.

2. Whisk yogurt, egg yolk, and lemon zest together in bowl. Pat cod dry with paper towels and sprinkle with ¼ teaspoon salt and ⅛ teaspoon pepper. Brush tops of fillets evenly with yogurt mixture. Working with 1 fillet at a time, dredge brushed side in nut mixture, pressing gently to adhere.

3. Transfer cod, crumb side up, to prepared rack and bake until cod flakes apart when gently prodded with paring knife and registers 140 degrees, 20 to 25 minutes, rotating sheet halfway through baking. Carefully transfer fish to individual serving plates and serve with lemon wedges.

PER SERVING

Cal 290 • **Total Fat** 13g • **Sat Fat** 1.5g • **Chol** 120mg
Sodium 320mg • **Total Carbs** 8g • **Fiber** 2g • **Total Sugar** 2g
Added Sugar 0g • **Protein** 34g • **Total Carbohydrate Choices** 0.5

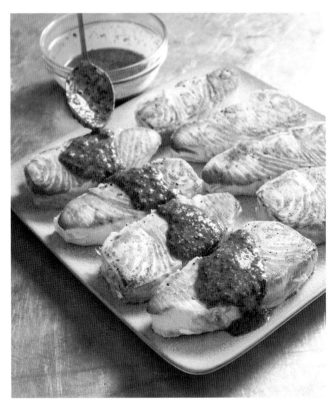

Mild halibut gets a big flavor boost from a classic sauce packed with mineral-rich cilantro.

Pan-Roasted Halibut with Chermoula
SERVES 8

WHY THIS RECIPE WORKS Cooks often pan-roast or sauté halibut because browning adds great flavor, but it can be a challenge to keep the fish from drying out. We didn't want to compromise on either texture or flavor, so we set out to develop a technique for cooking halibut that would produce perfectly cooked and tender fish with good browning. A combination of pan searing and oven roasting proved best. When they were done, the steaks were browned but still moist inside. We took our fish to the next level by serving it with chermoula, a zesty Moroccan dressing featuring a hefty amount of cilantro leaves, a great source of essential minerals and more. If 2 full halibut steaks aren't available, you can substitute four 6-ounce steaks. If halibut isn't available, you can substitute eight 6-ounce skin-on swordfish steaks, 1 to 1½ inches thick; be sure to adjust the cooking time in step 3 as needed. You will need a 12-inch ovensafe nonstick skillet for this recipe.

CHERMOULA
- ¾ cup fresh cilantro leaves
- ¼ cup extra-virgin olive oil
- 2 tablespoons lemon juice
- 4 garlic cloves, minced
- ½ teaspoon ground cumin
- ½ teaspoon paprika
- ¼ teaspoon salt
- ⅛ teaspoon cayenne pepper

HALIBUT
- 2 (1½-pound) skin-on full halibut steaks, 1 to 1½ inches thick and 10 to 12 inches long, trimmed of cartilage at both ends (see page 254)
- ¼ teaspoon salt
- ⅛ teaspoon pepper
- 2 tablespoons extra-virgin olive oil

1. FOR THE CHERMOULA Process all ingredients in food processor until smooth, about 1 minute, scraping down sides of bowl as needed; set aside for serving.

2. FOR THE HALIBUT Adjust oven rack to middle position and heat oven to 325 degrees. Pat halibut dry with paper towels and sprinkle with salt and pepper. Heat oil in 12-inch ovensafe nonstick skillet over medium-high heat until just smoking. Place halibut in skillet and cook until well browned on first side, about 5 minutes.

3. Gently flip halibut using 2 spatulas and transfer skillet to oven. Roast until halibut flakes apart when gently prodded with paring knife and registers 140 degrees, 6 to 9 minutes.

4. Carefully transfer halibut to cutting board. Remove skin from steaks and separate each quadrant of meat from bones by slipping knife or spatula between them (see page 254). Divide chermoula evenly among steaks and serve.

PER SERVING
Cal 230 • **Total Fat** 12g • **Sat Fat** 2g • **Chol** 70mg
Sodium 230mg • **Total Carbs** 1g • **Fiber** 0g • **Total Sugar** 0g
Added Sugar 0g • **Protein** 26g • **Total Carbohydrate Choices** <0.5

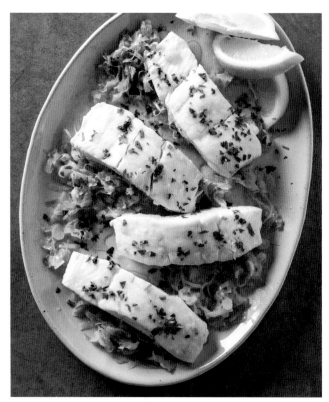

We jazz up halibut fillets with pungent mustard and aromatic leeks in this simple and delicious braise.

Braised Halibut with Leeks and Mustard
SERVES 4

WHY THIS RECIPE WORKS When it comes to methods for cooking fish, braising is often overlooked. But the approach, which requires cooking the fish in a small amount of liquid so that it gently simmers and steams, has a lot going for it. As a moist-heat cooking method, braising is gentle and thus forgiving, all but guaranteeing tender fish. Plus, it makes a great one-pot meal since it's easy to add vegetables to the pan to cook at the same time, and the cooking liquid becomes a sauce. We chose halibut for its sweet, delicate flavor and its firm texture, which made for easier handling, and paired it with the classic French flavors of leeks, white wine, and Dijon mustard. Because the portion of the fillets submerged in liquid cooks more quickly than the upper half that cooks in the steam, we cooked the fillets for a few minutes in the pan on just one side and then braised them parcooked side up to even out the cooking. For the cooking liquid, wine supplemented by the juices released by the fish and leeks during cooking delivered a sauce with balanced flavor and just the right amount of brightness. You can substitute cod, haddock, red snapper, or sea bass for the halibut.

4 (6-ounce) skinless halibut fillets, ¾ to 1 inch thick
   Salt and pepper
¼ cup extra-virgin olive oil
1 pound leeks, white and light green parts only, halved lengthwise, sliced thin, and washed thoroughly
1 teaspoon Dijon mustard
¾ cup dry white wine
1 tablespoon minced fresh parsley
   Lemon wedges

1. Pat halibut dry with paper towels and sprinkle with ¼ teaspoon salt. Heat oil in 12-inch skillet over medium heat until warm, about 15 seconds. Place halibut skinned side up in skillet and cook until bottom half of halibut begins to turn opaque (halibut should not brown), about 4 minutes. Using 2 spatulas, carefully transfer halibut raw side down to large plate.

2. Add leeks, mustard, and ⅛ teaspoon salt to oil left in skillet and cook over medium heat, stirring frequently, until softened, 10 to 12 minutes. Stir in wine and bring to simmer. Place halibut raw side down on top of leeks. Reduce heat to medium-low, cover, and simmer gently until halibut flakes apart when gently prodded with paring knife and registers 140 degrees, 6 to 10 minutes. Carefully transfer halibut to serving platter, tent loosely with aluminum foil, and let rest while finishing leeks.

3. Return leeks to high heat and simmer briskly until mixture is thickened slightly, 2 to 4 minutes. Season with pepper to taste. Arrange leek mixture around halibut and sprinkle with parsley. Serve with lemon wedges.

PER SERVING

Cal 350 • **Total Fat** 16g • **Sat Fat** 2.5g • **Chol** 85mg
Sodium 380mg • **Total Carbs** 8g • **Fiber** 1g • **Total Sugar** 2g
Added Sugar 0g • **Protein** 32g • **Total Carbohydrate Choices** 1

VARIATIONS
Braised Halibut with Carrots and Coriander
Substitute 1 pound carrots, peeled and shaved with vegetable peeler into ribbons, and 4 shallots, halved and sliced thin, for leeks. Substitute ½ teaspoon ground coriander for Dijon mustard and stir 1½ teaspoons lemon juice into carrot mixture in step 3 before seasoning with pepper. Substitute minced fresh cilantro for parsley.

PER SERVING

Cal 390 • **Total Fat** 17g • **Sat Fat** 2.5g • **Chol** 85mg
Sodium 420mg • **Total Carbs** 17g • **Fiber** 4g • **Total Sugar** 8g
Added Sugar 0g • **Protein** 33g • **Total Carbohydrate Choices** 1

Braised Halibut with Fennel and Tarragon

Substitute two 10-ounce fennel bulbs, stalks discarded, bulbs halved, cored, and sliced thin, and 4 shallots, halved and sliced thin, for leeks. Omit Dijon mustard and stir 1 teaspoon lemon juice into fennel mixture in step 3 before seasoning with pepper. Substitute minced fresh tarragon for parsley.

PER SERVING

Cal 380 • **Total Fat** 17g • **Sat Fat** 2.5g • **Chol** 85mg
Sodium 410mg • **Total Carbs** 17g • **Fiber** 5g • **Total Sugar** 8g
Added Sugar 0g • **Protein** 34g • **Total Carbohydrate Choices** 1

Halibut Baked in Foil with Tomatoes and Zucchini
SERVES 4

WHY THIS RECIPE WORKS Baking halibut *en papillote*—in a tightly sealed package to steam in its own juices—is a quick, mess-free way to enhance the fish's mild flavor, and including vegetables in the pouch is a surefire path to a healthful satisfying meal. Using aluminum foil rather than parchment made packet construction easy. For vegetables, we started with zucchini (salted to remove excess moisture), which would cook in the same amount of time as the fish. To give our packets plenty of flavor without overpowering the halibut, we made a tomato salsa, which added just the right kick. A splash of white wine boosted the flavor even more. The sealed packets needed only 15 to 20 minutes in the oven to steam and baste the fish and soften the zucchini. You can substitute cod, haddock, red snapper, or sea bass for the halibut. To prevent overcooking, open each packet promptly after baking.

1 pound zucchini, sliced crosswise into ¼-inch-thick rounds
  Salt and pepper
3 plum tomatoes, cored, seeded, and cut into ½-inch pieces
2 tablespoons extra-virgin olive oil
2 garlic cloves, minced
1 teaspoon minced fresh oregano or ¼ teaspoon dried
⅛ teaspoon red pepper flakes
4 (6-ounce) skinless halibut fillets, 1 to 1½ inches thick
¼ cup dry white wine
¼ cup chopped fresh basil
  Lemon wedges

1. Toss zucchini with ⅛ teaspoon salt and let drain in colander for 30 minutes; pat zucchini dry with paper towels, pressing firmly to remove as much liquid as possible. Adjust oven rack to middle position and heat oven to 450 degrees.

2. Combine tomatoes, oil, garlic, oregano, pepper flakes, and ⅛ teaspoon pepper in bowl. Pat halibut dry with paper towels and sprinkle with ¼ teaspoon salt and ⅛ teaspoon pepper.

3. Cut eight 12-inch sheets of aluminum foil; arrange 4 flat on counter. Shingle zucchini in center of foil sheets and sprinkle with wine. Place halibut on top of zucchini, then top halibut with tomato mixture. Place remaining pieces of foil on top. Press edges of foil together and fold together several times until each packet is well sealed and measures about 7 inches square. (Packets can be refrigerated for up to 3 hours before cooking. Increase baking time to 20 to 25 minutes when made ahead.)

4. Place packets on rimmed baking sheet, overlapping as needed, and bake until halibut flakes apart when gently prodded with paring knife and registers 140 degrees, 15 to 20 minutes. (To check temperature, poke thermometer through foil into halibut.)

MAKING A FOIL PACKET

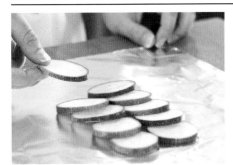

1. Shingle vegetables in center of foil.

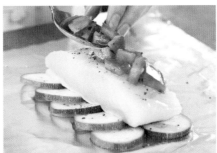

2. Place halibut on top of zucchini, then spoon tomato mixture over fish.

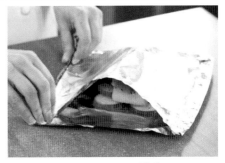

3. Place remaining pieces of foil on top and fold edges of foil together to create well-sealed packet.

5. Carefully open packets, allowing steam to escape away from you, and gently slide halibut, vegetables, and any accumulated juices onto individual serving plates. Sprinkle with basil and serve with lemon wedges.

PER SERVING

Cal 260 • **Total Fat** 10g • **Sat Fat** 1.5g • **Chol** 85mg
Sodium 320mg • **Total Carbs** 7g • **Fiber** 2g • **Total Sugar** 4g
Added Sugar 0g • **Protein** 34g • **Total Carbohydrate Choices** 0.5

Halibut en Cocotte with Cherry Tomatoes
SERVES 8

WHY THIS RECIPE WORKS Pairing fresh fish with olive oil and nutritionally valuable cherry tomatoes has many benefits, including the fact that the cherry tomatoes soften into a nearly spoonable, delicious sauce during the cooking time. Here we cook our fish *en cocotte,* a time-honored French approach to cooking meat and even fish in a large covered pot in a very low oven. Essentially, the fish is braised low and slow for the ultimate tender texture while being infused with aromatics and herbs. For our recipe we selected two similar-size halibut steaks (the steaks have cartilage at either end that contains small bones). After we cut off the cartilage, the steaks were ready to be braised. We started by pan-roasting garlic in olive oil to draw out its flavor, then stirred in cherry tomatoes and placed the halibut on top. As the fish cooked, the tomatoes began to break down, releasing their juices and helping to build a sauce. If 2 full halibut steaks aren't available, you can substitute eight 6-ounce steaks. If halibut isn't available, you can substitute four 6-ounce skin-on swordfish steaks, 1 to 1½ inches thick; be sure to adjust the cooking time in step 2 as needed.

> 2 tablespoons extra-virgin olive oil
> 2 garlic cloves, sliced thin
> ⅛ teaspoon red pepper flakes
> 12 ounces cherry tomatoes, quartered
> 1 tablespoon capers, rinsed
> 1 teaspoon minced fresh thyme or ¼ teaspoon dried
> 2 (1½-pound) skin-on full halibut steaks, 1 to 1½ inches thick and 10 to 12 inches long, trimmed of cartilage at both ends
> Salt and pepper

1. Adjust oven rack to lowest position and heat oven to 250 degrees. Cook 1 tablespoon oil, garlic, and pepper flakes in Dutch oven over medium-low heat until garlic is light golden, 2 to 4 minutes. Off heat, stir in tomatoes, capers, and thyme.

2. Pat halibut steaks dry with paper towels and sprinkle with ⅛ teaspoon salt and ⅛ teaspoon pepper. Lay halibut on top of tomatoes in pot. Place large sheet of aluminum foil over pot and press to seal, then cover with lid. Transfer pot to oven and cook until halibut flakes apart when gently prodded with paring knife and registers 140 degrees, 35 to 40 minutes.

3. Gently transfer halibut to serving platter and tent loosely with foil. Simmer tomato mixture over medium-high heat until thickened slightly, about 2 minutes. Off heat, stir in remaining 1 tablespoon oil and season with pepper to taste. Spoon sauce evenly over halibut and serve.

PER SERVING

Cal 170 • **Total Fat** 5g • **Sat Fat** 1g • **Chol** 70mg
Sodium 160mg • **Total Carbs** 2g • **Fiber** 1g • **Total Sugar** 1g
Added Sugar 0g • **Protein** 27g • **Total Carbohydrate Choices** <0.5

TRIMMING AND SERVING FULL HALIBUT STEAKS

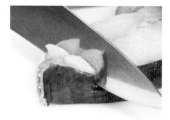 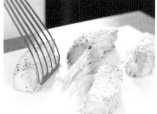

1. BEFORE COOKING Cut off the cartilage at the ends of the steaks so they will fit neatly in the pan and to eliminate the risk that small bones will end up on your dinner plate.

2. TO SERVE Remove the skin from the cooked steaks and separate the quadrants of meat from the bone by slipping a spatula or knife gently between them.

Pan-Roasted Sea Bass with Wild Mushrooms
SERVES 4

WHY THIS RECIPE WORKS This flavorful recipe is a great way to pack mushrooms into your meal—a very good thing as they provide B vitamins and are rich sources of minerals. And dried mushrooms, which are in the mix here as well, just concentrate those nutrients. For a sea bass and mushroom dinner, we liked a combination of full-flavored cremini and portobellos, with a small amount of dried porcini for a deep, woodsy flavor. We first tried sautéing the mushrooms and fish separately, but the result lacked unity. We decided to add the fish to the sautéed mushrooms in a

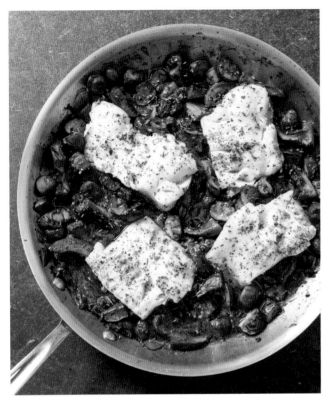

Fresh sea bass and a trio of nutrient-dense mushrooms make for a powerhouse dinner.

hot skillet and then slide the pan into the oven, so the fish and the mushrooms melded in flavor, and the porcini liquid reduced to a light, flavorful sauce. You can substitute cod, halibut, haddock, or red snapper for the sea bass.

½ cup water

⅓ ounce dried porcini mushrooms, rinsed

4 (6-ounce) skinless sea bass fillets, 1 to 1½ inches thick

¼ cup extra virgin olive oil
   Salt and pepper

1 sprig fresh rosemary

1 pound cremini mushrooms, trimmed and halved
   if small or quartered if large

12 ounces portobello mushroom caps, halved and sliced
   ½ inch thick

1 red onion, halved and sliced thin

2 garlic cloves, minced

1 tablespoon minced fresh parsley
   Lemon wedges

1. Adjust oven rack to lower-middle position and heat oven to 475 degrees. Microwave water and porcini mushrooms in covered bowl until steaming, about 1 minute. Let sit until softened, about 5 minutes. Drain mushrooms in fine-mesh strainer lined with coffee filter, reserving porcini liquid, and mince mushrooms.

2. Pat sea bass dry with paper towels, rub with 2 tablespoons oil, and sprinkle with ¼ teaspoon salt and ⅛ teaspoon pepper.

3. Heat remaining 2 tablespoons oil and rosemary in 12-inch ovensafe skillet over medium-high heat until shimmering. Add cremini mushrooms, portobello mushrooms, onion, and ¼ teaspoon salt. Cook, stirring occasionally, until mushrooms have released their liquid and are beginning to brown, 8 to 10 minutes. Stir in garlic and minced porcini mushrooms and cook until fragrant, about 30 seconds.

4. Off heat, stir in reserved porcini liquid. Nestle sea bass skinned side down into skillet, transfer to oven, and roast until sea bass flakes apart when gently prodded with paring knife and registers 140 degrees, 10 to 12 minutes. Sprinkle with parsley. Serve with lemon wedges.

PER SERVING

Cal 360 • **Total Fat** 18g • **Sat Fat** 3g • **Chol** 70mg
Sodium 430mg • **Total Carbs** 11g • **Fiber** 2g • **Total Sugar** 6g
Added Sugar 0g • **Protein** 36g • **Total Carbohydrate Choices** 1

NOTES FROM THE TEST KITCHEN

Reheating Fish

Fish is notoriously susceptible to overcooking, so reheating previously cooked fillets is something that makes nearly all cooks balk. But since almost everyone has leftover fish from time to time, we decided to figure out the best approach to warming it up.

As we had suspected, we had far more success reheating thick fillets and steaks than thin ones. Both swordfish and halibut steaks reheated nicely, retaining their moisture well and with no detectable change in flavor. But there was little we could do to prevent mackerel from drying out and overcooking when heated a second time; so we recommend serving leftover cooked thin fish in cold applications like salads.

To reheat thicker fish fillets, use this gentle approach: Place the fillets on a wire rack set in a rimmed baking sheet, cover them with foil (to prevent the exteriors of the fish from drying out), and heat them in a 275-degree oven until they register 125 to 130 degrees, about 15 minutes for 1-inch-thick fillets (timing varies according to fillet size).

Buying and Storing Fish

WHAT TO LOOK FOR Always buy fish from a trusted source (preferably one with high volume to help ensure freshness). The store, and the fish in it, should smell like the sea, not fishy or sour. And all the fish should be on ice or properly refrigerated. Fillets and steaks should look bright, shiny, and firm, not dull or mushy. Whole fish should have moist, taut skin, clear eyes, and bright red gills.

WHAT TO ASK FOR It is always better to have your fishmonger slice steaks and fillets to order rather than buying precut pieces that may have been sitting around. Don't be afraid to be picky at the seafood counter; a ragged piece of hake or a tail end of sea bass will be difficult to cook properly. It is important to keep your fish cold, so if you have a long ride home, ask your fishmonger for a bag of ice.

BUYING FROZEN FISH Thin fish fillets like flounder and sole are the best choice if you have to buy your fish frozen, because they freeze quickly, minimizing moisture loss. Firm fillets like halibut, snapper, and swordfish are acceptable to buy frozen if cooked beyond medium-rare, but at lower degrees of doneness they will have a dry, stringy texture. When buying frozen fish, make sure it is frozen solid, with no signs of freezer burn or excessive crystallization around the edges and no blood in the packaging. The ingredients should include only the name of the fish you are buying.

DEFROSTING FISH To defrost fish in the refrigerator overnight, remove the fish from its packaging, place it in a single layer on a rimmed plate or dish, and cover it with plastic wrap. You can also do a "quick thaw" by leaving the vacuum-sealed bags under cool running tap water for 30 minutes. Do not use a microwave to defrost fish; it will alter the texture of the fish or, worse, partially cook it. Dry the fish thoroughly with paper towels before seasoning and cooking it.

HOW TO STORE FISH Because fish is so perishable, it's best to buy it the day it will be cooked. If that's not possible, it's important to store it properly. When you get home, unwrap the fish, pat it dry, put it in a zipper-lock bag, press out the air, and seal the bag. Then set the fish on a bed of ice in a bowl that can hold the water once the ice melts, and place it in the back of the fridge, where it is coldest. If the ice melts before you use the fish, replenish it. The fish should keep for one day.

Grilled Sea Bass with Citrus and Black Olive Salad
SERVES 4

WHY THIS RECIPE WORKS: At its best, grilled sea bass boasts firm, moist flesh under a crisp, seared exterior, but many recipes turn out underdone, fishy-tasting fillets. To bring out the best in our grilled sea bass, we started by seeking out thick fillets. Sea bass skin is too tough to eat, so we removed it and rubbed the fish with oil to keep it from sticking to the grill. Unlike other meaty cuts of fish, grilling this fillet all the way through—cooking over the hottest part of the grill for up to 10 minutes before finishing on the cooler side—produced the best flavor; salting the fish before grilling also helped prevent any off-flavors. In under 20 minutes, the sea bass had taken on great flavorful char, but these rich fillets deserved a bright, fresh accompaniment. A zesty, fiber-rich citrus salad of orange and grapefruit segments, balanced out with chopped kalamata olives and a blend of cumin and paprika, paired perfectly with the fish. You can substitute cod, halibut, haddock, or red snapper for the sea bass. Use only the citrus pieces in the relish, not the juices, which will water down the flavor and texture.

2 oranges
1 red grapefruit
¼ cup pitted kalamata olives, chopped
2 tablespoons minced fresh parsley
½ teaspoon ground cumin
½ teaspoon paprika
  Pinch cayenne pepper
4 (6-ounce) skinless sea bass fillets,
  1 to 1½ inches thick
2 tablespoons extra-virgin olive oil
¼ teaspoon salt
⅛ teaspoon pepper

1. Cut away peel and pith from oranges and grapefruit. Quarter oranges, then slice crosswise into ½-inch-thick pieces. Cut grapefruit into 8 wedges, then slice wedges crosswise into ½-inch-thick pieces. Combine oranges, grapefruit, olives, parsley, cumin, paprika, and cayenne in bowl. Cover and set aside for serving.

2. Pat sea bass dry with paper towels, rub with oil, and sprinkle with salt and pepper.

3A. FOR A CHARCOAL GRILL Open bottom vent completely. Light large chimney starter filled with charcoal briquettes (6 quarts). When top coals are partially covered with ash, pour evenly over half of grill. Set cooking grate in place, cover, and open lid vent completely. Heat grill until hot, about 5 minutes.

3B. FOR A GAS GRILL Turn all burners to high, cover, and heat grill until hot, about 15 minutes. Leave primary burner on high and turn other burner(s) to medium-low.

4. Clean cooking grate, then repeatedly brush grate with well oiled paper towels until grate is black and glossy, 5 to 10 times. Place sea bass on hotter part of grill and cook, uncovered, until well browned, about 10 minutes, gently flipping fillets using 2 spatulas halfway through cooking.

5. Gently move sea bass to cooler part of grill and cook, uncovered, until sea bass flakes apart when gently prodded with paring knife and registers 140 degrees, 3 to 6 minutes. Transfer to serving platter and serve with salad.

PER SERVING

Cal 300 • **Total Fat** 11g • **Sat Fat** 2g • **Chol** 70mg
Sodium 270mg • **Total Carbs** 16g • **Fiber** 5g • **Total Sugar** 11g
Added Sugar 0g • **Protein** 33g • **Total Carbohydrate Choices** 1

Poached Snapper with Sherry-Tomato Vinaigrette
SERVES 4

WHY THIS RECIPE WORKS Poaching fish fillets in olive oil is a popular Italian and French technique that delivers supermoist, delicately cooked fish that makes the most of heart-healthy oil as a cooking medium. In our recipe the oil pulled double duty: We poached the fish in it, and then blended the oil into a bright tomato vinaigrette for serving. We placed half an onion in the skillet to displace the oil so it would come up higher in the pan— and we could use less of it. After adding the fish, we moved the skillet to the even heat of the oven. You can substitute sea bass, cod, halibut, or haddock for the snapper. You will need a 10-inch ovensafe nonstick skillet with a lid for this recipe.

- 4 **(6-ounce) skinless red snapper fillets, 1 inch thick**
  Salt and pepper
- ½ **cup extra-virgin olive oil**
- ½ **onion, peeled**
- 6 **ounces cherry tomatoes (2 ounces cut into ⅛-inch-thick rounds)**
- ½ **small shallot, peeled**
- 4 **teaspoons sherry vinegar**
- 1 **tablespoon minced fresh parsley**

1. Adjust oven rack to middle position and heat oven to 250 degrees. Pat snapper dry with paper towels and sprinkle with ¼ teaspoon salt. Let sit at room temperature for 20 minutes.

2. Heat oil in 10-inch ovensafe nonstick skillet over medium heat until registers 180 degrees. Off heat, place onion half in center of skillet. Arrange fillets skinned side up around onion (oil

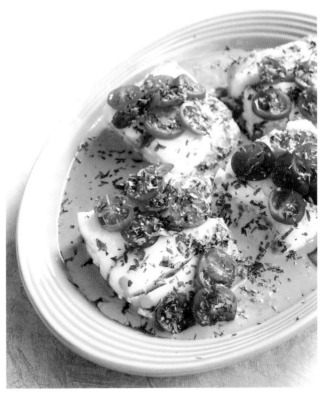

Tomatoes have substantial health benefits—here they are pureed into a sauce and sliced raw as a topping for poached snapper.

should come roughly halfway up fillets) and spoon some oil over each fillet. Cover, transfer skillet to oven, and cook for 15 minutes.

3. Remove skillet from oven (skillet handle will be hot), then carefully flip fillets using 2 spatulas. Cover and continue to bake snapper until it registers 130 to 135 degrees, 9 to 14 minutes. Carefully transfer snapper to serving platter, reserving ¼ cup oil, and tent loosely with aluminum foil.

4. Process reserved ¼ cup fish cooking oil, whole tomatoes, shallot, vinegar, ⅛ teaspoon salt, and ½ teaspoon pepper in blender until smooth, about 2 minutes, scraping down sides of bowl as needed. Add any accumulated fish juices and blend for 10 seconds. Strain sauce through fine-mesh strainer into bowl; discard solids. To serve, spoon vinaigrette around fish. Garnish each fillet with parsley and tomato rounds. Serve.

PER SERVING

Cal 310 • **Total Fat** 16g • **Sat Fat** 2.5g • **Chol** 65mg
Sodium 330mg • **Total Carbs** 2g • **Fiber** 1g • **Total Sugar** 1g
Added Sugar 0g • **Protein** 35g • **Total Carbohydrate Choices** <0.5

Swordfish en Cocotte with Shallots, Cucumber, and Mint
SERVES 4

WHY THIS RECIPE WORKS The premise behind the French method of cooking *en cocotte* (or casserole roasting) is to slow down the cooking process in order to concentrate flavor. Fish cooked for an extended period of time usually winds up dry, but a combination of low oven temperature, moist-heat environment, and the right cut of fish allows it to remain juicy and tender. We found that meaty swordfish steaks were particularly well suited to cooking en cocotte. The fresh Mediterranean flavors of mint, parsley, lemon, and garlic easily combined with sliced cucumber to make an insulating layer on which to cook the fish; we then turned the cucumber mixture into a complementary, flavorful topping for serving. It is important to choose steaks that are similar in size and thickness to ensure that each piece cooks at the same rate. You can substitute skin-on halibut for the swordfish.

¾ cup fresh mint leaves
¼ cup fresh parsley leaves
5 tablespoons extra-virgin olive oil
2 tablespoons lemon juice
4 garlic cloves, minced
1 teaspoon ground cumin
¼ teaspoon cayenne pepper
    Salt and pepper
3 shallots, sliced thin
1 cucumber, peeled, seeded, and sliced thin
4 (6-ounce) skin-on swordfish steaks,
    1 to 1½ inches thick

1. Adjust oven rack to lowest position and heat oven to 250 degrees. Process mint, parsley, 3 tablespoons oil, lemon juice, garlic, cumin, cayenne, and ⅛ teaspoon salt in food processor until smooth, about 20 seconds, scraping down sides of bowl as needed.

2. Heat remaining 2 tablespoons oil in Dutch oven over medium-low heat until shimmering. Add shallots, cover, and cook, stirring occasionally, until softened, about 5 minutes. Off heat, stir in processed mint mixture and cucumber.

3. Pat swordfish dry with paper towels and sprinkle with ¼ teaspoon salt and ⅛ teaspoon pepper. Place swordfish on top of cucumber-mint mixture. Place large sheet of aluminum foil over pot and press to seal, then cover with lid. Transfer pot to oven and cook until swordfish flakes apart when gently prodded with paring knife and registers 140 degrees, 35 to 40 minutes.

4. Transfer swordfish to serving platter. Season cucumber-mint mixture with pepper to taste, then spoon evenly over swordfish. Serve.

PER SERVING

Cal 440 • **Total Fat** 29g • **Sat Fat** 5g • **Chol** 110mg
Sodium 300mg • **Total Carbs** 8g • **Fiber** 3g • **Total Sugar** 3g
Added Sugar 0g • **Protein** 35g • **Total Carbohydrate Choices** 0.5

Grilled Swordfish with Eggplant, Tomato, and Chickpea Salad
SERVES 4

WHY THIS RECIPE WORKS Here grilled swordfish is paired with a salad packed with nutrients and fiber from a trio of eggplant, tomatoes, and nutty chickpeas. Since meaty swordfish stands up so well to grilling, we decided to grill swordfish steaks simultaneously with some eggplant for a quick and elegant grilled dinner. We gave a flavor boost to the fish by coating it with a paste of cilantro, onion, garlic, and warm spices (reserving part of the paste to dress the eggplant salad), which then bloomed over the hot fire. We removed the fish when the interior was just opaque since it would cook a little more from residual heat as it rested while we prepared the accompanying vegetables. After grilling the eggplant until soft and charred, we chopped it into chunks and mixed it with juicy cherry tomatoes and canned chickpeas, then dressed it with the remaining cilantro mixture for an easy and vibrant salad. You can substitute halibut for the swordfish.

1 cup fresh cilantro leaves
½ red onion, chopped coarse
5 tablespoons extra-virgin olive oil
3 tablespoons lemon juice
4 garlic cloves, chopped
1 teaspoon ground cumin
1 teaspoon paprika
¼ teaspoon cayenne pepper
⅛ teaspoon ground cinnamon
    Salt and pepper
4 (6-ounce) skin-on swordfish steaks, 1 to 1½ inches thick
1 large eggplant, sliced into ½-inch-thick rounds
6 ounces cherry tomatoes, halved
1 (15-ounce) can no-salt added chickpeas, rinsed

1. Process cilantro, onion, 3 tablespoons oil, lemon juice, garlic, cumin, paprika, cayenne, cinnamon, and ¼ teaspoon salt in food processor until smooth, about 2 minutes, scraping down sides of bowl as needed. Measure out and reserve ½ cup cilantro mixture. Transfer remaining cilantro mixture to large bowl and set aside.

2. Brush swordfish with reserved ½ cup cilantro mixture. Brush eggplant with remaining 2 tablespoons oil and sprinkle with ⅛ teaspoon salt and ⅛ teaspoon pepper.

3A. FOR A CHARCOAL GRILL Open bottom vent completely. Light large chimney starter filled with charcoal briquettes (6 quarts). When top coals are partially covered with ash, pour two-thirds evenly over half of grill, then pour remaining coals over other half of grill. Set cooking grate in place, cover, and open lid vent completely. Heat grill until hot, about 5 minutes.

3B. FOR A GAS GRILL Turn all burners to high, cover, and heat grill until hot, about 15 minutes. Leave primary burner on high and turn other burner(s) to medium-high.

4. Clean cooking grate, then repeatedly brush grate with well-oiled paper towels until black and glossy, 5 to 10 times. Place swordfish and eggplant on hotter part of grill. Cook swordfish, uncovered, until streaked with dark grill marks, 6 to 9 minutes, gently flipping steaks using 2 spatulas halfway through cooking. Cook eggplant, flipping as needed, until softened and lightly charred, about 8 minutes; transfer to bowl and cover with aluminum foil.

5. Gently move swordfish to cooler part of grill and continue to cook, uncovered, until swordfish flakes apart when gently prodded with paring knife and registers 140 degrees, 1 to 3 minutes per side; transfer to serving platter and tent loosely with foil.

6. Coarsely chop eggplant and add to bowl with cilantro mixture along with tomatoes and chickpeas. Gently toss to combine and season with pepper to taste. Serve.

PER SERVING

Cal 530 • **Total Fat** 30g • **Sat Fat** 5g • **Chol** 110mg
Sodium 380mg • **Total Carbs** 25g • **Fiber** 8g • **Total Sugar** 7g
Added Sugar 0g • **Protein** 40g • **Total Carbohydrate Choices** 1.5

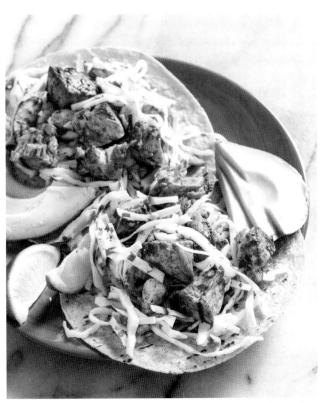

When making grilled fish tacos, we found sturdy swordfish to be the most reliable choice.

Grilled Fish Tacos
SERVES 6

WHY THIS RECIPE WORKS Flavorful grilled fish tacos can be a crowd-pleasing dinner option when done right. Unfortunately, many home cooks fall into a classic pitfall by either overcooking the fish or drowning the fresh flavor in a thick sauce. To make a flavorful, and foolproof, recipe we started by examining the classic cooking issues. Flaky fish like cod or snapper often ends up sticking to the grill, so we turned to meatier swordfish. Cutting the fish into even 1-inch strips ensured that each piece would finish cooking at the same time, and avoided dry, tough meat. To give our fish complex flavor in the time it took to set up the grill, we made a marinade of chile powders, garlic, oregano, coriander, and tomato paste. For a delicious pairing to our spiced swordfish we made an aromatic slaw and added a hefty amount of avocado slices. You can substitute halibut for the swordfish.

2 tablespoons plus 1 teaspoon canola oil
1 tablespoon ancho chile powder
2 teaspoons chipotle chile powder
2 garlic cloves, minced
1 teaspoon dried oregano
1 teaspoon ground coriander
  Salt
2 tablespoons no-salt-added tomato paste
½ cup orange juice
¼ cup lime juice (2 limes), plus wedges for serving
1½ pounds skinless swordfish steaks, 1 inch thick, cut lengthwise into 1-inch-wide strips
½ small head green cabbage, cored and sliced thin (4 cups)
¼ cup minced fresh cilantro
3 scallions, sliced thin
12 (6-inch) corn tortillas
2 avocados, halved, pitted, and sliced thin

1. Heat 2 tablespoons oil, ancho chile powder, and chipotle chile powder in 8-inch skillet over medium heat, stirring constantly, until fragrant and some bubbles form, 2 to 3 minutes. Add garlic, oregano, coriander, and ¾ teaspoon salt and continue to cook until fragrant, about 30 seconds longer. Add tomato paste and, using spatula, mash tomato paste with spice mixture until combined, about 20 seconds. Stir in orange juice and 2 tablespoons lime juice. Cook, stirring constantly, until thoroughly mixed and reduced slightly, about 2 minutes. Transfer chile mixture to large bowl and let cool for 15 minutes.

2. Add swordfish to bowl with chile mixture and stir gently with rubber spatula to coat fish. Cover and refrigerate for at least 30 minutes or up to 2 hours.

3. Meanwhile, combine cabbage, cilantro, scallions, remaining 2 tablespoons lime juice, remaining 1 teaspoon oil, and ¼ teaspoon salt in bowl.

4A. FOR A CHARCOAL GRILL Open bottom vent completely. Light large chimney starter mounded with charcoal briquettes (7 quarts). When top coals are partially covered with ash, pour evenly over grill. Set cooking grate in place, cover, and open lid vent completely. Heat grill until hot, about 5 minutes.

4B. FOR A GAS GRILL Turn all burners to high, cover, and heat grill until hot, about 15 minutes. Turn all burners to medium-high.

5. Clean and oil cooking grate. Arrange swordfish over grill. Cover and cook until fish has begun to brown, 3 to 5 minutes. Using thin spatula, turn fish. Cover and continue to cook until swordfish flakes apart when gently prodded with paring knife and registers 140 degrees, 3 to 5 minutes. Transfer to large platter, flake into pieces, and tent with aluminum foil.

6. Clean cooking grate. Place half of tortillas on grill. Cook on each side until softened and speckled with brown spots, 30 to 45 seconds per side. Wrap tortillas in dish towel or foil to keep warm. Repeat with remaining tortillas. Divide flaked fish, avocado, and slaw evenly among tortillas. Serve with lime wedges.

PER SERVING
Cal 500 • **Total Fat** 25g • **Sat Fat** 3.5g • **Chol** 75mg **Sodium** 530mg • **Total Carbs** 44g • **Fiber** 12g • **Total Sugar** 9g **Added Sugar** 0g • **Protein** 29g • **Total Carbohydrate Choices** 3

Pan-Seared Sesame-Crusted Tuna Steaks
SERVES 4

WHY THIS RECIPE WORKS Moist and rare in the middle with a seared crust, pan-seared tuna is a popular entrée in restaurants. We set out to determine the best method for preparing this simple dish at home. The consensus in the test kitchen was to create a master recipe for four 6-ounce steaks cooked in one batch in one pan. Starting with high-quality tuna—sushi grade if possible—is paramount; we prefer the flavor of yellowfin. After testing ¾-inch-thick steaks, we found that a thickness of at least 1 inch is necessary to achieve both good browning on the exterior of the tuna and a rare center. We started with a very hot skillet and 2 tablespoons of oil. Unfortunately, the tuna did not develop the deep brown crust that we were after. We tried using more fat to cook the very lean fish, as well as dipping the tuna in balsamic vinegar (in hopes that the sugar in the vinegar would help caramelize the crust), which gave our fish a darker color, but the crunch was still missing. We realized that we would need some sort of coating for the steaks in order to get a crispy, crunchy crust. Crushed peppercorns and spice rubs interfered with the tuna's flavor, but neutral sesame seeds were a big hit with tasters. Before searing the tuna in a nonstick skillet, we rubbed the steaks with oil and then coated them with sesame seeds; the oil helped the seeds stick to the fish. The sesame seeds browned in the skillet and formed a beautiful, nutty-tasting crust. We learned that tuna, like beef, will continue to cook from residual heat when removed from the stove, so when the interior of the tuna was near the desired degree of doneness (about 110 degrees on an instant-read thermometer), we transferred it to a platter. We prefer our tuna cooked rare. If you like yours medium-rare, cook the fish in step 2 until it is opaque at the perimeter and reddish pink at the center when checked with the tip of a paring knife and it registers 125 degrees, 2 to 3 minutes per side.

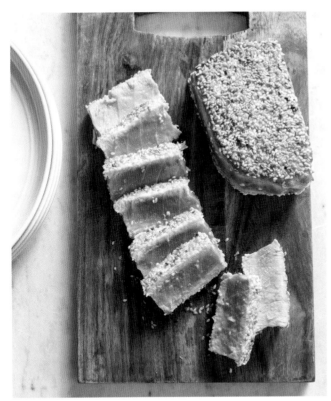

For an ultraflavorful and high-protein coating for our pan-seared tuna steaks we first coat them with oil and sesame seeds.

¾ cup sesame seeds
4 (6-ounce) skinless tuna steaks, 1 inch thick
2 tablespoons canola oil
¼ teaspoon salt
⅛ teaspoon pepper

1. Spread sesame seeds in shallow baking dish. Pat tuna steaks dry with paper towels, rub steaks all over with 1 tablespoon oil, then sprinkle with salt and pepper. Press both sides of each steak in sesame seeds to coat.

2. Heat remaining 1 tablespoon oil in 12-inch nonstick skillet over medium-high heat until just smoking. Place steaks in skillet and cook until seeds are golden and tuna is translucent red at center when checked with tip of paring knife and registers 110 degrees (for rare), 1 to 2 minutes per side. Transfer tuna to cutting board and slice ½ inch thick. Serve.

PER SERVING
Cal 330 • **Total Fat** 15g • **Sat Fat** 1g • **Chol** 65mg
Sodium 250mg • **Total Carbs** 2g • **Fiber** 1g • **Total Sugar** 0g
Added Sugar 0g • **Protein** 45g • **Total Carbohydrate Choices** <0.5

Seared Tuna with Harissa and Mushrooms
SERVES 4

WHY THIS RECIPE WORKS Harissa is a traditional bright and spicy North African condiment that adds a jolt of potent flavor to any recipe it's used in. It works well with the meaty tuna steaks and earthy mushrooms in this dish. Use harissa paste rather than harissa sauce here. Note that spiciness will vary greatly by brand. White mushrooms can be substituted for the cremini, if you prefer. We prefer our tuna cooked rare. If you like yours medium-rare, cook the fish in step 4 until it is opaque at the perimeter and reddish pink at the center when checked with the tip of a paring knife and it registers 125 degrees, 2 to 3 minutes per side.

5 tablespoons extra-virgin olive oil
3 tablespoons harissa
1 tablespoon lemon juice, plus lemon wedges for serving
1–3 tablespoons hot water
1 shallot, halved and sliced thin
1¼ pounds cremini mushrooms, trimmed and halved if small or quartered if large
12 ounces shiitake mushrooms, stemmed and sliced ½ inch thick
   Salt and pepper
1 head frisée (6 ounces), cored and cut into 1-inch pieces
4 (6-ounce) tuna steaks, 1 inch thick
2 tablespoons minced fresh mint

1. Combine 1 tablespoon oil, 2 tablespoons harissa, and lemon juice in bowl. Whisk in hot water, 1 tablespoon at a time, until sauce is pourable; set aside.

2. Heat 1 tablespoon oil in 12-inch nonstick skillet over medium heat until shimmering. Add shallot and cook until softened, about 2 minutes. Add cremini mushrooms, shiitake mushrooms, and ⅛ teaspoon salt, cover, and cook, stirring occasionally, until mushrooms have released their liquid, 8 to 10 minutes.

3. Uncover skillet, add 2 tablespoons oil, and cook, stirring occasionally, until mushrooms are deep golden brown and tender, 10 to 12 minutes. Add remaining 1 tablespoon harissa and cook until fragrant, about 30 seconds. Transfer mushrooms to bowl, add frisée, and toss to combine; set aside. Wipe skillet clean with paper towels.

4. Pat tuna dry with paper towels and sprinkle with ⅛ teaspoon salt and ⅛ teaspoon pepper. Heat remaining 1 tablespoon oil in now-empty skillet over medium-high heat until just smoking. Place steaks in skillet and cook until translucent red at center when checked with tip of paring knife and register 110 degrees (for rare), 1 to 2 minutes per side.

5. Transfer tuna to cutting board and slice ½ inch thick. Sprinkle mint over mushroom mixture and season with pepper to taste. Drizzle tuna evenly with reserved harissa sauce and serve with mushrooms and lemon wedges.

PER SERVING

Cal 490 • **Total Fat** 27g • **Sat Fat** 4g • **Chol** 65mg
Sodium 360mg • **Total Carbs** 12g • **Fiber** 3g • **Total Sugar** 6g
Added Sugar 0g • **Protein** 47g • **Total Carbohydrate Choices** 1

Pan-Seared Shrimp with Tomato and Avocado
SERVES 4

WHY THIS RECIPE WORKS Shrimp plus heart-healthy avocado, fresh cilantro, chopped tomatoes, and scallions equal a delicious, colorful, and nutrient-dense dish with satisfying Mexican flavors. Searing the shrimp quickly in batches produced the ultimate combination of well-caramelized exteriors and moist, tender interiors. This cooking method also preserved the shrimp's juiciness and trademark briny sweetness. After the second batch was seared and removed from the pan, we made our smoky, slightly spicy sauce. Later, we returned the shrimp to the pan with the sauce to heat them through with the other elements of the dish. The cooking times are for extra-large shrimp. If this size is not available in your market, buy large shrimp and shorten the cooking time slightly. For information on shopping for shrimp, see page 263. This dish is fairly spicy; to make it milder, use less chipotle.

1½ pounds extra-large shrimp (21 to 25 per pound),
    peeled and deveined
    Salt and pepper
 4 teaspoons canola oil
 1 pound tomatoes, cored, seeded, and cut into
    ½-inch pieces
 6 scallions, white and green parts separated and sliced thin
¼ cup minced fresh cilantro
 3 garlic cloves, minced
 1 tablespoon lime juice, plus lime wedges for serving
 1 teaspoon minced canned chipotle chile in adobo sauce
 1 avocado, halved, peeled, and cut into ½-inch pieces

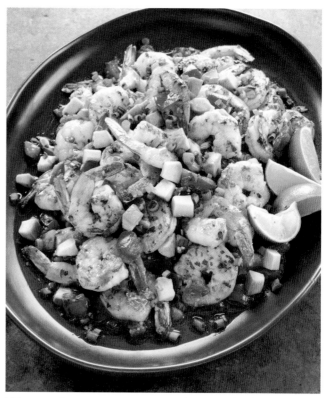

This appealing recipe is a Mexican take on stir-fried shrimp and is both super flavorful and heart-healthy.

1. Pat shrimp dry with paper towels and sprinkle with ¼ teaspoon salt and ⅛ teaspoon pepper. Heat 2 teaspoons oil in 12-inch nonstick skillet over medium-high heat until just smoking. Add half of shrimp and cook until opaque throughout, about 2 minutes. Transfer to bowl. Repeat with remaining 2 teaspoons oil and remaining shrimp.

2. Add tomatoes, scallion whites, cilantro, garlic, lime juice, and chipotle to now-empty skillet and cook until tomatoes soften slightly, about 1 minute. Off heat, return shrimp to skillet and toss to coat. Transfer to serving platter, season with pepper to taste, and sprinkle with scallion greens and avocado. Serve with lime wedges.

PER SERVING

Cal 240 • **Total Fat** 14g • **Sat Fat** 2g • **Chol** 160mg
Sodium 350mg • **Total Carbs** 12g • **Fiber** 5g • **Total Sugar** 4g
Added Sugar 0g • **Protein** 20g • **Total Carbohydrate Choices** 1

Grilled Marinated Shrimp Skewers
SERVES 6

WHY THIS RECIPE WORKS Jolts of grill flavor and subtle heat can enhance the delicately sweet and briny flavor of shrimp, but it's easy to overdo it. Most recipes overcook the shrimp and finish them in a bath of mouth-numbing sauce; we wanted juicy shrimp with a smoky crust and flavor that was more than just superficial. We looked to the spices of Morocco and found just the right blend: lime zest for tang, paprika to accent the smoky grill flavor, ginger and cayenne for complex heat, and cumin and plenty of garlic for a rounded earthy-sharp flavor. We left the fresh lime juice for finishing, since an acidic marinade can degrade shrimp's texture. Once lightly charred, we flipped the skewers to finish gently cooking on the cooler side of the grill. Butterflying the shrimp before marinating and grilling them opened up more shrimp flesh for the marinade to flavor. We also packed the shrimp very tightly onto the skewers so they would cook more slowly. For information on shopping for shrimp, see box at right. You will need four 12-inch metal skewers for this recipe.

MARINADE
- 3 tablespoons extra-virgin olive oil
- 6 garlic cloves, minced
- 1 teaspoon grated lime zest
- ½ teaspoon smoked paprika
- ½ teaspoon ground ginger
- ½ teaspoon ground cumin
- ¼ teaspoon salt
- ¼ teaspoon cayenne pepper

SHRIMP
- 1½ pounds extra-large shrimp (21 to 25 per pound), peeled and deveined
  Pepper
- 1 tablespoon minced fresh cilantro
  Lime wedges

1. FOR THE MARINADE Whisk all ingredients together in medium bowl.

2. FOR THE SHRIMP Pat shrimp dry with paper towels. Using paring knife, cut shrimp ½ inch deep down outside curve of shrimp, take care not to cut in half completely. Add shrimp to bowl with marinade and toss to coat. Cover and refrigerate for at least 30 minutes or up to 1 hour.

3A. FOR A CHARCOAL GRILL Open bottom vent completely. Light large chimney starter filled with charcoal briquettes (6 quarts). When top coals are partially covered with ash, pour evenly over half of grill. Set cooking grate in place, cover, and open lid vent completely. Heat grill until hot, about 5 minutes.

3B. FOR A GAS GRILL Turn all burners to high, cover, and heat grill until hot, about 15 minutes. Leave all burners on high.

4. Clean and oil cooking grate. Thread shrimp tightly onto four 12-inch metal skewers (about 8 shrimp per skewer), alternating direction of heads and tails. Place shrimp skewers on grill (on hotter side if using charcoal). Cook (covered if using gas), without moving them, until lightly charred on first side, 3 to 4 minutes. Flip skewers and move to cooler side of grill (if using charcoal) or turn all burners off (if using gas) and cook, covered, until shrimp are opaque throughout, 1 to 2 minutes. Using tongs, slide shrimp off skewers onto serving platter and season with pepper to taste. Sprinkle with cilantro and serve with lime wedges.

PER SERVING

Cal 130 • **Total Fat** 8g • **Sat Fat** 1g • **Chol** 105mg
Sodium 220mg • **Total Carbs** 2g • **Fiber** 0g • **Total Sugar** 0g
Added Sugar 0g • **Protein** 12g • **Total Carbohydrate Choices** <0.5

NOTES FROM THE TEST KITCHEN

Shopping for Shrimp: Buyer Beware

Most supermarket shrimp are frozen, so to prevent darkening or water loss during thawing, some manufacturers treat the shrimp with salt or sodium tripolyphosphate (STPP). We do not recommend cooking with STPP-treated shrimp. We have found that these preservatives can give shrimp an unpleasant, rubbery, or mushy texture and chemical flavor, as well as extra sodium. Check the ingredient list to see if your shrimp has been treated with salt or STPP; shrimp should be the only ingredient listed on the bag.

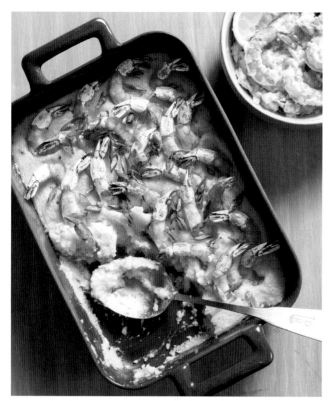

Our shrimp and grits casserole delivers big flavor and is easy to make—the shrimp cooks right on top of the grits at the end.

Cheesy Shrimp and Grits
SERVES 4

WHY THIS RECIPE WORKS This Southern favorite pairs creamy grits and sweet briny shrimp all in one casserole dish. To give the grits as much flavor as possible, we sautéed scallions, garlic, and spicy chipotle chile in the saucepan before cooking the grits. Using milk instead of heavy cream gave the grits a nice creaminess without making them too dense, and shredded cheddar cheese added rich flavor to the grits. As for the shrimp, we simply assembled the grits in a casserole dish and nestled in the shrimp so they could easily cook through, eliminating the need for another dish. Do not substitute instant grits here. For information on shopping for shrimp, see page 263.

  1 tablespoon extra-virgin olive oil
  3 scallions, white parts sliced thin, green parts
     sliced thin on bias
  2 garlic cloves, minced

  1 teaspoon minced canned chipotle chile in adobo sauce
  4 cups water
  ½ cup 1 percent low-fat milk
     Salt and pepper
  1 cup old-fashioned grits
  2 ounces sharp cheddar cheese, shredded (½ cup)
1½ pounds extra-large shrimp (21 to 25 per pound),
     peeled and deveined
     Lemon wedges

1. Adjust oven rack to middle position and heat oven to 450 degrees. Heat oil in medium saucepan over medium heat until shimmering. Add scallion whites and cook until softened, about 2 minutes. Stir in garlic and chipotle and cook until fragrant, about 30 seconds. Stir in water, milk, and pinch salt and bring to boil. Slowly whisk in grits. Reduce heat to low and cook, stirring often, until grits are thick and creamy, about 15 minutes.

2. Off heat, stir in cheese, ⅛ teaspoon salt, and ⅛ teaspoon pepper, then transfer to 13 by 9-inch baking dish. Nestle shrimp into grits, leaving tails exposed. Bake until shrimp are cooked through, about 15 minutes. Let cool slightly, then sprinkle with scallion greens. Serve with lemon wedges.

PER SERVING

Cal 330 • **Total Fat** 10g • **Sat Fat** 4g • **Chol** 175mg
Sodium 380mg • **Total Carbs** 32g • **Fiber** 3g • **Total Sugar** 2g
Added Sugar 0g • **Protein** 25g • **Total Carbohydrate Choices** 2

PEELING AND DEVEINING SHRIMP

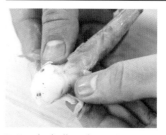 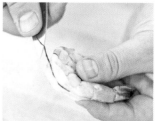

1. Break shell under swimming legs, which will come off as shell is removed. Leave tail intact, if desired, or tug tail to remove shell.

2. Use paring knife to make shallow cut along back of shrimp to expose vein. Use tip of paring knife to lift out vein. Discard vein by wiping blade against paper towel.

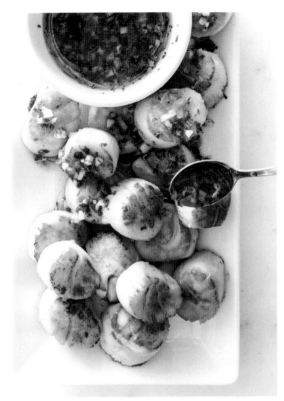

Drying the scallops really well before browning them in batches helps give them a perfect golden crust.

Seared Scallops with Orange-Lime Dressing
SERVES 4

WHY THIS RECIPE WORKS Seared scallops make for an ideal quick meal, as they cook in just a few minutes on the stovetop and have a mild flavor that works well with a wide variety of other ingredients. For this dish, we decided to punch up the scallops' mellow sweetness with a bold vinaigrette made with citrus, cilantro, and red pepper flakes. When searing the scallops, we found that trying to cook them all at once made the pan too crowded and caused them to steam. Waiting to add the scallops to the skillet until the oil was beginning to smoke, cooking the scallops in two batches instead of one, and using a nonstick skillet allowed them all to achieve a deep golden-brown crust. Sweet, bright, and tangy, these scallops are the perfect centerpiece for a light meal—even on a busy weeknight. For information on shopping for scallops, see page 267.

1½ pounds large sea scallops, tendons removed
⅛ teaspoon salt
⅛ teaspoon pepper
6 tablespoons extra-virgin olive oil
2 tablespoons orange juice
2 tablespoons lime juice
1 small shallot, minced
1 tablespoon minced fresh cilantro
⅛ teaspoon red pepper flakes

1. Place scallops in rimmed baking sheet lined with clean kitchen towel. Place second clean kitchen towel on top of scallops and press gently on towel to blot liquid. Let scallops sit at room temperature, covered with towel, for 10 minutes. Sprinkle scallops with salt and pepper.

2. Whisk ¼ cup oil, orange juice, lime juice, shallot, cilantro, and pepper flakes together in bowl. Set aside for serving.

3. Heat 1 tablespoon oil in 12-inch nonstick skillet over medium-high heat until just smoking. Add half of scallops to skillet and cook, without moving them, until well browned on first side, about 1½ minutes. Flip scallops and continue to cook, without moving them, until well browned on second side, sides are firm, and centers are opaque, about 1½ minutes. Transfer scallops to serving platter and tent loosely with aluminum foil. Repeat with remaining 1 tablespoon oil and remaining scallops. Whisk dressing to recombine and serve with scallops.

PER SERVING

Cal 310 • **Total Fat** 22g • **Sat Fat** 3g • **Chol** 40mg
Sodium 350mg • **Total Carbs** 7g • **Fiber** 0g • **Total Sugar** 1g
Added Sugar 0g • **Protein** 21g • **Total Carbohydrate Choices** 0.5

PREPPING SCALLOPS

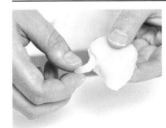

Use your fingers to peel away the small, crescent-shaped muscle that is sometimes attached to scallops, as this tendon becomes incredibly tough when cooked.

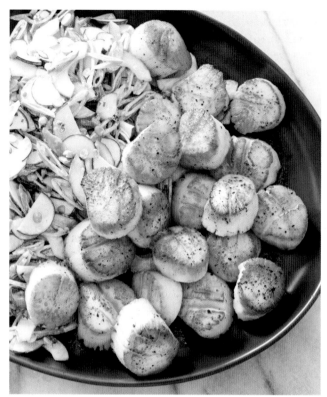

A vibrant three-vegetable slaw is a great accompaniment to simple seared scallops.

Seared Scallops with Snap Pea and Edamame Slaw
SERVES 4

WHY THIS RECIPE WORKS Scallops are a great lean protein source and make for a quick and easy summer meal. We seared the scallops quickly in canola oil, which allowed us to use the highest heat and achieve a beautifully browned exterior without overcooking the centers. For a nutrient-rich and delicious side dish, we paired our scallops with a fresh, vibrant slaw comprised of hearty edamame, crunchy snap peas and radishes, and cooling cucumber. To dress the slaw we created a blend of mayonnaise and yogurt for a lighter, cleaner-tasting dressing. A full 3 tablespoons of minced chives provided an oniony, herbal bite. For information on shopping for scallops, see page 267.

  3 tablespoons chopped fresh chives
  2 tablespoons plain low-fat yogurt
  2 tablespoons mayonnaise
 ½ teaspoon grated lemon zest plus 1 tablespoon juice
    Salt and pepper
 12 ounces sugar snap peas, strings removed and sliced thin on bias
 10 ounces frozen edamame, thawed
  1 English cucumber, halved lengthwise, seeded, and sliced thin
  6 radishes, trimmed, halved lengthwise, and sliced thin
 1½ pounds large sea scallops, tendons removed
  2 tablespoons canola oil

1. Whisk chives, yogurt, mayonnaise, lemon zest and juice, and ⅛ teaspoon salt together in large bowl. Add snap peas, edamame, cucumber, and radishes and stir to coat; set aside.

2. Place scallops in rimmed baking sheet lined with clean kitchen towel. Place second clean kitchen towel on top of scallops and press gently on towel to blot liquid. Let scallops sit at room temperature, covered with towel, for 10 minutes. Sprinkle scallops with ⅛ teaspoon salt and ⅛ teaspoon pepper.

3. Heat 1 tablespoon oil in 12-inch nonstick skillet over medium-heat until just smoking. Add half of scallops and cook, without moving them, until well browned on first side, about 1½ minutes. Flip scallops and continue to cook, without moving them, until well browned on second side, sides are firm, and centers are opaque, about 1½ minutes. Transfer scallops to serving platter and tent loosely with aluminum foil. Repeat with remaining 1 tablespoon oil and remaining scallops. Serve scallops with slaw.

PER SERVING
Cal 360 • **Total Fat** 16g • **Sat Fat** 1.5g • **Chol** 45mg
Sodium 480mg • **Total Carbs** 22g • **Fiber** 6g • **Total Sugar** 8g
Added Sugar 0g • **Protein** 32g • **Total Carbohydrate Choices** 1.5

Baked Scallops with Leeks and Lemon
SERVES 4

WHY THIS RECIPE WORKS This easy-to-make scallop dish is a healthier take on the classic French pairing of scallops and leeks in a cream sauce known as coquilles St. Jacques. First we sautéed sliced leeks until fully softened, then added garlic and thyme. To create our sauce, we added just a tablespoon of flour for thickening, whisking in a little white wine and milk. After seasoning our scallops, we simply placed them in the baking dish and topped them with this aromatic sauce. Once our scallops were perfectly done, which takes only about 15 minutes in the oven, we removed them from the pan and embellished the sauce left behind with lemon juice and parsley. For information on shopping for scallops, see box at right.

2 teaspoons canola oil
8 ounces leeks, white and light green parts only, halved lengthwise, sliced ¼ inch thick, and washed thoroughly
2 garlic cloves, minced
1 teaspoon minced fresh thyme or ¼ teaspoon dried
1 tablespoon all-purpose flour
¼ cup dry white wine
¾ cup 1 percent low-fat milk
¼ teaspoon grated lemon zest plus 1 tablespoon juice
Salt and pepper
1½ pounds large sea scallops, tendons removed
2 teaspoons minced fresh parsley

1. Adjust oven rack to middle position and heat oven to 450 degrees. Heat oil in medium saucepan over medium heat until shimmering. Add leeks and cook until softened, about 5 minutes.

2. Stir in garlic and thyme and cook until fragrant, about 30 seconds. Stir in flour and cook for 30 seconds. Slowly whisk in wine and milk and simmer until sauce is thickened, 2 to 3 minutes. Off heat, stir in lemon zest and season with pepper to taste.

3. Pat scallops dry with paper towels, then sprinkle with ⅛ teaspoon salt and ⅛ teaspoon pepper. Arrange scallops in single layer in 8-inch square baking dish and pour sauce over top. Bake until sides are firm and centers are opaque, 15 to 20 minutes.

4. Carefully transfer scallops to serving platter, leaving sauce behind in dish. Whisk lemon juice and parsley into sauce, pour evenly over scallops, and serve.

PER SERVING

Cal 190 • **Total Fat** 3.5 • **Sat Fat** 0.5g • **Chol** 45mg
Sodium 370mg • **Total Carbs** 14g • **Fiber** 1g • **Total Sugar** 3g
Added Sugar 0g • **Protein** 23g • **Total Carbohydrate Choices** 1

VARIATION
Baked Scallops with Leeks and Saffron

Add ⅛ teaspoon saffron threads with garlic and thyme. Omit lemon zest and reduce amount of lemon juice to 1½ teaspoons.

PER SERVING

Cal 190 • **Total Fat** 3.5g • **Sat Fat** 0.5g • **Chol** 45mg
Sodium 370mg • **Total Carbs** 14g • **Fiber** 1g • **Total Sugar** 3g
Added Sugar 0g • **Protein** 23g • **Total Carbohydrate Choices** 1

NOTES FROM THE TEST KITCHEN

Buying Scallops

In general, most recipes use only one type of scallop—sea scallops. The other scallop varieties, bay and Calico (the latter often mislabeled as bay), are much smaller and often too rare and expensive or very cheap and rubbery.

DRY VERSUS WET SCALLOPS Wet scallops are dipped in preservatives (a solution of water and sodium tripolyphosphate, known as STPP) to extend their shelf life. Unfortunately, these watery preservatives dull the scallops' flavor, ruin their texture, and add lots of extra sodium. Unprocessed, or dry, scallops have much more flavor and a creamy, smooth texture, plus they brown very nicely and don't contribute as much sodium. Dry scallops look ivory or pinkish; wet scallops are bright white.

DISTINGUISHING DRY FROM WET If your scallops are not labeled, you can find out if they are wet or dry with this quick microwave test: Place one scallop on a paper towel–lined plate and microwave for 15 seconds. A dry scallop will exude very little water, but a wet scallop will leave a sizable ring of moisture on the paper towel. (The microwaved scallop can be cooked as is.)

TREATING WET SCALLOPS When you can find only wet scallops, you can hide the off-putting taste of the preservative by soaking the scallops in a solution of 1 quart of cold water, ¼ cup of lemon juice, and 2 tablespoons of salt for 30 minutes. Be sure to pat the scallops very dry after soaking them. Even after this treatment, these scallops will be harder to brown than untreated dry scallops. Note that these scallops will also be higher in sodium.

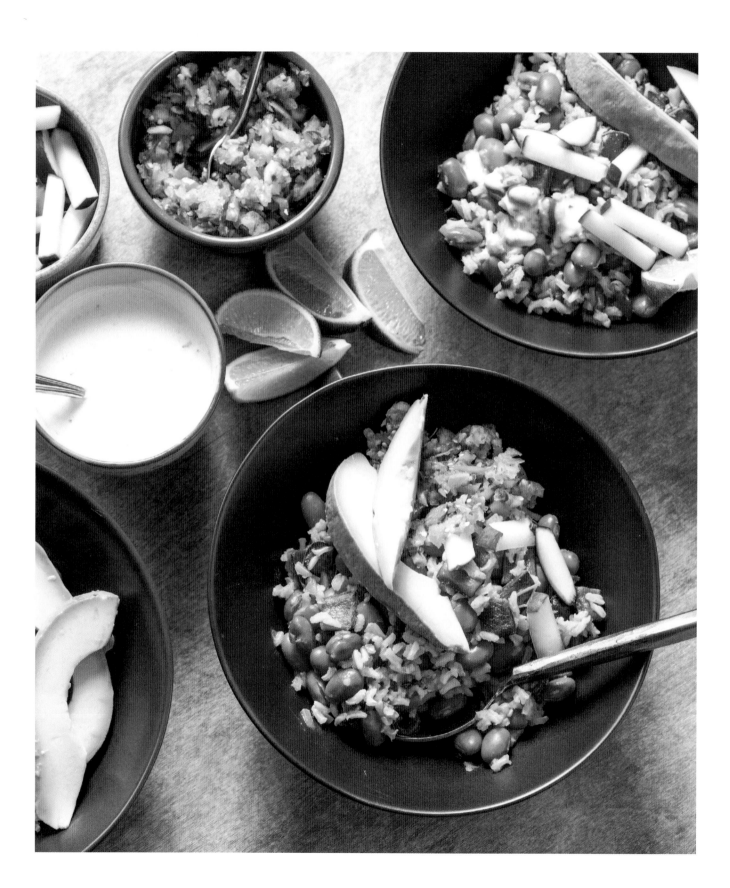

VEGETARIAN MAINS

Photo: Southwestern Brown Rice and Pinto Bean Bowl

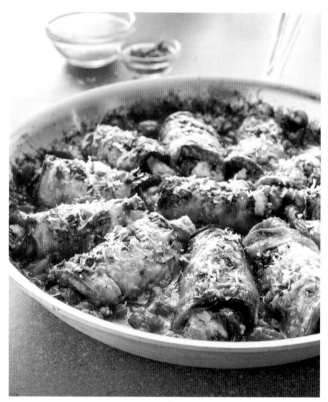

There is no need to salt or fry the eggplant to make these delicious ricotta-filled eggplant rolls.

Eggplant Involtini
SERVES 4

WHY THIS RECIPE WORKS Eggplant involtini is like a lighter and more summery version of eggplant Parmesan, with the flavorful and fiber-rich eggplant planks rolled around a creamy ricotta filling. Traditional recipes require a two-step process of salting the eggplant, and then breading and frying it; we found a way to avoid the work of both the breading and the frying. This method allowed the eggplant's flavor and meaty texture to take center stage in the dish: We could simply bake the eggplant until its excess moisture evaporated. Adding some Pecorino Romano to the ricotta meant we could use less filling without sacrificing flavor. Lastly, we threw together a simple but bright tomato sauce in a skillet, added the eggplant bundles to it, and finished the dish under the broiler so we could skip dirtying a casserole dish. Select shorter, wider eggplants for this recipe.

2 large eggplants (1½ pounds each), peeled and sliced lengthwise into ½-inch-thick planks (about 12 planks), end pieces trimmed to lie flat
6 tablespoons canola oil
Salt and pepper
2 garlic cloves, minced
¼ teaspoon dried oregano
Pinch red pepper flakes
1 (28-ounce) can no-salt-added whole peeled tomatoes, drained, juice reserved, and tomatoes chopped coarse
8 ounces (1 cup) whole-milk ricotta cheese
1 ounce Pecorino Romano cheese, grated (½ cup)
¼ cup plus 1 tablespoon chopped fresh basil
1 tablespoon lemon juice

1. Adjust 1 oven rack to lower-middle position and second rack 8 inches from broiler element. Heat oven to 375 degrees. Line 2 rimmed baking sheets with parchment paper and spray generously with vegetable oil spray. Brush 1 side of eggplant slices with 2½ tablespoons oil, then season with ⅛ teaspoon salt and ¼ teaspoon pepper. Flip slices over and repeat on second side with another 2½ tablespoons oil, ⅛ teaspoon salt, and ¼ teaspoon pepper. Arrange eggplant slices in single layer on prepared sheets. Bake until tender and lightly browned, 30 to 35 minutes, switching and rotating sheets halfway through baking. Let eggplant cool for 5 minutes, then flip each slice over using thin spatula.

2. Heat remaining 1 tablespoon oil in 12-inch broiler-safe skillet over medium-low heat until shimmering. Add garlic, ⅛ teaspoon salt, oregano, and pepper flakes and cook, stirring occasionally, until fragrant, about 30 seconds. Stir in tomatoes and their juice, bring to simmer, and cook until thickened, about 15 minutes. Cover to keep warm.

3. Combine ricotta, ¼ cup Pecorino, ¼ cup basil, and lemon juice in bowl. With widest short side facing you, spoon about 1 tablespoon ricotta mixture over bottom third of each eggplant slice (use slightly more filling for larger slices and slightly less for smaller slices). Gently roll up each eggplant slice and place seam side down in tomato sauce in skillet.

4. Heat broiler. Place skillet over medium heat, bring sauce to simmer, and cook for 5 minutes. Transfer skillet to oven and broil until eggplant is well browned and cheese is heated through, 5 to 10 minutes. Sprinkle with remaining ¼ cup Pecorino and let rest for 5 minutes. Sprinkle with remaining 1 tablespoon basil and serve.

PER SERVING
Cal 430 • **Total Fat** 31g • **Sat Fat** 7g • **Chol** 30mg
Sodium 430mg • **Total Carbs** 28g • **Fiber** 12g • **Total Sugar** 15g
Added Sugar 0g • **Protein** 14g • **Total Carbohydrate Choices** 2

Summer Squash "Spaghetti" with Roasted Cherry Tomato Sauce

SERVES 4

WHY THIS RECIPE WORKS Spiralizing vegetables is all the rage and for good reason: It offers lots of new ways to incorporate vitamin- and fiber-rich vegetables into your diet. Here we paired spiralized yellow squash with an aromatic, deeply flavorful tomato sauce. We halved and roasted cherry tomatoes, which drove off extra moisture and intensified their natural sweetness. Tossing the tomatoes with a bit of tomato paste and olive oil before roasting encouraged caramelization and gave the sauce a rounded flavor. Roasting the spiralized squash and then transferring it to a colander allowed us to get rid of any excess moisture. Seasoned ricotta brought much needed creaminess—and protein—to our dish. You can substitute zucchini for the summer squash, if desired. Our favorite spiralizer model is the Paderno World Cuisine Tri-Blade Plastic Spiral Vegetable Slicer.

- 6 ounces (¾ cup) whole-milk ricotta cheese
- 6 tablespoons chopped fresh basil
  Salt and pepper
- 3 pounds yellow summer squash, trimmed
- 2 pounds cherry tomatoes, halved
- 1 shallot, sliced thin
- 3 tablespoons extra-virgin olive oil
- 5 garlic cloves, minced
- 1 tablespoon minced fresh oregano or 1 teaspoon dried
- 1 tablespoon no-salt-added tomato paste
- ¼ teaspoon red pepper flakes

1. Adjust oven racks to upper-middle and lower-middle positions and heat oven to 375 degrees. Line rimmed baking sheet with aluminum foil. Combine ricotta, 2 tablespoons basil, ⅛ teaspoon salt, and ¼ teaspoon pepper in bowl; set aside for serving. Using spiralizer, cut squash into ⅛-inch-thick noodles, then cut noodles into 12-inch lengths.

2. Toss tomatoes, shallot, 2 tablespoons oil, garlic, oregano, tomato paste, pepper flakes, ⅛ teaspoon salt, and ¼ teaspoon pepper together in bowl. Spread tomato mixture in lined baking sheet and roast, without stirring, on lower rack until tomatoes are softened and skins begin to shrivel, about 30 minutes.

3. Meanwhile, toss squash with ⅛ teaspoon salt and remaining 1 tablespoon oil on second rimmed baking sheet and roast on upper rack until tender, 20 to 25 minutes. Transfer squash to colander and shake to remove any excess liquid; transfer to large serving bowl. (If tomatoes are not finished cooking, cover bowl with aluminum foil to keep warm.)

4. Add roasted tomato mixture and any accumulated juices to bowl with squash and gently toss to combine. Season with ⅛ teaspoon salt and pepper to taste. Dollop individual portions with 3 tablespoons ricotta mixture and sprinkle with remaining ¼ cup basil before serving.

PER SERVING
Cal 280 • **Total Fat** 17g • **Sat Fat** 5g • **Chol** 20mg
Sodium 390mg • **Total Carbs** 24g • **Fiber** 7g • **Total Sugar** 15g
Added Sugar 0g • **Protein** 13g • **Total Carbohydrate Choices** 1.5

MAKING SQUASH NOODLES

Depending on your spiralizer, the amount of trimming required will vary. You can also make noodles using a mandoline or V-slicer fitted with an ⅛-inch julienne attachment. Make sure to position the zucchini or summer squash vertically so the noodles are as long as possible.

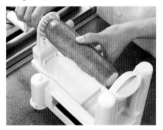

1. Trim yellow summer squash or zucchini so it will fit on prongs and blade.

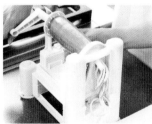

2. Set to ⅛-inch thickness and spiralize by turning crank.

3. Pull noodles straight and cut into 12-inch lengths.

Mexican-Style Spaghetti Squash Casserole

SERVES 4

WHY THIS RECIPE WORKS Spaghetti squash makes a great pasta replacement or a fun side dish, but we wanted to showcase this versatile vegetable's ability to work as a casserole by jazzing it up with bright Mexican flavors. We roasted the oblong yellow squash in the traditional method, simply halving it and roasting until the sweet strands could be easily shredded from the skins with a fork. While the squash roasted, we built a flavorful base for our casserole by blooming minced garlic, smoked paprika, and cumin in the microwave. Incorporating black beans, corn, and tomatoes added protein and heft while reinforcing the Mexican flavors. Scallions lent a subtle oniony flavor without overpowering the sweet squash, as well as a nice pop of color. Minced jalapeño gave just the right amount of gentle heat. We sampled a variety of toppings, but creamy, heart-healthy avocado and mellow, slightly briny queso fresco won us over. We also enjoyed serving our squash with a squeeze of lime juice. For more spice, include the seeds from the jalapeño chile.

1 (2½- to 3-pound) spaghetti squash, halved lengthwise and seeded
3 tablespoons extra-virgin olive oil
 Salt and pepper
2 garlic cloves, minced
½ teaspoon smoked paprika
½ teaspoon ground cumin
1 (15-ounce) can no-salt-added black beans, rinsed
1 cup frozen corn
6 ounces cherry tomatoes, quartered
6 scallions (4 minced, 2 sliced thin)
1 jalapeño chile, stemmed, seeded, and minced
1 avocado, halved, pitted, and cut into ½-inch pieces
2 ounces queso fresco, crumbled (½ cup)
 Lime wedges

1. Adjust oven rack to middle position and heat oven to 375 degrees. Lightly spray 8-inch square baking dish with vegetable oil spray. Brush cut sides of squash with 1 tablespoon oil and sprinkle with ⅛ teaspoon salt and ¼ teaspoon pepper. Place squash cut side down in prepared dish (squash will not sit flat in dish) and roast until just tender, 40 to 45 minutes. Flip squash cut side up and let sit until cool enough to handle, about 20 minutes. Do not turn off oven.

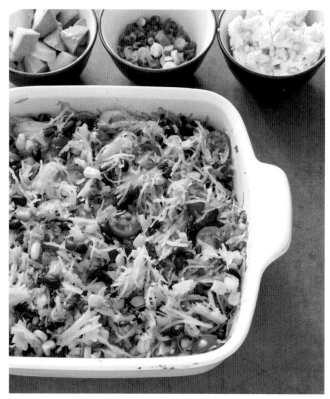

Shredded spaghetti squash makes a great base for a vegetable and bean-packed casserole.

2. Combine remaining 2 tablespoons oil, garlic, paprika, cumin, and ½ teaspoon salt in large bowl and microwave until fragrant, about 30 seconds. Stir in beans, corn, tomatoes, minced scallions, and jalapeño.

3. Using fork, scrape squash into strands in bowl with bean mixture. Stir to combine, then spread mixture evenly in now-empty dish and cover tightly with aluminum foil. Bake until heated through, 20 to 25 minutes. Sprinkle with avocado, queso fresco, and sliced scallions. Serve with lime wedges.

PER SERVING

Cal 400 • **Total Fat** 24g • **Sat Fat** 4.5g • **Chol** 10mg
Sodium 520mg • **Total Carbs** 41g • **Fiber** 11g • **Total Sugar** 9g
Added Sugar 0g • **Protein** 11g • **Total Carbohydrate Choices** 3

Stuffed Eggplant with Bulgur
SERVES 4

WHY THIS RECIPE WORKS Italian eggplants are the perfect size for stuffing, and they take on a rich, creamy texture when baked. Roasting the eggplants prior to stuffing was the key to preventing them from turning watery and tasteless. The slight caramelizing effect of roasting them on a preheated baking sheet added depth of flavor, too. We then drained the eggplants briefly on paper towels (which got rid of excess liquid) before adding the stuffing. Hearty, nutty bulgur, which requires only soaking before it's ready to eat, made a perfect filling base. Pecorino Romano cheese added richness while tomatoes lent bright flavor and a bit of moisture. When shopping, do not confuse bulgur with cracked wheat, which has a much longer cooking time and will not work in this recipe.

- 4 (10-ounce) Italian eggplants, halved lengthwise
- ¼ cup extra-virgin olive oil
-   Salt and pepper
- ½ cup medium-grind bulgur, rinsed
- ¼ cup water
- 1 onion, chopped fine
- 3 garlic cloves, minced
- 2 teaspoons minced fresh oregano or ½ teaspoon dried
- ¼ teaspoon ground cinnamon
- ⅛ teaspoon cayenne pepper
- 1 pound plum tomatoes, cored, seeded, and chopped
- 2 ounces Pecorino Romano cheese, grated (1 cup)
- 2 tablespoons pine nuts, toasted
- ¼ teaspoon grated lemon zest plus 1 tablespoon juice
- 2 tablespoons minced fresh parsley
-   Lemon wedges

PREPARING EGGPLANT FOR STUFFING

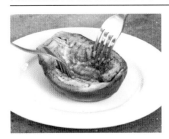

Using 2 forks, gently push flesh to sides of each eggplant half to make room in center for filling.

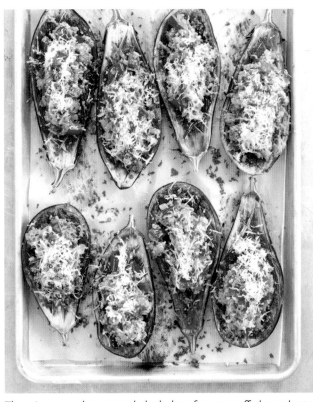

There is no need to precook the bulgur for our stuffed eggplants which also contain fresh tomatoes, pine nuts, and seasonings.

1. Adjust oven racks to upper-middle and lowest positions, place parchment paper–lined rimmed baking sheet on lowest rack, and heat oven to 400 degrees.

2. Score flesh of each eggplant half in 1-inch crosshatch pattern, about 1 inch deep. Brush scored sides of eggplant with 1 tablespoon oil and sprinkle with ⅛ teaspoon salt and ¼ teaspoon pepper. Lay eggplant cut side down on hot sheet and roast until flesh is tender, 40 to 50 minutes. Transfer eggplant cut side down to paper towel–lined baking sheet and let drain. Do not wash rimmed baking sheet.

3. Meanwhile, toss bulgur with water in bowl and let sit until grains are softened and liquid is fully absorbed, 20 to 40 minutes.

4. Heat 1 tablespoon oil in 12-inch skillet over medium heat until shimmering. Add onion and cook until softened, 5 minutes. Stir in garlic, oregano, cinnamon, cayenne, and ¼ teaspoon salt

All About Tofu

Tofu is high in protein as well as iron and calcium. We love it in the test kitchen because it is an ideal canvas for bold or aromatic sauces. It also takes to a wide variety of preparations from stir-frying and sautéing to roasting, braising, grilling, and scrambling. There are many recipes that include tofu throughout this book.

So what is tofu, exactly? Tofu is the result of a process that is similar to cheese making: curds, the result of coagulating soy milk, are set in a mold and pressed to extract as much, or as little, of the liquid whey as desired. Depending on how long the tofu is pressed, and how much coagulant is used, the amount of whey released will vary, creating a range of textures from soft to firm.

Choosing the Right Tofu

Tofu is available in a variety of textures: extra-firm, firm, medium-firm, soft, and silken. We use all these varieties throughout this book, and reaching for the right variety will be key to the success of any given recipe. In general, firmer varieties hold their shape when cooking, while softer varieties do not, so it follows that each type of tofu is best when used in specific ways.

Extra-Firm and Firm Tofu

We prefer extra-firm or firm tofu for stir-fries and noodle dishes as they hold their shape in high heat cooking applications or when tossed with pasta. These two varieties of tofu are also great marinated (they absorb marinade better than softer varieties) or tossed raw into salads.

Medium and Soft Tofu

Medium and soft tofu boast a creamy texture; we love to pan-fry these kinds of tofu, often coated with cornstarch, to achieve a crisp outside, which makes a nice textural contrast to the silky interior. Soft tofu is great scrambled like eggs.

Silken Tofu

Silken tofu has a soft, ultracreamy texture and is often used as a base for smoothies and dips, in desserts such as puddings, or as an egg replacement in vegan baked goods.

Storing Tofu

Tofu is highly perishable, so look for a package with the latest expiration date possible. To store an opened package, cover the tofu with water and store, refrigerated, in a covered container, changing the water daily.

and cook until fragrant, about 30 seconds. Stir in bulgur, tomatoes, ¾ cup Pecorino, pine nuts, and lemon zest and juice and cook until heated through, about 1 minute. Season with pepper to taste.

5. Return eggplant cut side up to rimmed baking sheet. Using 2 forks, gently push eggplant flesh to sides to make room for filling. Mound bulgur mixture into eggplant halves and pack lightly with back of spoon. Sprinkle with remaining ¼ cup Pecorino. Bake on upper-middle rack until cheese is melted, 5 to 10 minutes. Drizzle with remaining 2 tablespoons oil, sprinkle with parsley, and serve with lemon wedges.

PER SERVING

Cal 370 • **Total Fat** 22g • **Sat Fat** 5g • **Chol** 15mg
Sodium 320mg • **Total Carbs** 39g • **Fiber** 12g • **Total Sugar** 14g
Added Sugar 0g • **Protein** 11g • **Total Carbohydrate Choices** 2.5

Farro Bowl with Tofu, Mushrooms, and Spinach
SERVES 4

WHY THIS RECIPE WORKS Hearty, nutty farro is traditionally associated with Italy, but it also adapts well to bold Asian ingredients, as in this bowl featuring crispy seared tofu and a simple miso-ginger sauce. We found through testing that farro is best prepared using a pasta cooking method—boiled until tender and drained. Neutral-tasting tofu seemed like an easy way to incorporate a great source of plant-based protein into the bowl. Next came vegetables. Mushrooms were a must—we chopped some cremini and tossed them into the skillet after cooking the crispy tofu. They tasted meaty and rich, and a hit of sherry brought in some nutty flavor. To incorporate some greenery, we looked to baby spinach. After cooking the mushrooms, we cleared out the skillet, heated up some oil, and began wilting the quick-cooking spinach in batches. These tender leaves cooked down in no time and brought some colorful nutrients to the dish. To assemble the bowls, we piled the farro high with crisp tofu, earthy cremini, and spinach. A sprinkling of scallions made for a fresh finish, but the winning touch came with the sauce flavored with red miso, sesame oil, sherry vinegar, and ginger. With that, we had a soul-satisfying bowl worth craving. We prefer the flavor and texture of whole farro; pearled farro can be used, but the texture may be softer. Do not use quick-cooking or presteamed farro (read the ingredient list on the package to determine this) in this recipe. The cooking time for farro can vary greatly among different brands, so we recommend beginning to check for doneness after 10 minutes.

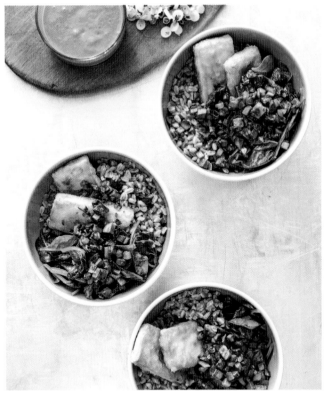

We swapped out rice for farro in this protein-packed bowl featuring tofu, earthy spinach, and cremini mushrooms.

2 tablespoons mayonnaise
5 teaspoons toasted sesame oil
1 tablespoon red miso
2 teaspoons sherry vinegar
1 teaspoon grated fresh ginger
1 cup whole farro
  Salt
14 ounces firm tofu
3 tablespoons cornstarch
¼ cup canola oil
10 ounces cremini mushrooms, trimmed and chopped coarse
2 tablespoons dry sherry
10 ounces (10 cups) baby spinach
2 scallions, sliced thin

1. Whisk mayonnaise, 1 tablespoon sesame oil, miso, 1 tablespoon water, 1 teaspoon vinegar, and ginger together in small bowl; set sauce aside for serving.

2. Bring 4 quarts water to boil in large pot. Add farro and 1 teaspoon salt and cook until grains are tender with slight chew, 15 to 30 minutes. Drain farro well and return to now-empty pot. Stir in remaining 2 teaspoons sesame oil and remaining 1 teaspoon vinegar and cover to keep warm.

3. Meanwhile, cut tofu crosswise into 8 equal slabs, arrange over paper towel–lined baking sheet, and let drain for 20 minutes. Gently press dry with paper towels.

4. Spread cornstarch in shallow dish. Coat tofu thoroughly in cornstarch, pressing gently to adhere; transfer to plate. Heat 2 tablespoons canola oil in 12-inch nonstick skillet over medium-high heat until just smoking. Add tofu and cook until crisp and browned, about 4 minutes per side. Transfer to paper towel–lined plate and tent with aluminum foil. Wipe skillet clean with paper towels.

5. Heat 1 tablespoon canola oil in now-empty skillet over medium-high heat until shimmering. Add mushrooms and ⅛ teaspoon salt and cook until beginning to brown, 5 to 8 minutes. Stir in sherry and cook, scraping up any browned bits, until skillet is nearly dry, about 1 minute; transfer to bowl.

6. Heat remaining 1 tablespoon canola oil in again-empty skillet over medium-high heat until shimmering. Add spinach, 1 handful at a time, and cook until just wilted, about 1 minute. Divide farro among individual serving bowls, then top with tofu, mushrooms, and spinach. Drizzle with miso-ginger sauce, sprinkle with scallions, and serve.

PER SERVING

Cal 530 • **Total Fat** 31g • **Sat Fat** 3g • **Chol** 5mg
Sodium 420mg • **Total Carbs** 48g • **Fiber** 7g • **Total Sugar** 5g
Added Sugar 0g • **Protein** 18g • **Total Carbohydrate Choices** 3

Southwestern Brown Rice and Pinto Bean Bowl
SERVES 6

WHY THIS RECIPE WORKS The sustaining combination of rice and beans is a staple in many cuisines. We wanted to make a simple hearty and nutritious dish with a bold Latin American profile. We preferred the texture and robust flavor of brown rice, not to mention that it is higher in fiber than white rice. After sautéing onion and poblano pepper, we added zesty aromatics and cooked them until fragrant. We then stirred in the rice and broth and simmered until the rice was tender. Canned pinto beans instead of dried beans simplified the dish; and to keep them from getting mushy we stirred them in partway through cooking the rice. A fresh and flavorful tomatillo salsa and a spicy crema added a welcomed fresh counterpart to this rich rice-and-beans dish.

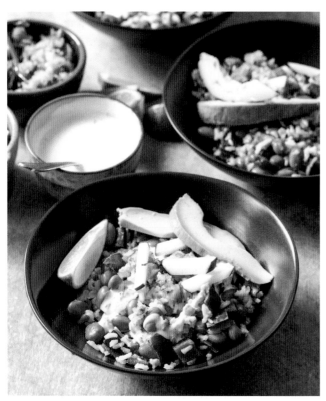

The key to this Southwestern bowl is a spice- and aromatic-infused brown rice base plus salsa, crema, and vegetables.

TOMATILLO SALSA

    1 pound tomatillos, husks and stems removed,
      rinsed, dried, and halved
    1 jalapeño chile, stemmed, seeded, and chopped
 ¼ cup fresh cilantro leaves
    1 garlic clove, peeled
    1 tablespoon extra-virgin olive oil
 ¼ teaspoon salt

CHIPOTLE CREMA

 ¼ cup mayonnaise
 ¼ cup plain low-fat yogurt
    1 tablespoon lime juice, plus lime wedges for serving
    2 teaspoons minced canned chipotle chile in adobo sauce
    1 garlic clove, minced

RICE

    1 tablespoon extra-virgin olive oil
    3 poblano chiles, stemmed, seeded,
      and cut into ½-inch pieces
    1 onion, chopped fine
    4 garlic cloves, minced
 2½ teaspoons ground cumin
 1½ teaspoons ground coriander
 ⅛ teaspoon cayenne pepper
    1 cup long-grain brown rice, rinsed
 3¼ cups low-sodium vegetable broth
 ½ teaspoon salt
    2 (15-ounce) cans no-salt-added pinto beans, rinsed
 10 radishes, trimmed and cut into matchsticks
    1 avocado, halved, pitted, and sliced ½-inch-thick

1. FOR THE TOMATILLO SALSA Pulse tomatillos, jalapeño, cilantro, and garlic in food processor until chopped, about 8 pulses. Transfer to fine-mesh strainer set over bowl and let drain for 10 minutes, discard liquid. Stir in oil and salt and set aside for serving.

2. FOR THE CHIPOTLE CREMA Combine mayonnaise, yogurt, lime juice, chipotle, and garlic in small bowl; set aside for serving.

3. FOR THE RICE Heat oil in 12-inch nonstick skillet over medium-high heat until shimmering. Add poblanos and onion and cook until softened and lightly browned, 5 to 7 minutes. Stir in minced garlic, cumin, coriander, and cayenne and cook until fragrant, about 30 seconds.

4. Stir in rice, broth, and ½ teaspoon salt and bring to simmer. Cover, reduce heat to medium-low, and cook, stirring occasionally, for 25 minutes. Stir in beans and cook, covered, until liquid is absorbed and rice is tender, 20 to 25 minutes.

5. Divide rice mixture among individual serving bowls, then top with salsa, crema, radishes, and avocado. Serve with lime wedges.

PER SERVING

Cal 410 • **Total Fat** 20g • **Sat Fat** 2.5g • **Chol** 5mg
Sodium 460mg • **Total Carbs** 53g • **Fiber** 13g • **Total Sugar** 8g
Added Sugar 0g • **Protein** 12g • **Total Carbohydrate Choices** 3.5

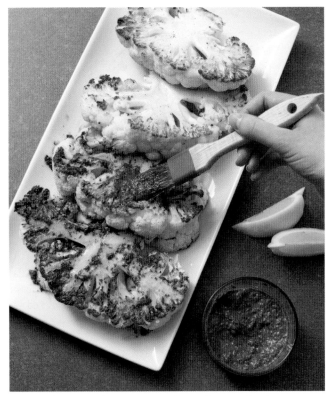

For cauliflower steaks that are tender and caramelized, we roast them first covered and then uncovered.

Cauliflower Steaks with Chimichurri Sauce

SERVES 4

WHY THIS RECIPE WORKS Cauliflower is a nutritional hero: It's full of fiber and a rich source of vitamins B6 and C and potassium. So making the most of this vegetable is a good thing for everyone. Enter cauliflower steaks. When you roast thick planks of cauliflower, they develop a meaty texture and become nutty, sweet, and caramelized. Many recipes, however, are fussy, involving transitions between stovetop and oven. We wanted a simpler method that produced four perfectly cooked cauliflower steaks simultaneously, so we opted for a rimmed baking sheet and a scorching oven. Steaming the cauliflower briefly under foil followed by high-heat uncovered roasting produced well-caramelized steaks with tender interiors. To elevate the cauliflower to centerpiece status, we paired it with a vibrant Chimichurri Sauce. We brushed the hot steaks with the bright sauce so they'd soak up its robust flavor. Look for fresh, firm, bright white heads of cauliflower that feel heavy for their size and are free of blemishes or soft spots; florets are more likely to separate from older heads of cauliflower.

2 heads cauliflower (2 pounds each)
¼ cup extra-virgin olive oil
    Salt and pepper
1 recipe Chimichurri (page 207)
    Lemon wedges

1. Adjust oven rack to lowest position and heat oven to 500 degrees. Working with 1 head cauliflower at a time, discard outer leaves and trim stem flush with bottom florets. Halve cauliflower lengthwise through core. Cut one 1½-inch-thick slab lengthwise from each half, trimming any florets not connected to core. Repeat with remaining cauliflower. (You should have 4 steaks; reserve remaining cauliflower for another use.)

2. Place steaks on rimmed baking sheet and drizzle with 2 tablespoons oil. Sprinkle with pinch salt and ⅛ teaspoon pepper and rub to distribute. Flip steaks and repeat.

3. Cover sheet tightly with foil and roast for 5 minutes. Remove foil and continue to roast until bottoms of steaks are well browned, 8 to 10 minutes. Gently flip and continue to roast until cauliflower is tender and second sides are well browned, 6 to 8 minutes.

4. Transfer steaks to serving platter and brush tops evenly with ¼ cup chimichurri. Serve with lemon wedges and remaining chimichurri.

PER SERVING
Cal 370 • **Total Fat** 29g • **Sat Fat** 4.5g • **Chol** 0mg
Sodium 300mg • **Total Carbs** 24g • **Fiber** 10g • **Total Sugar** 9g
Added Sugar 0g • **Protein** 9g • **Total Carbohydrate Choices** 1.5

CUTTING CAULIFLOWER STEAKS

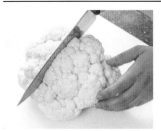 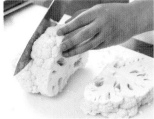

1. Halve the cauliflower lengthwise through the core.

2. Cut one 1½-inch-thick slab from each cauliflower half.

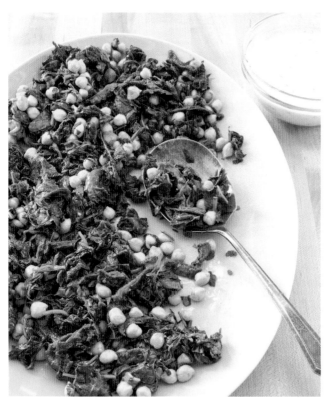

This dish puts spinach front and center and builds layers of flavor that will have your family reaching for seconds.

Sautéed Spinach with Chickpeas and Garlicky Yogurt

SERVES 4

WHY THIS RECIPE WORKS It is good to have a hearty spinach-based main course in your repertoire given that this leafy green is so nutrient dense. Here we turned to convenient and tender baby spinach and added hearty protein-rich chickpeas and an aromatic yogurt sauce. The trickiest part of cooking spinach is getting it tender but not mushy, so we knew we'd need a strategy for ridding the spinach of excess liquid. Parcooking it in the microwave and then draining it turned out to be the best solution. We pressed the microwaved spinach in a colander to eliminate water, coarsely chopped it, and pressed it again. Then all we had to do was quickly sauté it. As for seasonings, we started by toasting a good amount of sliced garlic in oil, then added coriander and turmeric to the

skillet to bloom. Canned chickpeas bulked up this dish without adding any more work, and thinly sliced sun-dried tomatoes contributed another layer of bright flavor. For the final touch to this dish, we put together a quick garlicky yogurt sauce with a dash of fresh mint for brightness.

- 1 cup plain low-fat yogurt
- 2 tablespoons chopped fresh mint
- 5 garlic cloves (4 sliced thin, 1 minced)
- 18 ounces (18 cups) baby spinach
- 2 tablespoons extra-virgin olive oil
- 1 teaspoon ground coriander
- 1 teaspoon ground turmeric
- ¼ teaspoon grated lemon zest
- ⅛ teaspoon red pepper flakes
- 2 (15-ounce) cans no-salt-added chickpeas, rinsed
- ½ cup oil-packed sun-dried tomatoes, sliced thin
  Salt and pepper

1. Combine yogurt, mint, and minced garlic in bowl; cover and refrigerate sauce until ready to serve.

2. Microwave spinach and ¼ cup water in covered bowl until spinach is wilted and has reduced in volume by half, 3 to 4 minutes. Remove bowl from microwave and keep covered for 1 minute. Carefully transfer spinach to colander and, using back of rubber spatula, gently press spinach to release excess liquid. Transfer spinach to cutting board and chop coarsely. Return spinach to colander and press again.

3. Cook 1 tablespoon oil and sliced garlic in 12-inch skillet over medium heat, stirring constantly, until garlic is light golden brown and beginning to sizzle, 3 to 6 minutes. Stir in coriander, turmeric, lemon zest, and pepper flakes and cook until fragrant, about 30 seconds. Stir in chickpeas, tomatoes, and 2 tablespoons water. Cook, stirring occasionally, until water evaporates and tomatoes are softened, 1 to 2 minutes.

4. Stir in spinach and ¼ teaspoon salt and cook until uniformly wilted and glossy green, about 2 minutes. Transfer spinach mixture to serving platter, drizzle with remaining 1 tablespoon oil, and season with pepper to taste. Serve with yogurt sauce.

PER SERVING

Cal 310 • **Total Fat** 11g • **Sat Fat** 2g • **Chol** 5mg
Sodium 360mg • **Total Carbs** 37g • **Fiber** 10g • **Total Sugar** 5g
Added Sugar 0g • **Protein** 15g • **Total Carbohydrate Choices** 2.5

Tunisian-Style Grilled Vegetables with Couscous and Eggs

SERVES 6

WHY THIS RECIPE WORKS For our take on the robustly flavored grilled vegetable salad known as *mechouia*, we started by prepping the vegetables for the grill. To maximize surface area for flavorful charring, we halved eggplant, zucchini, and plum tomatoes lengthwise and stemmed and flattened bell peppers. We also scored the eggplant and zucchini so they would release their excess moisture as they cooked.

DRESSING

- 2 teaspoons coriander seeds
- 1½ teaspoons caraway seeds
- 1 teaspoon cumin seeds
- 5 tablespoons extra-virgin olive oil
- ½ teaspoon paprika
- ⅛ teaspoon cayenne pepper
- 3 garlic cloves, minced
- ¼ cup chopped fresh parsley
- ¼ cup chopped fresh cilantro
- 2 tablespoons chopped fresh mint
- 1 teaspoon grated lemon zest plus 2 tablespoons juice
  Salt

COUSCOUS AND VEGETABLES

- 1 tablespoon extra-virgin olive oil
- 1 cup whole-wheat couscous
- ¾ cup water
- ¾ cup low-sodium vegetable broth
  Salt and pepper
- 2 red or green bell peppers, tops and bottoms trimmed, stemmed and seeded, and peppers flattened
- 1 small eggplant, halved lengthwise and scored on cut sides
- 1 zucchini (8 to 10 ounces), halved lengthwise and scored on cut sides
- 4 plum tomatoes, cored and halved lengthwise
- 2 shallots, unpeeled
- 6 hard-cooked eggs, peeled and halved

1. FOR THE DRESSING Grind coriander seeds, caraway seeds, and cumin seeds in spice grinder until finely ground. Whisk ground spices, oil, paprika, and cayenne together in bowl. Reserve 3 tablespoons spiced oil mixture for brushing vegetables before grilling. Heat remaining spiced oil and garlic in 8-inch skillet over low heat, stirring occasionally, until fragrant and small bubbles appear, 8 to 10 minutes. Transfer to large bowl, let cool for 10 minutes, then whisk in parsley, cilantro, mint, lemon zest and juice, and ¼ teaspoon salt; set aside for serving.

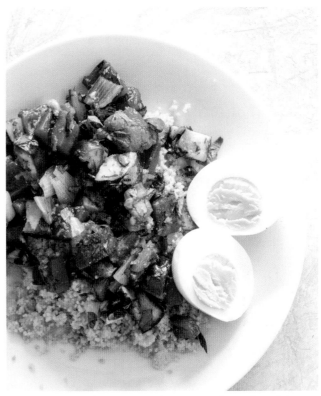

Our Tunisian salad relies on multiple spices for its flavorful dressing that enhances a variety of grilled vegetables.

2. FOR THE COUSCOUS AND VEGETABLES Heat oil in saucepan over medium heat until shimmering. Add couscous and toast, stirring often, until a few grains begin to brown, about 3 minutes. Transfer couscous to large bowl. Add water, broth, and pinch salt to saucepan and bring to boil. Once boiling, immediately pour broth mixture over couscous, cover tightly with plastic wrap, and let sit until grains are tender, about 12 minutes. Fluff gently with fork to combine. Season with pepper to taste.

3. Meanwhile, brush interior of bell peppers and cut sides of eggplant, zucchini, and tomatoes with reserved oil mixture and sprinkle with ¼ teaspoon salt.

4A. FOR A CHARCOAL GRILL Open bottom vent completely. Light large chimney starter three-quarters filled with charcoal briquettes (4½ quarts). When top coals are partially covered with ash, pour evenly over grill. Set cooking grate in place, cover, and open lid vent completely. Heat grill until hot, about 5 minutes.

4B. FOR A GAS GRILL Turn all burners to high, cover, and heat grill until hot, about 15 minutes. Turn all burners to medium-high.

5. Clean and oil cooking grate. Place bell peppers, eggplant, zucchini, tomatoes, and shallots cut side down on grill. Cook (covered if using gas), turning as needed, until tender and slightly charred, 8 to 16 minutes. Transfer eggplant, zucchini, tomatoes, and shallots to baking sheet as they finish cooking; place bell peppers in bowl, cover with plastic wrap, and let steam to loosen skins.

6. Let vegetables cool slightly. Peel bell peppers, tomatoes, and shallots. Chop all vegetables into ½-inch pieces, then toss gently with dressing in bowl. Season with pepper to taste. Serve vegetables and hard-cooked eggs over couscous.

PER SERVING

Cal 380 • **Total Fat** 20g • **Sat Fat** 3.5g • **Chol** 185mg
Sodium 300mg • **Total Carbs** 37g • **Fiber** 9g • **Total Sugar** 10g
Added Sugar 0g • **Protein** 13g • **Total Carbohydrate Choices** 2.5

Stir-Fried Tofu with Shiitakes and Green Beans
SERVES 4

WHY THIS RECIPE WORKS There are many reasons to love stir-fries: They're quick, healthful, and open to endless variations. We wanted to develop a classic stir-fry that captured our infatuation with the dish, so we refreshed ourselves on the wisdom we've collected over the years. For a cooking vessel, we use a nonstick skillet (a wok is designed for a pit-style stove). Patience is on our ingredient list; despite the name, if you overstir your stir-fry, you'll lose that coveted sear. And the process is fast; you must have your ingredients ready before you start cooking. We paired sturdy green beans and meaty, mineral-rich shiitake mushrooms with cornstarch-coated tofu, which developed a slightly crunchy sheath. Although we often cook the vegetables in batches, here we were able to stir-fry them at the same time; the moisture released from the mushrooms nicely steamed the green beans. For a balanced brown sauce, we combined soy sauce, sesame oil, rice vinegar, and pepper flakes, and we thickened it with cornstarch.

SAUCE
- ¾ cup low-sodium vegetable broth
- 3 tablespoons low-sodium soy sauce
- 2 tablespoons rice vinegar
- 2 teaspoons cornstarch
- 1 tablespoon toasted sesame oil
- ⅛ teaspoon red pepper flakes

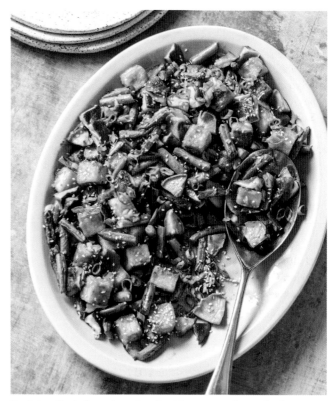

Draining the tofu and coating it with cornstarch are the keys to a stir-fry where the tofu is crispy on the outside and creamy inside.

STIR-FRY
- 14 ounces extra-firm tofu, cut into ¾-inch pieces
- 3 tablespoons cornstarch
- 3 tablespoons canola oil
- 2 scallions, white and green parts separated and sliced thin on bias
- 3 garlic cloves, minced
- 1 tablespoon grated fresh ginger
- 12 ounces green beans, trimmed and cut on bias into 1-inch lengths
- 12 ounces shiitake mushrooms, stemmed and quartered
- 1 tablespoon toasted sesame seeds (optional)

1. FOR THE SAUCE Whisk all ingredients together in bowl.

2. FOR THE STIR-FRY Spread tofu on paper towel–lined baking sheet and let drain for 20 minutes. Gently pat dry with paper towels. Toss drained tofu with cornstarch in bowl.

3. Combine 1 teaspoon oil, scallion whites, garlic, and ginger in bowl. Heat 2 tablespoons oil in 12-inch nonstick skillet over high heat until shimmering. Add tofu and cook, turning as needed, until crisp and well browned on all sides, 12 to 15 minutes; transfer to paper towel–lined plate.

4. Add remaining 2 teaspoons oil to now-empty skillet and heat over medium-high heat until shimmering. Add green beans and mushrooms, cover, and cook until mushrooms release their liquid and green beans are bright green and beginning to soften, 4 to 5 minutes. Uncover and continue to cook until vegetables are spotty brown, about 3 minutes.

5. Push vegetables to sides of skillet. Add garlic mixture to center and cook, mashing mixture into skillet, until fragrant, about 30 seconds. Stir garlic mixture into vegetables, then stir in tofu. Whisk sauce to recombine, then add to skillet and cook, stirring constantly, until sauce is thickened, about 30 seconds. Transfer to serving platter and sprinkle with scallion greens and sesame seeds, if using. Serve.

PER SERVING

Cal 310 • **Total Fat** 21g • **Sat Fat** 2g • **Chol** 0mg
Sodium 470mg • **Total Carbs** 19g • **Fiber** 4g • **Total Sugar** 5g
Added Sugar 0g • **Protein** 14g • **Total Carbohydrate Choices** 1.5

Indian-Style Vegetable Curry
SERVES 6

WHY THIS RECIPE WORKS Vegetable curries are a great hearty choice for a vegetarian meal. Filled with bold flavors and a good variety of vegetables, they can be healthy, satisfying, and delicious—as long as the vegetables are well cooked and the flavors are balanced. To nail the bold flavor we turned to a few pantry-friendly items like curry powder, garam masala, garlic, and tomato paste while fresh ginger and a serrano chile pumped up the flavor even more. A combination of sweet potatoes, canned diced tomatoes, eggplant, green beans, and chickpeas guaranteed everyone would walk away from the table satiated. We started by cooking the sweet potatoes since they would take the longest to become tender, followed by the eggplant and green beans. We also found that 20 minutes of simmering eliminated any tinny taste in the tomatoes and allowed the chickpeas to turn from crumbly to creamy. Finishing the dish with a generous handful of cilantro and a dollop of Greek yogurt helped to add brightness and brought our flavors into balance. You can adjust the spice level of this dish by either including less of the serrano chile or adding its seeds.

1 (14.5-ounce) can no-salt-added diced tomatoes
3 tablespoons canola oil
4 teaspoons curry powder
1½ teaspoons garam masala
2 onions, chopped fine

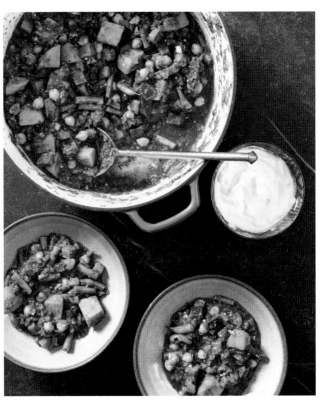

This curry is a satisfying combination of vitamin-rich sweet potatoes, meaty eggplant, earthy green beans, and chickpeas.

12 ounces sweet potatoes, peeled and cut into 1-inch pieces
Salt and pepper
3 garlic cloves, minced
1 serrano chile, stemmed, seeded, and minced
1 tablespoon grated fresh ginger
1 tablespoon no-salt-added tomato paste
1 pound eggplant, cut into ½-inch pieces
8 ounces green beans, trimmed and cut into 1-inch lengths
2 cups water
1 (15-ounce) can no-salt-added chickpeas, rinsed
¼ cup minced fresh cilantro
⅔ cup 2 percent Greek yogurt

1. Pulse tomatoes with their juice in food processor until nearly smooth, with some ¼-inch pieces visible, about 3 pulses.

2. Heat oil in Dutch oven over medium heat until shimmering. Add curry powder and garam masala and cook until fragrant, about 10 seconds. Add onions, sweet potatoes, and ¼ teaspoon salt and cook, stirring occasionally, until onions are browned and sweet potatoes are golden brown at edges, about 10 minutes.

3. Stir in garlic, chile, ginger, and tomato paste and cook until fragrant, about 30 seconds. Add eggplant and green beans and cook, stirring constantly, until vegetables are coated with spices, about 2 minutes.

4. Gradually stir in water, scraping up any browned bits. Stir in tomatoes and chickpeas and bring to simmer. Cover, reduce heat to low, and cook until vegetables are tender, 20 to 25 minutes. Off heat, stir in cilantro and ½ teaspoon salt and season with pepper to taste. Serve with yogurt.

PER SERVING

Cal 240 • **Total Fat** 8g • **Sat Fat** 1g • **Chol** 0mg
Sodium 380mg • **Total Carbs** 34g • **Fiber** 9g • **Total Sugar** 12g
Added Sugar 0g • **Protein** 8g • **Total Carbohydrate Choices** 2

Curried Tempeh with Cauliflower and Peas
SERVES 6

WHY THIS RECIPE WORKS With its deep, intense flavors, curry makes a perfect pairing for strong-tasting tempeh. To create truly complex curry flavor, we started by toasting curry powder and garam masala in oil. A serrano chile delivered the right combination of flavor and spice. Blooming glutamate-rich tomato paste with our seasonings added a meaty, savory element to the curry. Canned diced tomatoes pulsed in a food processor formed the base of the sauce. Simmering the tempeh in the curry for 15 minutes helped to infuse it with the curry's flavor. To round out our curry, we added cauliflower, simmering it in the sauce until tender, and convenient frozen peas. Finishing our tempeh curry with a dash of light coconut milk imparted a little extra richness while still staying healthy. You can adjust the spice level of this dish by either including less of the serrano chile or adding its seeds.

1 (14.5-ounce) no-salt-added can diced tomatoes
¼ cup canola oil
2 tablespoons curry powder
1½ teaspoons garam masala
2 onions, chopped fine
   Salt and pepper
3 garlic cloves, minced
1 tablespoon grated fresh ginger
1 serrano chile, stemmed, seeded, and minced
1 tablespoon no-salt-added tomato paste
½ head cauliflower (1 pound), cored and cut into 1-inch florets
8 ounces tempeh, cut into 1-inch pieces
1¼ cups water

1 cup frozen peas
¼ cup light coconut milk
2 tablespoons minced fresh cilantro
   Lime wedges

1. Pulse diced tomatoes with their juice in food processor until nearly smooth, with some ¼-inch pieces visible, about 3 pulses.

2. Heat oil in Dutch oven over medium-high heat until shimmering. Add curry powder and garam masala and cook until fragrant, about 10 seconds. Add onions and ¼ teaspoon salt and cook, stirring occasionally, until softened and browned, about 10 minutes.

3. Reduce heat to medium. Stir in garlic, ginger, serrano, and tomato paste and cook until fragrant, about 30 seconds. Add cauliflower and tempeh and cook, stirring constantly, until florets are coated with spices, about 2 minutes.

4. Gradually stir in water, scraping up any browned bits. Stir in tomatoes and bring to simmer. Cover, reduce heat to low, and cook until vegetables are tender, 10 to 15 minutes.

5. Stir in peas, coconut milk, and ¾ teaspoon salt and cook until heated through, 1 to 2 minutes. Off heat, stir in cilantro and season with pepper to taste. Serve with lime wedges.

PER SERVING

Cal 240 • **Total Fat** 15g • **Sat Fat** 2.5g • **Chol** 0mg
Sodium 430mg • **Total Carbs** 19g • **Fiber** 6g • **Total Sugar** 6g
Added Sugar 0g • **Protein** 12g • **Total Carbohydrate Choices** 1.5

NOTES FROM THE TEST KITCHEN

Getting to Know Tempeh

While tofu has hit the mainstream, tempeh might not be as familiar. Tempeh is made by fermenting cooked soybeans, then forming the mixture into a firm, dense cake. Some versions also contain beans, grains, and flavorings. It serves as a good meat substitute and is a mainstay of many vegetarian diets—it's particularly popular in Southeast Asia. It has a strong nutty flavor, but it also will absorb flavors easily. And because it's better than tofu at holding its shape when cooked, it's a versatile choice for many dishes, from sandwiches and tacos to curry. It's also a healthy choice, since it's high in protein, cholesterol-free, and contains many essential vitamins and minerals. Tempeh is sold refrigerated in most supermarkets and can be found with different grain and flavoring combinations. We use five-grain tempeh in our recipes, but any plain variety will work. If you are gluten-free, be sure to look for a gluten-free brand of tempeh.

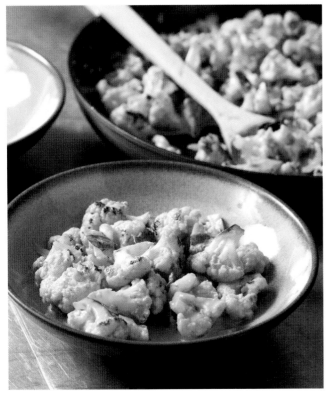

A sauce that combines coconut milk and store-bought red curry paste makes it easy to whip up this nutritious cauliflower curry.

Thai-Style Red Curry with Cauliflower
SERVES 4

WHY THIS RECIPE WORKS Thai cooking is all about balance, so when we set out to make a red curry with cauliflower, we knew that developing the deep, nutty flavor of the cauliflower was important. Typically, we turn to the oven to achieve this, but for a curry dish that could otherwise be on the table in about 15 minutes, this felt like an unnecessary step. Instead, we confined ourselves to the skillet. Achieving tender, golden-brown cauliflower without scorching turned out to be a two-step process that took just about 10 minutes. First, we cooked the cauliflower along with water in a covered skillet for about 5 minutes, steaming it until it was just tender, then we uncovered the skillet to finish the cooking in canola oil. This final uncovered cooking time drove off any remaining water left in the skillet, tenderized the cauliflower further, and allowed it to develop deep golden browning without any charring. A few minutes in the skillet at the very end of cooking was all the red curry sauce needed to bloom its flavors and thicken enough to coat the cauliflower nicely.

1 (13.5-ounce) can light coconut milk
1 tablespoon fish sauce
1 teaspoon grated lime zest plus 1 tablespoon juice
2 teaspoons Thai red curry paste
⅛ teaspoon red pepper flakes
2 tablespoons plus 1 teaspoon canola oil
2 garlic cloves, minced
1 teaspoon grated fresh ginger
1 large head cauliflower (3 pounds), cored and cut into ¾-inch florets
¼ cup fresh basil leaves, torn into rough ½-inch pieces

1. Whisk coconut milk, fish sauce, lime zest and juice, curry paste, and pepper flakes together in bowl. In separate bowl, combine 1 teaspoon oil, garlic, and ginger.

2. Heat remaining 2 tablespoons oil in 12-inch nonstick skillet over high heat until shimmering. Add cauliflower and ¼ cup water, cover, and cook until cauliflower is just tender and translucent, about 5 minutes. Uncover and continue to cook, stirring occasionally, until liquid is evaporated and cauliflower is tender and well browned, 8 to 10 minutes.

3. Push cauliflower to sides of skillet. Add garlic mixture and cook, mashing mixture into skillet, until fragrant, about 30 seconds. Stir garlic mixture into cauliflower and reduce heat to medium-high. Whisk coconut milk mixture to recombine, add to skillet, and simmer until slightly thickened, about 4 minutes. Off heat, stir in basil. Serve.

PER SERVING

Cal 200 • Total Fat 13g • Sat Fat 4g • Chol 0mg
Sodium 380mg • Total Carbs 20g • Fiber 7g • Total Sugar 7g
Added Sugar 0g • Protein 7g • Total Carbohydrate Choices 1

VARIATION
Thai-Style Red Curry with Bell Peppers and Tofu

Omit cauliflower, water, and salt. Toss 14 ounces extra-firm tofu, pressed dry with paper towels and cut into ¾-inch cubes, with ⅓ cup cornstarch; transfer tofu to strainer and shake gently to remove excess cornstarch. Add coated tofu to heated oil in step 2 and cook until crisp and browned on all sides, 10 to 15 minutes; transfer tofu to clean bowl. Add 2 red bell peppers, cut into 2-inch-long matchsticks, to oil left in skillet and cook until crisp-tender, about 2 minutes, before adding garlic mixture. Return tofu to skillet with sauce.

PER SERVING

Cal 260 • Total Fat 17g • Sat Fat 4.5g • Chol 0mg
Sodium 280mg • Total Carbs 14g • Fiber 3g • Total Sugar 3g
Added Sugar 0g • Protein 11g • Total Carbohydrate Choices 1

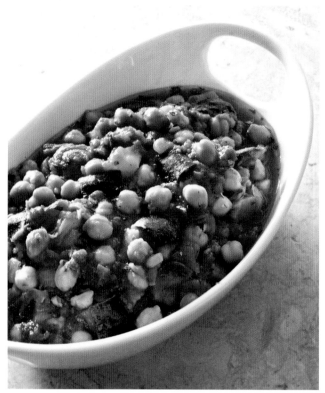

After building a flavor base on the stovetop, we add the eggplant, tomatoes, and chickpeas and braise them in the oven.

Stewed Chickpeas with Eggplant and Tomatoes
SERVES 6

WHY THIS RECIPE WORKS There is a reason so many vegetarian dishes feature eggplant: It takes well to many cooking mediums and pairs well with beans, grains, and tomatoes. Here fresh eggplant and canned chickpeas create a hearty stew with deep savory flavor. The soft and creamy texture of the eggplant is complemented by the firm-tender chickpeas, and chopped canned tomatoes give the dish a rustic texture and tomatoey backbone. We tested cooking methods and times and landed on a combination stovetop-oven method that worked to create the texture we were after. To jump-start the cooking process, we sautéed onions, bell pepper, garlic, oregano, and bay leaves to create an aromatic base. We added our chickpeas, tomatoes, and eggplant (cutting it into 1-inch pieces ensured that it softened but didn't completely break down) and transferred the pot to the oven. Baking the mixture uncovered concentrated the flavors and allowed any unwanted liquid to evaporate, eliminating the need to pretreat the eggplant. Stirring a couple of times during cooking ensured that the top layer didn't dry out. Some fresh oregano, added at the end, gave

this dish a welcome burst of herbaceous flavor. We were happy to find that this versatile dish tasted equally good when served warm or at room temperature.

¼ cup extra-virgin olive oil
2 onions, chopped
1 green bell pepper, stemmed, seeded, and chopped fine
Salt and pepper
3 garlic cloves, minced
1 tablespoon minced fresh oregano or 1 teaspoon dried
2 bay leaves
1 pound eggplant, cut into 1-inch pieces
1 (28-ounce) can no-salt-added whole peeled tomatoes, drained with juice reserved, chopped coarse
2 (15-ounce) cans no-salt-added chickpeas, drained with 1 cup liquid reserved

1. Adjust oven rack to lower-middle position and heat oven to 400 degrees. Heat oil in Dutch oven over medium heat until shimmering. Add onions, bell pepper, ½ teaspoon salt, and ¼ teaspoon pepper and cook until softened, about 5 minutes. Stir in garlic, 1 teaspoon oregano, and bay leaves and cook until fragrant, about 30 seconds.

2. Stir in eggplant, tomatoes and reserved juice, and chickpeas and reserved liquid and bring to boil. Transfer pot to oven and cook, uncovered, until eggplant is very tender, 45 to 60 minutes, stirring twice during cooking.

3. Discard bay leaves. Stir in remaining 2 teaspoons oregano and season with pepper to taste. Serve.

PER SERVING
Cal 270 • **Total Fat** 10g • **Sat Fat** 1.5g • **Chol** 0mg
Sodium 470mg • **Total Carbs** 34g • **Fiber** 9g • **Total Sugar** 9g
Added Sugar 0g • **Protein** 9g • **Total Carbohydrate Choices** 2

NOTES FROM THE TEST KITCHEN

Using Bay Leaves

Bay leaves are a key seasoning in many soups and stews. In the test kitchen, we use fresh herbs more often than dried— bay leaves being an exception. We prefer dried bay leaves to fresh; they work just as well in long-cooked recipes, are cheaper, and will keep for 3 months in the freezer in an airtight container. We prefer Turkish bay leaves to those from California. The California bay leaf has a medicinal and potent, eucalyptus-like flavor, but the Turkish bay leaf has a mild, green, and slightly clovelike flavor.

Vegan Black Bean Burgers
SERVES 6

WHY THIS RECIPE WORKS Satisfying black beans seem like a natural base for a hearty burger, but most black bean burgers are mushy or fall apart when flipped. We managed to harness the sticking power of the beans' natural starches and, with just a few additions, create a great vegan burger. For a dry binder, we used tortilla chips that we ground in the food processor; their corn flavor added a pleasing Southwestern flair to our burgers, which we enhanced with scallions, fresh cilantro, garlic, ground cumin and coriander, and hot sauce. As for a moist binder, instead of an egg we found that the liquid from the black bean can provided the necessary cohesion, and the beans were sticky enough to hold together without an additional binder. The black bean liquid also boosted the overall flavor of the burgers. We dried the rinsed beans well to ensure we had control over the moisture content of our burgers. When forming the patties, it's important to pack them together firmly.

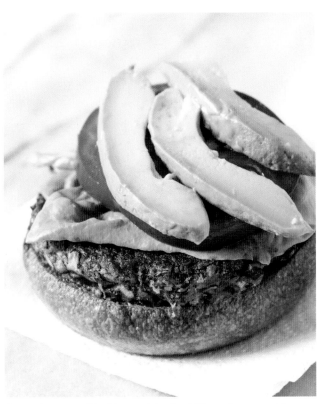

Ground corn tortilla chips and the liquid from the canned beans ensure cohesive and tasty black bean burgers that are also vegan.

2 (15-ounce) cans no-salt-added black beans, drained, with 6 tablespoons bean liquid reserved, and rinsed
2 tablespoons all-purpose flour
4 scallions, minced
3 tablespoons minced fresh cilantro
2 garlic cloves, minced
1 teaspoon ground cumin
1 teaspoon hot sauce (optional)
½ teaspoon ground coriander
½ teaspoon salt
¼ teaspoon pepper
1 ounce corn tortilla chips, crushed (½ cup)
¼ cup canola oil
6 100 percent whole-wheat burger buns, lightly toasted (optional)
2 avocados, halved, pitted, and sliced ¼ inch thick
1 head Bibb lettuce (8 ounces), leaves separated
2 tomatoes, cored and sliced ¼ inch thick

1. Line rimmed baking sheet with triple layer of paper towels, spread beans over towels, and let sit for 15 minutes.

2. Whisk reserved bean liquid and flour in large bowl until well combined and smooth. Stir in scallions, cilantro, garlic, cumin, hot sauce, if using, coriander, salt, and pepper until well combined. Process tortilla chips in food processor until finely ground, about 30 seconds. Add black beans and pulse until beans are coarsely ground, about 5 pulses. Transfer bean mixture to bowl with flour mixture and mix until well combined.

3. Adjust oven rack to middle position and heat oven to 200 degrees. Divide mixture into 6 equal portions and pack firmly into 3½-inch-wide patties.

4. Heat 1 tablespoon oil in 10-inch nonstick skillet over medium heat until shimmering. Gently lay 3 patties in skillet and cook until crisp and well browned on first side, about 5 minutes. Gently flip patties, add 1 tablespoon oil, and cook until crisp and well browned on second side, 3 to 5 minutes.

5. Transfer burgers to wire rack set in rimmed baking sheet and place in oven to keep warm. Wipe out skillet with paper towels and repeat with remaining 2 tablespoons oil and remaining patties. Serve burgers on buns, if using, and top with avocado, lettuce, and tomatoes.

PER SERVING WITH BUN

Cal 450 • **Total Fat** 24g • **Sat Fat** 2.5g • **Chol** 0mg
Sodium 460mg • **Total Carbs** 52g • **Fiber** 15g • **Total Sugar** 6g
Added Sugar 0g • **Protein** 13g • **Total Carbohydrate Choices** 3.5

PER SERVING WITHOUT BUN

Cal 340 • **Total Fat** 21g • **Sat Fat** 2.5g • **Chol** 0mg
Sodium 240mg • **Total Carbs** 30g • **Fiber** 11g • **Total Sugar** 2g
Added Sugar 0g • **Protein** 9g • **Total Carbohydrate Choices** 2

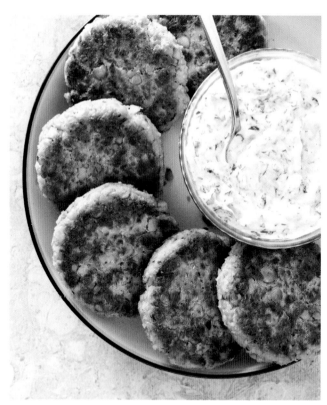

We use extra-virgin olive oil and Greek yogurt to make both the chickpea cakes and the flavorful sauce that goes with them.

Chickpea Cakes with Cucumber-Yogurt Sauce

SERVES 4

WHY THIS RECIPE WORKS Buttery, nutty chickpeas make a great foundation for a light yet filling vegetarian patty. They are protein-rich and just as satisfying as a beef burger, and they can be mixed and formed ahead of time and stored overnight for a quick dinner. To keep our recipe easy, we decided to use canned beans rather than dried, which would require an overnight soak before we could prep and form the patties. Pulsing the chickpeas in the food processor was quick and gave us just the right coarse texture for cohesive cakes. For the flavors, we started with the fragrant Indian spice mix garam masala. Tasters liked the aromatic flavor of onion, but it released moisture as it sat, making the cakes gummy. Swapping the onion for scallions fixed the problem, lending a nice onion flavor without excess moisture. Fresh cilantro added a bright complexity. For a cool, creamy counterpoint, we made a simple cucumber-yogurt sauce to top the cakes. Be careful to avoid overprocessing the bean mixture, as it will cause the cakes to become mealy in texture.

CUCUMBER-YOGURT SAUCE

- 1 cucumber, peeled, halved lengthwise, seeded, and shredded
- Salt and pepper
- 1 cup 2 percent Greek yogurt
- 2 tablespoons extra-virgin olive oil
- 2 tablespoons minced fresh cilantro
- 1 garlic clove, minced

CHICKPEA CAKES

- 2 (15-ounce) cans no-salt-added chickpeas, rinsed
- ½ cup 2 percent Greek yogurt
- 2 large eggs
- 5 tablespoons extra-virgin olive oil
- 1 teaspoon garam masala
- ¼ teaspoon salt
- ⅛ teaspoon cayenne pepper
- 1 cup 100 percent whole-wheat panko bread crumbs
- 5 scallions, sliced thin
- 3 tablespoons minced fresh cilantro
- 1 shallot, minced

1. FOR THE CUCUMBER-YOGURT SAUCE Toss cucumber with ½ teaspoon salt in fine-mesh strainer and let drain for 15 minutes. Combine drained cucumber with yogurt, oil, cilantro, and garlic and season with pepper to taste. (Sauce can be refrigerated for up to 1 day.)

2. FOR THE CHICKPEA CAKES Line rimmed baking sheet with parchment paper. Pulse chickpeas in food processor to coarse puree with few large pieces remaining, about 8 pulses.

3. In medium bowl, whisk yogurt, eggs, 2 tablespoons oil, garam masala, salt, and cayenne together. Stir in chickpeas, panko, scallions, cilantro, and shallot until combined. Divide mixture into 8 equal portions, pack firmly into 1-inch-thick patties, and place on prepared sheet. Cover and refrigerate patties for at least 1 hour and up to 24 hours.

4. Heat 1½ tablespoons oil in 12-inch nonstick skillet over medium heat until shimmering. Gently lay 4 patties in skillet and cook until well browned on first side, 6 to 8 minutes. Gently flip patties and cook until golden brown on second side, 6 to 8 minutes. Transfer patties to serving platter and tent with aluminum foil. Return now-empty skillet to medium heat and repeat with remaining 1½ tablespoons oil and remaining patties. Serve with cucumber-yogurt sauce.

PER SERVING
Cal 540 • **Total Fat** 30g • **Sat Fat** 5g • **Chol** 95mg
Sodium 410mg • **Total Carbs** 44g • **Fiber** 9g • **Total Sugar** 7g
Added Sugar 0g • **Protein** 22g • **Total Carbohydrate Choices** 3

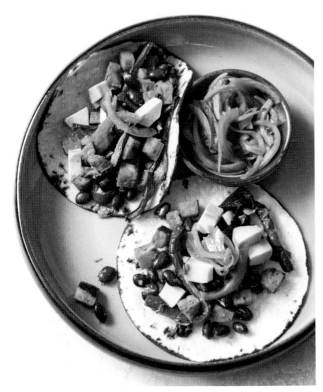

These vegetarian tacos feature sweet potatoes, which provide a wealth of vitamin A, and very little saturated fat.

Sweet Potato, Poblano, and Black Bean Tacos

SERVES 6

WHY THIS RECIPE WORKS Tacos are often focused on rich meats, but we wanted a delicious version that was all about vegetables. Our favorite combination turned out to be sweet potatoes and poblano chiles, which we seasoned with fragrant garlic, cumin, coriander, and oregano. Roasting produced caramelized exteriors and tender interiors. Adding black beans turned the tacos into a satiating meal packed with vitamins and fiber.

½ cup red wine vinegar
½ teaspoon red pepper flakes
1 red onion, halved and sliced thin
3 tablespoons extra-virgin olive oil
3 garlic cloves, minced
1½ teaspoons ground cumin
1½ teaspoons ground coriander
1 teaspoon minced fresh oregano or ¼ teaspoon dried
  Salt and pepper
1 pound sweet potatoes, peeled and cut into ½-inch pieces

4 poblano chiles, stemmed, seeded, and cut into ½-inch-wide strips
1 (15-ounce) can no-salt added black beans, rinsed
¼ cup chopped fresh cilantro
12 (6-inch) corn tortillas, warmed
1 avocado, halved, pitted, and cut into ½-inch pieces

1. Adjust oven racks to upper-middle and lower-middle positions and heat oven to 450 degrees. Line 2 rimmed baking sheets with aluminum foil. Microwave vinegar and pepper flakes in medium bowl until steaming, about 2 minutes. Stir in onion and let sit until ready to serve.

2. Whisk oil, garlic, cumin, coriander, oregano, ½ teaspoon salt, and ½ teaspoon pepper together in large bowl. Add potatoes and poblanos to oil mixture and toss to coat.

3. Spread vegetable mixture in even layer in lined baking sheets. Roast vegetables until tender and golden brown, about 30 minutes, stirring vegetables and switching and rotating sheets halfway through baking.

4. Return vegetables to now-empty bowl, add black beans and cilantro, and gently toss to combine. Divide vegetables evenly among warm tortillas and top with avocado and pickled onions. Serve.

PER SERVING

Cal 350 • **Total Fat** 14g • **Sat Fat** 2g • **Chol** 0mg
Sodium 250mg • **Total Carbs** 51g • **Fiber** 11g • **Total Sugar** 7g
Added Sugar 0g • **Protein** 8g • **Total Carbohydrate Choices** 3.5

NOTES FROM THE TEST KITCHEN

Sweet Potato or Yam?

You often hear "yam" and "sweet potato" used interchangeably, but they actually belong to completely different botanical families. Yams, generally sold in Latin and Asian markets, are often sold in chunks (they can grow to be several feet long) and can be found in dozens of varieties, with flesh ranging from white to light yellow to pink, and skin from off-white to brown. They all have very starchy flesh. Sweet potatoes are also found in several varieties and can have firm or soft flesh, but it's the soft varieties that have in the past been mislabeled as "yams," and the confusion continues to this day. The U.S. Department of Agriculture now requires labels with the term "yam" to be accompanied by the term "sweet potato" when appropriate. We typically buy the conventional sweet potato, a longish, knobby tuber with dark orange-brown skin and vivid flesh. Beauregard is our favorite variety.

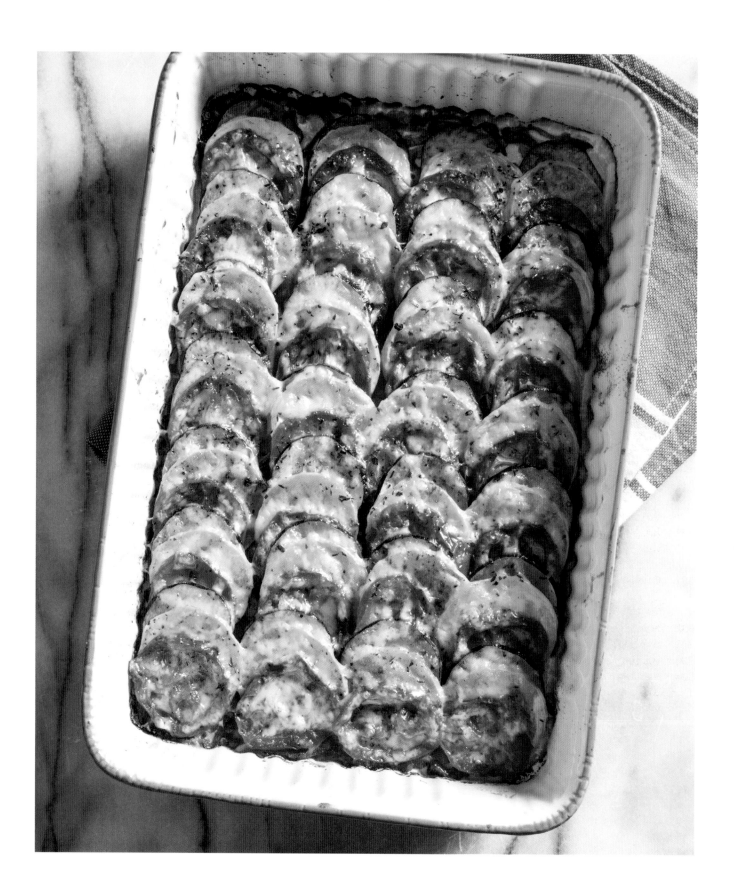

Photo: Squash and Tomato Tian

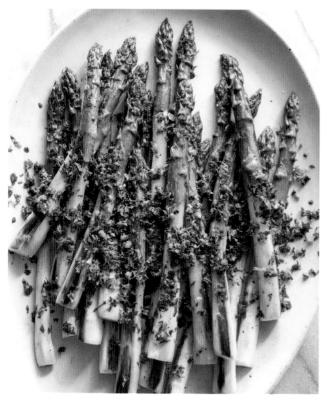

Whether you choose to make the simplest version of roasted asparagus or dress it up, our method ensures perfect results.

Roasted Asparagus
SERVES 6

WHY THIS RECIPE WORKS Roasting is a delicious and easy way to prepare asparagus. But simply tossing the spears with oil, salt, and pepper and spreading them on a baking sheet doesn't always produce reliably crisp-tender spears. After a few tests, we discovered that thicker spears (½ inch in diameter) held up better to roasting, but they required some prep. Trimming off the woody stems wasn't even a question, but what to do with the tough skins? Though it seemed a little fussy, we found that peeling the bottom halves of the stalks—just enough to expose the creamy white flesh—delivered consistently tender and visually appealing asparagus. To ensure a hard sear on our spears, we preheated the baking sheet and resisted the urge to give it a shake during roasting. The result? Intense, flavorful browning on one side of the asparagus and vibrant green on the other. For a variation with complementary seasoning, gremolata, a bright garnish of minced fresh mint and fresh parsley, orange zest, minced garlic, and a hit of cayenne, reinforced the stalks' vibrant flavor and gave our simple side a distinct presence. This recipe works best with thick asparagus spears that are between ½ and ¾ inch in diameter. Do not use pencil-thin asparagus; it overcooks too easily.

> 2 pounds thick asparagus, trimmed
> 2 tablespoons plus 2 teaspoons extra-virgin olive oil
> ½ teaspoon salt
> ¼ teaspoon pepper

1. Adjust oven rack to lowest position, place rimmed baking sheet on rack, and heat oven to 500 degrees. Peel bottom halves of asparagus spears until white flesh is exposed, then toss with 2 tablespoons oil, salt, and pepper.

2. Transfer asparagus to preheated sheet and spread into single layer. Roast, without moving asparagus, until undersides of spears are browned, tops are bright green, and tip of paring knife inserted at base of largest spear meets little resistance, 8 to 10 minutes. Transfer asparagus to serving platter and drizzle with remaining 2 teaspoons oil. Serve.

PER SERVING
Cal 80 • Total Fat 6g • Sat Fat 1g • Chol 0mg
Sodium 190mg • Total Carbs 4g • Fiber 2g • Total Sugar 2g
Added Sugar 0g • Protein 3g • Total Carbohydrate Choices <0.5

VARIATIONS
Roasted Asparagus with Mint-Orange Gremolata
Combine 2 tablespoons minced fresh mint, 2 tablespoons minced fresh parsley, 2 teaspoons grated orange zest, 1 minced garlic clove, and pinch cayenne pepper in bowl. Sprinkle gremolata over asparagus before serving.

PER SERVING
Cal 80 • Total Fat 6g • Sat Fat 1g • Chol 0mg
Sodium 190mg • Total Carbs 5g • Fiber 2g • Total Sugar 2g
Added Sugar 0g • Protein 3g • Total Carbohydrate Choices <0.5

PEELING ASPARAGUS

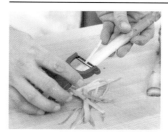

Trim woody ends of asparagus spears. Peel bottom halves of spears until white flesh is exposed.

Roasted Asparagus with Tarragon-Lemon Gremolata

Combine 2 tablespoons minced fresh tarragon, 2 tablespoons minced fresh parsley, 2 teaspoons grated lemon zest, and 1 minced garlic clove in bowl. Sprinkle gremolata over asparagus before serving.

PER SERVING

Cal 80 • **Total Fat** 6g • **Sat Fat** 1g • **Chol** 0mg
Sodium 190mg • **Total Carbs** 5g • **Fiber** 2g • **Total Sugar** 2g
Added Sugar 0g • **Protein** 3g • **Total Carbohydrate Choices** <0.5

Roasted Beets
SERVES 4

WHY THIS RECIPE WORKS This recipe delivers perfectly roasted beets with a bright vinaigrette. And since beets have been shown to offer many health benefits, including lowering blood pressure, it's good to have a simple, hands-off method for cooking them. This method is great too if you want to cook up beets to add to your leafy green or grain salads. Foil-wrapped roasted beets were more moist than unwrapped roasted beets, but the latter had more flavor. We minimized bleeding by not peeling the skin or slicing off the tops of the beets prior to cooking. To ensure even cooking, we recommend using beets that are similar in size—roughly 3 inches in diameter.

1½ **pounds beets, trimmed**
1 **tablespoon extra-virgin olive oil**
1 **tablespoon sherry vinegar**
1 **tablespoon minced fresh parsley**
 Salt and pepper

1. Adjust oven rack to middle position and heat oven to 400 degrees. Wrap beets individually in aluminum foil and place on rimmed baking sheet. Roast beets until skewer inserted into center meets little resistance (you will need to unwrap beets to test them), 45 to 60 minutes.

2. Remove beets from oven and slowly open foil packets (being careful of rising steam). When beets are cool enough to handle but still warm, gently rub off skins using paper towels.

3. Slice beets into ½-inch-thick wedges, then toss with oil, vinegar, parsley, and ¼ teaspoon salt. Season with pepper to taste and serve warm or at room temperature. (Beets can be refrigerated for up to 3 days; return to room temperature before serving.)

PER SERVING

Cal 80 • **Total Fat** 3.5g • **Sat Fat** 0.5g • **Chol** 0mg
Sodium 240mg • **Total Carbs** 11g • **Fiber** 3g • **Total Sugar** 8g
Added Sugar 0g • **Protein** 2g • **Total Carbohydrate Choices** 1

VARIATIONS
Roasted Beets with Ricotta Salata

Feta cheese can be substituted for the ricotta salata.

Substitute lime juice for vinegar and add ¼ teaspoon ground cumin with oil in step 3. Reduce salt to ⅛ teaspoon. Sprinkle with ¼ cup crumbled ricotta salata before serving.

PER SERVING

Cal 100 • **Total Fat** 5g • **Sat Fat** 1.5g • **Chol** 5mg
Sodium 280mg • **Total Carbs** 12g • **Fiber** 3g • **Total Sugar** 8g
Added Sugar 0g • **Protein** 3g • **Total Carbohydrate Choices** 1

Roasted Beets with Garlic and Walnuts

Wrap 1 head garlic tightly in aluminum foil and roast along with beets. Once roasted, squeeze garlic cloves from skins and mince. Toss minced roasted garlic and ¼ cup toasted and chopped walnuts with beets in step 3.

PER SERVING

Cal 140 • **Total Fat** 9g • **Sat Fat** 1g • **Chol** 0mg
Sodium 240mg • **Total Carbs** 14g • **Fiber** 4g • **Total Sugar** 8g
Added Sugar 0g • **Protein** 3g • **Total Carbohydrate Choices** 1

AVOIDING BEET STAINS

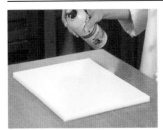

To prevent beet juice from staining your cutting board, spray the surface lightly with vegetable oil spray before prepping the beets.

Vegetable Cooking Times

Vegetables are a great way to fill out your plate and amp up fiber and nutrients at any meal. And while it is nice to have stand-alone recipes for a variety of interesting vegetable side dishes, this handy chart shows how to prepare vegetables in the simplest (and quickest) ways.

TYPE OF VEGETABLE	AMOUNT/ YIELD	PREPARATION	BOILING TIME (AMOUNT OF WATER AND SALT)	STEAMING TIME	MICROWAVING TIME (AMOUNT OF WATER)
Asparagus	1 bunch (1 pound)/ serves 3	tough ends trimmed	2 to 4 minutes (4 quarts water plus 1 tablespoon salt)	3 to 5 minutes	3 to 6 minutes (3 tablespoons water)
Beets	1½ pounds (6 medium)/serves 4	greens discarded and beets scrubbed well	X	35 to 55 minutes	18 to 24 minutes (¾ cup water)
Broccoli	1 bunch (1½ pounds)/ serves 4	florets cut into 1- to 1½-inch pieces and stalks peeled and cut into ¼-inch-thick pieces	2 to 4 minutes (4 quarts water plus 1 tablespoon salt)	4 to 6 minutes	4 to 6 minutes (3 tablespoons water)
Brussels Sprouts	1 pound/serves 4	stem ends trimmed, discolored leaves removed, and halved through stem	6 to 8 minutes (4 quarts water plus 1 tablespoon salt)	7 to 9 minutes	X
Carrots	1 pound/serves 4	peeled and sliced ¼ inch thick on bias	3 to 4 minutes (4 quarts water plus 1 tablespoon salt)	5 to 6 minutes	4 to 7 minutes (2 tablespoons water)
Cauliflower	1 head (2 pounds)/ serves 4 to 6	cored and florets cut into 1-inch pieces	5 to 7 minutes (4 quarts water plus 1 tablespoon salt)	7 to 9 minutes	4 to 7 minutes (¼ cup water)
Green Beans	1 pound/ serves 4	stem ends trimmed	3 to 5 minutes (4 quarts water plus 1 tablespoon salt)	6 to 8 minutes	4 to 6 minutes (3 tablespoons water)
Red Potatoes	2 pounds (6 medium)/ serves 4	scrubbed and poked several times with fork	16 to 22 minutes (4 quarts water plus 1 tablespoon salt)	18 to 24 minutes	6 to 10 minutes (no water and uncovered)
Russet Potatoes	2 pounds (4 medium)/ serves 4	scrubbed and poked several times with fork	X	X	8 to 12 minutes (no water and uncovered)
Snap Peas	1 pound/serves 4	stems trimmed and strings removed	2 to 4 minutes (4 quarts water plus 1 tablespoon salt)	4 to 6 minutes	3 to 6 minutes (3 tablespoons water)
Snow Peas	1 pound/serves 4	stems trimmed and strings removed	2 to 3 minutes (4 quarts water plus 1 tablespoon salt)	4 to 6 minutes	3 to 6 minutes (3 tablespoons water)
Squash (Winter)	2 pounds/serves 4	peeled, seeded, and cut into 1-inch chunks	X	12 to 14 minutes	8 to 11 minutes (¼ cup water)
Sweet Potatoes	2 pounds (3 medium)/serves 4	peeled and cut into 1-inch chunks	X	12 to 14 minutes	8 to 10 minutes (¼ cup water)

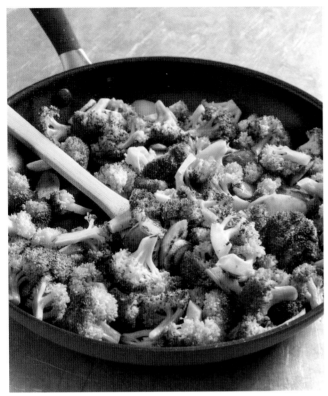

Broccoli stalks are highly nutritious so be sure to peel and slice them and add them to the skillet first so they cook through.

Pan-Roasted Broccoli
SERVES 6

WHY THIS RECIPE WORKS Forget about dull, waterlogged steamed broccoli. Once you discover this pan-roasting method, you'll be serving up a variety of broccoli side dishes regularly. For pan-roasted broccoli with bright green florets and toasty-brown stalks, we trimmed the florets into small pieces and the stalks into oblong coins for maximum browning. For broccoli that was nicely browned but also cooked through properly, we layered the stalks evenly in a hot, lightly oiled skillet. Once they began to brown we added the florets along with water and allowed the mixture to steam until nearly tender. Stirring the salt and pepper right into the steaming water kept things simple and allowed us to infuse the broccoli with flavor. Avoid buying broccoli with stalks that are cracked or bend easily, or with florets that are yellow or brown. If your broccoli stalks are especially thick, split them in half lengthwise before slicing.

¼ teaspoon salt
⅛ teaspoon pepper
2 tablespoons extra-virgin olive oil
1¾ pounds broccoli, florets cut into 1½-inch pieces, stalks peeled and cut on bias into ¼-inch-thick slices

1. Stir 3 tablespoons water, salt, and pepper together in small bowl until salt dissolves; set aside. Heat oil in 12-inch nonstick skillet over medium-high heat until just smoking. Add broccoli stalks in even layer and cook, without stirring, until browned on bottoms, about 2 minutes. Add florets to skillet and toss to combine. Cook, without stirring, until bottoms of florets just begin to brown, 1 to 2 minutes.

2. Add water mixture and cover skillet. Cook until broccoli is bright green but still crisp, about 2 minutes. Uncover and continue to cook until water has evaporated, broccoli stalks are tender, and florets are crisp-tender, about 2 minutes. Serve.

PER SERVING

Cal 70 • **Total Fat** 5g • **Sat Fat** 0.5g • **Chol** 0mg
Sodium 125mg • **Total Carbs** 5g • **Fiber** 2g • **Total Sugar** 1g
Added Sugar 0g • **Protein** 2g • **Total Carbohydrate Choices** <0.5

VARIATIONS
Pan-Roasted Broccoli with Roasted Red Peppers
Add ¼ cup thinly sliced jarred roasted red peppers to skillet after uncovering in step 2. Sprinkle broccoli with ¼ cup grated Pecorino Romano cheese before serving.

PER SERVING

Cal 80 • **Total Fat** 6g • **Sat Fat** 1g • **Chol** 0mg
Sodium 180mg • **Total Carbs** 6g • **Fiber** 2g • **Total Sugar** 2g
Added Sugar 0g • **Protein** 3g • **Total Carbohydrate Choices** 0.5

Pan-Roasted Broccoli with Garlic and Anchovy
Add 1 minced anchovy fillet and 2 minced garlic cloves to skillet after uncovering in step 2.

PER SERVING

Cal 70 • **Total Fat** 5g • **Sat Fat** 0.5g • **Chol** 0mg
Sodium 150mg • **Total Carbs** 6g • **Fiber** 2g • **Total Sugar** 1g
Added Sugar 0g • **Protein** 3g • **Total Carbohydrate Choices** 0.5

All About Garlic

Here's everything you need to know about buying, storing, and cooking with garlic.

Buying Garlic

Pick heads without spots, mold, or sprouting. Squeeze them to make sure they are not rubbery or missing cloves. The garlic shouldn't have much of a scent. Of the various garlic varieties, your best bet is soft-neck garlic, since it stores well and is heat-tolerant. This variety features a circle of large cloves surrounding a small cluster at the center. Hard-neck garlic has a stiff center staff surrounded by large, uniform cloves and boasts a more intense flavor. But since it's easily damaged and doesn't store as well as soft-neck garlic, wait to buy it at the farmers' market.

Storing Garlic

Whole heads of garlic should last at least a few weeks if stored in a cool, dark place with plenty of air circulation to prevent spoiling and sprouting.

Preparing Garlic

Keep in mind that garlic's pungency emerges only after its cell walls are ruptured, triggering the creation of a compound called allicin. The more a clove is broken down, the more allicin that is produced. Thus you can control the amount of bite garlic contributes to a recipe by how fine or coarse you cut it. It's also best not to cut garlic in advance; the longer cut garlic sits, the harsher its flavor.

Cooking Garlic

Garlic's flavor is sharpest when raw. Once it is heated above 150 degrees, its enzymes are destroyed and no new flavor is produced. This is why roasted garlic, which is cooked slowly and takes longer to reach 150 degrees, has a mellow, slightly sweet flavor. Garlic browned at very high temperatures (300 to 350 degrees) results in a more bitter flavor. To avoid the creation of bitter compounds, wait to add garlic to the pan until other ingredients have softened. And don't cook garlic over high heat for much longer than 30 seconds.

Roasted Broccoli
SERVES 6

WHY THIS RECIPE WORKS Broccoli's awkward shape, tough stems, and shrubby florets may seem to make it a poor candidate for roasting, but we found a method that delivered incredible results. Success in roasting this oddly shaped vegetable came down to how we cut it up. To maximize its direct contact with the sheet pan (thereby increasing its flavor-boosting browning), we cut the crowns into wedges and the trimmed stalks into thick planks. Preheating a baking sheet on the lowest rack of a 500-degree oven meant our broccoli pieces would begin to sizzle and sear on contact, delivering crisp-tipped florets and blistered and browned stalks that were subtly sweet and perfectly seasoned. Make sure to trim away the outer peel from the broccoli stalks as directed; otherwise, they will turn tough when roasted.

1¾ pounds broccoli
3 tablespoons extra-virgin olive oil
3 garlic cloves, minced
½ teaspoon salt
Pinch pepper
Lemon wedges

1. Adjust oven rack to lowest position, place rimmed baking sheet on rack, and heat oven to 500 degrees. Cut broccoli horizontally at juncture of crowns and stalks. Cut crowns into 4 wedges (if 3 to 4 inches in diameter) or 6 wedges (if 4 to 5 inches in diameter). Trim tough outer peel from stalks, then cut into ½-inch-thick planks that are 2 to 3 inches long.

2. Combine oil, garlic, salt, and pepper in large bowl. Add broccoli and toss to coat. Working quickly, lay broccoli in single layer, flat sides down, on preheated sheet. Roast until stalks are well browned and tender and florets are lightly browned, 9 to 11 minutes. Transfer to serving dish and serve with lemon wedges.

PER SERVING

Cal 90 • **Total Fat** 7g • **Sat Fat** 1g • **Chol** 0mg
Sodium 220mg • **Total Carbs** 6g • **Fiber** 2g • **Total Sugar** 1g
Added Sugar 0g • **Protein** 2g • **Total Carbohydrate Choices** 0.5

VARIATION
Roasted Broccoli with Shallots, Fennel Seeds, and Parmesan

Omit garlic and reduce salt to ¼ teaspoon. While broccoli roasts, heat 1 tablespoon extra-virgin olive oil in 8-inch skillet over medium heat until shimmering. Add 3 thinly sliced shallots and cook, stirring often, until shallots soften and are beginning to brown, 5 to 6 minutes. Stir in 1 teaspoon coarsely chopped fennel seeds and cook until shallots are golden brown, 1 to 2 minutes; remove from heat. Toss roasted broccoli with shallot mixture and garnish with ½ ounce shaved Parmesan cheese before serving.

PER SERVING

Cal 130 • **Total Fat** 10g • **Sat Fat** 1.5g • **Chol** 0mg
Sodium 170mg • **Total Carbs** 8g • **Fiber** 3g • **Total Sugar** 3g
Added Sugar 0g • **Protein** 4g • **Total Carbohydrate Choices** 0.5

Broiled Broccoli Rabe
SERVES 4

WHY THIS RECIPE WORKS Most recipes for broccoli rabe call for blanching and shocking the greens before cooking in order to tame its bitterness—a fussy method that also washes out all of its distinctive flavor. When we learned that most of the vegetable's bitterness comes from an enzymatic reaction triggered when the florets are cut or chewed, we kept the leafy parts of the vegetable whole. Because the heat from cooking then deactivated the enzyme, much of the bitterness was tamed. We also skipped stovetop methods and broiled the rabe, which created deep caramelization without overcooking the pieces. Plus, broiling the rabe took just minutes and required nothing more than a rimmed baking sheet. Because the amount of heat generated by a broiler varies from oven to oven, we recommend keeping an eye on the broccoli rabe as it cooks. If the leaves are getting too dark or not browning in the time specified in the recipe, adjust the distance of the oven rack from the broiler element.

- 3 **tablespoons extra-virgin olive oil**
- 1 **pound broccoli rabe**
- 1 **garlic clove, minced**
- ¼ **teaspoon salt**
- ¼ **teaspoon red pepper flakes**
     Lemon wedges

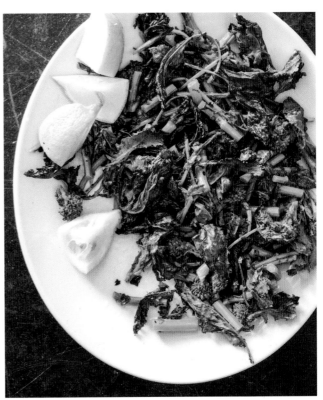

To tame broccoli rabe's legendary bitterness, don't cut the leaves, toss it with a garlic-oil mixture, and broil it for mere minutes.

1. Adjust oven rack 4 inches from broiler element and heat broiler. Brush rimmed baking sheet with 1 tablespoon oil.

2. Trim and discard bottom 1 inch of broccoli rabe stems. Wash broccoli rabe with cold water, then dry with clean dish towel. Cut tops (leaves and florets) from stems, then cut stems into 1-inch pieces (keep tops whole). Transfer broccoli rabe to prepared sheet.

3. Combine remaining 2 tablespoons oil, garlic, salt, and pepper flakes in small bowl. Pour oil mixture over broccoli rabe and toss to combine.

4. Broil until half of leaves are well browned, 2 to 2½ minutes. Using tongs, toss to expose unbrowned leaves. Return sheet to oven and continue to broil until most leaves are lightly charred and stems are crisp-tender, 2 to 2½ minutes. Transfer to serving platter and serve, passing lemon wedges.

PER SERVING

Cal 120 • **Total Fat** 11g • **Sat Fat** 1.5g • **Chol** 0mg
Sodium 180mg • **Total Carbs** 4g • **Fiber** 3g • **Total Sugar** 0g
Added Sugar 0g • **Protein** 4g • **Total Carbohydrate Choices** <0.5

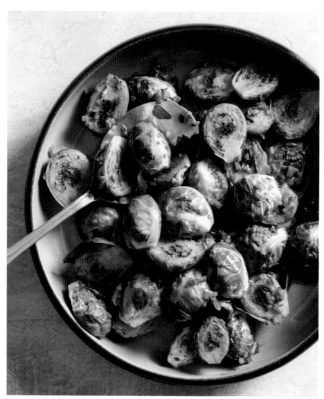

A brown-and-braise method yields sprouts with caramelization and a tender bite.

1 tablespoon extra-virgin olive oil
1 pound Brussels sprouts, trimmed and halved
2 shallots, minced
1 teaspoon minced fresh thyme
  Salt and pepper
¾ cup unsalted chicken broth
¼ cup balsamic vinegar
1 tablespoon unsalted butter

1. Heat oil in 12-inch nonstick skillet over medium heat until shimmering. Arrange Brussels sprouts cut side down in skillet and cook until browned, about 5 minutes. Stir in shallots, thyme, and ¼ teaspoon salt and cook until shallots are softened, about 2 minutes.

2. Stir in broth and vinegar, cover, and cook until sprouts are bright green and nearly tender, about 9 minutes. Uncover and continue to cook until sprouts are tender and liquid is slightly thickened, about 2 minutes. Off heat, stir in butter and season with pepper to taste. Serve.

PER SERVING
Cal 130 • **Total Fat** 7g • **Sat Fat** 2.5g • **Chol** 10mg
Sodium 200mg • **Total Carbs** 15g • **Fiber** 5g • **Total Sugar** 6g
Added Sugar 0g • **Protein** 5g • **Total Carbohydrate Choices** 1

Skillet-Braised Brussels Sprouts with Balsamic Vinegar
SERVES 4

WHY THIS RECIPE WORKS Brussels sprouts are finally receiving favorable attention with chefs dishing them up in a wide variety of interesting ways. For a simple method for cooking these nutrient-dense little cabbages at home, skillet braising is just the ticket as it allows you to brown them first for flavorful caramelizing and then braise them with a little chicken broth to ensure that they are tender but not mushy. First we made sure to halve the sprouts through the stem end, which ensured they would not fall apart and we'd get that desirable browning on the cut sides. Then we heated up a little extra-virgin olive oil in the skillet and browned our sprouts. Shallots and fresh thyme went in next for flavoring. Then we added chicken broth and a little balsamic vinegar, covered the skillet, and cooked until the sprouts were tender and all the liquid had been absorbed. The vinegar added a tartness that is always a great foil for the strong, earthy taste of Brussels sprouts. To finish, just a touch of butter added silky richness.

Sautéed Cabbage with Parsley and Lemon
SERVES 6

WHY THIS RECIPE WORKS We wanted a simple preparation for humble green cabbage that would bring out the vegetable's natural sweetness and maintain its crisp-tender texture. Instead of boiling or braising, we pan-steamed and then sautéed the cabbage over relatively high heat to cook it quickly and add an extra layer of flavor from browning. A precooking step of soaking the cabbage reduced bitterness while providing extra moisture to help the cabbage steam. Cooked onion helped reinforce sweetness, and lemon juice provided punch. Fresh parsley offered a bright finish.

1 small head green cabbage (1¼ pounds), cored and sliced thin
2 tablespoons extra-virgin olive oil
1 onion, halved and sliced thin
  Salt and pepper
¼ cup chopped fresh parsley
1½ teaspoons lemon juice

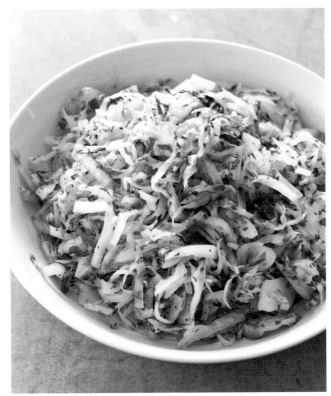

Despite its simplicity, this humble sautéed cabbage dish is a flavorful and comforting way to make the most of this superfood.

1. Place cabbage in large bowl and cover with cold water. Let sit for 3 minutes; drain well.

2. Heat 1 tablespoon oil in 12-inch nonstick skillet over medium-high heat until shimmering. Add onion and ¼ teaspoon salt and cook until softened and lightly browned, 5 to 7 minutes; transfer to bowl.

3. Heat remaining 1 tablespoon oil in now-empty skillet over medium-high heat until shimmering. Add cabbage and sprinkle with ¼ teaspoon salt and ¼ teaspoon pepper. Cover and cook, without stirring, until cabbage is wilted and lightly browned on bottom, about 3 minutes. Stir and continue to cook, uncovered, until cabbage is crisp-tender and lightly browned in places, about 4 minutes, stirring once halfway through cooking. Off heat, stir in onion, parsley, and lemon juice. Season with pepper to taste and serve.

PER SERVING

Cal 80 • **Total Fat** 4.5g • **Sat Fat** 0.5g • **Chol** 0mg
Sodium 220mg • **Total Carbs** 8g • **Fiber** 3g • **Total Sugar** 4g
Added Sugar 0g • **Protein** 1g • **Total Carbohydrate Choices** 0.5

Boiled Carrots with Paprika and Mint
SERVES 4

WHY THIS RECIPE WORKS In our recipe for boiled carrots, we cut 1 pound of carrots into 1½- to 2-inch lengths and then halved or quartered them lengthwise, depending on thickness, so that they all cooked at the same rate. We cooked them in 2 cups of water with just a tiny amount of salt. After 6 minutes, we drained the carrots and added oil for richness and some vinegar for brightness. A bit of spice and some fresh herbs completed this simple side dish. For even cooking, it is important that the carrot pieces are of similar size. This recipe was developed using carrots with diameters between 1 and 1½ inches at the thick ends. If you are using larger carrots, you may have to cut them into more pieces.

1 pound carrots, peeled
Salt
1 tablespoon extra-virgin olive oil
1 teaspoon sherry vinegar, plus extra for serving
½ teaspoon paprika
1 tablespoon chopped fresh mint

1. Cut carrots into 1½- to 2-inch lengths. Leave thin pieces whole, halve medium pieces lengthwise, and quarter thick pieces lengthwise.

2. Bring 2 cups water to boil in medium saucepan over high heat. Add carrots and ⅛ teaspoon salt, cover, and cook until tender throughout, about 6 minutes (start timer as soon as carrots go into water).

3. Drain carrots and return them to now-empty saucepan. Add oil, vinegar, paprika, and pinch salt and stir until combined. Stir in mint. Season with extra vinegar to taste. Serve.

PER SERVING

Cal 70 • **Total Fat** 4g • **Sat Fat** 0.5g • **Chol** 0mg
Sodium 140mg • **Total Carbs** 10g • **Fiber** 3g • **Total Sugar** 5g
Added Sugar 0g • **Protein** 1g • **Total Carbohydrate Choices** 0.5

VARIATION
Boiled Carrots with Scallions and Ginger
Substitute 1 teaspoon toasted sesame oil for extra-virgin olive oil, rice vinegar for sherry vinegar, ¼ teaspoon grated fresh ginger for paprika, and 1 minced scallion for mint.

PER SERVING

Cal 50 • **Total Fat** 1.5g • **Sat Fat** 0g • **Chol** 0mg
Sodium 140mg • **Total Carbs** 10g • **Fiber** 3g • **Total Sugar** 5g
Added Sugar 0g • **Protein** 1g • **Total Carbohydrate Choices** 0.5

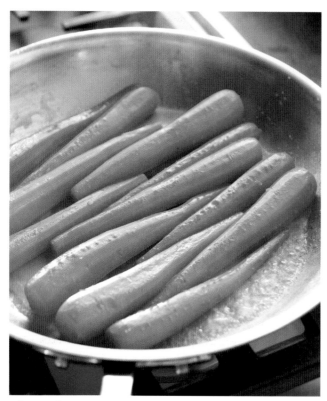

When cooking carrots whole in a skillet, we trap the moisture and steam by topping them with a parchment round.

Slow-Cooked Whole Carrots
SERVES 6

WHY THIS RECIPE WORKS Cooking whole carrots slowly brings out a new dimension of sweetness and flavor. Gently steeping the carrots in warm water before cooking them firmed up the vegetable's cell walls so that the carrots could be cooked for a long time without falling apart. We also topped the carrots with a cartouche (a circle of parchment that sits directly on the food) during cooking to ensure that the moisture in the pan cooked the carrots evenly. Finishing cooking at a simmer evaporated the liquid and concentrated the carrots' flavor so that they tasted great when served on their own or with a flavorful relish. Use carrots that measure ¾ to 1¼ inches across at the thickest end.

- 1 tablespoon extra-virgin olive oil
- ½ teaspoon salt
- 1½ pounds carrots, peeled

1. Cut parchment paper into 11-inch circle, then cut 1-inch hole in center, folding paper as needed.

2. Bring 3 cups water, oil, and salt to simmer in 12-inch skillet over high heat. Off heat, add carrots, top with parchment, cover skillet, and let sit for 20 minutes.

3. Uncover, leaving parchment in place, and bring to simmer over high heat. Reduce heat to medium-low and cook until most of water has evaporated and carrots are very tender, about 45 minutes.

4. Discard parchment, increase heat to medium-high, and cook, shaking skillet often, until carrots are lightly glazed and no water remains, 2 to 4 minutes. Serve.

PER SERVING

Cal 60 • **Total Fat** 2.5g • **Sat Fat** 0g • **Chol** 0mg
Sodium 100mg • **Total Carbs** 10g • **Fiber** 3g • **Total Sugar** 5g
Added Sugar 0g • **Protein** 1g • **Total Carbohydrate Choices** 0.5

FOLDING PARCHMENT FOR SLOW-COOKED CARROTS

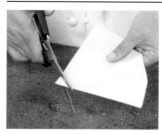

1. Cut parchment into 11-inch circle, then cut 1-inch hole in center, folding paper as needed to cut out hole.

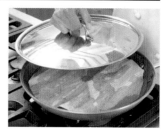

2. Lay parchment circle on top of carrots, underneath lid, to help retain and evenly distribute moisture during cooking.

Roasted Spiralized Carrots
SERVES 6

WHY THIS RECIPE WORKS We set out to create a simple and versatile yet interesting carrot side dish. Using a spiralizer to cut the carrots into uniform ⅛-inch-thick "noodles" ensured that the carrots cooked evenly, and roasting them covered for half the roasting time steamed them slightly and prevented them from drying out. We then uncovered the baking sheet and returned it to the oven to allow the noodles' surface moisture to evaporate, encouraging light caramelization and creating perfectly tender noodles. We kept the flavorings simple to allow the carrots' flavor to shine—just a handful of fresh thyme for earthy notes. For the best noodles, use carrots that measure at least ¾ inch across at the thinnest end and 1½ inches across at the thickest end. Our favorite spiralizer model is the Paderno World Cuisine Tri-Blade Plastic Spiral Vegetable Slicer.

2 pounds carrots, trimmed and peeled
2 tablespoons extra-virgin olive oil
2 teaspoons minced fresh thyme
   Salt and pepper

1. Adjust oven rack to middle position and heat oven to 375 degrees. Using spiralizer, cut carrots into ⅛-inch-thick noodles, then cut noodles into 12-inch lengths. Toss carrots with 1 tablespoon oil, thyme, ½ teaspoon salt, and ¼ teaspoon pepper on rimmed baking sheet. Cover baking sheet tightly with aluminum foil and roast for 15 minutes. Remove foil and continue to roast until carrots are tender, 10 to 15 minutes.

2. Transfer carrots to serving platter, drizzle with remaining 1 tablespoon oil, and season with pepper to taste. Serve.

PER SERVING

Cal 100 • **Total Fat** 5g • **Sat Fat** 0.5g • **Chol** 0mg
Sodium 290mg • **Total Carbs** 13g • **Fiber** 4g • **Total Sugar** 6g
Added Sugar 0g • **Protein** 1g • **Total Carbohydrate Choices** 1

Roasted Cauliflower
SERVES 6

WHY THIS RECIPE WORKS Many people think cauliflower is bland because its common preparations—steamed or served raw as crudités—do not do this sweet, nutty vegetable any justice. Roasting, on the other hand, highlights those appealing traits at every turn. To maximize the dense head's direct contact with the baking sheet, we sliced it into wedges, creating plenty of flat surfaces for browning. To keep the cauliflower from drying out in a hot oven, we started it covered and allowed it to steam in its own moisture until barely tender. Then we removed the foil and returned the pan to the oven until the wedges were caramelized and browned. Flipping each wedge halfway through roasting ensured even cooking and color. Thanks to its natural sweetness and rich flavor, our roasted cauliflower needed little enhancement—just a touch of salt and pepper did the trick. This dish stands well on its own or drizzled with additional extra-virgin olive oil.

1 head cauliflower (2 pounds)
¼ cup extra-virgin olive oil
   Salt and pepper

1. Adjust oven rack to lowest position and heat oven to 475 degrees. Line a rimmed baking sheet with aluminum foil. Trim outer leaves off cauliflower and cut stem flush with bottom of head. Cut head into 8 equal wedges. Place wedges, with either cut side down, on lined baking sheet, drizzle with 2 tablespoons oil, and sprinkle with ¼ teaspoon salt and ⅛ teaspoon pepper. Gently rub oil and seasonings into cauliflower. Gently flip cauliflower and repeat on second cut side with remaining 2 tablespoons oil, ¼ teaspoon salt, and ⅛ teaspoon pepper.

2. Cover baking sheet tightly with foil and roast for 10 minutes. Remove foil and continue to roast until bottoms of cauliflower wedges are golden, 8 to 12 minutes.

3. Remove sheet from oven, carefully flip wedges using spatula, and continue to roast until cauliflower is golden all over, 8 to 12 minutes. Transfer to serving dish, season with pepper to taste, and serve.

PER SERVING

Cal 120 • **Total Fat** 10g • **Sat Fat** 1.5g • **Chol** 0mg
Sodium 240mg • **Total Carbs** 8g • **Fiber** 3g • **Total Sugar** 3g
Added Sugar 0g • **Protein** 3g • **Total Carbohydrate Choices** 0.5

VARIATION
Spicy Roasted Cauliflower
Stir 2 teaspoons curry powder or chili powder into oil in bowl before seasoning cauliflower in step 1.

PER SERVING

Cal 120 • **Total Fat** 10g • **Sat Fat** 1.5g • **Chol** 0mg
Sodium 240mg • **Total Carbs** 8g • **Fiber** 3g • **Total Sugar** 3g
Added Sugar 0g • **Protein** 3g • **Total Carbohydrate Choices** 0.5

Braised Cauliflower with Garlic and White Wine
SERVES 6

WHY THIS RECIPE WORKS When properly cooked and imaginatively flavored, braised cauliflower can be toothsome, nutty, and slightly sweet. However, too many recipes result in cauliflower that is waterlogged and bland or, worse, sulfurous and unappealing. To avoid these problems (which stem from overcooking), we knew we would need to quickly braise the florets. To this end, we cut the florets into small, 1½-inch pieces, which reduced the total cooking time. Sautéing the cauliflower in olive oil imparted nuttiness. Because we wanted the cauliflower to cook in our braising liquid for only a short amount of time, we maximized its impact by creating an ultraflavorful broth that the porous vegetable could absorb. White wine and broth made for a complexly flavored base, and a generous amount of garlic along with a pinch of red pepper flakes added punch and deeper flavor. For the best texture and taste, make sure to brown the cauliflower well in step 1.

3 garlic cloves, minced

1 teaspoon plus 3 tablespoons extra-virgin olive oil

⅛ teaspoon red pepper flakes

1 head cauliflower (2 pounds), cored and cut into 1½-inch florets
    Salt and pepper

⅓ cup unsalted chicken broth

⅓ cup dry white wine

2 tablespoons minced fresh parsley

1. Combine garlic, 1 teaspoon oil, and pepper flakes in small bowl. Heat remaining 3 tablespoons oil in 12-inch skillet over medium-high heat until shimmering. Add cauliflower and ½ teaspoon salt and cook, stirring occasionally, until florets are golden brown, 7 to 9 minutes.

2. Push cauliflower to sides of skillet. Add garlic mixture to center and cook, mashing mixture into skillet, until fragrant, about 30 seconds. Stir garlic mixture into cauliflower.

3. Stir in broth and wine and bring to simmer. Reduce heat to medium-low, cover, and cook until cauliflower is crisp-tender, 4 to 6 minutes. Off heat, stir in parsley and season with pepper to taste. Serve.

PER SERVING

Cal 120 • **Total Fat** 8g • **Sat Fat** 1.5g • **Chol** 0mg
Sodium 250mg • **Total Carbs** 9g • **Fiber** 3g • **Total Sugar** 3g
Added Sugar 0g • **Protein** 3g • **Total Carbohydrate Choices** 0.5

VARIATIONS
Braised Cauliflower with Capers and Anchovies
Add 2 anchovy fillets, rinsed and minced, and 1 tablespoon rinsed and minced capers to oil mixture in step 1. Reduce salt to ¼ teaspoon. Stir 1 tablespoon lemon juice into cauliflower with parsley.

PER SERVING

Cal 130 • **Total Fat** 8g • **Sat Fat** 1.5g • **Chol** 0mg
Sodium 230mg • **Total Carbs** 9g • **Fiber** 3g • **Total Sugar** 3g
Added Sugar 0g • **Protein** 4g • **Total Carbohydrate Choices** 0.5

Braised Cauliflower with Sumac and Mint
Substitute 2 teaspoons ground sumac for pepper flakes. In step 3, increase broth to ½ cup and omit wine. Once cauliflower is crisp-tender, uncover and continue to cook until liquid is almost evaporated, about 1 minute. Substitute chopped fresh mint for parsley and stir ¼ cup plain low-fat yogurt into cauliflower with mint.

PER SERVING

Cal 120 • **Total Fat** 8g • **Sat Fat** 1.5g • **Chol** 0mg
Sodium 260mg • **Total Carbs** 9g • **Fiber** 3g • **Total Sugar** 4g
Added Sugar 0g • **Protein** 4g • **Total Carbohydrate Choices** 0.5

CUTTING CAULIFLOWER INTO FLORETS

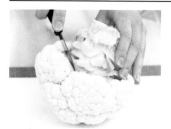

1. Pull off any leaves, then cut out core of cauliflower using paring knife.

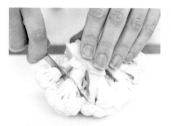

2. Separate florets from inner stem using tip of knife.

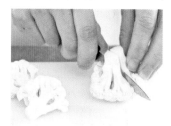

3. Cut larger florets into smaller pieces by slicing through stem end.

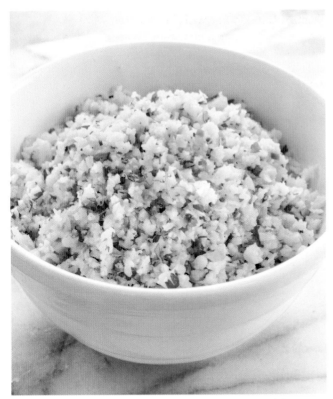

Processing cauliflower florets in the food processor yields pieces similar to rice that turn tender and flavorful when sautéed.

Cauliflower Rice
SERVES 4

WHY THIS RECIPE WORKS Cauliflower is a popular go-to for a low-carb rice replacement, since it's easy to process the florets into rice-size granules that cook up pleasantly fluffy. To make our cauliflower rice foolproof, we first needed to figure out the best way to chop the florets to the right size. We found that using the food processor made quick work of breaking down the florets and created a fairly consistent texture. Working in batches helped to ensure that all of the florets broke down evenly. Next, we needed to give our neutral-tasting cauliflower a boost in flavor; a shallot and a small amount of chicken broth did the trick. To ensure that the cauliflower was tender but still retained a pleasant, rice-like chew, we first steamed the "rice" in a covered pot, then finished cooking it uncovered to evaporate any remaining moisture. A mere ¼ teaspoon of salt and a splash of lemon juice just before serving brought plenty of seasoning to our simple rice side. We also decided to develop a couple of flavorful variations so that our cauliflower rice could accompany any number of meals. For the first one, we opted for a generously spiced curry profile and added sliced almonds for crunch and nuttiness. We also created a Tex-Mex version with spicy fresh jalapeños, cumin, and cilantro. This recipe can be doubled; use a Dutch oven and increase the cooking time to about 25 minutes in step 2.

1 head cauliflower (2 pounds), cored and cut into
  1-inch florets (6 cups)
2 tablespoons extra-virgin olive oil
1 shallot, minced
½ cup unsalted chicken broth
  Salt and pepper
2 tablespoons minced fresh parsley
1 teaspoon lemon juice

1. Working in 2 batches, pulse cauliflower in food processor until finely ground into ¼- to ⅛-inch pieces, 6 to 8 pulses, scraping down sides of bowl as needed; transfer to bowl.

2. Heat oil in large saucepan over medium-low heat until shimmering. Add shallot and cook until softened, about 3 minutes. Stir in processed cauliflower, broth, and ¼ teaspoon salt. Cover and cook, stirring occasionally, until cauliflower is tender, 12 to 15 minutes.

3. Uncover and continue to cook until cauliflower rice is almost completely dry, about 3 minutes. Off heat, stir in parsley, lemon juice, and ⅛ teaspoon salt. Season with pepper to taste. Serve.

PER SERVING

Cal 130 • **Total Fat** 8g • **Sat Fat** 1.5g • **Chol** 0mg
Sodium 300mg • **Total Carbs** 13g • **Fiber** 5g • **Total Sugar** 5g
Added Sugar 0g • **Protein** 5g • **Total Carbohydrate Choices** 1

VARIATIONS
Curried Cauliflower Rice

Add ¼ teaspoon ground cardamom, ¼ teaspoon ground cinnamon, and ¼ teaspoon ground turmeric to saucepan with shallot. Substitute 1 tablespoon shredded fresh mint for parsley and stir ¼ cup toasted sliced almonds into cauliflower rice with mint.

PER SERVING

Cal 160 • **Total Fat** 11g • **Sat Fat** 1.5g • **Chol** 0mg
Sodium 300mg • **Total Carbs** 14g • **Fiber** 6g • **Total Sugar** 5g
Added Sugar 0g • **Protein** 6g • **Total Carbohydrate Choices** 1

Tex-Mex Cauliflower Rice

Add 2 jalapeños, stemmed, seeded, and minced, 1 minced garlic clove, 1 teaspoon ground cumin, and 1 teaspoon ground coriander to saucepan with shallot. In step 3, substitute cilantro for parsley and 1 tablespoon lime juice for lemon juice and omit salt.

PER SERVING

Cal 140 • **Total Fat** 8g • **Sat Fat** 1.5g • **Chol** 0mg
Sodium 300mg • **Total Carbs** 14g • **Fiber** 5g • **Total Sugar** 5g
Added Sugar 0g • **Protein** 5g • **Total Carbohydrate Choices** 1

Marinated Eggplant with Capers and Mint
SERVES 6

WHY THIS RECIPE WORKS Marinated eggplant, a highlight of antipasto platters, has a surprisingly creamy texture and a deep yet tangy flavor. However, many recipes we tried turned out overly greasy, with accompanying flavors that were either muted and dull or so strong that they overwhelmed the eggplant. We wanted a recipe that would keep the eggplant in the spotlight, with a complementary, brightly flavored marinade. To start, we experimented with cooking techniques: We tried frying but found that the eggplant absorbed too much oil; pan-frying in batches required too much time for a simple side dish; and roasting yielded either leathery eggplant skin or undercooked and tough flesh. We found that broiling was perfect; we could achieve flavorful browning on the eggplant and it cooked through perfectly. To encourage even more browning, we first salted the eggplant, which drew out excess moisture. As for the marinade, a Greek-inspired combination of extra-virgin olive oil (using only a few tablespoons kept the eggplant from turning greasy), red wine vinegar, capers, lemon zest, oregano, garlic, and mint worked perfectly. We prefer using kosher salt because residual grains can be easily wiped away from the eggplant; if using table salt, be sure to reduce all of the salt amounts in the recipe by half.

1½ pounds Italian eggplant, sliced into 1-inch-thick rounds
   Kosher salt and pepper
¼ cup extra-virgin olive oil
4 teaspoons red wine vinegar
1 tablespoon capers, rinsed and minced
1 garlic clove, minced
½ teaspoon grated lemon zest
½ teaspoon minced fresh oregano
3 tablespoons minced fresh mint

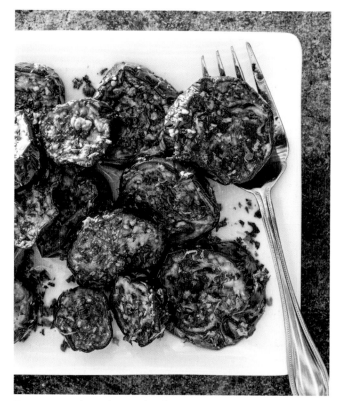

For marinated eggplant with a firm texture and a bit of flavorful browning, broiling is the perfect cooking method.

1. Spread eggplant on paper towel–lined baking sheet, sprinkle both sides with ½ teaspoon salt, and let sit for 30 minutes.

2. Adjust oven rack 4 inches from broiler element and heat broiler. Thoroughly pat eggplant dry with paper towels, arrange on aluminum foil–lined rimmed baking sheet in single layer, and lightly brush both sides with 1 tablespoon oil. Broil eggplant until mahogany brown and lightly charred, 6 to 8 minutes per side.

3. Whisk remaining 3 tablespoons oil, vinegar, capers, garlic, lemon zest, oregano, and ¼ teaspoon pepper together in large bowl. Add eggplant and mint and gently toss to combine. Let eggplant cool to room temperature, about 1 hour. Season with pepper to taste and serve.

PER SERVING

Cal 120 • **Total Fat** 10g • **Sat Fat** 1.5g • **Chol** 0mg
Sodium 85mg • **Total Carbs** 7g • **Fiber** 3g • **Total Sugar** 4g
Added Sugar 0g • **Protein** 1g • **Total Carbohydrate Choices** 0.5

Broiled Eggplant with Basil

SERVES 6

WHY THIS RECIPE WORKS This is a dead simple method for preparing eggplant, which can get soggy and mushy in many applications. If you simply slice and broil eggplant, it will steam in its own juice rather than brown. So to get broiled eggplant with great color and texture, we started by salting the eggplant to draw out its moisture. After 30 minutes, we patted the eggplant slices dry, moved them to a baking sheet (lined with aluminum foil for easy cleanup), and brushed them with oil. With the excess moisture taken care of, a few minutes per side under the blazing-hot broiler turned the eggplant a beautiful mahogany color. With its concentrated roasted flavor, all the eggplant needed was a sprinkling of fresh basil. It is important to slice the eggplant thin so that the interior will cook through by the time the exterior is browned. We prefer using kosher salt because residual grains can be easily wiped away from the eggplant; if using table salt, be sure to reduce the salt amount in the recipe by half.

1½ pounds eggplant, sliced into ¼-inch-thick rounds
    Kosher salt and pepper
3 tablespoons extra-virgin olive oil
2 tablespoons chopped fresh basil

1. Spread eggplant on paper towel–lined baking sheet, sprinkle both sides with 1½ teaspoons salt, and let sit for 30 minutes.

2. Adjust oven rack 4 inches from broiler element and heat broiler. Thoroughly pat eggplant dry with paper towels, arrange on aluminum foil–lined rimmed baking sheet in single layer, and brush both sides with oil. Broil eggplant until mahogany brown and lightly charred, about 4 minutes per side. Transfer eggplant to serving platter, season with pepper to taste, and sprinkle with basil. Serve.

PER SERVING
Cal 90 • **Total Fat** 7g • **Sat Fat** 1g • **Chol** 0mg
Sodium 140mg • **Total Carbs** 7g • **Fiber** 3g • **Total Sugar** 4g
Added Sugar 0g • **Protein** 1g • **Total Carbohydrate Choices** 0.5

All About Eggplant

Though it's commonly thought of as a vegetable, eggplant is actually a fruit. Eggplants are available year-round. When shopping, look for eggplants that are firm, with smooth skin and no soft or brown spots. They should feel heavy for their size. Eggplants are very perishable and will get bitter if they overripen, so aim to use them within a day or two. They can be stored in a cool, dry place short-term, but for more than one or two days, refrigeration is best. There are many varieties of eggplant, ranging anywhere from 2 to 12 inches long, from round to oblong, and from dark purple to white. Here are a few of the most common varieties:

Globe

The most common variety in the United States, globe eggplant has a mild flavor and a tender texture that works well in most cooked applications. It can be sautéed, broiled, grilled, and pureed. Because of its high water content, it's often best to lightly salt and drain it before cooking.

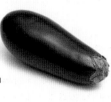

Italian

Also called baby eggplant, Italian eggplant looks like a smaller version of a globe eggplant. It has moderately moist flesh and a distinct spicy flavor and can be sautéed, broiled, grilled, and more.

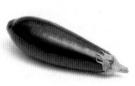

Chinese

Chinese eggplant has firm, somewhat dry flesh with an intense, slightly sweet taste. It is best for sautéing, stewing, or stir-frying.

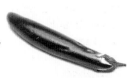

Thai

With crisp, applelike flesh and a bright, grassy flavor with a hint of spiciness, Thai eggplant can be eaten raw. It's also good sautéed or stir-fried.

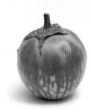

Braised Fennel with White Wine and Parmesan
SERVES 4

WHY THIS RECIPE WORKS While fennel is excellent served raw in salads and antipasti, its crisp anise flavor turns mild and sweet once cooked. We wanted a recipe for braised fennel that would infuse the fennel with rich, savory flavor. The problem with cooking fennel lies in trying to achieve uniformly tender pieces. A combination of proper vegetable prep and cooking technique turned out to be the key to evenly cooked fennel. Fan-shaped wedges proved good for braising because the thin slices cooked through quickly and evenly. It was important to cook the fennel slowly to deliver tender but not mushy results. A combination of butter, white wine, and Parmesan gave the fennel rich, balanced flavor.

   3 tablespoons extra-virgin olive oil
   2 fennel bulbs, stalks discarded, bulbs cut vertically
     into ½-inch-thick slices
     Salt and pepper
   ⅓ cup dry white wine
   ¼ cup grated Parmesan cheese

1. Heat 2 tablespoons oil in 12-inch nonstick skillet over medium heat until shimmering. Add fennel and sprinkle with ⅛ teaspoon salt and ⅛ teaspoon pepper. Add wine, cover, and simmer for 15 minutes.

2. Turn slices over and continue to simmer, covered, until fennel is nearly tender, has absorbed most of liquid, and starts to turn golden, about 10 minutes.

3. Turn fennel again and continue to cook until golden on second side, about 4 minutes. Transfer to serving platter, drizzle with remaining 1 tablespoon oil, and sprinkle with Parmesan. Serve.

PER SERVING

Cal 160 • **Total Fat** 12g • **Sat Fat** 2g • **Chol** 5mg
Sodium 200mg • **Total Carbs** 9g • **Fiber** 4g • **Total Sugar** 5g
Added Sugar 0g • **Protein** 3g • **Total Carbohydrate Choices** 0.5

SLICING FENNEL FOR BRAISING

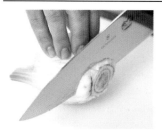 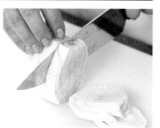

1. Cut off tops and feathery fronds, trim very thin slice from bottom of base, and remove any tough or blemished outer layers.

2. Place trimmed fennel bulb upright on base and cut vertically into ½-inch-thick slabs.

Sautéed Green Beans with Garlic and Herbs
SERVES 4

WHY THIS RECIPE WORKS To get tender, lightly browned, fresh-tasting green beans using just one pan, we turned to sautéing. But simply sautéing raw beans in hot oil resulted in blackened exteriors and undercooked interiors. Cooking the beans in water in a covered pan, then removing the lid to evaporate the liquid and brown the beans was better, but not foolproof. For the best results, we sautéed the beans until spotty brown, then added water to the pan and covered it so the beans could cook through. Once the beans were bright green but still crisp, we lifted the lid to evaporate the water and promote additional browning. A little olive oil added to the pan at this stage lent richness and promoted even more browning. A few additional ingredients, such as garlic and herbs, added flavor without overcomplicating our recipe. This recipe yields beans that are crisp-tender. If you prefer beans that are a little softer or if you are using large, tough beans, increase the amount of water by 1 tablespoon and cook, covered, for 1 minute longer.

   4 teaspoons extra-virgin olive oil
   3 garlic cloves, minced
   1 teaspoon minced fresh thyme
   1 pound green beans, trimmed and cut into 2-inch lengths
     Salt and pepper
   2 teaspoons lemon juice
   1 tablespoon minced fresh parsley, basil, and/or mint

1. Combine 1 tablespoon oil, garlic, and thyme in bowl. Heat remaining 1 teaspoon oil in 12-inch nonstick skillet over medium heat until just smoking. Add beans, ¼ teaspoon salt, and ⅛ teaspoon pepper and cook, stirring occasionally, until spotty brown, 4 to 6 minutes. Add ¼ cup water, cover, and cook until beans are bright green and still crisp, about 2 minutes.

2. Uncover, increase heat to high, and cook until water evaporates, 30 to 60 seconds. Add oil mixture and cook, stirring often, until beans are crisp-tender, lightly browned, and beginning to wrinkle, 1 to 3 minutes. Off heat, stir in lemon juice and parsley and season with pepper to taste. Serve.

PER SERVING

Cal 80 • **Total Fat** 5g • **Sat Fat** 0.5g • **Chol** 0mg
Sodium 150mg • **Total Carbs** 8g • **Fiber** 3g • **Total Sugar** 3g
Added Sugar 0g • **Protein** 2g • **Total Carbohydrate Choices** 0.5

VARIATIONS
Sautéed Green Beans with Thyme, Coriander, and Sesame Seeds

Add ¼ teaspoon ground coriander and ¼ teaspoon ground cumin to oil with garlic. Substitute 1 tablespoon toasted sesame seeds for parsley.

PER SERVING

Cal 90 • **Total Fat** 6g • **Sat Fat** 1g • **Chol** 0mg
Sodium 150mg • **Total Carbs** 9g • **Fiber** 3g • **Total Sugar** 3g
Added Sugar 0g • **Protein** 2g • **Total Carbohydrate Choices** 0.5

Sautéed Green Beans with Feta and Oregano

Omit thyme. Substitute 2 teaspoons minced fresh oregano for parsley and sprinkle with ¼ cup crumbled feta cheese before serving.

PER SERVING

Cal 100 • **Total Fat** 6g • **Sat Fat** 2g • **Chol** 5mg
Sodium 220mg • **Total Carbs** 8g • **Fiber** 3g • **Total Sugar** 4g
Added Sugar 0g • **Protein** 3g • **Total Carbohydrate Choices** 0.5

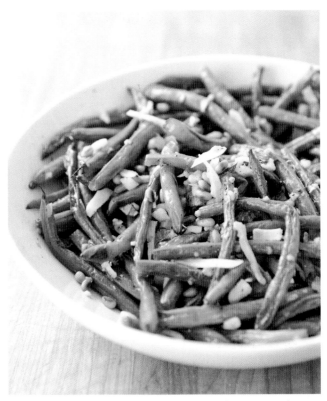

Roasting is a great way to add flavor to everyday supermarket green beans, and the method is fast and easy.

Roasted Green Beans with Pecorino and Pine Nuts
SERVES 6

WHY THIS RECIPE WORKS Roasted green beans can be dry and leathery; we wanted earthy, sweet beans with moist interiors and just the right amount of browning. We started by roasting the beans covered to allow them to steam and soften slightly. A mixture of flavorful extra-virgin olive oil, salt, and pepper was enough to season them thoroughly. To add a lively bite to the blistered beans, we tossed them with a lemony vinaigrette, microwaving garlic and lemon zest with oil to bloom their flavors and tame the garlic's raw bite. We topped the beans with salty, sharp Pecorino and crunchy toasted pine nuts. Use the large holes of a box grater to shred the Pecorino.

1½ pounds green beans, trimmed
¼ cup extra-virgin olive oil
Salt and pepper
2 garlic cloves, minced
1 teaspoon grated lemon zest plus 1 tablespoon juice
1 teaspoon Dijon mustard
2 tablespoons chopped fresh basil
¼ cup shredded Pecorino Romano cheese
2 tablespoons pine nuts, toasted

1. Adjust oven rack to lowest position and heat oven to 475 degrees. Toss green beans with 1 tablespoon oil, ¼ teaspoon salt, and ½ teaspoon pepper. Transfer to rimmed baking sheet and spread into single layer.

2. Cover sheet tightly with aluminum foil and roast for 10 minutes. Remove foil and continue to roast until green beans are spotty brown, about 10 minutes, stirring halfway through roasting.

3. Meanwhile, combine remaining 3 tablespoons oil, garlic, and lemon zest in medium bowl and microwave until bubbling, about 1 minute. Let mixture steep for 1 minute, then whisk in lemon juice, mustard, ⅛ teaspoon salt, and ¼ teaspoon pepper until combined.

4. Transfer green beans to bowl with dressing, add basil, and toss to combine. Season with pepper to taste. Transfer green beans to serving platter and sprinkle with Pecorino and pine nuts. Serve.

PER SERVING
Cal 150 • Total Fat 12g • Sat Fat 2g • Chol 0mg
Sodium 200mg • Total Carbs 8g • Fiber 3g • Total Sugar 3g
Added Sugar 0g • Protein 3g • Total Carbohydrate Choices 0.5

VARIATION
Roasted Green Beans with Almonds and Mint
Substitute lime zest and juice for lemon zest and juice, ¼ cup torn fresh mint leaves for basil, and toasted and chopped whole blanched almonds for pine nuts. Omit Pecorino.

PER SERVING
Cal 140 • Total Fat 11g • Sat Fat 1.5g • Chol 0mg
Sodium 170mg • Total Carbs 8g • Fiber 3g • Total Sugar 3g
Added Sugar 0g • Protein 3g • Total Carbohydrate Choices 0.5

Garlicky Braised Kale
SERVES 8

WHY THIS RECIPE WORKS For a one-pot recipe that would make the most of a generous harvest or market haul of hearty kale, we first briefly cooked it with broth. Onion and a substantial amount of garlic gave the greens some aromatic character. Adding the greens in three batches allowed them to wilt down so they fit in the pot. When the kale had reached the tender texture we wanted, we removed the lid and raised the heat to allow the liquid to cook off. This will look like a mountain of raw kale before it's cooked, but it wilts down and will eventually all fit into the pot.

6 tablespoons extra-virgin olive oil
1 large onion, chopped fine
10 garlic cloves, minced
¼ teaspoon red pepper flakes
2 cups unsalted chicken broth
Salt and pepper
4 pounds kale, stemmed and cut into 3-inch pieces
1 tablespoon lemon juice, plus extra for seasoning

1. Heat 3 tablespoons oil in Dutch oven over medium heat until shimmering. Add onion and cook until softened and lightly browned, 5 to 7 minutes. Stir in garlic and pepper flakes and cook until fragrant, about 1 minute. Stir in broth, 1 cup water, and ½ teaspoon salt and bring to simmer.

2. Add one-third of kale, cover, and cook, stirring occasionally, until wilted, 2 to 4 minutes. Repeat with remaining kale in 2 batches. Continue to cook, covered, until kale is tender, 13 to 15 minutes.

3. Remove lid and increase heat to medium-high. Cook, stirring occasionally, until most liquid has evaporated and greens begin to sizzle, 10 to 12 minutes. Off heat, stir in remaining 3 tablespoons oil and lemon juice. Season with pepper and extra lemon juice to taste. Serve.

PER SERVING
Cal 190 • Total Fat 12g • Sat Fat 1.5g • Chol 0mg
Sodium 240mg • Total Carbs 17g • Fiber 6g • Total Sugar 5g
Added Sugar 0g • Protein 8g • Total Carbohydrate Choices 1

Hearty Greens

Super-versatile hearty greens can be prepared in many ways, or added to a whole host of recipes to boost flavor and nutrition. Their sturdy leaves offer earthy flavor and texture as well as an abundance of nutrients—iron, fiber, vitamins K, A, and C, and magnesium, just to name a few. The season for hearty greens spans from early fall until late spring, sometimes stretching into summer. A large bunch of greens will reduce dramatically when cooked, so don't be intimidated if the greens initially dominate the pan.

Selecting Hearty Greens

There are many types of hearty greens, but the ones below are the ones we use most often since they are widely available in American markets.

Swiss Chard

Swiss chard has dark, ruffled leaves and tough stems that can be crimson red, orange, yellow, or white. The leaves and stems need to be cooked separately as the stems take much longer to soften. Look for bunches with bright stems and leaves that are firm and undamaged.

Collard Greens

Collard greens have dark green, very wide leaves and thick stems. Look for bunches with trimmed stems and no sign of yellowing or wilting. Unless you plan to slice the leaves thinly, it is best to braise collard greens until tender. They pair well with strongly flavored ingredients. Be sure to strip the leaves from the stems, which are tough and woody.

Kale

Kale comes in many varieties: curly green kale, red kale, more delicate Tuscan kale, and baby kale. The hearty leaves have a surprisingly sweet undertone. Kale is easy to find both in bunches and in prewashed bags. Tender baby kale can be eaten raw in salads without any special treatment, but mature kale is tougher. To eat it raw, cut it into pieces, then vigorously knead it for about 5 minutes.

Mustard Greens

There are many varieties of mustard greens, but the most common has crisp, bright green leaves and thin stems. These greens have a medium-hot flavor with a fairly strong bite.

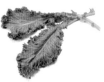

Storing Hearty Greens

To preserve freshness, store greens loosely in a dry plastic bag in the refrigerator. Kept this way, the greens can last for five to seven days.

PREPPING HEARTY GREENS

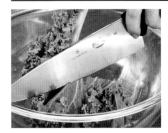

1A. To stem, hold leaf at base of stem and use knife to slash leafy portion from either side of tough stem.

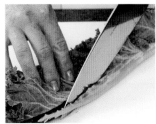

1B. Alternatively, fold each leaf in half and cut along edge of rib to remove the thickest part of rib and stem.

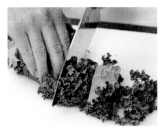

2. After separating leaves, stack several and either cut into strips or roll pile into cigar shape and coarsely chop.

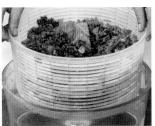

3. Fill salad spinner bowl with cool water, add cut greens, and gently swish them around. Let grit settle to bottom of bowl, then lift greens out and drain water. Repeat until greens no longer release any dirt.

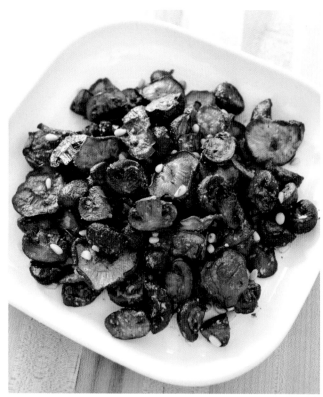

A light salt-water brine before roasting ensures evenly salted mushrooms; we then season with flavorings before serving.

Roasted Mushrooms with Parmesan and Pine Nuts

SERVES 4

WHY THIS RECIPE WORKS From earthy and smoky to deep and woodsy, mushrooms have an amazing range of flavors and textures. We decided to develop a simple side that showcased this versatile ingredient along with some bold flavors. A combination of full-flavored cremini and meaty shiitakes gave us the deepest, most well-rounded flavor. Sautéing the mushrooms required cooking them in multiple batches to achieve good browning, so we opted instead to roast them in a hot oven. But this presented a new problem: Since roasting concentrates flavor, it became clear that our mushrooms were unevenly seasoned—some were inedibly salty, and others were quite bland. To remedy this, we brined the mushrooms briefly before roasting. The salted water ensured even and thorough seasoning, and the excess water easily evaporated during cooking. Finally, we dressed the mushrooms in olive oil and lemon juice before adding flavorful Italian-inspired mix-ins: Parmesan, parsley, and pine nuts.

Salt and pepper
1½ pounds cremini mushrooms, trimmed and left whole if small, halved if medium, or quartered if large
1 pound shiitake mushrooms, stemmed, caps larger than 3 inches halved
3 tablespoons extra-virgin olive oil
1 teaspoon lemon juice
1 ounce Parmesan cheese, grated (½ cup)
2 tablespoons pine nuts, toasted
2 tablespoons chopped fresh parsley

1. Adjust oven rack to lowest position and heat oven to 450 degrees. Dissolve 5 teaspoons salt in 2 quarts room-temperature water in large container. Add cremini and shiitake mushrooms, cover with plate or bowl to submerge, and soak at room temperature for 10 minutes.

2. Drain mushrooms and pat dry with paper towels. Toss mushrooms with 2 tablespoons oil, then spread into single layer in rimmed baking sheet. Roast until liquid from mushrooms has completely evaporated, 35 to 45 minutes.

3. Remove sheet from oven (be careful of escaping steam when opening oven) and, using metal spatula, carefully stir mushrooms. Return to oven and continue to roast until mushrooms are deeply browned, 5 to 10 minutes.

4. Whisk remaining 1 tablespoon oil and lemon juice together in large bowl. Add mushrooms and toss to coat. Stir in Parmesan, pine nuts, and parsley and season with pepper to taste. Serve immediately.

PER SERVING
Cal 220 • **Total Fat** 16g • **Sat Fat** 2.5g • **Chol** 5mg
Sodium 190mg • **Total Carbs** 10g • **Fiber** 0.5g • **Total Sugar** 7g
Added Sugar 0g • **Protein** 9g • **Total Carbohydrate Choices** 0.5

VARIATIONS
Roasted Mushrooms with Harissa and Mint
In step 4, increase lemon juice to 2 teaspoons and whisk 1 minced garlic clove, 2 teaspoons harissa, ¼ teaspoon ground cumin, and ⅛ teaspoon salt into oil mixture. Omit Parmesan and pine nuts and substitute mint for parsley.

PER SERVING
Cal 180 • **Total Fat** 13g • **Sat Fat** 1.5g • **Chol** 0mg
Sodium 160mg • **Total Carbs** 11g • **Fiber** 1g • **Total Sugar** 7g
Added Sugar 0g • **Protein** 5g • **Total Carbohydrate Choices** 1

Roasted Mushrooms with Roasted Garlic and Smoked Paprika

Add 3 unpeeled whole garlic cloves to sheet with mushrooms. Remove garlic from sheet in step 3 when stirring mushrooms. When garlic is cool enough to handle, peel and mash. In step 4, substitute 2 teaspoons sherry vinegar for lemon juice and whisk mashed garlic, ½ teaspoon smoked paprika, and ⅛ teaspoon salt into oil mixture. Omit Parmesan and pine nuts.

PER SERVING

Cal 160 • **Total Fat** 11g • **Sat Fat** 1.5g • **Chol** 0mg
Sodium 140mg • **Total Carbs** 11g • **Fiber** 0.5g • **Total Sugar** 7g
Added Sugar 0g • **Protein** 5g • **Total Carbohydrate Choices** 1

PREPARING MUSHROOMS

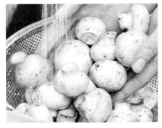

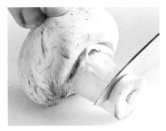

1. Rinse mushrooms under cold water just before cooking. Don't wash mushrooms that will be eaten raw; simply brush dirt away with soft pastry brush or cloth.

2. Tender stems on white button and cremini mushrooms should be trimmed, then prepped and cooked alongside caps. Tough, woody stems on shiitakes and portobellos should be removed.

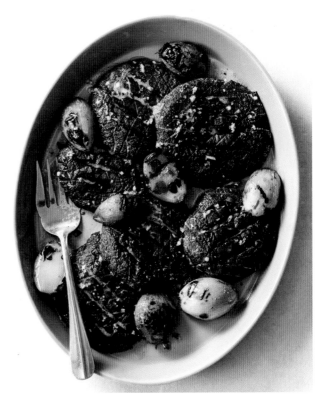

Cutting a crosshatch pattern into meaty portobello mushrooms helps them release moisture and absorb smoky flavor.

Grilled Portobello Mushrooms and Shallots with Rosemary-Dijon Vinaigrette
SERVES 6

WHY THIS RECIPE WORKS Meaty portobello mushrooms are a great match for the heat and smoke of the grill, which concentrates their flavor and produces perfect charred-on-the-outside, tender-on-the-inside mushrooms. To give these meaty mushrooms some extra interest, we decided to grill some aromatic shallots alongside and serve both with a lively dressing. We were happy to find that the shallots and mushrooms cooked in the same amount of time and had just enough smoky flavor after roughly 15 minutes on the grill. We drizzled our vegetables with the vinaigrette while they were still warm. You will need two 12-inch metal skewers for this recipe.

6 tablespoons extra-virgin olive oil
1 small garlic clove, minced
2 teaspoons lemon juice
1 teaspoon Dijon mustard
1 teaspoon minced fresh rosemary
  Salt and pepper
8 shallots, peeled
6 portobello mushroom caps (4 to 5 inches in diameter), gills removed

1. Whisk 2 tablespoons oil, garlic, lemon juice, mustard, rosemary, and ½ teaspoon salt together in small bowl. Season with pepper to taste; set aside for serving.

2. Thread shallots through roots and stem ends onto two 12-inch metal skewers. Using paring knife, cut ½-inch crosshatch pattern, ¼ inch deep, on tops of mushroom caps. Brush shallots and mushroom caps with remaining ¼ cup oil and season with pepper.

3A. FOR A CHARCOAL GRILL Open bottom vent completely. Light large chimney starter half filled with charcoal briquettes (3 quarts). When top coals are partially covered with ash, pour evenly over grill. Set cooking grate in place, cover, and open lid vent completely. Heat grill until hot, about 5 minutes.

3B. FOR A GAS GRILL Turn all burners to high, cover, and heat grill until hot, about 15 minutes. Turn all burners to medium.

4. Clean and oil cooking grate. Place shallots and mushrooms, gill side up, on grill. Cook (covered if using gas) until mushrooms have released their liquid and vegetables are charred on first side, about 8 minutes. Flip mushrooms and shallots and continue to cook (covered if using gas) until vegetables are tender and charred on second side, about 8 minutes. Transfer vegetables to serving platter. Remove skewers from shallots and discard any charred outer layers, if desired. Whisk vinaigrette to recombine and drizzle over vegetables. Serve.

PER SERVING

Cal 170 • **Total Fat** 14g • **Sat Fat** 2g • **Chol** 0mg
Sodium 230mg • **Total Carbs** 9g • **Fiber** 2g • **Total Sugar** 5g
Added Sugar 0g • **Protein** 3g • **Total Carbohydrate Choices** 0.5

PREPARING PORTOBELLOS FOR THE GRILL

Removing gills prevents muddy flavor, and scoring mushroom caps helps them release excess moisture.

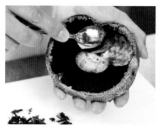 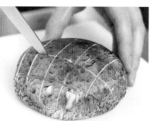

1. To prepare portobellos, use spoon to scrape gills off underside of mushroom cap.

2. Using tip of sharp knife, lightly score top of each mushroom cap in crosshatch pattern.

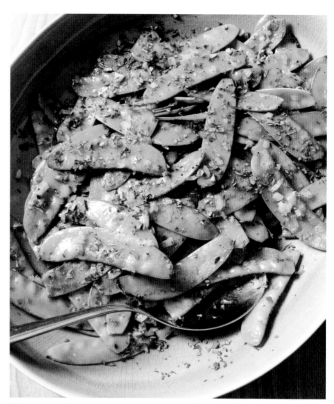

We mash a fragrant mixture of oil, shallot, and lemon zest into the center of the skillet after briefly cooking the snow peas.

Sautéed Snow Peas with Lemon and Parsley
SERVES 4

WHY THIS RECIPE WORKS If you simply toss delicate snow peas into a hot skillet with a little oil you will end up with a limp, army-green side dish that no one wants to eat. Our easy sauté method is a game changer, and with the variations below, you'll never be bored. To highlight and amplify the delicate flavor of the peas, we knew we needed to brown them to caramelize their flavor. We tried a traditional stir-fry technique, but the constant stirring gave us greasy, overcooked pods without any browning. Cooking the peas without stirring for a short time helped to achieve a flavorful sear, then we continued to cook them, stirring constantly, until they were just crisp-tender. To boost flavor, we cleared the center of the pan and quickly sautéed a mixture of minced shallot, oil, and lemon zest before stirring everything together. A squeeze of lemon juice and a sprinkling of parsley added just before serving kept this dish fresh and bright.

1 tablespoon canola oil
1 small shallot, minced
1 teaspoon finely grated lemon zest plus 1 teaspoon juice
12 ounces snow peas, strings removed
Salt and pepper
1 tablespoon minced fresh parsley

1. Combine 1 teaspoon oil, shallot, and lemon zest in bowl. Heat remaining 2 teaspoons oil in 12-inch nonstick skillet over high heat until just smoking. Add snow peas and sprinkle with ¼ teaspoon salt and ⅛ teaspoon pepper. Cook, without stirring, for 30 seconds. Stir briefly, then cook, without stirring, for 30 seconds. Continue to cook, stirring constantly, until peas are crisp-tender, 1 to 2 minutes.

2. Clear center of skillet, add shallot mixture, and cook, mashing mixture into skillet, until fragrant, about 30 seconds. Stir shallot mixture into peas. Stir in lemon juice and parsley and season with pepper to taste. Transfer to bowl and serve.

PER SERVING
Cal 70 • **Total Fat** 3.5g • **Sat Fat** 0g • **Chol** 0mg
Sodium 150mg • **Total Carbs** 7g • **Fiber** 2g • **Total Sugar** 4g
Added Sugar 0g • **Protein** 2g • **Total Carbohydrate Choices** 0.5

VARIATIONS
Sautéed Snow Peas with Ginger, Garlic, and Scallion
Substitute 2 minced garlic cloves, 2 teaspoons grated fresh ginger, and 2 minced scallion whites for shallot and lemon zest, and red pepper flakes for black pepper. Substitute rice vinegar for lemon juice, and 2 sliced scallion greens for parsley.

PER SERVING
Cal 70 • **Total Fat** 3.5g • **Sat Fat** 0g • **Chol** 0mg
Sodium 150mg • **Total Carbs** 7g • **Fiber** 2g • **Total Sugar** 3g
Added Sugar 0g • **Protein** 3g • **Total Carbohydrate Choices** 0.5

Sautéed Snow Peas with Garlic, Cumin, and Cilantro
Add 2 minced garlic cloves and ½ teaspoon toasted and lightly crushed cumin seeds to shallot mixture in step 1. Substitute ½ teaspoon lime zest for lemon zest, lime juice for lemon juice, and cilantro for parsley.

PER SERVING
Cal 70 • **Total Fat** 3.5g • **Sat Fat** 0g • **Chol** 0mg
Sodium 150mg • **Total Carbs** 7g • **Fiber** 2g • **Total Sugar** 4g
Added Sugar 0g • **Protein** 3g • **Total Carbohydrate Choices** 0.5

Sautéed Snow Peas with Lemon Grass and Basil
Substitute 2 teaspoons minced fresh lemon grass for lemon zest, lime juice for lemon juice, and basil for parsley.

PER SERVING
Cal 70 • **Total Fat** 3.5g • **Sat Fat** 0g • **Chol** 0mg
Sodium 150mg • **Total Carbs** 7g • **Fiber** 2g • **Total Sugar** 3g
Added Sugar 0g • **Protein** 2g • **Total Carbohydrate Choices** 0.5

REMOVING STRINGS FROM SNOW PEAS

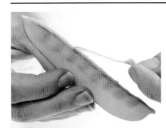

To remove the fibrous string from snow peas, simply snap off the tip of the snow pea while pulling down along the flat side of the pod. The same method also works for snap peas.

Roasted Smashed Potatoes
SERVES 6

WHY THIS RECIPE WORKS The majority of a potato's fiber is contained in the skin. Our unpeeled roasted smashed potatoes yield a creamy interior and satisfyingly crunchy exterior. We chose Red Bliss potatoes for their moist texture and thin skin. To soften the potatoes, we parcooked them on a baking sheet covered in foil on the oven's bottom rack, with a splash of water in the pan; this gave us creamy flesh that tasted sweet, deep, and earthy. Letting the hot potatoes rest after they parcooked meant they wouldn't crumble apart when smashed, and drizzling the potatoes with olive oil before and after smashing ensured that the oil reached every nook and cranny. And finally, using another baking sheet balanced on top of the parcooked potatoes to smash them gave us perfect cracked patties in one fell swoop. With a little chopped fresh thyme, that second drizzle of olive oil, and another stint in the oven, we had perfectly browned and crisp-skinned potatoes. This recipe is designed to work with potatoes 1½ to 2 inches in diameter; do not use potatoes any larger. It is important to thoroughly cook the potatoes so that they will smash easily. Remove the potatoes from the baking sheet as soon as they are done browning—they will toughen if left too long. A potato masher can also be used to "smash" the potatoes. We prefer to use kosher salt in this recipe. If using table salt, reduce salt to ½ teaspoon.

Understanding Potato Types

Though potatoes are considered a starchy vegetable and contain a fair amount of carbohydrates, they are also full of potassium, fiber, and other beneficial nutrients (especially if left unpeeled) and can be included in a diabetic diet as part of the starch and grain part of your plate. Different varieties of potatoes have varying textures (determined by starch level), so you can't just reach for any potato and expect great results. Potatoes fall into three main categories—baking, boiling, and all-purpose—depending on texture.

Baking Potatoes

Dry, floury baking potatoes contain more total starch (20 to 22 percent) than potatoes in other categories, giving them a dry, mealy texture. They are the best choice when baking and frying, and work well when you want to thicken a stew or soup, but not when you want distinct chunks of potatoes. Common varieties: russet, russet Burbank, and Idaho.

All-Purpose Potatoes

These potatoes contain less total starch (18 to 20 percent) than baking potatoes but more than firm boiling potatoes. All-purpose potatoes can be mashed or baked but won't be as fluffy as baking potatoes. They can also be used in salads and soups but won't be quite as firm as boiling potatoes. Common varieties: Yukon Gold, Yellow Finn, Purple Peruvian, Kennebec, and Katahdin.

Boiling Potatoes

Boiling potatoes contain a relatively low amount of total starch (16 to 18 percent), which means they have a firm, smooth, and waxy texture. Often they are called "new" potatoes because they are less-mature potatoes harvested in late spring and summer. They are less starchy than "old" potatoes because they haven't had time to convert their sugar to starch. They also have thinner skins. Firm, waxy potatoes are perfect when you want the potatoes to hold their shape, as with potato salad. They are also a good choice when roasting or boiling. Common varieties: Red Bliss, French fingerling, red creamer, and White Rose.

2 pounds small Red Bliss potatoes (about 18), scrubbed
¼ cup extra-virgin olive oil
1 teaspoon chopped fresh thyme
1 teaspoon kosher salt
⅛ teaspoon pepper

1. Adjust oven racks to top and bottom positions and heat oven to 500 degrees. Arrange potatoes on rimmed baking sheet, pour ¾ cup water into baking sheet, and wrap tightly with aluminum foil. Cook on bottom rack until paring knife or skewer slips in and out of potatoes easily (poke through foil to test), 25 to 30 minutes. Remove foil and cool 10 minutes. If any water remains on baking sheet, blot dry with paper towel.

2. Drizzle 2 tablespoons oil over potatoes and roll to coat. Space potatoes evenly on baking sheet and place second baking sheet on top; press down firmly on baking sheet, flattening potatoes until ⅓ to ½ inch thick. Remove top sheet and sprinkle potatoes evenly with thyme, salt, and pepper. Drizzle evenly with remaining 2 tablespoons oil.

3. Roast potatoes on top rack for 15 minutes. Transfer potatoes to bottom rack and continue to roast until well browned, 20 to 30 minutes longer. Serve immediately.

PER SERVING
Cal 190 • **Total Fat** 10g • **Sat Fat** 1.5g • **Chol** 0mg
Sodium 210mg • **Total Carbs** 24g • **Fiber** 3g • **Total Sugar** 2g
Added Sugar 0g • **Protein** 3g • **Total Carbohydrate Choices** 1.5

FLATTENING POTATOES EVENLY

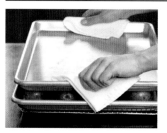 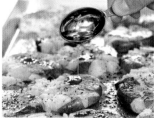

1. Place second baking sheet on top of partially cooled and oiled potatoes. Press down firmly and evenly on top sheet until potatoes are ⅓ to ½ inch thick.

2. Sprinkle flattened potatoes evenly with fresh thyme, kosher salt, and pepper, then drizzle with more olive oil before final stint in oven.

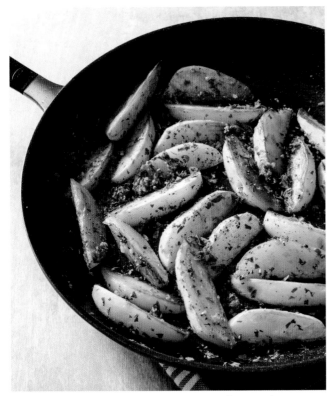

Greek-inspired potatoes feature bold lemon flavor and come together quickly in a skillet on the stovetop.

Greek-Style Garlic-Lemon Potatoes
SERVES 6

WHY THIS RECIPE WORKS In Greece, potato wedges are cooked in plenty of olive oil until browned and crisp and then accented with classic Greek flavors like lemon and oregano. For our version, we chose Yukon Golds, which hold their shape nicely and cook up with pleasantly fluffy interiors, and browned them in a nonstick skillet in olive oil to give them deep flavor and color. We then covered the pan to allow the potatoes to finish cooking through. A combination of juice and zest gave them full lemon flavor, and a modest amount of garlic contributed an aromatic backbone. Letting the lemon, garlic, and oregano cook briefly with the potatoes gave the dish a rounded, cohesive flavor profile. A final sprinkling of parsley added welcome freshness.

3 tablespoons extra-virgin olive oil
3 Yukon Gold potatoes (about 8 ounces each), peeled and cut lengthwise into 8 wedges
1½ tablespoons minced fresh oregano
3 garlic cloves, minced

2 teaspoons grated lemon zest plus 1½ tablespoons juice
Salt and pepper
1½ tablespoons minced fresh parsley

1. Heat 2 tablespoons oil in 12-inch nonstick skillet over medium-high heat until shimmering. Add potatoes cut side down in single layer and cook until golden brown on first side (skillet should sizzle but not smoke), about 6 minutes. Using tongs, flip potatoes onto second cut side and cook until golden brown, about 5 minutes. Reduce heat to medium-low, cover, and cook until potatoes are tender, 8 to 12 minutes.

2. Meanwhile, whisk remaining 1 tablespoon oil, oregano, garlic, lemon zest and juice, ½ teaspoon salt, and ½ teaspoon pepper together in small bowl. When potatoes are tender, gently stir in garlic mixture and cook, uncovered, until fragrant, about 2 minutes. Off heat, gently stir in parsley and season with pepper to taste. Serve.

PER SERVING
Cal 160 • **Total Fat** 7g • **Sat Fat** 1g • **Chol** 0mg
Sodium 200mg • **Total Carbs** 21g • **Fiber** 2g • **Total Sugar** 0g
Added Sugar 0g • **Protein** 3g • **Total Carbohydrate Choices** 1.5

Roasted Spiralized Sweet Potatoes with Walnuts and Feta
SERVES 6

WHY THIS RECIPE WORKS This nutritious side dish features spiralized sweet potatoes cut into beautiful ⅛-inch-thick noodles that cook quickly. We found that simply roasting the potatoes in a hot oven, uncovered, for about 12 minutes gave us the result we were after: sweet potatoes that were tender but not mushy, with just a bit of caramelization. To finish the dish, we sprinkled on ¼ cup each of tangy feta and earthy, omega-3-rich walnuts, plus a generous sprinkle of fresh parsley. Sweet potato noodles are quite delicate; be careful when tossing them with the oil and seasonings in step 2, and again when transferring them to the serving platter. If you do not have a spiralizer, you can use a mandoline or V-slicer fitted with a ⅛-inch julienne attachment. Make sure to position the vegetables on the mandoline vertically so that the resulting noodles are as long as possible. We do not recommend cutting vegetable noodles by hand.

2 pounds sweet potatoes, peeled
2 tablespoons extra-virgin olive oil
Salt and pepper

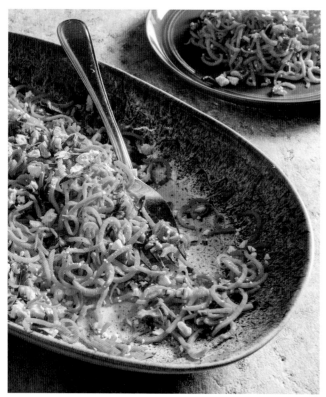

Roasted spiralized sweet potatoes take center stage when topped with briny feta cheese and omega-3-rich walnuts.

¼ cup walnuts, toasted and chopped coarse
1 ounce feta cheese, crumbled (¼ cup)
2 tablespoons chopped fresh parsley

1. Adjust oven rack to middle position and heat oven to 450 degrees. Using spiralizer, cut sweet potatoes into ⅛-inch-thick noodles, then cut noodles into 12-inch lengths.

2. Toss potato noodles with 1 tablespoon oil, ¼ teaspoon salt, and ⅛ teaspoon pepper and spread on rimmed baking sheet. Roast until potatoes are just tender, 12 to 14 minutes, stirring once halfway through roasting.

3. Season potatoes with pepper to taste and transfer to serving platter. Sprinkle walnuts, feta, and parsley over top, then drizzle with remaining 1 tablespoon oil. Serve.

PER SERVING
Cal 180 • **Total Fat** 8g • **Sat Fat** 1.5g • **Chol** 5mg
Sodium 210mg • **Total Carbs** 24g • **Fiber** 4g • **Total Sugar** 7g
Added Sugar 0g • **Protein** 3g • **Total Carbohydrate Choices** 1.5

Best Baked Sweet Potatoes
SERVES 4

WHY THIS RECIPE WORKS The goal when baking sweet potatoes is entirely different than when baking russets: creamy not fluffy flesh with deeply complex flavor. Sweet potatoes roast differently than russets due to their lower starch level and higher sugar content. We learned that to roast a whole sweet potato to the point where its exterior was nicely tanned and its interior was silky and sweetly caramelized, the potatoes needed to reach 200 degrees and stay there for an hour, long enough for the starches to gelatinize and moisture to evaporate for concentrated flavor. To keep our recipe efficient, we microwaved the potatoes until they hit 200 degrees and then transferred them to a hot oven to linger. Putting them on a wire rack set in a rimmed baking sheet allowed air to circulate around the potatoes and also caught any sugar that oozed from the potatoes as they roasted. Any variety of orange- or red-skinned, orange-fleshed sweet potato can be used in this recipe, but we highly recommend using Garnet (also sold as Diane). Avoid varieties with tan or purple skin, which are starchier and less sweet than those with orange and red skins. We prefer to use sweet potatoes that are smaller, about 8 ounces.

4 (8-ounce) sweet potatoes, unpeeled, each lightly pricked with fork in 3 places

1. Adjust oven rack to middle position and heat oven to 425 degrees. Place wire rack in aluminum foil–lined rimmed baking sheet and spray rack with vegetable oil spray. Place potatoes on large plate and microwave until potatoes yield to gentle pressure and reach internal temperature of 200 degrees, 6 to 9 minutes, flipping potatoes every 3 minutes.

2. Transfer potatoes to prepared rack and bake for 1 hour (exteriors of potatoes will be lightly browned and potatoes will feel very soft when squeezed).

3. Slit each potato lengthwise; using clean dish towel, hold ends and squeeze slightly to push flesh up and out. Transfer potatoes to serving dish. Serve.

PER SERVING
Cal 170 • **Total Fat** 0g • **Sat Fat** 0g • **Chol** 0mg
Sodium 120mg • **Total Carbs** 40g • **Fiber** 7g • **Total Sugar** 12g
Added Sugar 0g • **Protein** 3g • **Total Carbohydrate Choices** 2.5

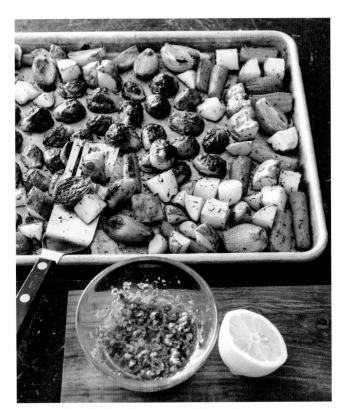

For roasted vegetables that are out of the ordinary, we serve them with a dressing bright with capers and lemon.

Roasted Root Vegetables with Lemon-Caper Sauce
SERVES 6

WHY THIS RECIPE WORKS We set out to create a hearty winter side that would elevate humble root vegetables. We chose a combination of Brussels sprouts, red potatoes, and carrots to create a balance of flavors and textures. To ensure that the vegetables would roast evenly, we cut them into equal-size pieces. Arranging the Brussels sprouts in the center of the baking sheet, with the hardier potatoes and carrots around the perimeter, kept the more delicate sprouts from charring in the hot oven. Before roasting, we tossed the vegetables with olive oil, thyme, and rosemary. Whole garlic cloves and halved shallots softened and mellowed in the oven, lending great flavor to the finished dish. Once all of the vegetables were perfectly tender and caramelized, we tossed them with a bright, Mediterranean-inspired dressing of lemon juice, capers, and parsley.

Starchy Versus Non-Starchy Vegetables

Vegetables are important to a diabetic diet—they are high in nutrients, fiber, and water content. Unfortunately, not all vegetables are created equal and for a diabetic diet it is important to distinguish non-starchy vegetables from their starchy counterparts.

Starchy vegetables are considered a carbohydrate food and must be accounted for when planning meals. They are nutrient-rich carb options; just make sure the portion is strictly controlled. The most common starchy vegetables include:

- Potatoes (keep on the skin to maximize the fiber)
- Sweet Potatoes and Yams
- Winter Squash (Acorn and Butternut)
- Beans (Pinto, Navy, Kidney, etc.)
- Peas
- Corn

On the flip side, non-starchy vegetables are low in carbohydrate content, high in fiber, and low in calories. Overall they do not affect blood sugar as much as starchy vegetables and can be eaten more liberally. Non-starchy vegetables are a great way to fill up your plate, balance out your meal, and get an infusion of various nutrients. There is a large variety of non-starchy vegetables with as many ways to cook them. Non-starchy vegetables include:

- Artichokes
- Asparagus
- Beets
- Broccoli
- Brussels Sprouts
- Cabbage
- Carrots
- Cauliflower
- Celery
- Cucumbers
- Eggplant
- Green Beans and Wax Beans
- Jícama
- Leafy Greens (Spinach, Kale, Chard, Collard Greens, etc.)
- Leeks
- Mushrooms
- Onions and Scallions
- Peapods
- Peppers
- Radishes
- Salad Greens (Romaine, Mixed Greens, Arugula)
- Tomatoes
- Turnips

1 pound Brussels sprouts, trimmed and halved
1 pound red potatoes, unpeeled, cut into 1-inch pieces
8 shallots, peeled and halved
4 carrots, peeled and cut into 2-inch lengths, thick ends halved lengthwise
6 garlic cloves, peeled
3 tablespoons extra-virgin olive oil
2 teaspoons minced fresh thyme
1 teaspoon minced fresh rosemary
Salt and pepper
2 tablespoons minced fresh parsley
1½ tablespoons capers, rinsed and minced
1 tablespoon lemon juice, plus extra for seasoning

1. Adjust oven rack to middle position and heat oven to 450 degrees. Toss Brussels sprouts, potatoes, shallots, and carrots with garlic, 1 tablespoon oil, thyme, rosemary, ½ teaspoon salt, and ¼ teaspoon pepper.

2. Spread vegetables into single layer on rimmed baking sheet, arranging Brussels sprouts cut side down in center of sheet. Roast until vegetables are tender and golden brown, 30 to 35 minutes, rotating sheet halfway through roasting.

3. Whisk parsley, capers, lemon juice, and remaining 2 tablespoons oil together in large bowl. Add roasted vegetables and toss to combine. Season with pepper and extra lemon juice to taste. Serve.

PER SERVING

Cal 200 • **Total Fat** 8g • **Sat Fat** 1g • **Chol** 0mg
Sodium 310mg • **Total Carbs** 31g • **Fiber** 7g • **Total Sugar** 8g
Added Sugar 0g • **Protein** 5g • **Total Carbohydrate Choices** 2

Sautéed Spinach with Yogurt and Dukkah
SERVES 4

WHY THIS RECIPE WORKS This stellar recipe pairs earthy spinach with a lemony yogurt sauce. To make a successful side dish using this pair of ingredients, we started with the spinach. We found that we greatly preferred the hearty flavor and texture of curly-leaf spinach to baby spinach, which wilted down into mush. We cooked the spinach in extra-virgin olive oil and, once it was cooked, used tongs to squeeze out the excess moisture. Lightly

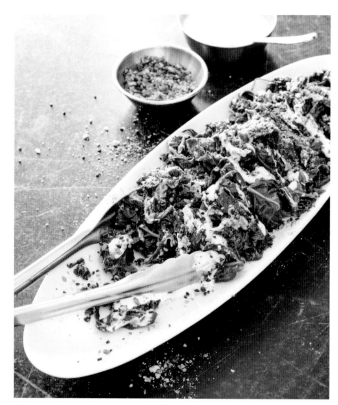

This modern take on spinach features a zesty yogurt sauce and a sprinkling of dukkah, a super-flavorful spice and nut blend.

toasted minced garlic, cooked after the spinach in the same pan, added a sweet nuttiness. We emphasized the yogurt's tanginess with lemon zest and juice and drizzled it over our garlicky spinach, but tasters thought the dish seemed incomplete. To elevate the flavor and give it some textural contrast, we sprinkled on some dukkah, an Egyptian blend of ground chickpeas, nuts, and spices. Two pounds of flat-leaf spinach (about three bunches) can be substituted for the curly-leaf spinach. When shopping for dukkah, look for a blend that doesn't include salt.

½ cup plain low-fat yogurt
1½ teaspoons grated lemon zest plus 1 teaspoon juice
3 tablespoons extra-virgin olive oil
20 ounces curly-leaf spinach, stemmed
2 garlic cloves, minced
Salt and pepper
¼ cup dukkah

1. Combine yogurt and lemon zest and juice in bowl; set aside for serving. Heat 1 tablespoon oil in Dutch oven over high heat until shimmering. Add spinach, 1 handful at a time, stirring and tossing each handful to wilt slightly before adding more. Cook spinach, stirring constantly, until uniformly wilted, about 1 minute. Transfer spinach to colander and squeeze between tongs to release excess liquid.

2. Wipe pot dry with paper towels. Add remaining 2 tablespoons oil and garlic to now-empty pot and cook over medium heat until fragrant, about 30 seconds. Add spinach and ⅛ teaspoon salt and toss to coat, gently separating leaves to evenly coat with garlic oil. Off heat, season with pepper to taste. Transfer spinach to serving platter, drizzle with yogurt sauce, and sprinkle with dukkah. Serve.

PER SERVING

Cal 180 • **Total Fat** 13g • **Sat Fat** 2g • **Chol** 0mg
Sodium 320mg • **Total Carbs** 10g • **Fiber** 4g • **Total Sugar** 2g
Added Sugar 0g • **Protein** 6g • **Total Carbohydrate Choices** <0.5

Sautéed Swiss Chard with Garlic
SERVES 6

WHY THIS RECIPE WORKS The key to sautéing hearty chard is to get the stems to finish cooking at the same time as the leaves. Unlike spinach's quick-cooking stems and kale's inedibly tough ribs, Swiss chard stems fall somewhere in the middle. To encourage the stems to cook efficiently and evenly, we sliced them thin on the bias and gave them a head start by sautéing them with garlic over relatively high heat, creating a crisp-tender texture and complex, lightly caramelized flavor. We introduced the tender leaves later and in two stages, allowing the first batch to begin wilting before adding the rest. Served with a squeeze of lemon, the result was a bright, nuanced side of greens with a range of appealing textures in every bite. You can use any variety of Swiss chard for this recipe.

2 tablespoons extra-virgin olive oil
3 garlic cloves, sliced thin
1½ pounds Swiss chard, stems sliced ¼ inch thick on bias, leaves sliced into ½-inch-wide strips
2 teaspoons lemon juice
    Pepper

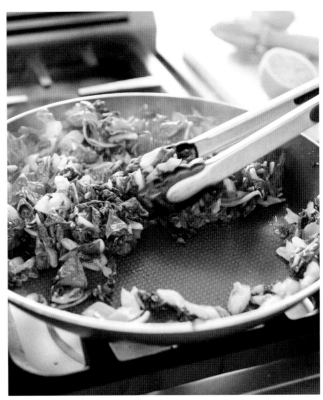

Swiss chard is a nutrition powerhouse so it's handy to have a simple recipe for how to cook it perfectly.

1. Heat oil in 12-inch nonstick skillet over medium-high heat until just shimmering. Add garlic and cook, stirring constantly, until lightly browned, 30 to 60 seconds. Add chard stems and cook, stirring occasionally, until spotty brown and crisp-tender, about 6 minutes.

2. Add two-thirds of chard leaves and cook, tossing with tongs, until just starting to wilt, 30 to 60 seconds. Add remaining chard leaves and continue to cook, stirring frequently, until leaves are tender, about 3 minutes. Off heat, stir in lemon juice and season with pepper to taste. Serve.

PER SERVING

Cal 60 • **Total Fat** 5g • **Sat Fat** 0.5g • **Chol** 0mg
Sodium 220mg • **Total Carbs** 5g • **Fiber** 2g • **Total Sugar** 1g
Added Sugar 0g • **Protein** 2g • **Total Carbohydrate Choices** 0.5

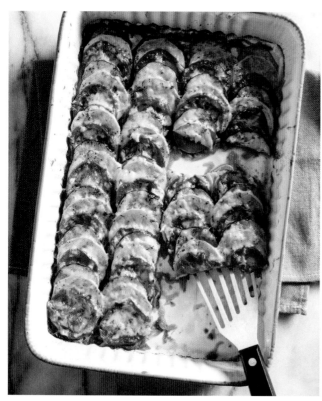

A topping of nutty Gruyère adds big flavor to this hearty tian featuring a trio of fresh vegetables.

Squash and Tomato Tian
SERVES 6

WHY THIS RECIPE WORKS Hailing from Provence and named for the region's popular terra-cotta dishes, a tian is a layered casserole of summer vegetables perfumed with olive oil and thyme and crusted with Gruyère cheese. The trick to a great tian is figuring out how to ensure perfectly cooked vegetables; mushy or under-cooked vegetables will not do. We started with a layer of caramelized onions, which we cooked with minced garlic to achieve full aromatic flavor. Similar-sized slices of zucchini and summer squash—and plum tomatoes, which have a similar diameter to squash—made up the rest of the vegetables. Cutting them all on a mandoline gave us perfect slices in seconds. Alternating the vegetables and keeping them fairly tightly shingled gave us the look we wanted and kept the whole dish sliceable.

As for cooking the tian, we found that covering the baking dish with foil trapped the heat and partially steamed the vegetables, allowing them to keep their moisture. After they'd steamed for 30 minutes, we sprinkled cheese over the top and returned the dish to the oven for the second phase of cooking. We like a mix of yellow summer squash and zucchini, but you can use just one or the other. Try to buy vegetables that are the same size, roughly 2 inches in diameter. Slicing the vegetables ⅛ inch thick is crucial for the success of this dish; use a mandoline, V-slicer, or food processor fitted with a ⅛-inch-thick slicing blade.

- 2 **tablespoons extra-virgin olive oil**
- 4 **onions, halved and sliced thin**
  Salt and pepper
- 2 **garlic cloves, minced**
- 1 **zucchini, trimmed and sliced ⅛ inch thick**
- 1 **yellow squash, trimmed and sliced ⅛ inch thick**
- I **pound plum tomatoes, cored and sliced ⅛ inch thick**
- 1 **teaspoon minced fresh thyme**
- 2 **ounces Gruyère cheese, shredded (½ cup)**

1. Heat 1 tablespoon oil in 12-inch nonstick skillet over medium-high heat until shimmering. Add onions and ¼ teaspoon salt and cook, stirring often, until softened, about 5 minutes. Reduce heat to medium-low and continue to cook, stirring frequently, until onions are golden and caramelized, about 30 minutes. Stir in garlic and cook until fragrant, about 30 seconds, then remove from heat.

2. Lightly spray 13 by 9-inch baking dish with vegetable oil spray. Adjust oven rack to middle position and heat oven to 375 degrees. Spread onion mixture in prepared dish. Alternately shingle zucchini, yellow squash, and tomatoes on top of onions.

3. Brush tops of vegetables with remaining 1 tablespoon oil. Sprinkle with thyme and season with pepper to taste. Cover dish tightly with foil and bake until vegetables are almost tender, about 30 minutes.

4. Remove foil, sprinkle with Gruyère, and continue to bake until bubbling around edges and lightly browned on top, 20 to 30 minutes. Let rest for 10 minutes before serving.

PER SERVING
Cal 140 • **Total Fat** 8g • **Sat Fat** 2.5g • **Chol** 10mg
Sodium 170mg • **Total Carbs** 12g • **Fiber** 3g • **Total Sugar** 7g
Added Sugar 0g • **Protein** 5g • **Total Carbohydrate Choices** 1

Zucchini, Tomato, and Potato Tian
Substitute 1 pound russet potatoes, peeled and sliced ⅛ inch thick, for yellow squash.

PER SERVING
Cal 190 • **Total Fat** 8g • **Sat Fat** 2.5g • **Chol** 10mg
Sodium 180mg • **Total Carbs** 25g • **Fiber** 3g • **Total Sugar** 6g
Added Sugar 0g • **Protein** 6g • **Total Carbohydrate Choices** 1.5

Squash, Tomato, and Eggplant Tian
We like to use thin, Japanese eggplant here because its narrow diameter matches that of other vegetables in dish. Large globe eggplant cannot be substituted.

Substitute 8 ounces Japanese eggplant, trimmed and sliced ⅛ inch thick, for zucchini.

PER SERVING
Cal 140 • **Total Fat** 8g • **Sat Fat** 2.5g • **Chol** 10mg
Sodium 170mg • **Total Carbs** 13g • **Fiber** 4g • **Total Sugar** 7g
Added Sugar 0g • **Protein** 5g • **Total Carbohydrate Choices** 1

ASSEMBLING A SUMMER VEGETABLE TIAN

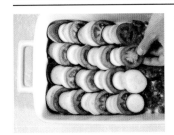

Alternately shingle the vegetables—zucchini, yellow squash, and tomatoes—tightly on top of the onions in tidy, attractive rows.

Spaghetti Squash with Garlic and Parmesan
SERVES 6

WHY THIS RECIPE WORKS The delicate flavor and creamy flesh of spaghetti squash make it a great addition to any meal, but many recipes bury the squash underneath too many competing flavors. We kept our recipe simple so the delicate and earthy flavor of the squash would shine through. Brushing the squash halves with oil, seasoning them with salt and pepper, and roasting them cut side down brought out the sweetness of the flesh. Once the squash was cooked, shredding it was as simple as holding the halves over a bowl and scraping them with a fork. After draining the excess

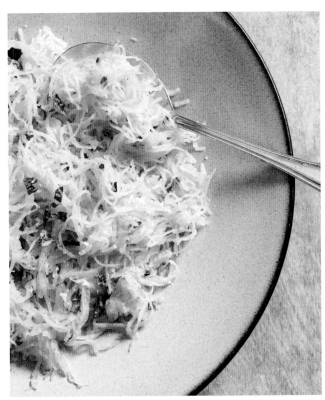

This spaghetti squash side dish gets a flavor boost from a mix of Parmesan, basil, lemon juice, and garlic.

liquid, we dressed the squash with Parmesan, fresh basil, lemon juice, and garlic for an easy, flavorful side dish that tasted like summer. Choose a firm squash with an even, pale-yellow color. Avoid greenish-tinged squashes, which are immature, and those that yield to gentle pressure, which are old.

1 spaghetti squash (2½ pounds), halved lengthwise and seeded
2 tablespoons extra-virgin olive oil
Salt and pepper
¼ cup grated Parmesan cheese
1 tablespoon chopped fresh basil
1 teaspoon lemon juice
1 garlic clove, minced

1. Adjust oven rack to middle position and heat oven to 450 degrees. Brush cut sides of squash with 1 tablespoon oil and sprinkle with ½ teaspoon salt and ¼ teaspoon pepper. Lay squash cut side down in 13 by 9-inch baking dish. Roast squash until just tender and tip of paring knife can be slipped into flesh with slight resistance, 25 to 30 minutes.

All About Squash

Generally, squash is divided into two categories: winter squash and summer squash. Zucchini and yellow squash are the most common varieties of summer squash. They both have thin, edible skins and a high moisture content, so they cook quickly whether steamed, baked, or sautéed. Winter squashes have hard, thick peels and firm flesh that requires longer cooking to turn tender. The flesh can vary from deep yellow to orange in color.

Buying Winter Squash

Whether acorn, butternut, delicata, or another variety, winter squash should feel hard; soft spots are an indication that the squash has been mishandled. Squash should also feel heavy for its size, a sign that the flesh is moist and ripe. Most supermarkets sell butternut squash that has been completely or partially prepped. Whole squash you peel yourself has the best flavor and texture, but if you are looking to save a few minutes of prep, we have found that the peeled and halved squash is fine. We don't like the butternut squash sold in chunks; while it's a timesaver, the flavor is wan and the texture stringy.

Buying Zucchini and Yellow Summer Squash

Choose zucchini and summer squash that are firm and without soft spots. Smaller squashes are more flavorful and less watery than larger specimens; they also have fewer seeds. Look for zucchini and summer squash no heavier than 8 ounces, and preferably just 6 ounces.

Storing Squash

You can store winter squash in a cool, well-ventilated spot for several weeks. Zucchini and summer squash are more perishable; store them in the refrigerator in a partially sealed zipper-lock bag for up to five days.

2. Flip squash over and let cool slightly. Holding squash with clean dish towel over large bowl, use fork to scrape squash flesh from skin while shredding it into fine pieces.

3. Drain excess liquid from bowl, then gently stir Parmesan, basil, lemon juice, garlic, and remaining 1 tablespoon oil into squash. Season with pepper to taste and serve.

PER SERVING

Cal 100 • **Total Fat** 6g • **Sat Fat** 1g • **Chol** 0mg
Sodium 260mg • **Total Carbs** 10g • **Fiber** 2g • **Total Sugar** 4g
Added Sugar 0g • **Protein** 2g • **Total Carbohydrate Choices** 0.5

SHREDDING SPAGHETTI SQUASH

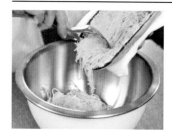

Holding roasted squash half with clean dish towel over large bowl, use fork to scrape squash flesh from skin, shredding flesh into fine pieces.

Roasted Winter Squash with Tahini and Feta
SERVES 6

WHY THIS RECIPE WORKS We wanted a savory recipe for roasted butternut squash that was simple but beyond the ordinary. We peeled the squash to remove not only the tough outer skin but also the rugged fibrous layer of white flesh just beneath, ensuring supremely tender squash. To encourage the squash slices to caramelize, we used a hot 425-degree oven, placed the squash on the lowest oven rack, and increased the baking time to evaporate moisture. Finally, we selected a mix of Greek-inspired toppings that added healthy crunch, creaminess, and fresh flavor: pistachios, feta, mint, and tahini spiked with lemon juice. This dish can be served warm or at room temperature. For the best texture, be sure to peel the squash thoroughly to remove all of the fibrous flesh just below the skin.

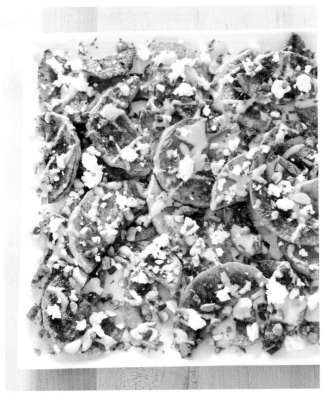

This dressed-up version of roasted squash has a hearty amount of fiber and protein and little saturated fat.

3 pounds butternut squash
3 tablespoons extra-virgin olive oil
Salt and pepper
1 tablespoon tahini
1½ teaspoons lemon juice
1 ounce feta cheese, crumbled (¼ cup)
¼ cup shelled pistachios, toasted and chopped fine
2 tablespoons chopped fresh mint

1. Adjust oven rack to lowest position and heat oven to 425 degrees. Using sharp vegetable peeler or chef's knife, remove squash skin and fibrous threads just below skin (squash should be completely orange with no white flesh). Halve squash lengthwise and scrape out seeds. Place squash cut side down on cutting board and slice crosswise into ½-inch-thick pieces.

2. Toss squash with 2 tablespoons oil, ½ teaspoon salt, and ½ teaspoon pepper and arrange in rimmed baking sheet in single layer. Roast squash until sides touching sheet toward back of oven are well browned, 25 to 30 minutes. Rotate sheet and continue to roast until sides touching sheet toward back of oven are well browned, 6 to 10 minutes.

3. Use metal spatula to flip each piece and continue to roast until squash is very tender and sides touching sheet are browned, 10 to 15 minutes.

4. Transfer squash to serving platter. Whisk tahini, lemon juice, remaining 1 tablespoon oil, and pinch salt together in bowl. Drizzle squash with tahini dressing and sprinkle with feta, pistachios, and mint. Serve.

PER SERVING
Cal 210 • **Total Fat** 12g • **Sat Fat** 2g • **Chol** 5mg
Sodium 250mg • **Total Carbs** 25g • **Fiber** 5g • **Total Sugar** 5g
Added Sugar 0g • **Protein** 4g • **Total Carbohydrate Choices** 1.5

CUTTING UP SQUASH FOR ROASTING

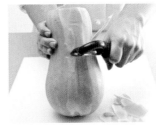

1. Using sharp vegetable peeler or chef's knife, remove squash skin and fibrous threads just below skin.

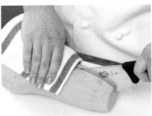

2. Carefully drive tip of chef's knife into center of peeled squash. Place folded dish towel on top of squash, over tip of knife.

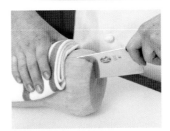

3. Drive rest of knife down through end of squash. Turn squash around and repeat from opposite side to cut squash in half.

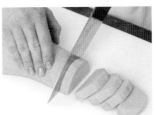

4. Scrape out seeds using spoon, then place squash flat side down on cutting board and slice into ½-inch-thick pieces.

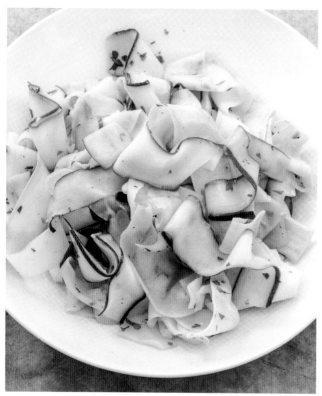

Thin ribbons of zucchini cook quickly in a little olive oil; a bright vinaigrette makes them irresistible.

Sautéed Zucchini Ribbons
SERVES 6

WHY THIS RECIPE WORKS Quick-cooking and delicately flavored, yellow summer squash and zucchini are ubiquitous in farmers' markets so it's good to have a variety of ways to use them. To create a fresh, simple recipe, we started with very thinly sliced squash, using a peeler to make even "ribbons" and discarding the waterlogged seeds. The ultrathin ribbons browned and cooked so quickly that they didn't have time to break down and release their liquid, eliminating the need to salt them before cooking. The cooked squash needed little embellishment; a quick, tangy vinaigrette of extra-virgin olive oil, garlic, and lemon and a sprinkle of fresh parsley rounded out the flavors. We like a mix of yellow summer squash and zucchini, but you can use just one or the other. The thickness of the squash ribbons may vary depending on the peeler used; we developed this recipe with our winning Kuhn Rikon Original Swiss Peeler, which produces ribbons that are 1/32 inch thick. Steeping the minced garlic in lemon juice mellows the garlic's bite; do not skip this step. To avoid overcooking the squash, start checking for doneness at the lower end of the cooking time.

1 small garlic clove, minced
1 teaspoon grated lemon zest plus 1 tablespoon juice
4 (6- to 8-ounce) zucchini and/or yellow summer squash, trimmed
2 tablespoons plus 1 teaspoon extra-virgin olive oil
Salt and pepper
1½ tablespoons chopped fresh parsley

1. Combine garlic and lemon juice in large bowl and set aside for at least 10 minutes. Using vegetable peeler, shave off 3 ribbons from 1 side of summer squash, then turn squash 90 degrees and shave off 3 more ribbons. Continue to turn and shave ribbons until you reach seeds; discard core. Repeat with remaining squash.

2. Whisk 2 tablespoons oil, 1/4 teaspoon salt, 1/8 teaspoon pepper, and lemon zest into garlic–lemon juice mixture.

3. Heat remaining 1 teaspoon oil in 12-inch nonstick skillet over medium-high heat until just smoking. Add squash and cook, tossing occasionally with tongs, until squash has softened and is translucent, 3 to 4 minutes. Transfer squash to bowl with dressing, add parsley, and gently toss to coat. Season with pepper to taste. Serve.

PER SERVING
Cal 70 • **Total Fat** 6g • **Sat Fat** 1g • **Chol** 0mg
Sodium 105mg • **Total Carbs** 4g • **Fiber** 1g • **Total Sugar** 2g
Added Sugar 0g • **Protein** 1g • **Total Carbohydrate Choices** <0.5

VARIATION
Sautéed Zucchini Ribbons with Mint and Pistachios
Substitute 1½ teaspoons cider vinegar for lemon juice and omit zest. Substitute 1/3 cup chopped fresh mint for parsley and sprinkle squash with 2 tablespoons toasted and chopped pistachios before serving.

PER SERVING
Cal 90 • **Total Fat** 7g • **Sat Fat** 1g • **Chol** 0mg
Sodium 105mg • **Total Carbs** 5g • **Fiber** 2g • **Total Sugar** 3g
Added Sugar 0g • **Protein** 2g • **Total Carbohydrate Choices** <0.5

Grilled Zucchini and Red Onion with Lemon-Basil Dressing
SERVES 4

WHY THIS RECIPE WORKS Perfectly tender grilled zucchini makes a great pairing for just about any grilled fish or meat. To double up on flavor, we wanted to combine zucchini with another vegetable. Mindful of their complementary cooking times, we paired our mild-flavored zucchini with sweet red onion. We cooked the onion slices on skewers to make sure they wouldn't fall apart. For a bright finish, we whisked up a quick lemon dressing to flavor the vegetables after they came off the grill, then topped them with fresh basil. After about 5 minutes, faint grill marks should begin to appear on the undersides of the vegetables; if necessary, adjust their position on the grill or adjust the heat level. The vegetables can be served hot, warm, or at room temperature. You will need two 12-inch metal skewers for this recipe.

1 large red onion, peeled and sliced into ½-inch-thick rounds
1 pound zucchini, sliced lengthwise into ¾-inch-thick planks
¼ cup extra-virgin olive oil
  Salt and pepper
1 teaspoon grated lemon zest plus 1 tablespoon juice
1 small garlic clove, minced
¼ teaspoon Dijon mustard
1 tablespoon chopped fresh basil

1. Thread onion rounds from side to side onto two 12-inch metal skewers. Brush onion and zucchini with 2 tablespoons oil, sprinkle with ⅛ teaspoon salt, and season with pepper. Whisk remaining 2 tablespoons oil, lemon zest and juice, garlic, mustard, and ¼ teaspoon salt together in bowl; set aside for serving.

2A. FOR A CHARCOAL GRILL Open bottom vent completely. Light large chimney starter half filled with charcoal briquettes (3 quarts). When top coals are partially covered with ash, pour evenly over grill. Set cooking grate in place, cover, and open lid vent completely. Heat grill until hot, about 5 minutes.

2B. FOR A GAS GRILL Turn all burners to high, cover, and heat grill until hot, about 15 minutes. Turn all burners to medium.

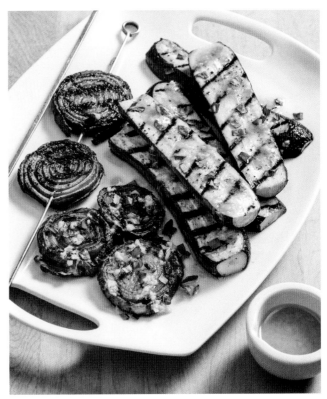

The key to cooking onions on the grill is to cut them into thick rounds and thread them onto skewers.

3. Clean and oil cooking grate. Place vegetables cut side down on grill. Cook (covered if using gas), turning as needed, until tender and caramelized, 18 to 22 minutes; transfer vegetables to serving platter as they finish cooking. Remove skewers from onion and discard any charred outer rings. Whisk dressing to recombine, then drizzle over vegetables. Sprinkle with basil and serve.

PER SERVING
Cal 160 • **Total Fat** 14g • **Sat Fat** 2g • **Chol** 0mg
Sodium 240mg • **Total Carbs** 7g • **Fiber** 2g • **Total Sugar** 4g
Added Sugar 0g • **Protein** 2g • **Total Carbohydrate Choices** 0.5

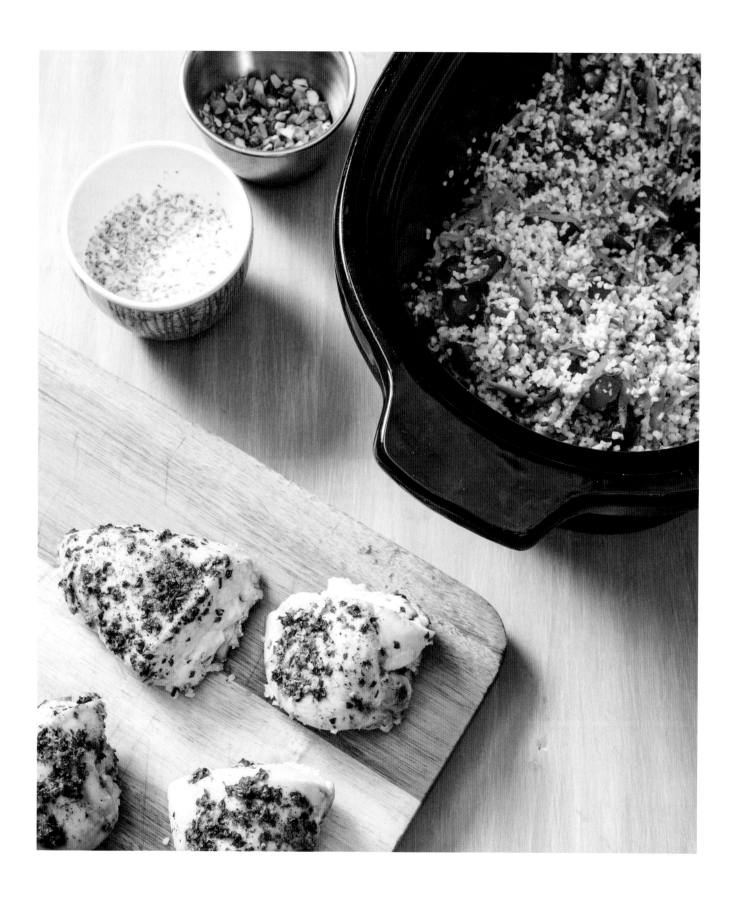

SLOW COOKER FAVORITES

NOTE: All recipes in this chapter require a 4- to 7-quart slow cooker. Some recipes require an oval slow cooker.

Photo: Herbed Chicken with Warm Bulgur Salad and Yogurt Sauce

Hearty Turkey Soup with Swiss Chard

SERVES 6

COOKING TIME 6 to 7 hours on Low

WHY THIS RECIPE WORKS Turkey thighs deliver a full-flavored soup without a lot of extra steps. To complement the meaty turkey, we microwaved leeks and colorful chard stems to bring out their sweetness, which added valuable depth to the broth. Nutritious chopped chard leaves were added during the last 20 minutes of cooking for an earthy contrast. Orzo was the perfect addition to the soup, adding substance. For the turkey, you can substitute an equal amount of bone-in chicken thighs; reduce the cooking time to 4 to 5 hours.

1½ pounds leeks, white and light green parts only, halved lengthwise, sliced ¼ inch thick, and washed thoroughly
8 ounces Swiss chard, stems chopped and leaves cut into 1-inch pieces
4 teaspoons extra-virgin olive oil
1 teaspoon no-salt-added tomato paste
1 teaspoon minced fresh thyme or ¼ teaspoon dried
Salt and pepper
8 cups unsalted chicken broth
2 carrots, peeled and cut into ½-inch pieces
2 bay leaves
2 pounds bone-in turkey thighs, skin removed, trimmed of all visible fat
¼ cup 100 percent whole-wheat orzo

1. Microwave leeks, chard stems, 1 tablespoon oil, tomato paste, thyme, and ½ teaspoon salt in bowl, stirring occasionally, until vegetables are softened, about 5 minutes; transfer to slow cooker. Stir in broth, carrots, and bay leaves. Nestle turkey thighs into slow cooker. Cover and cook until turkey is tender, 6 to 7 hours on low.

2. Meanwhile, bring 2 quarts water to boil in large saucepan. Add orzo and ½ teaspoon salt and cook, stirring often, until al dente. Drain orzo, rinse with cold water, then toss with remaining 1 teaspoon oil in bowl; set aside.

3. Transfer turkey to cutting board, let cool slightly, then shred into bite-size pieces using 2 forks; discard bones. Discard bay leaves.

4. Stir chard leaves into soup, cover, and cook on high until tender, 20 to 30 minutes. Stir in orzo and turkey and let sit until heated through, about 5 minutes. Season with pepper to taste. Serve.

PER 2-CUP SERVING
Cal 210 • **Total Fat** 6g • **Sat Fat** 1g • **Chol** 60mg
Sodium 600mg • **Total Carbs** 17g • **Fiber** 4g • **Total Sugar** 5g
Added Sugar 0g • **Protein** 24g • **Total Carbohydrate Choices** 1

SHREDDING MEAT

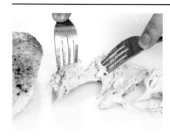

To shred chicken, turkey, beef, or pork into bite-size pieces, hold a fork in each hand, with the tines facing down. Insert the tines into the cooked meat and gently pull the forks away from each other, breaking the meat apart.

PREPARING LEEKS

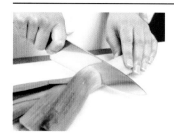

1. Trim and discard root and dark green leaves.

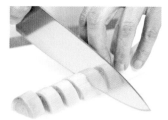

2. Cut trimmed leek in half lengthwise, then slice into pieces according to recipe.

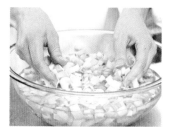

3. Rinse cut leeks thoroughly using salad spinner or bowl of water to remove dirt and sand.

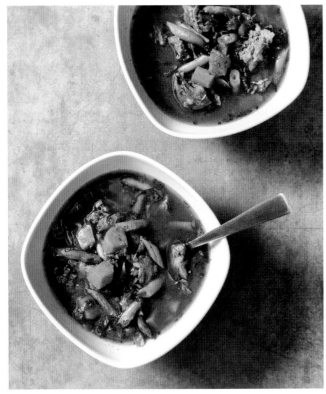

Lean and easy-to-prep, blade steaks lend great beefy flavor to this vegetable-packed soup.

Beef and Garden Vegetable Soup
SERVES 6
COOKING TIME 9 to 10 hours on Low or 6 to 7 hours on High

WHY THIS RECIPE WORKS It's rare that you find a vegetable-packed soup that also features tender, juicy chunks of beef, but this slow-cooker version does just that. Because the meat simmers for hours in the slow cooker, it infuses the fragrant broth with beefy flavor. To build flavor, we doctored chicken broth with dried porcini mushrooms, tomato paste, and soy sauce for depth and sweetness. While most beef soups go heavy on the meat and light on the vegetables, we increased the amount of vegetables to add substance and fiber to the soup. One final touch perfected our beef and vegetable soup recipe: Steaming green beans in the microwave with a little bit of water and adding them at the end of cooking ensured that they were not overcooked and stayed crisp and green.

2 onions, chopped fine
3 tablespoons no-salt-added tomato paste
4 garlic cloves, minced
1 tablespoon minced fresh thyme or 1 teaspoon dried
¼ ounce dried porcini mushrooms, rinsed and minced
1 tablespoon canola oil
  Salt and pepper
6 cups unsalted chicken broth
4 carrots, peeled and cut into ½-inch pieces
1 (14.5-ounce) can no-salt-added diced tomatoes
2 teaspoons low-sodium soy sauce
2 pounds beef blade steaks, ¾ to 1 inch thick, trimmed of all visible fat and gristle
8 ounces green beans, trimmed and cut on bias into 1-inch lengths
¼ cup chopped fresh basil

1. Microwave onions, tomato paste, garlic, thyme, porcini, oil, and ½ teaspoon salt in bowl, stirring occasionally, until onions are softened, about 5 minutes; transfer to slow cooker. Stir in broth, carrots, tomatoes and their juice, and soy sauce. Nestle steaks into slow cooker. Cover and cook until beef is tender, 9 to 10 hours on low or 6 to 7 hours on high.

2. Transfer steaks to cutting board, let cool slightly, then shred into bite-size pieces using 2 forks; discard gristle.

3. Microwave green beans with 1 tablespoon water in covered bowl, stirring occasionally, until crisp-tender, 4 to 6 minutes. Drain green beans, then stir into soup along with beef; let sit until heated through, about 5 minutes. Stir in basil and season with pepper to taste. Serve.

PER 2-CUP SERVING
Cal 330 • **Total Fat** 12g • **Sat Fat** 4.5g • **Chol** 105mg
Sodium 560mg • **Total Carbs** 19g • **Fiber** 6g • **Total Sugar** 10g
Added Sugar 0g • **Protein** 38g • **Total Carbohydrate Choices** 1

TRIMMING BLADE STEAKS

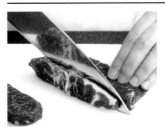

To trim blade steaks, halve each steak lengthwise, leaving the gristle on one half. Then simply cut the gristle away.

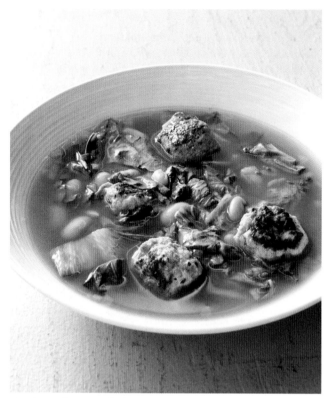

Thanks to the escarole, beans, and turkey, this meatball soup is loaded with protein and low in saturated fat.

Italian Meatball and Escarole Soup

SERVES 6

COOKING TIME 4 to 6 hours on Low or 3 to 5 hours on High

WHY THIS RECIPE WORKS Hearty beans, delicate meatballs, and wilted greens make for a classic and healthy Italian soup, but timing the dish in a slow cooker took extra care. While most bean-based soups start with cooking dried beans for hours before adding the meatballs, this just would not work in the slow cooker. So rather than settle for a soup with tough meatballs or under-cooked beans, we reached for canned beans and broth. To create our rich Italian-style broth we added some classic ingredients: onion, garlic, and red pepper flakes. For the meatballs we decided to use flavorful ground turkey. To protect the lean meat from drying out, we mixed it with a panade (a combination of bread and milk) as well as some Parmesan cheese and an egg yolk for flavor and richness. Searing the meatballs in a skillet before adding them to the slow cooker allowed them to keep their shape and added a browned, meaty flavor to the broth. Since we had the skillet out, we took the opportunity to brown our aromatics to

further enhance their flavor. Escarole, which is rich in fiber, vitamins, and minerals, ramped up the nutritional profile of this hearty soup. We sliced a whole head and stirred it in toward the end. Be sure to use ground turkey, not ground turkey breast (also labeled 99 percent fat-free), in this recipe.

> 2 slices 100 percent whole-wheat sandwich bread, torn into quarters
> ¼ cup 1 percent low-fat milk
> 1 ounce Parmesan cheese, grated (½ cup)
> 3 tablespoons minced fresh parsley
> 1 large egg yolk
> 1½ teaspoons minced fresh oregano or ½ teaspoon dried
> 4 garlic cloves, minced
> Salt and pepper
> 1 pound ground turkey
> 2 teaspoons canola oil
> 1 onion, chopped fine
> ¼ teaspoon red pepper flakes
> 6 cups unsalted chicken broth
> 1 (15-ounce) can no-salt-added cannellini beans, rinsed
> 1 head escarole (1 pound), trimmed and sliced 1 inch thick
> 1 tablespoon lemon juice

1. Mash bread, milk, Parmesan, parsley, egg yolk, oregano, half of garlic, and ½ teaspoon pepper into paste in large bowl using fork. Add ground turkey and hand-knead until well combined. Pinch off and roll turkey mixture into tablespoon-size meatballs (about 24 meatballs).

2. Heat 1 teaspoon oil in 12-inch nonstick skillet over medium heat until shimmering. Brown half of meatballs on all sides, about 5 minutes; transfer to slow cooker. Repeat with remaining 1 teaspoon oil and remaining meatballs; transfer to slow cooker.

3. Add onion and ½ teaspoon salt to fat left in skillet and cook over medium heat until onion is softened, about 5 minutes. Stir in pepper flakes and remaining garlic and cook until fragrant, about 30 seconds; transfer to slow cooker. Gently stir in broth and beans, cover, and cook until meatballs are tender, 4 to 6 hours on low or 3 to 5 hours on high.

4. Stir escarole into soup, 1 handful at a time, cover, and cook on high until tender, 15 to 20 minutes. Stir in lemon juice and season with pepper to taste. Serve.

PER 2-CUP SERVING

Cal 250 • **Total Fat** 6g • **Sat Fat** 2.5g • **Chol** 65mg
Sodium 540mg • **Total Carbs** 14g • **Fiber** 7g • **Total Sugar** 5g
Added Sugar 0g • **Protein** 30g • **Total Carbohydrate Choices** 1

Spring Vegetable and Barley Soup

SERVES 6

COOKING TIME 4 to 6 hours on Low or 3 to 5 hours on High

WHY THIS RECIPE WORKS For a light spring soup, we paired asparagus and summer squash with hearty pearl barley. To build flavor in such a simple soup, we found we needed to get out our skillet and sauté a hefty amount of shallots until softened and just starting to brown, then add garlic and red pepper flakes before transferring them to the slow cooker along with broth, barley, and lemon zest. The barley itself added a filling texture and a nutty taste, and as it simmered with the rest of the ingredients, it acquired the flavor of the aromatic broth. A sprinkling of Parmesan before serving added welcome richness to this light, fragrant soup. Do not substitute hulled, hull-less, quick-cooking, or presteamed barley for the pearled barley in this recipe.

- 1 tablespoon extra-virgin olive oil
- 4 shallots, minced
- 4 garlic cloves, minced
- ¼ teaspoon red pepper flakes
- 8 cups unsalted chicken broth
- ¾ cup pearled barley
- 2 (2-inch) strips lemon zest
  Salt and pepper
- 8 ounces thin asparagus, trimmed and cut on bias into 1-inch lengths
- 1 yellow summer squash, quartered lengthwise and sliced ½ inch thick
- 2 ounces (2 cups) baby arugula
- ¼ cup grated Parmesan cheese

1. Heat oil in 12-inch skillet over medium heat until shimmering. Add shallots and cook until softened and lightly browned, about 5 minutes. Stir in garlic and pepper flakes and cook until fragrant, about 30 seconds. Stir in 1 cup broth, scraping up any browned bits; transfer to slow cooker. Stir in remaining 7 cups broth, barley, lemon zest, and ½ teaspoon salt. Cover and cook until barley is tender, 4 to 6 hours on low or 3 to 5 hours on high.

2. Stir asparagus and squash into soup, cover, and cook on high until tender, 20 to 30 minutes. Stir in arugula and let sit until slightly wilted, about 3 minutes. Season with pepper to taste. Sprinkle individual portions with Parmesan before serving.

PER 2-CUP SERVING

Cal 190 • **Total Fat** 4.5g • **Sat Fat** 1g • **Chol** 5mg
Sodium 460mg • **Total Carbs** 28g • **Fiber** 7g • **Total Sugar** 5g
Added Sugar 0g • **Protein** 12g • **Total Carbohydrate Choices** 2

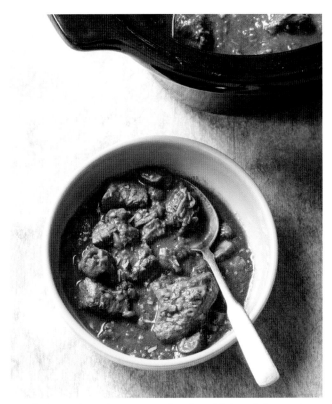

Smoked paprika and cinnamon plus the addition of chopped almonds and parsley help give this stew its Catalan identity.

Catalan Beef Stew

SERVES 6

COOKING TIME 9 to 10 hours on Low or 6 to 7 hours on High

WHY THIS RECIPE WORKS This super-flavorful Spanish-style stew features tender chunks of beef, mushrooms, and tomatoes. Chopped almonds and parsley contribute more flavor while adding crunch and a nutritional boost. To streamline the preparation, we browned only half the beef, which gave us the same flavor without a lot of work. We then bolstered the base of the stew with hearty tomato paste, garlic, and spices to achieve maximum impact, using flour as the thickener. Deglazing the pan with beef broth and wine preserved all of our precious flavors.

- 2 pounds boneless beef chuck-eye roast, trimmed of all visible fat, and cut into 1½-inch pieces
  Salt and pepper
- 4 teaspoons canola oil
- 1 pound cremini mushrooms, trimmed and quartered
- 2 onions, chopped fine
- 3 tablespoons all-purpose flour

¼ cup no-salt-added tomato paste

3 garlic cloves, minced

1 teaspoon smoked paprika

¾ teaspoon ground cinnamon

2 cups low-sodium beef broth

½ cup dry white wine

2 (14.5-ounce) cans no-salt-added diced tomatoes, drained

¼ cup slivered almonds, toasted and chopped fine

2 tablespoons minced fresh parsley

1 tablespoon sherry vinegar

1. Pat beef dry with paper towels and sprinkle with ½ teaspoon salt and ¼ teaspoon pepper. Heat 1 teaspoon oil in 12-inch skillet over medium-high heat until just smoking. Brown half of beef on all sides, about 8 minutes; transfer to slow cooker along with remaining uncooked beef.

2. Add mushrooms, onions, and remaining 1 tablespoon oil to fat left in skillet and cook over medium heat until softened and lightly browned, about 10 minutes. Stir in flour, tomato paste, garlic, paprika, and cinnamon and cook until fragrant, about 1 minute. Slowly whisk in broth and wine, scraping up any browned bits and smoothing out any lumps; transfer to slow cooker.

3. Stir tomatoes into slow cooker, cover, and cook until beef is tender, 9 to 10 hours on low or 6 to 7 hours on high. Stir in almonds, parsley, and vinegar. Season with pepper to taste. Serve.

PER 1²/₃-CUP SERVING

Cal 350 • **Total Fat** 13g • **Sat Fat** 3.5g • **Chol** 100mg
Sodium 460mg • **Total Carbs** 16g • **Fiber** 3g • **Total Sugar** 6g
Added Sugar 0g • **Protein** 38g • **Total Carbohydrate Choices** 1

NOTES FROM THE TEST KITCHEN

Testing Slow Cookers

Previous experience testing slow cookers taught us that glass lids were a must; so were oval-shaped crocks, as these can accommodate large roasts and offer more versatility than round crocks. The **KitchenAid 6-Quart Slow Cooker with Solid Glass Lid** ($99.99) met all our criteria. We also liked its well-designed control panel with a countdown timer that was simple and unambiguous to set and allowed us to monitor progress.

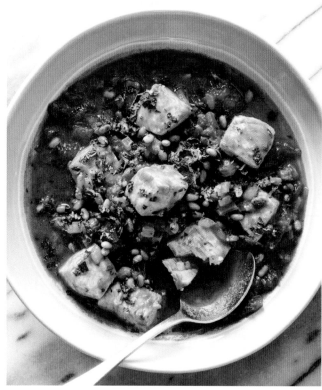

Sturdy swordfish steaks, cut into pieces, are added to the slow cooker for the last 30 minutes in this flavorful Sicilian stew.

Sicilian Fish Stew
SERVES 6
COOKING TIME 4 to 6 hours on Low or 3 to 5 hours on High

WHY THIS RECIPE WORKS In Sicily, fish is combined with tomatoes and local ingredients to create a simple stew that relies on the intermingling of salty, sweet, and sour flavors. For our slow cooker riff on this stew we created a balanced tomatoey broth base from a basic trio of ingredients: onions, celery, and garlic, which we bloomed in the microwave along with tomato paste and thyme. Some clam juice gave us the brininess of the sea, and a little white wine gave us much needed acidity. Golden raisins and capers imparted nice punches of sweet and salty flavor. Cooking the swordfish for only the last half-hour ensured tender, flaky fish that remained moist. And since many fish stews feature a nutty herb topping for a hit of texture and flavor, we went with a slight twist on gremolata, a classic Italian herb condiment, swapping in mint and orange for the usual lemon and parsley to give us nuanced freshness. Halibut is a good substitute for the swordfish.

2 onions, chopped fine
1 celery rib, chopped fine
2 tablespoons extra-virgin olive oil
2 tablespoons no-salt-added tomato paste
4 garlic cloves, minced
1 teaspoon minced fresh thyme or ¼ teaspoon dried
　Salt and pepper
　Pinch red pepper flakes
2 (8-ounce) bottles clam juice
1 (14.5-ounce) can no-salt-added diced tomatoes, drained
¼ cup dry white wine
2 tablespoons golden raisins
2 tablespoons capers, rinsed
1½ pounds skinless swordfish steaks, 1 to 1½ inches thick, cut into 1-inch pieces
¼ cup pine nuts, toasted and chopped
¼ cup minced fresh mint
1 teaspoon grated orange zest

1. Microwave onions, celery, oil, tomato paste, three-quarters of garlic, thyme, ½ teaspoon salt, ¼ teaspoon pepper, and pepper flakes in bowl, stirring occasionally, until vegetables are softened, about 5 minutes; transfer to slow cooker. Stir in clam juice, tomatoes, wine, raisins, and capers, cover, and cook until flavors meld, 4 to 6 hours on low or 3 to 5 hours on high.

2. Stir swordfish into stew, cover, and cook on high until swordfish flakes apart when gently prodded with paring knife, about 30 minutes.

3. Combine pine nuts, mint, orange zest, and remaining garlic in bowl. Season stew with pepper to taste. Serve, topping individual portions with pine nut mixture.

PER 1-CUP SERVING

Cal 300 • **Total Fat** 16g • **Sat Fat** 3g • **Chol** 75mg
Sodium 500mg • **Total Carbs** 12g • **Fiber** 2g • **Total Sugar** 6g
Added Sugar 0g • **Protein** 25g • **Total Carbohydrate Choices** 1

CUTTING UP SWORDFISH FOR STEW

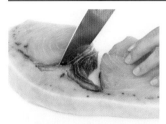 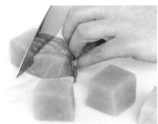

1. Using sharp knife, trim skin and dark lines from flesh.　**2.** Cut trimmed flesh into 1-inch pieces.

Turkey Chili
SERVES 8
COOKING TIME 4 to 5 hours on Low

WHY THIS RECIPE WORKS Turkey chili is a great alternative to classic beef chili, providing a leaner but no less flavorful meal for the dinner table. To keep the turkey moist and tender while slow cooking, we treat it with salt and baking soda. Both ingredients help the meat hold on to moisture, so it doesn't shed liquid during cooking. We also found the addition of broth and a little low-sodium soy sauce helped reinforce the meatiness of the leaner meat. Be sure to use ground turkey, not ground turkey breast (also labeled 99 percent fat-free), in this recipe.

2 pounds ground turkey
2 tablespoons water
　Salt and pepper
½ teaspoon baking soda
¼ cup canola oil
3 onions, chopped fine
1 red bell pepper, stemmed, seeded, and chopped
¼ cup no-salt-added tomato paste
3 tablespoons chili powder
6 garlic cloves, minced
1 tablespoon ground cumin
¾ teaspoon dried oregano
1¼ cups unsalted chicken broth, plus extra as needed
2 tablespoons low-sodium soy sauce
2 (15-ounce) cans no-salt-added kidney beans, rinsed
1 (28-ounce) can no-salt-added diced tomatoes, drained
1 (15-ounce) can no-salt-added tomato sauce
2 teaspoons minced canned chipotle chile in adobo sauce
¼ cup chopped fresh cilantro
　Lime wedges

1. Toss turkey with water, ¼ teaspoon salt, and baking soda in bowl until thoroughly combined. Set aside for 20 minutes.

2. Heat oil in 12-inch skillet over medium heat until shimmering. Add onions and bell pepper and cook until softened and lightly browned, 8 to 10 minutes. Stir in tomato paste, chili powder, garlic, cumin, and oregano and cook until fragrant, about 1 minute.

3. Add half of turkey mixture and cook, breaking up turkey with wooden spoon, until no longer pink, about 5 minutes. Repeat with remaining turkey mixture. Stir in broth and soy sauce, scraping up any browned bits; transfer to slow cooker.

4. Stir beans, tomatoes, tomato sauce, and chipotle into slow cooker. Cover and cook until turkey is tender, 4 to 5 hours on low. Break up any remaining large pieces of turkey with spoon. Adjust consistency with extra hot broth as needed. Season with pepper to taste. Sprinkle individual portions with cilantro and serve with lime wedges.

PER 1½-CUP SERVING

Cal 320 • **Total Fat** 9g • **Sat Fat** 2.5g • **Chol** 45mg
Sodium 500mg • **Total Carbs** 25g • **Fiber** 10g • **Total Sugar** 8g
Added Sugar 0g • **Protein** 36g • **Total Carbohydrate Choices** 2

NOTES FROM THE TEST KITCHEN

Chipotle Chiles in Adobo

Chipotle chiles are jalapeños that have been ripened until red, then smoked and dried. They are sold as is, ground to a powder, or packed in *adobo*, a tomato-based sauce (which we prefer). Once opened, canned chipotles in adobo will keep for two weeks in the refrigerator, or can be frozen for up to two months. To freeze, puree the chiles and quick-freeze teaspoonfuls on a plastic wrap–covered plate. Once hard, transfer the frozen pieces to a zipper-lock freezer bag.

Latin-Style Chicken with Tomatoes and Olives

SERVES 4
COOKING TIME 2 to 3 hours on Low

WHY THIS RECIPE WORKS This classic Latin-style chicken features tender chicken breasts braised in a chunky tomato sauce; gently simmering the chicken in the sauce helps it to remain moist while enriching the flavors of both. Our testing revealed that canned diced tomatoes with their juice had the fresh tomato taste we wanted but created too much liquid during cooking. Draining the diced tomatoes, plus adding tomato paste, created the thickened sauce we were after. Finishing the sauce with green olives gave our dish a briny contrast, and a sprinkling of fresh cilantro and lime juice tied it all together. Check the chicken's temperature after 2 hours of cooking and continue to monitor until it registers 160 degrees. You will need an oval slow cooker for this recipe.

1 onion, halved and sliced thin
4 garlic cloves, sliced thin
2 tablespoons extra-virgin olive oil
1 tablespoon no-salt-added tomato paste
2 teaspoons minced fresh oregano or ½ teaspoon dried
¼ teaspoon ground cumin
1 (14.5-ounce) can no-salt-added diced tomatoes, drained
2 (12-ounce) bone-in split chicken breasts, skin removed, trimmed of all visible fat, and halved crosswise
 Salt and pepper
⅓ cup pitted large brine-cured green olives, chopped coarse
2 tablespoons chopped fresh cilantro
1 tablespoon lime juice

1. Microwave onion, garlic, oil, tomato paste, oregano, and cumin in bowl, stirring occasionally, until onion is softened, about 5 minutes; transfer to oval slow cooker. Stir in tomatoes. Sprinkle chicken with ¼ teaspoon salt and ⅛ teaspoon pepper and nestle into slow cooker. Cover and cook until chicken registers 160 degrees, 2 to 3 hours on low.

2. Transfer chicken to serving platter. Stir olives, cilantro, lime juice, and ¼ teaspoon salt into sauce and season with pepper to taste. Spoon sauce over chicken and serve.

PER SERVING

Cal 270 • **Total Fat** 11g • **Sat Fat** 2g • **Chol** 100mg
Sodium 410mg • **Total Carbs** 9g • **Fiber** 2g • **Total Sugar** 5g
Added Sugar 0g • **Protein** 32g • **Total Carbohydrate Choices** 1

Chicken with Warm Potato and Radish Salad

SERVES 4
COOKING TIME 2 to 3 hours on Low

WHY THIS RECIPE WORKS For a fresh take on the classic chicken and potato dinner, we wanted to pair tender bone-in chicken with a warm, vinaigrette-based potato salad. We had to make sure that the potatoes and chicken cooked through in the same amount of time, as the lean meat can quickly overcook and turn dry. We seasoned the breasts simply with a mix of fresh thyme, salt, and pepper. To get the potatoes to cook at the same rate, we quartered small potatoes and gave them a head start in the microwave before adding them to the slow cooker along with the chicken. While

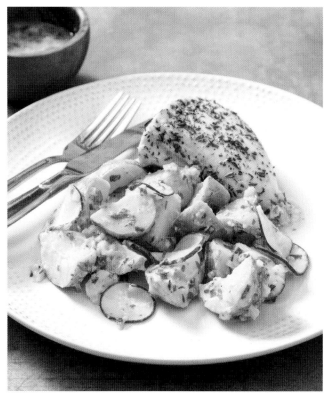

A fresh take on a chicken and potato dinner, our recipe delivers herb-topped chicken and a vinaigrette-style potato salad.

the chicken rested, we turned the tender potatoes into a delicious side dish by tossing them with a simple zesty dressing flavored with minced shallot, Dijon mustard, and parsley. Fresh radishes added great color and crunch as well as a nutritional boost. Look for potatoes measuring 1 to 2 inches in diameter; do not substitute full-size Yukon Gold potatoes as they will not cook through properly. You will need an oval slow cooker for this recipe. Check the chicken's temperature after 2 hours of cooking and continue to monitor until it registers 160 degrees.

1¾ pounds small Yukon Gold potatoes, unpeeled, quartered
2 (12-ounce) bone-in split chicken breasts, skin removed, trimmed of all visible fat, and halved crosswise
1 tablespoon minced fresh thyme or 1 teaspoon dried
Salt and pepper
3 tablespoons extra-virgin olive oil
3 tablespoons minced fresh parsley
1 shallot, minced

1 tablespoon Dijon mustard
2 teaspoons grated lemon zest plus 2 tablespoons juice
5 radishes, trimmed and sliced thin

1. Microwave potatoes and ¼ cup water in covered bowl, stirring occasionally, until almost tender, about 15 minutes; transfer to oval slow cooker. Sprinkle chicken with thyme, ¼ teaspoon salt, and ⅛ teaspoon pepper and nestle into slow cooker. Cover and cook until chicken registers 160 degrees, 2 to 3 hours on low.

2. Transfer chicken to serving platter. Whisk oil, parsley, shallot, 2 tablespoons water, mustard, lemon zest and juice, and ⅛ teaspoon salt together in large bowl. Measure out and reserve ¼ cup dressing. Drain potatoes and transfer to bowl with remaining dressing. Add radishes and toss to combine. Season with pepper to taste. Serve chicken with potato salad and reserved dressing.

PER SERVING

Cal 440 • **Total Fat** 14g • **Sat Fat** 2.5g • **Chol** 100mg **Sodium** 320mg • **Total Carbs** 38g • **Fiber** 3g • **Total Sugar** 1g **Added Sugar** 0g • **Protein** 36g • **Total Carbohydrate Choices** 2.5

Herbed Chicken with Warm Bulgur Salad and Yogurt Sauce
SERVES 4
COOKING TIME 2 to 3 hours on Low

WHY THIS RECIPE WORKS Fiber- and protein-rich bulgur is a great pairing for tender herbed chicken, and we found that the two cooked perfectly together in the slow cooker. We used an aromatic mixture of garlic, oregano, and lemon zest as a rub on the chicken, and saved a portion to mix in with the bulgur as well. We drained the bulgur at the end of cooking to remove excess liquid and seasoned it with olive oil, lemon juice, parsley, tomatoes, and carrots to turn the hearty grain into a vibrant salad. Then we topped the chicken and bulgur with a simple yogurt sauce and a sprinkling of pistachio nuts. When shopping, don't confuse bulgur with cracked wheat, which has a much longer cooking time and will not work in this recipe. You will need an oval slow cooker for this recipe. Check the chicken's temperature after 2 hours of cooking and continue to monitor until it registers 160 degrees.

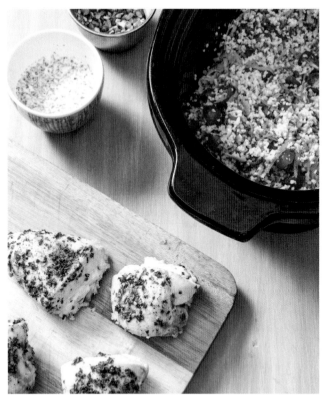

We remove the skin from the chicken before adding it to the slow cooker, which cuts down on saturated fat.

1 cup medium-grind bulgur, rinsed
1 cup unsalted chicken broth
Salt and pepper
¼ cup extra-virgin olive oil
4 teaspoons minced fresh oregano
1¼ teaspoons grated lemon zest plus 2 tablespoons juice
1 garlic clove, minced
Salt and pepper
⅛ teaspoon ground cardamom
2 (12-ounce) bone-in split chicken breasts, skin removed, trimmed of all visible fat, and halved crosswise
½ cup 2 percent Greek yogurt
½ cup minced fresh parsley
3 tablespoons water
8 ounces cherry tomatoes, quartered
1 carrot, peeled and shredded
¼ cup chopped toasted pistachios

1. Lightly coat oval slow cooker with vegetable oil spray. Combine bulgur, broth, and ⅛ teaspoon salt in prepared slow cooker. Microwave 1 tablespoon oil, 1 tablespoon oregano, 1 teaspoon lemon zest, garlic, ¼ teaspoon salt, ¼ teaspoon pepper, and cardamom in bowl until fragrant, about 30 seconds; let cool slightly. Rub chicken with oregano mixture, then arrange, skinned side up, in even layer in prepared slow cooker. Cover and cook until chicken registers 160 degrees, 2 to 3 hours on low.

2. Whisk yogurt, 1 tablespoon parsley, water, remaining 1 teaspoon oregano, remaining ¼ teaspoon lemon zest, and ⅛ teaspoon salt together in bowl. Season sauce with pepper to taste.

3. Transfer chicken to serving platter, brushing any bulgur that sticks to breasts back into slow cooker. Drain bulgur mixture, if necessary, and return to now-empty slow cooker. Add remaining 3 tablespoons oil, remaining 7 tablespoons parsley, lemon juice, tomatoes, carrot, and ⅛ teaspoon salt and fluff with fork to combine. Season with pepper to taste. Sprinkle bulgur salad with pistachios. Serve chicken with salad and yogurt sauce.

PER SERVING

Cal 500 • **Total Fat** 23g • **Sat Fat** 4g • **Chol** 100mg
Sodium 440mg • **Total Carbs** 36g • **Fiber** 7g • **Total Sugar** 5g
Added Sugar 0g • **Protein** 41g • **Total Carbohydrate Choices** 2.5

Chicken Thighs with Black-Eyed Pea Ragout
SERVES 6
COOKING TIME 4 to 5 hours on Low

WHY THIS RECIPE WORKS Juicy chicken, tender black-eyed peas, and earthy kale are a great combination for a healthy and comforting supper. We found that dry mustard and hot sauce were the keys to getting the right balance between heat and spice in this recipe. Dry mustard added to the slow cooker at the beginning of cooking infused the chicken with a subtle flavor, while finishing the peas with hot sauce punched up the heat and acidity of the dish. Pureeing a portion of the peas also helped to thicken the juices released from the chicken during cooking. You will need an oval slow cooker for this recipe.

1 pound kale, stemmed and chopped coarse
1 onion, chopped fine
4 garlic cloves, minced
1 tablespoon extra-virgin olive oil
1 teaspoon dry mustard
2 teaspoons minced fresh thyme or ½ teaspoon dried
2 (15-ounce) cans no-salt-added black-eyed peas, rinsed
½ cup unsalted chicken broth
Salt and pepper

6 (5-ounce) bone-in chicken thighs, skin removed, trimmed of all visible fat

2 teaspoons hot sauce, plus extra for serving
   Lemon wedges

1. Lightly coat oval slow cooker with vegetable oil spray. Microwave kale, onion, garlic, oil, mustard, and thyme in covered bowl, stirring occasionally, until vegetables are softened, 5 to 7 minutes; transfer to prepared slow cooker.

2. Process one-third of peas, broth, and ¼ teaspoon salt in food processor until smooth, about 30 seconds; transfer to slow cooker. Stir in remaining peas. Sprinkle chicken with ¼ teaspoon salt and ¼ teaspoon pepper and nestle into slow cooker. Cover and cook until chicken is tender, 4 to 5 hours on low.

3. Transfer chicken to serving platter. Stir hot sauce into ragout and season with pepper to taste. Serve chicken with ragout and lemon wedges, passing extra hot sauce separately.

PER SERVING

Cal 240 • **Total Fat** 8g • **Sat Fat** 1.5g • **Chol** 80mg
Sodium 380mg • **Total Carbs** 20g • **Fiber** 6g • **Total Sugar** 4g
Added Sugar 0g • **Protein** 24g • **Total Carbohydrate Choices** 1.5

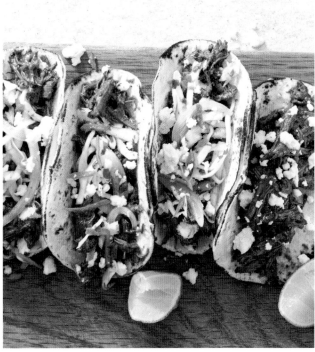

The slow cooker renders chuck roast meltingly tender and perfectly spiced for a batch of almost hands-off taco filling.

Shredded Beef Tacos with Cabbage-Carrot Slaw

SERVES 6
COOKING TIME 7 to 8 hours on Low or 4 to 5 hours on High

WHY THIS RECIPE WORKS Spiced shredded beef tacos topped with a healthy, vibrant slaw are both filling and nutritious. To make our red sauce we built a flavorful mixture of dried ancho chiles, chipotle chiles, tomato paste, and a hint of cinnamon. The different types of chiles created layers of heat without turning the sauce overly spicy. We bloomed the aromatics, including the dried chiles, with oil in the microwave to bring out their full flavor and added them to the slow cooker with a little water to distribute the spices evenly. Once the beef was pull-apart tender, we simply pureed the braising liquid into a rich, smooth sauce and tossed it with the shredded beef.

½ onion, chopped fine

1 ounce (2 to 3) dried ancho chiles, stemmed, seeded, and torn into 1-inch pieces (½ cup)

3 garlic cloves, minced

1 tablespoon no-salt-added tomato paste

1 tablespoon canola oil

1 teaspoon minced canned chipotle chile in adobo sauce

½ teaspoon ground cinnamon

¾ cup water, plus extra as needed
   Salt

2 pounds boneless beef chuck-eye roast, trimmed of all visible fat and cut into 1½-inch pieces

½ head napa cabbage, cored and sliced thin (6 cups)

1 carrot, peeled and shredded

1 jalapeño chile, stemmed, seeded, and sliced thin

¼ cup lime juice (2 limes), plus lime wedges for serving

¼ cup chopped fresh cilantro

12 (6-inch) corn tortillas, warmed

1 ounce queso fresco, crumbled (¼ cup)

1. Microwave onion, anchos, garlic, tomato paste, oil, chipotle, and cinnamon in bowl, stirring occasionally, until onion is softened, about 5 minutes; transfer to slow cooker. Stir in water and ½ teaspoon salt. Stir beef into slow cooker. Cover and cook until beef is tender, 7 to 8 hours on low or 4 to 5 hours on high.

2. Combine cabbage, carrot, jalapeño, lime juice, cilantro, and ¼ teaspoon salt in large bowl. Cover slaw and refrigerate until ready to serve.

3. Using slotted spoon, transfer beef to another large bowl. Using 2 forks, shred beef into bite-size pieces; cover to keep warm.

4. Process cooking liquid in blender until smooth, about 1 minute. Adjust sauce consistency with hot water as needed. Toss beef with 1 cup sauce. Toss slaw to recombine. Divide beef evenly among tortillas and top with slaw and queso fresco. Serve, passing lime wedges and remaining sauce separately.

PER SERVING

Cal 420 • **Total Fat** 14g • **Sat Fat** 3.5g • **Chol** 100mg
Sodium 500mg • **Total Carbs** 36g • **Fiber** 7g • **Total Sugar** 6g
Added Sugar 0g • **Protein** 39g • **Total Carbohydrate Choices** 2.5

NOTES FROM THE TEST KITCHEN

Warming Tortillas

Warming tortillas to soften them is crucial. If your tortillas are dry, pat each with a little water before warming them. Wrap warmed tortillas in aluminum foil or a clean dish towel to keep them warm and soft.

On the Stovetop

When warming tortillas on the stovetop, work with one tortilla at a time. For a gas stove, place the tortilla over a medium flame until slightly charred, about 30 seconds per side. For an electric stove, toast the tortilla in a skillet over medium-high heat until it is softened and speckled with brown spots, 20 to 30 seconds per side. Transfer the toasted tortillas to a plate and cover with a dish towel to keep them warm.

In the Oven

Wrap up to six tortillas in aluminum foil and place them in a 350-degree oven for about 5 minutes. To keep the tortillas warm, simply leave them wrapped in foil until ready to use.

WARMING TORTILLAS ON THE STOVETOP

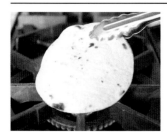

Warm tortilla directly on cooking grate over medium gas flame until slightly charred around edges, about 30 seconds per side. Or warm, one at a time, in dry skillet over medium-high heat until softened and speckled brown, 20 to 30 seconds per side.

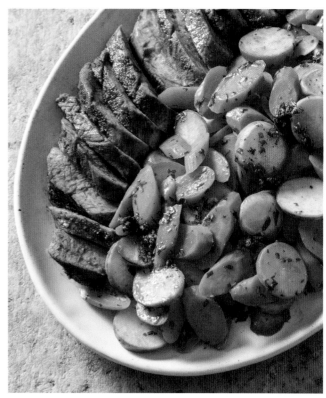

Carrots and radishes are a nutritious duo that makes a great side for our spiced, slow-cooker pork tenderloin.

Spiced Pork Tenderloin with Carrots and Radishes
SERVES 4
COOKING TIME 1 to 2 hours on Low

WHY THIS RECIPE WORKS We wanted to make tender spice-rubbed pork tenderloin with a healthy and easy side dish—all in the slow cooker. Carrots and radishes were an appealingly fresh combination that paired well with the simple spice combination that we used for the pork. First, we jump-started the carrots in the microwave so they would cook through by the time our tenderloin was done. Next, we seasoned the pork with fragrant cumin and paprika. Because it is cooked gently and not browned, the tenderloin will be rosy throughout. Check the tenderloin's temperature after 1 hour of cooking and continue to monitor until it registers 145 degrees. You will need an oval slow cooker for this recipe.

1½ pounds carrots, peeled and sliced ¼ inch thick on bias
10 radishes, trimmed and sliced ¼ inch thick
¼ cup unsalted chicken broth

3 tablespoons extra-virgin olive oil

1 teaspoon ground cumin

1 teaspoon paprika

1 (1-pound) pork tenderloin, trimmed of all visible fat
Salt and pepper

2 tablespoons lime juice

2 tablespoons minced fresh cilantro

1 teaspoon minced canned chipotle chile in adobo sauce

1. Microwave carrots and ¼ cup water in covered bowl, stirring occasionally, until crisp-tender, about 8 minutes. Drain carrots and transfer to oval slow cooker. Stir in radishes and broth.

2. Microwave 1 teaspoon oil, cumin, and paprika in bowl until fragrant, about 30 seconds; let cool slightly. Rub tenderloin with spice mixture and sprinkle with ¼ teaspoon salt and ⅛ teaspoon pepper. Nestle tenderloin into slow cooker, cover, and cook until pork registers 145 degrees, 1 to 2 hours on low.

3. Transfer tenderloin to carving board, tent with aluminum foil, and let rest for 5 minutes.

4. Whisk remaining 8 teaspoons oil, lime juice, cilantro, and chipotle together in bowl, then season dressing with pepper to taste. Drain vegetables from cooker and transfer to large bowl. Stir in 2 tablespoons of dressing and season with pepper to taste. Slice tenderloin ½ inch thick and serve with vegetables and remaining dressing.

PER SERVING

Cal 300 • **Total Fat** 14g • **Sat Fat** 2.5g • **Chol** 75mg
Sodium 350mg • **Total Carbs** 20g • **Fiber** 6g • **Total Sugar** 9g
Added Sugar 0g • **Protein** 26g • **Total Carbohydrate Choices** 1

Pork Loin with Fennel, Oranges, and Olives

SERVES 8
COOKING TIME 1 to 2 hours on Low

WHY THIS RECIPE WORKS Fennel, oranges, and olives are a classic Italian combination that we wanted to serve with a tender pork loin roast. After quickly searing the roast to give it a deep color and more satisfying flavor, we sautéed the fennel in white wine until softened. We uncovered the skillet and caramelized the fennel before transferring it to the slow cooker, then nestled the seared roast on top. While the roast rested, we stirred orange segments and chopped kalamata olives into the fennel. The bright citrus of the oranges and the brininess of the olives combined

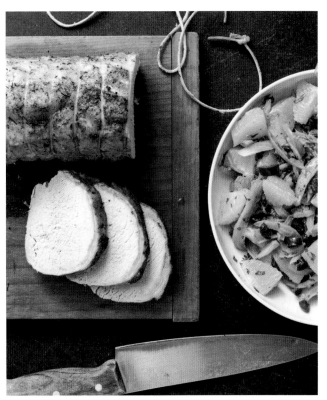

Every time you make a pork loin in your slow cooker you should take its temperature after one hour of cooking.

with the anise flavor of the fennel to create the perfect medley of Mediterranean flavors. Check the temperature of the pork loin after 1 hour of cooking and continue to monitor until it registers 140 degrees. We found that leaving a ⅛-inch-thick layer of fat on top of the roast is ideal; if your roast has a thicker fat cap, trim it to be about ⅛ inch thick. You will need an oval slow cooker for this recipe.

1 (2-pound) boneless center-cut pork loin roast,
 fat trimmed to ⅛ inch

1 teaspoon herbes de Provence
 Salt and pepper

1 tablespoon extra-virgin olive oil

3 fennel bulbs, stalks discarded, bulbs halved, cored,
 and sliced thin

½ cup dry white wine

2 garlic cloves, minced

4 oranges, plus 1 tablespoon grated orange zest

½ cup pitted kalamata olives, chopped

2 tablespoons minced fresh tarragon

1. Pat roast dry with paper towels and sprinkle with herbes de Provence, ½ teaspoon salt, and ¼ teaspoon pepper. Heat oil in 12-inch skillet over medium-high heat until just smoking. Brown roast on all sides, 7 to 10 minutes; transfer to plate.

2. Add fennel and wine to now-empty skillet, cover, and cook, stirring occasionally, until fennel begins to soften, about 5 minutes. Uncover and continue to cook until fennel is dry and lightly browned, about 5 minutes. Stir in garlic and cook until fragrant, about 30 seconds; transfer to oval slow cooker. Nestle roast fat side up into slow cooker. Cover and cook until pork registers 140 degrees, 1 to 2 hours on low.

3. Transfer roast to carving board, tent with aluminum foil, and let rest for 15 minutes. Meanwhile, cut away peel and pith from oranges. Quarter oranges, then slice crosswise into ½-inch-thick pieces. Stir orange segments, orange zest, olives, and ¼ teaspoon salt into fennel mixture and let sit until heated through, about 5 minutes. Stir in tarragon and season with pepper to taste. Slice pork ½ inch thick and serve with fennel-orange mixture.

PER SERVING

Cal 240 • **Total Fat** 7g • **Sat Fat** 1.5g • **Chol** 70mg
Sodium 350mg • **Total Carbs** 15g • **Fiber** 4g • **Total Sugar** 10g
Added Sugar 0g • **Protein** 27g • **Total Carbohydrate Choices** 1

NOTES FROM THE TEST KITCHEN

Buying Kalamata Olives

Although kalamata olives are often packed in olive oil in their native Greece, on American soil we almost always find them swimming in a vinegary brine. We prefer the fresher kalamatas from the refrigerated section of the supermarket (also packed in brine) over the jarred, shelf-stable ones, which are bland and mushy in comparison. If you can't find kalamatas in the refrigerator section of your market, look for them at the salad bar.

HOW TO PEEL BEETS

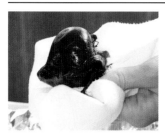

Peel roasted beets by rubbing them with paper towels. The skins should slide right off. For easy cleanup, do this over the foil used for roasting the beets.

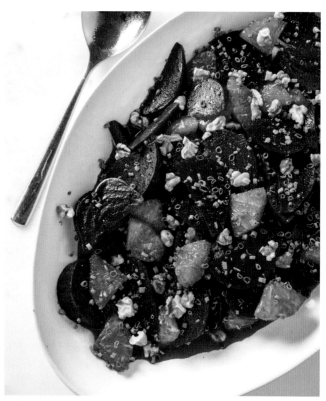

Packed with vitamins, minerals, and fiber, beets are easy to prepare in the slow cooker.

Beets with Oranges and Walnuts
SERVES 4
COOKING TIME 6 to 7 hours on Low or 4 to 5 hours on High

WHY THIS RECIPE WORKS Using a slow cooker is a great hands-off way to make many healthy side dishes, including vegetables. Cooking beets in the slow cooker guaranteed beets with an undiluted, earthy flavor, and freed up the oven. Wrapping the beets in aluminum foil and including ½ cup of water in the slow cooker ensured that they cooked through evenly. Cutting the cooked beets into fork-friendly wedges made them easy to eat, and a simple white wine vinaigrette added brightness. Orange pieces, toasted walnuts, and minced chives turned our slow-cooked vegetable into an impressive bistro-style side dish. To ensure even cooking, we recommend using beets that are similar in size—roughly 3 inches in diameter. You will need an oval slow cooker for this recipe.

1½ pounds beets, trimmed
  2 oranges
 ¼ cup white wine vinegar
1½ tablespoons extra-virgin olive oil

Salt and pepper
¼ cup walnuts, toasted and chopped coarse
2 tablespoons minced fresh chives

1. Wrap beets individually in aluminum foil and place in oval slow cooker. Add ½ cup water, cover, and cook until beets are tender, 6 to 7 hours on low or 4 to 5 hours on high.

2. Transfer beets to cutting board and carefully remove foil (watch for steam). When beets are cool enough to handle, rub off skins with paper towels and cut into ½-inch-thick wedges.

3. Cut away peel and pith from oranges. Quarter oranges and slice crosswise into ½-inch-thick pieces. Whisk vinegar, oil, ¼ teaspoon salt, and ¼ teaspoon pepper together in large bowl. Add beets and orange pieces and toss to coat. Season with pepper to taste. Sprinkle with walnuts and chives and serve.

PER SERVING

Cal 190 • **Total Fat** 10g • **Sat Fat** 1g • **Chol** 0mg
Sodium 260mg • **Total Carbs** 25g • **Fiber** 7g • **Total Sugar** 18g
Added Sugar 0g • **Protein** 4g • **Total Carbohydrate Choices** 1.5

Braised Fennel with Orange-Tarragon Dressing
SERVES 4
COOKING TIME 8 to 9 hours on Low or 5 to 6 hours on High

WHY THIS RECIPE WORKS We wanted a recipe for braised fennel that would infuse the vegetable with rich, savory flavor. Cutting the fennel into wedges turned out to be the key to evenly cooked pieces, and we made sure to braise them long enough to deliver uniformly tender but not mushy results. A combination of garlic, juniper berries, and thyme provided a base of seasoning for this appealing side dish, and we finished it off with a simple orange-tarragon dressing. Don't core the fennel bulb when cutting it into wedges; the core helps hold the layers of fennel together during cooking. You will need an oval slow cooker for this recipe.

2 garlic cloves, peeled and smashed
2 sprigs fresh thyme
1 teaspoon juniper berries
2 fennel bulbs, stalks discarded, bulbs halved, each half cut into 4 wedges
2 tablespoons extra-virgin olive oil
2 teaspoons grated orange zest plus 1 tablespoon juice
1 teaspoon minced fresh tarragon
Salt and pepper

1. Combine 1 cup water, garlic, thyme sprigs, and juniper berries in oval slow cooker. Place fennel wedges cut side down in cooker (wedges may overlap). Cover and cook until fennel is tender, 8 to 9 hours on low or 5 to 6 hours on high.

2. Whisk oil, orange zest and juice, tarragon, ¼ teaspoon salt, and ¼ teaspoon pepper together in bowl. Using slotted spoon, transfer fennel to serving dish, brushing away any garlic cloves, thyme sprigs, or juniper berries that stick to fennel. Drizzle fennel with dressing. Serve.

PER SERVING

Cal 100 • **Total Fat** 7g • **Sat Fat** 1g • **Chol** 0mg
Sodium 210mg • **Total Carbs** 9g • **Fiber** 4g • **Total Sugar** 5g
Added Sugar 0g • **Protein** 2g • **Total Carbohydrate Choices** 0.5

Braised Swiss Chard with Shiitakes and Peanuts
SERVES 6
COOKING TIME 1 to 2 hours on High

WHY THIS RECIPE WORKS For an Asian take on nutrient-rich Swiss chard, we turned to toasted sesame oil, a good amount of grated fresh ginger, and minced garlic for our aromatic base. And for heartiness, as well as a lot of vitamins, minerals, and fiber, we added shiitake mushrooms, braising them along with the chard. Once the chard was perfectly tender, we stirred in rice vinegar and some additional ginger, keeping the flavors fresh and vibrant. Chopped peanuts and sliced scallions provided a healthy and colorful finish to the dish.

2 pounds Swiss chard, stems chopped fine, leaves cut into 1-inch pieces
4 ounces shiitake mushrooms, stemmed and sliced ¼ inch thick
3 garlic cloves, minced
2 teaspoons toasted sesame oil
2 teaspoons grated fresh ginger
⅛ teaspoon red pepper flakes
1 tablespoon rice vinegar
Pepper
¼ cup chopped dry-roasted peanuts
2 scallions, sliced thin

1. Lightly coat slow cooker with vegetable oil spray. Microwave chard stems, mushrooms, garlic, 1 teaspoon oil, 1 teaspoon ginger, and pepper flakes in bowl, stirring occasionally, until vegetables are softened, about 5 minutes; transfer to prepared slow cooker. Stir in chard leaves, cover, and cook until chard is tender, 1 to 2 hours on high.

2. Stir in vinegar, remaining 1 teaspoon oil, and remaining 1 teaspoon ginger. Season with pepper to taste. (Swiss chard can be held on warm or low setting for up to 2 hours.) Sprinkle with peanuts and scallions before serving.

PER SERVING

Cal 90 • **Total Fat** 5g • **Sat Fat** 1g • **Chol** 0mg
Sodium 330mg • **Total Carbs** 9g • **Fiber** 3g • **Total Sugar** 3g
Added Sugar 0g • **Protein** 5g • **Total Carbohydrate Choices** 0.5

Big-Batch Brown Rice with Parmesan and Herbs

SERVES 12
COOKING TIME 2 to 3 hours on High

WHY THIS RECIPE WORKS We wondered if the steady, gentle heat of the slow cooker would take the challenge out of cooking brown rice. After some experiments that resulted in burnt rice and undercooked grains, we learned that while brown rice needs a head start with boiling water in the slow cooker, it can indeed emerge with light and fluffy grains every time. Cooking on high was best, and we laid a piece of parchment paper over the rice to protect the grains on top from drying out as the water was absorbed. You will need an oval slow cooker for this recipe. For an accurate measurement of boiling water, bring a full kettle of water to a boil and then measure out the desired amount. Spraying the slow cooker with vegetable oil spray prevents the rice from sticking to the sides of the slow cooker.

CREATING A PARCHMENT SHIELD

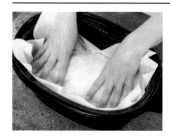

Press 16 by 12-inch sheet of parchment paper firmly onto rice, folding down edges as needed.

---

3 cups boiling water
2 cups long-grain brown rice, rinsed
1 tablespoon unsalted butter
  Salt and pepper
2 ounces Parmesan cheese, grated (1 cup)
½ cup chopped fresh basil, dill, or parsley
2 teaspoons lemon juice

1. Lightly coat oval slow cooker with vegetable oil spray. Combine boiling water, rice, butter, ½ teaspoon salt, and ½ teaspoon pepper in prepared slow cooker. Gently press 16 by 12-inch sheet of parchment paper onto surface of water, folding down edges as needed. Cover and cook until rice is tender and all water is absorbed, 2 to 3 hours on high.

2. Discard parchment. Fluff rice with fork, then gently fold in Parmesan, basil, and lemon juice. Season with pepper to taste. Serve.

PER SERVING

Cal 130 • **Total Fat** 4 • **Sat Fat** 1.5g • **Chol** 5mg
Sodium 180mg • **Total Carbs** 24g • **Fiber** 2g • **Total Sugar** 0g
Added Sugar 0g • **Protein** 4g • **Total Carbohydrate Choices** 1.5

No-Fuss Quinoa with Lemon

SERVES 6
COOKING TIME 3 to 4 hours on Low or 2 to 3 hours on High

WHY THIS RECIPE WORKS We love quinoa for its nutty taste, nutritional value, and ease of preparation. To keep the grains separate and fluffy during cooking, we toasted them in the microwave before adding the quinoa to the slow cooker. We dressed the quinoa simply with lemon and parsley to make a universally appealing side dish. Be sure to rinse the quinoa in a fine-mesh strainer before using; rinsing removes the quinoa's bitter protective coating (called saponin). Spraying the slow cooker with vegetable oil spray prevents the quinoa from sticking to the sides of the slow cooker.

1½ cups prewashed white quinoa, rinsed
  1 onion, chopped fine
  1 tablespoon extra-virgin olive oil
1¾ cups water
  2 (2-inch) strips lemon zest plus 1 tablespoon juice
    Salt and pepper
  2 tablespoons minced fresh parsley

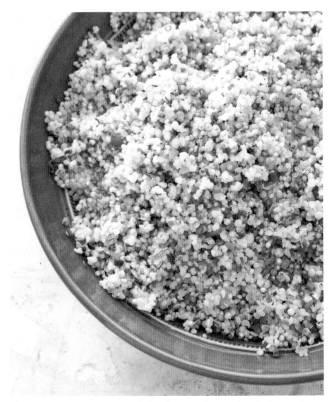

The steamy environment of the slow cooker makes it the perfect way to cook a big batch of flavorful quinoa with separate grains.

1. Lightly coat slow cooker with vegetable oil spray. Microwave quinoa, onion, and 1 teaspoon oil in bowl, stirring occasionally, until quinoa is lightly toasted and onion is softened, about 5 minutes; transfer to prepared slow cooker. Stir in water, lemon zest, and ½ teaspoon salt. Cover and cook until quinoa is tender and all water is absorbed, 3 to 4 hours on low or 2 to 3 hours on high.

2. Discard lemon zest. Fluff quinoa with fork, then gently fold in lemon juice, parsley, and remaining 2 teaspoons oil. Season with pepper to taste. Serve.

PER SERVING

Cal 190 • **Total Fat** 5g • **Sat Fat** 0.5g • **Chol** 0mg
Sodium 200mg • **Total Carbs** 30g • **Fiber** 4g • **Total Sugar** 3g
Added Sugar 0g • **Protein** 6g • **Total Carbohydrate Choices** 2

Lentil Salad with Radishes, Cilantro, and Pepitas

SERVES 6
COOKING TIME 3 to 4 hours on Low or 2 to 3 hours on High

WHY THIS RECIPE WORKS A lentil salad can be a hearty, impressive, and easy main course, and we found that the slow and even heat of the slow cooker was the perfect way to cook great lentils every time. We knew that cooking lentils with plenty of liquid was necessary to ensure even cooking. Adding a little salt and vinegar to the cooking liquid (we preferred water for a pure lentil flavor) gave us lentils that were firm yet creamy. In addition, aromatics in the cooking water created a flavorful backbone during cooking. Once the lentils were cooked to the ideal texture and drained, we added fresh and bright ingredients to create big flavor that turned this dish into a hearty side that could double as a vegetarian main course. *Lentilles du Puy*, also called French green lentils, are our first choice for this recipe, but brown, black, or regular green lentils are fine, too.

  1 **cup lentilles du Puy, picked over and rinsed**
  3 **tablespoons lime juice (2 limes)**
  3 **garlic cloves, minced**
  1 **tablespoon ground cumin**
1½ **teaspoons dried oregano**
    Salt and pepper
  6 **radishes, trimmed, halved, and sliced thin**
  1 **red bell pepper, stemmed, seeded, and cut into ½-inch pieces**
  ¼ **cup fresh cilantro leaves**
  1 **jalapeño chile, stemmed, seeded, and minced**
  1 **shallot, minced**
  ¼ **cup extra-virgin olive oil**
  2 **tablespoons roasted pepitas**
  2 **ounces queso fresco, crumbled (½ cup)**

1. Combine 4 cups water, lentils, 1 tablespoon lime juice, garlic, cumin, oregano, and ½ teaspoon salt in slow cooker. Cover and cook until lentils are tender, 3 to 4 hours on low or 2 to 3 hours on high.

2. Drain lentils and transfer to large serving bowl; let cool slightly. Add radishes, bell pepper, cilantro, jalapeño, shallot, oil, and remaining 2 tablespoons lime juice and gently toss to combine. Season with pepper to taste. Sprinkle with pepitas and queso fresco. Serve.

PER SERVING

Cal 250 • **Total Fat** 14g • **Sat Fat** 3g • **Chol** 5mg
Sodium 200mg • **Total Carbs** 23g • **Fiber** 6g • **Total Sugar** 2g
Added Sugar 0g • **Protein** 10g • **Total Carbohydrate Choices** 1.5

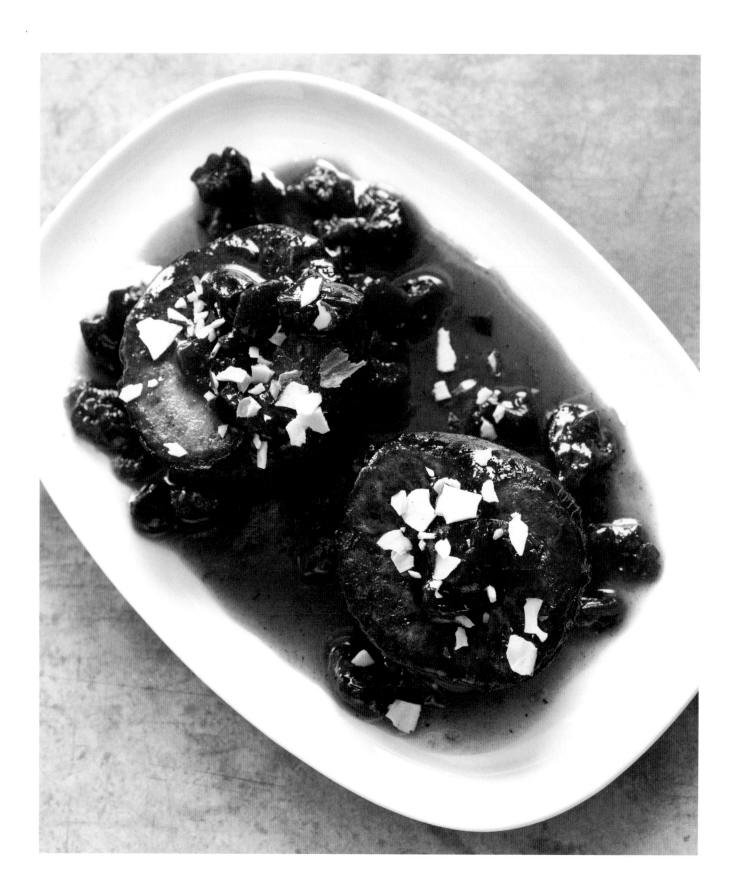

SPECIAL TREATS

Photo: Roasted Plums with Dried Cherries and Almonds

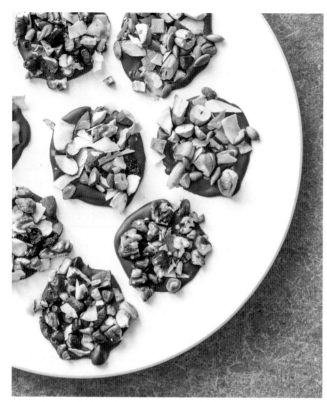

These low-carb chocolate treats are packed with healthy nuts, seeds, and dried fruit.

Pomegranate and Nut Chocolate Clusters
MAKES 12 CLUSTERS

WHY THIS RECIPE WORKS Chocolate-enrobed clusters of nuts, seeds, and fruit sound somewhat healthy, but their small size belies their high sugar content. For our lower-sugar version, we knew we couldn't use enough chocolate to create fully enrobed clusters, so we opted instead to simply top dollops of melted chocolate with a variety of nuts, seeds, and fruit. We found that semisweet chocolate had the best balance of deep, rich chocolate flavor without any bitterness. We tried quickly melting all of the chocolate in the microwave, but this resulted in melty, gooey chocolate that never fully hardened. To ensure that the chocolate resolidified, we needed to melt it slowly and gently. To do this, we microwaved most of the chocolate at 50 percent power until it was partially melted and then stirred in the remaining chocolate, relying on additional short bursts in the microwave to melt all of the chocolate. Finally, we came up with several colorful combinations of nuts, seeds, and fruit to give our clusters both dimension and textural contrast.

⅓ cup pecans, toasted and chopped
¼ cup shelled pistachios, toasted and chopped
2 tablespoons unsweetened flaked coconut, toasted
2 tablespoons pomegranate seeds
3 ounces semisweet chocolate, chopped fine

1. Line rimmed baking sheet with parchment paper. Combine pecans, pistachios, coconut, and pomegranate seeds in bowl.

2. Microwave 2 ounces chocolate in bowl at 50 percent power, stirring often, until about two-thirds melted, 45 to 60 seconds. Remove bowl from microwave; stir in remaining 1 ounce chocolate until melted. If necessary, microwave chocolate at 50 percent power for 5 seconds at a time until melted.

3. Working quickly, measure 1 teaspoon melted chocolate onto prepared sheet and spread into 2½-inch wide circle using back of spoon. Repeat with remaining chocolate, spacing circles 1½ inches apart.

4. Sprinkle pecan mixture evenly over chocolate and press gently to adhere. Refrigerate until chocolate is firm, about 30 minutes. Serve.

PER CLUSTER
Cal 80 • **Total Fat** 6g • **Sat Fat** 2g • **Chol** 0mg
Sodium 0mg • **Total Carbs** 6g • **Fiber** 1g • **Total Sugar** 5g
Added Sugar 0g • **Protein** 1g • **Total Carbohydrate Choices** 0.5

VARIATIONS
Mango and Nut Chocolate Clusters
Substitute cashews for pecans, pepitas for pistachios, and 4 teaspoons chopped unsweetened dried mango for pomegranate seeds.

PER CLUSTER
Cal 80 • **Total Fat** 6g • **Sat Fat** 2g • **Chol** 0mg
Sodium 0mg • **Total Carbs** 7g • **Fiber** 1g • **Total Sugar** 5g
Added Sugar 0g • **Protein** 2g • **Total Carbohydrate Choices** 0.5

Cherry and Nut Chocolate Clusters
Substitute almonds for pecans, walnuts for pistachios, and 4 teaspoons chopped dried unsweetened cherries for pomegranate seeds.

PER CLUSTER
Cal 80 • **Total Fat** 6g • **Sat Fat** 2g • **Chol** 0mg
Sodium 0mg • **Total Carbs** 6g • **Fiber** 1g • **Total Sugar** 5g
Added Sugar 0g • **Protein** 2g • **Total Carbohydrate Choices** 0.5

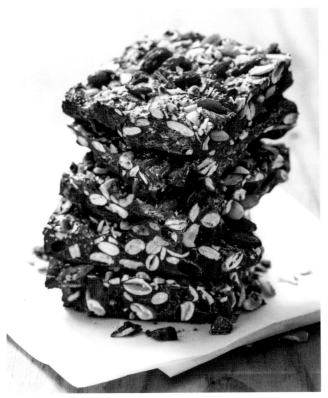

Dark chocolate of 70 percent cacao or higher is rich in nutrients and minerals and brings the most antioxidant benefits.

Dark Chocolate Bark with Pepitas and Goji Berries
SERVES 16

WHY THIS RECIPE WORKS Yes, a small amount of chocolate can be a part of a nutritious diet. The key, apart from portion size, is sticking to a higher cacao chocolate, which contains more antioxidants. A piece of chocolate bark makes the perfect alternative to a candy bar. We filled our bark with crunchy roasted pepitas and chewy, tart goji berries; cinnamon and spicy chipotle powder gave it a surprising depth and some heat, while a hit of sea salt brought out all the flavors. Stirring some grated chocolate into melted chocolate proved a simple but effective tempering technique, resulting in chocolate that set up shiny and crisp. We prefer the flavor of 70 percent dark chocolate; higher cacao percentages will also work (see page 361) but the flavor will be less sweet and more intense. To grate the chocolate, use the large holes of a box grater.

1 pound 70 percent dark chocolate, 12 ounces chopped fine, 4 ounces grated
2 teaspoons ground cinnamon
1 teaspoon chipotle chile powder
2 cups roasted pepitas, 1¾ cups left whole, ¼ cup chopped
1 cup dried goji berries, chopped
1 teaspoon coarse sea salt

1. Make parchment paper sling for 13 by 9-inch baking pan by folding 2 long sheets of parchment; first sheet should be 13 inches wide and second sheet should be 9 inches wide. Lay sheets in pan perpendicular to each other, with extra parchment hanging over edges of pan. Push parchment into corners and up sides of pan, smoothing parchment flush to pan.

2. Microwave 12 ounces finely chopped chocolate in large bowl at 50 percent power, stirring every 15 seconds, until melted but not much hotter than body temperature (check by holding in the palm of your hand), 2 to 3 minutes. Stir in 4 ounces grated chocolate, cinnamon, and chile powder until smooth and chocolate is completely melted (returning to microwave for no more than 5 seconds at a time to finish melting if necessary).

3. Stir 1¾ cups whole pepitas and ¾ cup goji berries into chocolate mixture. Working quickly, use rubber spatula to spread chocolate mixture evenly into prepared pan. Sprinkle with remaining ¼ cup chopped pepitas and remaining ¼ cup goji berries and gently press topping into chocolate. Sprinkle evenly with salt and refrigerate until chocolate is set, about 30 minutes.

4. Using parchment overhang, lift chocolate out of pan and transfer to cutting board; discard parchment. Using serrated knife and gentle sawing motion, cut chocolate into 16 even pieces. Serve.

PER SERVING
Cal 260 • **Total Fat** 21g • **Sat Fat** 9g • **Chol** 0mg
Sodium 140mg • **Total Carbs** 20g • **Fiber** 4g • **Total Sugar** 10g
Added Sugar 0g • **Protein** 8g • **Total Carbohydrate Choices** 1

VARIATION
Dark Chocolate Bark with Almonds and Cherries
Omit cinnamon and chipotle chile powder. Substitute toasted almonds for pepitas and unsweetened dried tart cherries for goji berries.

PER SERVING
Cal 280 • **Total Fat** 23g • **Sat Fat** 8g • **Chol** 0mg
Sodium 125mg • **Total Carbs** 22g • **Fiber** 4g • **Total Sugar** 11g
Added Sugar 0g • **Protein** 6g • **Total Carbohydrate Choices** 1.5

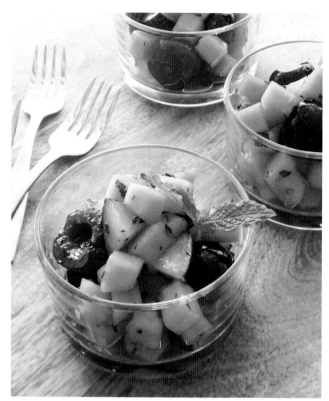

Mashing a little sugar with fresh mint before stirring it into the fruit gives this fruit salad balanced, complex flavor.

Melon, Plums, and Cherries with Mint and Vanilla
SERVES 6

WHY THIS RECIPE WORKS This composed fresh fruit salad makes a great snack but is beautiful enough as dessert after a nice meal. We found that a small amount of sugar encouraged the fruit to release its juices, creating a more cohesive salad. We balanced the sweetness with fresh lime juice, but tasters wanted more complexity. Mashing the sugar with fresh mint before stirring it into the fruit worked perfectly and ensured even distribution of flavor throughout the salad.

 2 teaspoons sugar
 1 tablespoon minced fresh mint
 3 cups cantaloupe cut into ½-inch pieces
 2 plums, halved, pitted, and cut into ½-inch pieces
 8 ounces fresh sweet cherries, pitted and halved
 ¼ teaspoon vanilla extract
 1 tablespoon lime juice, plus extra for seasoning

Combine sugar and mint in large bowl. Using rubber spatula, press mixture into side of bowl until sugar becomes damp, about 30 seconds. Add cantaloupe, plums, cherries, and vanilla and gently toss to combine. Let sit at room temperature, stirring occasionally, until fruit releases its juices, 15 to 30 minutes. Stir in lime juice and season with extra lime juice to taste. Serve.

PER ¾-CUP SERVING
Cal 70 • **Total Fat** 0g • **Sat Fat** 0g • **Chol** 0mg
Sodium 15mg • **Total Carbs** 19g • **Fiber** 2g • **Total Sugar** 16g
Added Sugar 1g • **Protein** 1g • **Total Carbohydrate Choices** 1

VARIATION
Peaches, Blackberries, and Strawberries with Basil and Pepper
SERVES 6
Nectarines can be substituted for the peaches.

 2 teaspoons sugar
 2 tablespoons chopped fresh basil
 ½ teaspoon pepper
 3 peaches, halved, pitted, and cut into ½-inch pieces
 10 ounces (2 cups) blackberries
 10 ounces strawberries, hulled and quartered (2 cups)
 1 tablespoon lime juice, plus extra for seasoning

Combine sugar, basil, and pepper in large bowl. Using rubber spatula, press mixture into side of bowl until sugar becomes damp, about 30 seconds. Add peaches, blackberries, and strawberries and gently toss to combine. Let sit at room temperature, stirring occasionally, until fruit releases its juices, 15 to 30 minutes. Stir in lime juice and season with extra lime juice to taste. Serve.

PER ¾-CUP SERVING
Cal 70 • **Total Fat** 0.5g • **Sat Fat** 0g • **Chol** 0mg
Sodium 0mg • **Total Carbs** 18g • **Fiber** 5g • **Total Sugar** 13g
Added Sugar 1g • **Protein** 2g • **Total Carbohydrate Choices** 1

Strawberries with Balsamic Vinegar
SERVES 6

WHY THIS RECIPE WORKS Strawberries with balsamic vinegar may sound a bit trendy, but this Italian combination actually dates back hundreds of years. We wanted to pay homage to this tradition and create our own dessert in which the vinegar enhanced, not overwhelmed, the flavor of bright summer berries. But high-end aged balsamic vinegars can cost a pretty penny, so we opted instead to use an inexpensive vinegar and employ a few tricks to coax more flavor from it. First, we simmered the vinegar with sugar to approximate the syrupy texture of an aged vinegar. Next we enhanced the flavor with a squirt of fresh lemon juice, which brought just the right amount of brightness. We tossed the berries with light brown sugar—rather than the traditional granulated—and a pinch of pepper for the most complex flavor. Once we mixed the sliced berries and sugar together, it took about 15 minutes for the berries to release their juice; if the strawberries sat any longer than this, they continued to soften and became quite mushy. If you don't have light brown sugar on hand, you can sprinkle the berries with an equal amount of granulated white sugar.

⅓ cup balsamic vinegar
2 teaspoons granulated sugar
½ teaspoon lemon juice
2 pounds strawberries, hulled and sliced lengthwise ¼ inch thick (5 cups)
1 tablespoon packed light brown sugar
Pinch pepper

1. Bring vinegar, granulated sugar, and lemon juice to simmer in small saucepan over medium heat and cook, stirring occasionally, until thickened and measures about 3 tablespoons, about 3 minutes. Transfer syrup to small bowl and let cool completely.

2. Gently toss strawberries with brown sugar and pepper in large bowl. Let sit at room temperature, stirring occasionally, until strawberries begin to release their juice, 10 to 15 minutes. Pour syrup over strawberries and gently toss to combine. Serve.

PER ¾-CUP SERVING
Cal 80 • **Total Fat** 0g • **Sat Fat** 0g • **Chol** 0mg
Sodium 0mg • **Total Carbs** 19g • **Fiber** 3g • **Total Sugar** 15g
Added Sugar 4g • **Protein** 1g • **Total Carbohydrate Choices** 1

Nectarines and Berries in Prosecco
SERVES 8

WHY THIS RECIPE WORKS For a celebratory yet light dessert, we wanted to combine fresh fruit with sparkling wine. After some enjoyable experimentation, we settled on nectarines and berries as our fruit and prosecco for the wine. But simply pouring prosecco over lightly sugared fruit resulted in disappointingly disparate flavors. Instead, we tossed the fruit with sugar and allowed the mixture to macerate. The nectarines and berries softened and released some of their juices, which, when combined with the chilled wine, contributed to a more cohesive flavor profile and a harmonious blend of fruit and fizz. Orange liqueur added some depth as well as some nice citrus notes. Peaches or plums can be substituted for the nectarines. While we prefer to use prosecco here, any young, fruity sparkling wine will work.

10 ounces (2 cups) blackberries or raspberries
10 ounces strawberries, hulled and quartered (2 cups)
1 pound nectarines, pitted and cut into ¼-inch wedges
1 tablespoon sugar
1 tablespoon orange liqueur, such as Grand Marnier or triple sec
2 tablespoons chopped fresh mint
¼ teaspoon grated lemon zest
¾ cup chilled prosecco

Gently toss blackberries, strawberries, nectarines, sugar, orange liqueur, mint, and lemon zest together in large bowl. Let sit at room temperature, stirring occasionally, until fruit begins to release its juices, about 15 minutes. Just before serving, pour prosecco over fruit.

PER 1¼-CUP SERVING
Cal 80 • **Total Fat** 0g • **Sat Fat** 0g • **Chol** 0mg
Sodium 0mg • **Total Carbs** 14g • **Fiber** 3g • **Total Sugar** 10g
Added Sugar 2g • **Protein** 1g • **Total Carbohydrate Choices** 1

NOTES FROM THE TEST KITCHEN

Washing and Storing Berries

Washing berries before you use them is always a safe practice. We think that the best way to wash them is to place the berries in a colander and rinse them gently under running water for at least 30 seconds. As for drying berries, we've tested a variety of methods and have found that a salad spinner lined with a buffering layer of paper towels is the best approach.

It's particularly important to store berries carefully, because they are prone to growing mold and rotting quickly. If the berries aren't going to be used immediately, we recommend cleaning them with a mild vinegar solution (3 cups of water mixed with 1 cup of distilled white vinegar), which will destroy the bacteria, then drying them and storing them in a paper towel–lined airtight container.

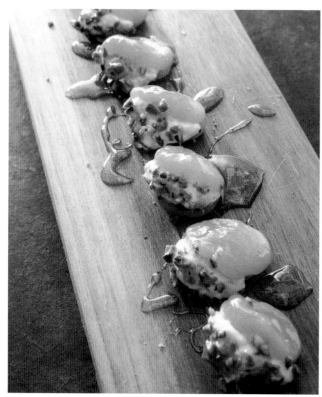

We simmer dried apricots in a bay- and cardamom-scented syrup to rehydrate them and infuse them with flavor.

Turkish Stuffed Apricots with Rose Water and Pistachios
SERVES 6

WHY THIS RECIPE WORKS Stuffed apricots are an iconic Turkish dessert. The authentic version calls for rehydrating dried apricots before candying them in a sugar syrup, filling them with a cream made from water buffalo milk, and topping them with pistachios. We found that by tweaking the sugar concentration of the syrup, we could simultaneously cook, candy, and rehydrate our apricots. This not only streamlined our recipe but also tempered any excessive sweetness. Bay leaves and cardamom pods steeped in our syrup contributed aromatic depth to the fruit. Thick Greek yogurt made a perfect substitute for the hard-to-find water buffalo cream; we added a bit of rose water to the yogurt to enhance the floral qualities of the apricots. Chopped toasted pistachios made for a traditional finish, and their crunch contrasted beautifully with the rich yogurt and tender fruit. Rose water can be found in Middle Eastern markets as well as in the international food aisle of many supermarkets; if you cannot find it, simply omit it. Look for whole dried apricots that are roughly 1½ inches in diameter.

½ cup 2 percent Greek yogurt
¼ cup sugar
½ teaspoon rose water
½ teaspoon grated lemon zest plus 1 tablespoon juice
   Salt
2 cups water
4 green cardamom pods, cracked
2 bay leaves
24 whole dried apricots
¼ cup shelled pistachios, toasted and chopped fine

1. Combine yogurt, 1 teaspoon sugar, rose water, lemon zest, and pinch salt in small bowl. Refrigerate filling until ready to use.

2. Bring water, cardamom pods, bay leaves, lemon juice, and remaining sugar to simmer in small saucepan over medium-low heat and cook, stirring occasionally, until sugar has dissolved, about 2 minutes. Stir in apricots, return to simmer, and cook, stirring occasionally, until plump and tender, 25 to 30 minutes. Using slotted spoon, transfer apricots to plate and let cool to room temperature.

3. Discard cardamom pods and bay leaves. Bring syrup to boil over high heat and cook, stirring occasionally, until thickened and measures about 3 tablespoons, 4 to 6 minutes; let cool to room temperature.

4. Place pistachios in shallow dish. Place filling in small zipper-lock bag and snip off 1 corner to create ½-inch opening. Pipe filling evenly into opening of each apricot and dip exposed filling into pistachios; transfer to serving platter. Drizzle apricots with syrup and serve.

PER SERVING (4 APRICOTS)
Cal 150 • **Total Fat** 3g • **Sat Fat** 0.5g • **Chol** 0mg
Sodium 40mg • **Total Carbs** 28g • **Fiber** 3g • **Total Sugar** 25g
Added Sugar 8g • **Protein** 3g • **Total Carbohydrate Choices** 2

STUFFING APRICOTS

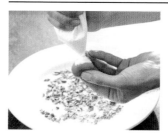 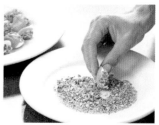

1. Transfer filling to small zipper-lock bag and snip off 1 corner to create ½-inch opening. Pipe filling evenly into opening of each apricot.

2. Dip exposed filling into pistachios; transfer to platter and drizzle with spiced syrup before serving.

Maple-Caramel Apples

SERVES 8

WHY THIS RECIPE WORKS Caramelizing apples until satiny and tender, then topping them with a warm, decadent caramel sauce is a perfect treatment for this often-humble fruit. But in many recipes, the apples turn out barely browned and anemic, or, by the time they're beautifully browned, they are mealy and fall apart. By cooking the apples in butter and a small amount of maple syrup, we could quickly achieve browning without risking overcooking the apples. In fact, the browning occurred a little too quickly: Tasters found these apples a bit underdone. We decided to introduce the maple syrup at a later stage in cooking to allow the apples more time to cook through. This produced perfectly tender apples with burnished amber exteriors. We made a caramel with some additional maple syrup and finished it with a bit of heavy cream and Calvados to create a rich, velvety sauce. We recommend using firm apples, such as Jonagold, Fuji, or Braeburn, in this recipe.

2 tablespoons unsalted butter
4 crisp apples (6½ ounces each), peeled, cored, and halved
6 tablespoons maple syrup
¼ cup heavy cream
1 tablespoon Calvados or apple brandy
¼ teaspoon salt
½ cup sliced almonds, toasted

1. Melt butter in 12-inch nonstick skillet over medium heat. Place apples cut side down in skillet and cook until beginning to brown, 8 to 10 minutes. Flip apples cut side up, add 2 tablespoons maple syrup to skillet, and cook until apples are just tender and tip of paring knife easily pierces fruit, 4 to 6 minutes, adjusting heat as needed to prevent syrup from getting too dark. Off heat, turn apples to coat with caramel, then transfer, cut side up, to platter.

2. Add remaining ¼ cup maple syrup to now-empty skillet and bring to boil over medium heat. Reduce heat to medium-low and cook until mixture thickens slightly and registers 260 degrees, 3 to 4 minutes. Off heat, carefully whisk in cream, Calvados, and salt. Return skillet to medium-low heat and simmer until alcohol has evaporated and mixture thickens again, about 1 minute.

3. Drizzle caramel evenly over apples and sprinkle with almonds. Serve.

PER ½ APPLE
Cal 170 • **Total Fat** 8g • **Sat Fat** 3.5g • **Chol** 15mg
Sodium 75mg • **Total Carbs** 23g • **Fiber** 3g • **Total Sugar** 18g
Added Sugar 9g • **Protein** 2g • **Total Carbohydrate Choices** 2

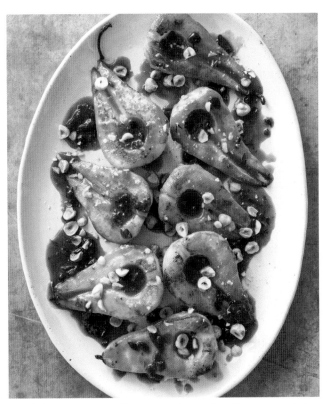

Our hybrid stovetop and oven-roasting method turns pears into an easy and elegant, deeply flavorful dessert.

Roasted Pears with Cider Sauce

SERVES 8

WHY THIS RECIPE WORKS Roasted pears can easily become a raft for a sticky-sweet caramel sauce that overpowers the flavor of the pears. Plus, the pears are often either colorless and mushy or burned and crunchy. We knew we had our work cut out for us if we wanted to achieve our goal: a low-sugar recipe for crisp-tender, beautifully caramelized roasted pears. By starting our fruit over the direct heat of the stovetop we were able to evaporate some of the juices that would otherwise inhibit proper browning. We finished the pears in the oven so they would cook and brown on the outsides. Once the pears were cooked through, we made a simple, flavorful sauce for them using apple cider. The cider picked up the flavorful browned bits left behind by the pears, and we boosted flavor further using ginger, cinnamon, and star anise—no extra sugar needed. Finally, a sprinkling of dried cranberries added a tart-sweet element, and chopped hazelnuts provided welcome crunch and nuttiness. We recommend using firm pears, such as Bartlett or Bosc, in this recipe. Other nuts, such as almonds, pecans, or walnuts, can be substituted for the hazelnuts.

3 tablespoons unsalted butter

4 firm but ripe pears (7 ounces each), peeled, halved, and cored

1 cup apple cider

½ teaspoon cornstarch

¼ cup dried cranberries, chopped

1 cinnamon stick

2 star anise pods

1 (2-inch) piece ginger, peeled and lightly crushed

⅛ teaspoon salt

2 tablespoons chopped toasted and skinned hazelnuts

1. Adjust oven rack to middle position and heat oven to 450 degrees. Melt 2 tablespoons butter in 12-inch ovensafe skillet over medium-high heat. Place pear halves cut side down in skillet and cook, without moving them, until just beginning to brown, about 3 minutes.

2. Transfer skillet to oven and roast pears for 15 minutes. Using tongs, carefully flip pears cut side up and continue to roast until tip of paring knife easily pierces fruit, about 10 minutes.

3. Carefully remove skillet from oven (skillet handle will be hot) and transfer pears to platter. Whisk cider and cornstarch together in bowl. Return now-empty skillet to medium-high heat and add cider mixture, cranberries, cinnamon, star anise, ginger, and salt. Simmer vigorously, scraping up any browned bits with spoon, until sauce is thickened slightly and measures ¾ cup, 5 to 7 minutes.

4. Off heat, discard cinnamon, star anise, and ginger and stir in remaining 1 tablespoon butter. Spoon sauce over pears, sprinkle with hazelnuts, and serve.

PER ½ PEAR

Cal 130 • **Total Fat** 6g • **Sat Fat** 2.5g • **Chol** 10mg
Sodium 40mg • **Total Carbs** 22g • **Fiber** 3g • **Total Sugar** 16g
Added Sugar 0g • **Protein** 1g • **Total Carbohydrate Choices** 1.5

Roasted Plums with Dried Cherries and Almonds
SERVES 8

WHY THIS RECIPE WORKS Plums, roasted until perfectly tender and bronzed, make an ideal after-dinner treat. Since they contain a lot of liquid, we needed to drive off some moisture before we could achieve any browning, so we started by cooking the fruit on the stovetop. Transferring the skillet to the oven for the remainder of the cooking time ensured consistent browning and fork-tender flesh. We made use of the flavorful browned bits in the pan by making a quick pan sauce. Just a little bit of sugar and some dried

cherries brought balanced sweetness, and toasted almonds lent textural contrast. Select plums that yield slightly when pressed. If your plums are small, use a total of 1 to 1¼ pounds. The fruit can be served as is or with plain Greek yogurt.

2 tablespoons unsalted butter

4 ripe but firm plums (4 to 6 ounces each), peeled, halved, and cored

1¼ cups dry white wine

½ cup dried unsweetened tart cherries

3 tablespoons sugar

¼ teaspoon ground cinnamon

⅛ teaspoon salt

1 teaspoon lemon juice

⅓ cup sliced almonds, toasted

1. Adjust oven rack to middle position and heat oven to 450 degrees. Melt butter in 12-inch ovensafe skillet over medium-high heat. Place plum halves cut side down in skillet and cook, without moving them, until just beginning to brown, 3 to 5 minutes.

2. Transfer skillet to oven and roast plums for 5 minutes. Using tongs, carefully flip plums and continue to roast until tip of paring knife easily pierces fruit, about 5 minutes.

3. Carefully remove skillet from oven (skillet handle will be hot) and transfer plums to platter. Add wine, cherries, sugar, cinnamon, and salt to now-empty skillet and bring to simmer over medium-high heat. Cook, whisking to scrape up any browned bits, until sauce is reduced and has consistency of maple syrup, 7 to 10 minutes.

4. Off heat, stir in lemon juice. Pour sauce over plums and sprinkle with almonds. Serve.

PER ½ PLUM

Cal 150 • **Total Fat** 5g • **Sat Fat** 2g • **Chol** 10mg
Sodium 40mg • **Total Carbs** 19g • **Fiber** 2g • **Total Sugar** 14g
Added Sugar 5g • **Protein** 1g • **Total Carbohydrate Choices** 1

Warm Figs with Goat Cheese and Honey
SERVES 6

WHY THIS RECIPE WORKS A piece of barely enhanced fresh fruit is an elegant and healthy end to any meal, and the sweet flesh and delicate flavor of figs need little adornment. We started by choosing the ripest, plumpest figs we could find. Halving them and topping them with a bit of tangy goat cheese offset their sweetness nicely. A brief stint in a hot oven was enough to warm the figs and

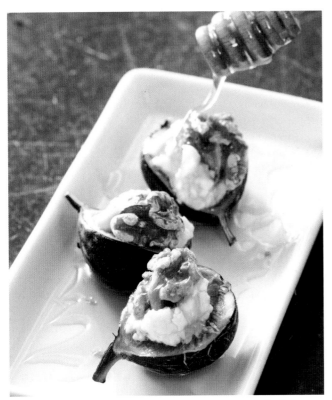

You can make an ultrasimple fruit dessert by pairing fresh figs with tangy goat cheese and toasted walnuts.

cheese through, and topping each one with a toasted walnut half offered pleasant crunchy contrast. Finally, a drizzle of mild honey brought all the elements together with a hit of floral sweetness.

2 ounces goat cheese
9 fresh figs, halved lengthwise
18 walnut halves, toasted
2 tablespoons honey

1. Adjust oven rack to middle position and heat oven to 500 degrees. Spoon heaping ½ teaspoon goat cheese onto each fig half and arrange on parchment paper–lined rimmed baking sheet. Bake figs until heated through, about 4 minutes; transfer to serving platter.

2. Place 1 walnut half on top of each fig half and drizzle with honey. Serve.

PER 3 FIG HALVES
Cal 140 • **Total Fat** 6g • **Sat Fat** 2g • **Chol** 5mg
Sodium 45mg • **Total Carbs** 21g • **Fiber** 3g • **Total Sugar** 18g
Added Sugar 5g • **Protein** 3g • **Total Carbohydrate Choices** 1.5

All About Nuts

With their meaty texture, great flavor, and abundant healthy fats and protein, nuts are welcome in the diabetic diet. We often use them to lend richness, flavor, and crunch to both sweet and savory recipes, and, of course, they make a great snack all on their own.

Storing Nuts

All nuts are high in oil and will become rancid rather quickly. In the test kitchen, we store all nuts in the freezer in freezer-safe zipper-lock bags. Frozen nuts will keep for months, and there's no need to defrost before toasting or chopping.

Toasting Nuts

Toasting nuts brings out their flavors and gives them a satisfying crunchy texture. To toast a small amount (under 1 cup), put the nuts (or seeds) in a dry, small skillet over medium heat. Shake the skillet occasionally to prevent scorching and toast until they are lightly browned and fragrant, 3 to 8 minutes. Watch them closely since they can go from golden to burnt very quickly. To toast more than 1 cup of nuts, spread the nuts in a single layer on a rimmed baking sheet and toast in a 350-degree oven. To promote even toasting, shake the baking sheet every few minutes, and toast until the nuts are lightly browned and fragrant, 5 to 10 minutes.

Skinning Nuts

The skins from some nuts, such as walnuts and hazelnuts, can impart a bitter flavor and undesirable texture in some dishes. To remove the skins, simply rub the hot toasted nuts inside a clean dish towel.

Almond Primer

Most nuts can be found either raw, toasted, or roasted, but almonds are sold in a dizzying array of varieties: raw, roasted, blanched, slivered, sliced, and smoked. So which almonds do we prefer? When it comes to decorating cookies, we like the clean presentation of whole skinless blanched almonds. For other baked goods, leafy salads, and simple side dishes, we find that thinly sliced raw almonds (with or without their skins) deliver a nice, light flavor and texture. In stir-fries and pilafs, we love the substantial crunch of thick-cut slivered almonds. Roasted almonds are best for eating out of hand. As for smoked almonds, we find their bold flavor and crunch are best in snacks like spiced nuts or party mixes.

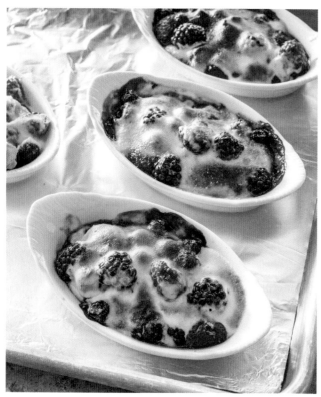

Our custard sauce uses honey and a little heavy cream to make a luxurious topping for fresh berries.

Individual Summer Berry Gratins

SERVES 6

WHY THIS RECIPE WORKS Often served over fresh berries, sabayon is a creamy, sugar-forward dessert sauce that makes for an elegant treat. To create a lower-sugar version with all the custardy appeal of the original, we decided to use honey as our sweetener, which we knew would keep the color clean and would be easy to incorporate with the other ingredients. Although many classic recipes call for wine, we found its flavor overpowering with so little sugar to balance it out. Instead, we opted to flavor our sabayon with just lemon juice and a little zest. Two egg yolks and a small amount of water produced just the light, airy consistency we were after. A moderate amount of honey sweetened the sabayon, tempering the lemon's tart bite without overwhelming it. For additional richness without unwanted eggy flavor, we made a quick whipped cream and folded it into the sabayon. For the berries, we selected a mixture of raspberries, blueberries, and blackberries and dressed them up with some honey and fresh tarragon, whose sweet anise notes complemented the berries nicely and gave the dessert a sophisticated and distinctive flavor. We then baked the berries briefly—just long enough for them to start releasing their juices. To finish, we dolloped the sabayon on top of the berries, then broiled, which browned the sabayon and offered pleasant caramel notes to our simple dessert. You will need six shallow 6-ounce broiler-safe gratin dishes for this recipe. Make sure to keep an eye on the sabayon while broiling as it can burn quickly. Do not use frozen berries for this recipe.

¼ cup honey
2 tablespoons water
2 large egg yolks
½ teaspoon grated lemon zest plus 2 tablespoons juice
  Salt
5 ounces (1 cup) raspberries
5 ounces (1 cup) blackberries
5 ounces (1 cup) blueberries
1 tablespoon minced fresh tarragon
3 tablespoons heavy cream

1. Adjust oven rack to upper-middle position and heat oven to 400 degrees. Line rimmed baking sheet with aluminum foil. Combine 3 tablespoons honey, water, egg yolks, lemon zest and juice, and ⅛ teaspoon salt together in medium bowl and set over saucepan filled with 1 inch of barely simmering water. Cook, whisking gently but constantly, until mixture is slightly thickened, creamy, and glossy, 5 to 10 minutes (mixture will form loose mounds when dripped from whisk).

2. Remove bowl from saucepan and whisk constantly for 30 seconds to cool slightly. Transfer bowl to refrigerator and chill until mixture is completely cool, about 10 minutes.

3. Meanwhile, gently combine raspberries, blackberries, blueberries, tarragon, and ⅛ teaspoon salt in bowl. Microwave remaining 1 tablespoon honey until loose, about 20 seconds. Drizzle warm honey over berry mixture and toss gently to coat evenly. Divide berry mixture evenly among six shallow 6-ounce gratin dishes set on prepared sheet. Bake berries until warm and just beginning to release their juices, about 8 minutes.

4. Transfer sheet to wire rack and heat broiler. Whisk heavy cream in medium bowl until it holds soft peaks, 30 to 90 seconds. Using rubber spatula, gently fold whipped cream into cooled egg mixture, then spoon mixture evenly over berries. Broil until topping is golden brown, 1 to 2 minutes, rotating sheet halfway through broiling. Serve immediately.

PER GRATIN
Cal 120 • **Total Fat** 4.5g • **Sat Fat** 2.5g • **Chol** 70mg
Sodium 105mg • **Total Carbs** 21g • **Fiber** 3g • **Total Sugar** 15g
Added Sugar 11g • **Protein** 2g • **Total Carbohydrate Choices** 1.5

Apple Cinnamon Rollups
MAKES 6 DANISH

WHY THIS RECIPE WORKS Apple Danish are often no-holds-barred confections, with sticky-sweet fillings that barely resemble fruit. They're also a production to make; the flaky dough alone can take hours, not to mention the time required to make the filling. Luckily, store-bought puff pastry proved to be a perfect base for our faux Danish: It's easy to work with, takes no time to prep, and contains very little sugar. But that was only half the battle. We also wanted a simple, fruit-forward filling that wasn't laden with sugar but still tasted pleasantly sweet. We decided to brush a small amount of apricot jelly onto the puff pastry to give the rollups a sweet-tart base. A sprinkle of cinnamon sugar gave us the sweetness we craved without going overboard. Sliced apples, tossed with ginger, lemon juice, and a bit more cinnamon, made a perfect filling. Rolling the puff pastry around the apple slices created rose-like treats that were as pretty as they were delicious. Parbaking the apple slices ensured that they were pliable enough to roll without breaking. To thaw frozen puff pastry, let it sit either in the refrigerator for 24 hours or on the counter for 30 minutes to 1 hour.

2 apples (6 ounces each), cored, halved, and sliced thin
1 tablespoon unsalted butter, melted and cooled
2 teaspoons lemon juice
1 teaspoon ground cinnamon
½ teaspoon ground ginger
¼ teaspoon salt
2 tablespoons sugar
1 (9½ by 9-inch) sheet puff pastry, thawed
2 tablespoons apricot preserves

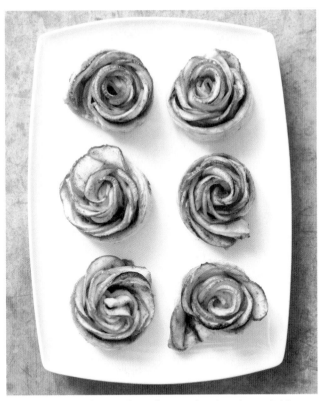

Parbaking apple slices softens them and makes them pliable enough to create a rose-shaped pastry without breaking.

1. Adjust oven rack to middle position and heat oven to 375 degrees. Toss apples with melted butter, lemon juice, ½ teaspoon cinnamon, ginger, and salt in bowl. Spread apples in single layer on parchment paper–lined rimmed baking sheet and bake until softened, about 10 minutes. Set aside until cool enough to handle, about 10 minutes.

ASSEMBLING APPLE CINNAMON ROLLUPS

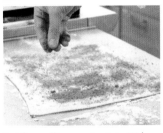

1. After rolling pastry into 12 by 10-inch rectangle, brush with preserves and sprinkle with cinnamon sugar.

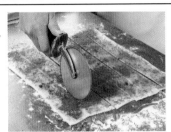

2. Using sharp knife or pizza wheel, cut pastry lengthwise into six 10 by 2-inch strips.

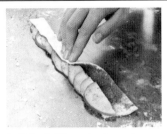

3. Shingle 12 apple slices down 1 length of dough, leaving 1-inch border of dough on one side, then fold bare inch of dough over bottom of apple slices.

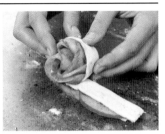

4. Roll up dough and apples into tight pinwheel.

2. Line clean baking sheet with parchment and lightly spray with canola oil spray. Combine sugar and remaining ½ teaspoon cinnamon in bowl.

3. Roll pastry into 12 by 10-inch rectangle on lightly floured counter, with long side parallel to counter edge. Brush preserves evenly over top and sprinkle with cinnamon sugar. Using sharp knife or pizza wheel, cut pastry lengthwise into six 10 by 2-inch strips.

4. Working with 1 strip of dough at a time, shingle 12 apple slices, peel side out, along length of dough, leaving 1-inch border of dough on one side. Fold bare inch of dough over bottom of apple slices, leaving top of apple slices exposed. Roll up dough and apples into tight pinwheel and place, apple side up, on prepared sheet.

5. Bake until golden brown and crisp, 22 to 26 minutes, rotating sheet halfway through baking. Let Danish cool on sheet for 15 minutes before serving.

PER DANISH

Cal 240 • **Total Fat** 12g • **Sat Fat** 6g • **Chol** 5mg
Sodium 240mg • **Total Carbs** 36g • **Fiber** 2g • **Total Sugar** 13g
Added Sugar 4g • **Protein** 3g • **Total Carbohydrate Choices** 2.5

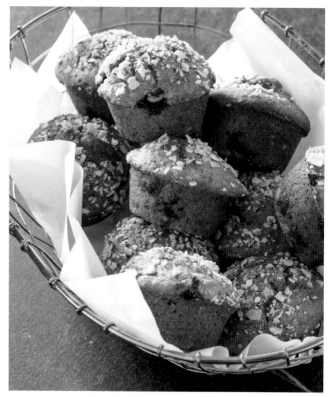

A combination of whole-wheat and all-purpose flours provides the ideal structure for these blueberry muffins.

Whole-Wheat Blueberry Muffins
MAKES 12 MUFFINS

WHY THIS RECIPE WORKS We wanted to build a healthier blueberry muffin using whole-wheat flour. Problem is, most whole-wheat muffins are dense, bland sinkers that nobody wants to eat. Could we create a version that was tender and delicious? First, we needed to address the cardboard-like flavor that plagues so many whole-wheat muffins. We replaced part of the whole-wheat flour with ground toasted almonds and loved how their richness and nuttiness complemented the whole wheat's own earthy, nutty flavor. But the muffins were still squat and dense. Switching gears, we combined two leaveners—baking soda and baking powder. We were surprised to find how tender our muffins became—too tender. Because whole-wheat flour forms a relatively weak gluten network (which was further weakened by the fat in the almonds), these muffins lacked the structure to even come out of the pan. Incorporating ¾ cup all-purpose flour into the mix brought structural integrity back to our muffins while keeping them tender.

1 cup sliced almonds, lightly toasted
1 cup (5½ ounces) whole-wheat flour
¾ cup (3¾ ounces) all-purpose flour
2 teaspoons baking powder
½ teaspoon baking soda
¾ teaspoon salt
1 cup low-fat buttermilk
⅔ cup packed (4⅔ ounces) dark brown sugar
2 large eggs
¼ cup canola oil
2 teaspoons vanilla extract
7½ ounces (1½ cups) fresh or frozen blueberries

1. Adjust oven rack to middle position and heat oven to 400 degrees. Spray 12-cup muffin tin, including top, generously with canola oil spray. Pulse ¼ cup almonds in food processor until coarsely chopped, 4 to 6 pulses; transfer to small bowl and set aside for topping.

2. Add whole-wheat flour, all-purpose flour, baking powder, baking soda, salt, and remaining ¾ cup almonds to now-empty processor and process until well combined and almonds are finely ground, about 30 seconds; transfer to large bowl.

3. In separate bowl, whisk buttermilk, sugar, eggs, oil, and vanilla until combined. Using rubber spatula, stir buttermilk mixture into almond-flour mixture until just combined (do not overmix). Gently fold in blueberries until incorporated.

4. Divide batter evenly among prepared muffin cups (cups will be filled to rim) and sprinkle with reserved chopped almonds. Bake until golden brown and toothpick inserted in center comes out with few crumbs attached, 16 to 18 minutes, rotating tin halfway through baking.

5. Let muffins cool in tin on wire rack for 10 minutes. Remove muffins from tin and let cool for 20 minutes before serving.

PER MUFFIN

Cal 240 • **Total Fat** 10g • **Sat Fat** 1g • **Chol** 30mg
Sodium 310mg • **Total Carbs** 32g • **Fiber** 3g • **Total Sugar** 14g
Added Sugar 11g • **Protein** 6g • **Total Carbohydrate Choices** 2

PORTIONING MUFFINS

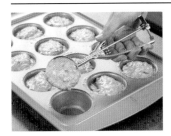

For neat, evenly sized muffins, portion batter into each cup using measuring cup or ice cream scoop, then circle back and evenly distribute remaining batter with spoon.

Oatmeal Cookies with Chocolate and Goji Berries
MAKES 24 COOKIES

WHY THIS RECIPE WORKS Few desserts are more appealing than warm cookies straight from the oven. Instead of depriving ourselves of this treat, we sought to create a "better for you" cookie that emphasized whole grains. As we love the soft chew and heartiness of the oatmeal-raisin variety, we used that as our starting point. A hefty 3 cups of fiber-rich rolled oats would ensure plenty of whole-grain benefits. Using solely oat flour resulted in a crumbly dough, so we ultimately stuck with all-purpose flour to provide the necessary structure. We wanted some nutritious mix-ins, so for an antioxidant boost, we stirred chopped dark chocolate and a

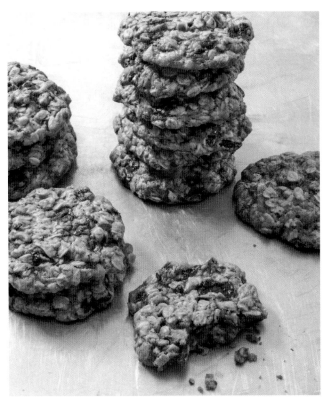

Nutrient-rich dried goji berries are a good source of vitamins, iron, and fiber, making them a good add-in to cookies.

cup of sweet-tart goji berries into the dough. Heart-healthy canola oil kept the cookies dense and chewy. A bit of salt complemented the oats and brought out their nuttiness, and a tablespoon of water helped the cookies spread to the perfect size. Do not use quick, instant, or thick-cut oats in this recipe. If you can't find goji berries, you can substitute dried unsweetened tart cherries. We prefer the flavor of 70 percent dark chocolate in this recipe, though higher cacao percentages will also work (see page 261).

- 1 cup (5 ounces) all-purpose flour
- ¾ teaspoon salt
- ½ teaspoon baking soda
- 1 cup packed (7 ounces) dark brown sugar
- ⅔ cup canola oil
- 1 tablespoon water
- 1 teaspoon vanilla extract
- 1 large egg plus 1 large yolk
- 3 cups (9 ounces) old-fashioned rolled oats
- 1 cup dried goji berries
- 3½ ounces 70 percent dark chocolate, chopped into ¼-inch pieces

1. Adjust oven rack to middle position and heat oven to 375 degrees. Line 2 rimmed baking sheets with parchment paper. Whisk flour, salt, and baking soda together in bowl; set aside.

2. Whisk sugar, oil, water, and vanilla together in large bowl until well combined. Add egg and yolk and whisk until smooth. Using rubber spatula, stir in flour mixture until fully combined. Add oats, goji berries, and chocolate and stir until evenly distributed (mixture will be stiff).

3. Divide dough into 24 portions, each about heaping 2 tablespoons. Using damp hands, tightly roll into balls and space 2 inches apart on prepared sheets, 12 balls per sheet. Press balls to ¾-inch thickness.

4. Bake, 1 sheet at a time, until edges are set and centers are soft but not wet, 8 to 10 minutes, rotating sheet halfway through baking. Let cookies cool on sheets for 5 minutes, then transfer to wire rack. Let cookies cool completely before serving.

PER COOKIE

Cal 190 • **Total Fat** 9g • **Sat Fat** 2g • **Chol** 15mg
Sodium 100mg • **Total Carbs** 24g • **Fiber** 2g • **Total Sugar** 11g
Added Sugar 8g • **Protein** 3g • **Total Carbohydrate Choices** 1.5

NOTES FROM THE TEST KITCHEN

Freezing Cookie Dough

By keeping unbaked cookie dough in the freezer, you can bake just a few cookies at a time. Portion out the dough as you would for baking right away—either on parchment-lined baking sheets or on large plates—and freeze the dough until solid, at least 30 minutes. Arrange the frozen unbaked cookies in a zipper-lock bag or in layers in an airtight storage container and place them back in the freezer for up to two months. You may need to increase the recipe's baking time, but no defrosting is necessary.

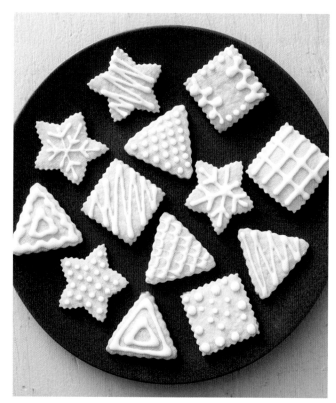

To achieve perfectly flat cookies, we strike the baking sheet against the oven door partway through baking.

Holiday Cookies
MAKES FORTY 2½-INCH COOKIES

WHY THIS RECIPE WORKS We were pleasantly surprised that halving the sugar of our holiday cookie recipe yielded buttery, sweet cookies. But without the added sugar, the cookies domed during baking, producing an unsightly (and undecoratable) hump on each cookie. Without the tenderizing power of the extra sugar, the cookies were developing too much gluten structure, and the initial burst of heat in the oven was causing water in the dough to quickly turn to steam, an effect called "oven spring." We tried lowering the oven temperature to diminish the oven spring, but the cookies still had noticeable domes. We tried manipulating the amount of butter and cream cheese, but it made no difference. We arrived at a solution through a happy accident: Halfway through baking, if we jostled the baking sheet, some of the cookies would deflate and bake up perfectly flat. By striking the pan against a surface partway through baking, we could create flat, uniform shapes every time. Using this simple but unconventional method, we were able to cut the sugar in half without sacrificing texture or aesthetics.

COOKIES

6 tablespoons (2⅔ ounces) granulated sugar

2½ cups (12½ ounces) all-purpose flour

⅛ teaspoon salt

16 tablespoons unsalted butter, cut into 16 pieces and softened

1 ounce cream cheese, softened

2 teaspoons vanilla extract

GLAZE

1 ounce cream cheese

1–2 tablespoons 1 percent low-fat milk

⅛ teaspoon salt

¾ cup (3 ounces) confectioners' sugar

1. FOR THE COOKIES Using stand mixer fitted with paddle, mix sugar, flour, and salt together on low speed until combined, about 1 minute. Add butter, 1 piece at a time, and mix until only pea-size pieces remain, about 1 minute. Add cream cheese and vanilla and mix until dough just begins to form large clumps, about 30 seconds.

2. Transfer dough to clean counter, knead until dough forms cohesive mass, then divide into 2 equal pieces. Shape each piece into 4-inch disk, then wrap in plastic wrap and refrigerate until firm, at least 30 minutes or up to 3 days.

3. Adjust oven rack to middle position and heat oven to 375 degrees. Working with 1 piece of dough at a time, roll ⅛ inch thick between 2 sheets of parchment paper. Slide dough, still between parchment, onto baking sheet and refrigerate until firm, about 20 minutes.

4. Line 2 baking sheets with parchment. Working with 1 sheet of dough at a time, remove top sheet of parchment and cut dough as desired using cookie cutters; space cookies ¾ inch apart on prepared sheets. (Dough scraps can be patted together, chilled, and rerolled once.)

5. Bake cookies, 1 sheet at a time, until lightly puffed but still underdone, about 5 minutes. Remove partially baked cookies from oven and, holding sheet firmly with both hands, rap pan flat against open oven door 3 to 5 times until puffed cookies flatten. Rotate pan, return cookies to oven, and continue to bake until light golden brown around edges, 4 to 6 minutes. Let cookies cool completely on sheet.

6. FOR THE GLAZE Whisk cream cheese, 1 tablespoon milk, and salt together in medium bowl until smooth. Whisk in confectioners' sugar until smooth, adding remaining 1 tablespoon

milk as needed until glaze is thin enough to drizzle. Drizzle or decorate each cookie with glaze as desired. Let glaze set for at least 6 hours before serving.

PER COOKIE

Cal 90 • **Total Fat** 5g • **Sat Fat** 3g • **Chol** 15mg
Sodium 20mg • **Total Carbs** 11g • **Fiber** 0g • **Total Sugar** 4g
Added Sugar 4g • **Protein** 1g • **Total Carbohydrate Choices** 1

NOTES FROM THE TEST KITCHEN

Using A Sugar Substitute

When it comes to making desserts, many diabetics turn to using sugar substitutes such as Splenda. Splenda is the brand name for granulated sucralose, which is sucrose plus chlorine. There is also a blend available that is a mix of granulated sucralose and granulated sugar. Keep in mind that these substitutes are not carbohydrate- or calorie-free.

Although many artificial sweeteners have been deemed "safe" for use by the FDA, their effect on the body and brain remains under continuous debate and research in the medical and nutrition communities. Regular use and reliance on artificial sweeteners may change the way we taste food by increasing the desire for intense sweetness, thus diminishing tolerance to more complex and less sweet (and oftentimes more nutritious) foods such as fruits and vegetables. Additionally, research suggests that regular use of artificial sweeteners may prevent us from associating sweetness with caloric intake, again leading us to eat more sweet foods over nutritious foods, ultimately increasing the risk of becoming overweight and obese.

We've tested some of our recipes using Splenda and found that not only were texture and structure less than desirable, but it left an artificial aftertaste. Baked goods also turned out unappealingly pale, since sugar encourages browning. So in the test kitchen we prefer to skip the fake stuff and just use sugar in moderation. Our goal is to use real foods—like granulated sugar—and to show that they can fit into a diabetes diet with careful meal planning and portion control. At the end of the day sweets should not play a big role in your diabetic meal plan. They are a form of carbohydrates and keeping tabs on your total carbohydrate intake and balancing those carbohydrates are what matters most.

Almond Biscotti
MAKES 15 COOKIES

WHY THIS RECIPE WORKS Our ideal lower-sugar biscotti had to meet the perfect afternoon coffee requirements: bold, nutty flavor; satisfying (but not tooth-breaking) crunch; good for dipping but equally delicious on their own. We found that cutting the sugar of our traditional recipe by half produced a satisfactory flavor, and we did not miss the extra sweetness. But while the cookies were certainly flavorful, they were drier and a bit harder than we wanted. With less sugar, the dough was unable to hold on to as much moisture. The typical two-step baking process—once to set the log, and a second time to toast the slices—only exacerbated the problem. To account for the loss in moisture, we reduced the baking time in both stages. The resulting biscotti were less dry and sandy, but they were still a bit hard to bite. Whipping the eggs helped alleviate this problem by imparting lift and aeration to the cookies. But too much gluten was still developing in the dough; in order to temper the gluten development and contribute a slight crumbliness, we cut the flour with ground toasted almonds— which gave the added benefit of extra nutty flavor. Be sure to toast the nuts lightly before making the dough, as they will continue to toast as the biscotti bake.

²/₃ cups whole almonds, lightly toasted
¾ cup plus 2 tablespoons (4⅓ ounces) all-purpose flour
1 teaspoon baking powder
⅛ teaspoon salt
1 large egg, plus 1 lightly beaten large egg white
¼ cup (1¾ ounces) sugar
2 tablespoons unsalted butter, melted and cooled
¾ teaspoon almond extract
¼ teaspoon vanilla extract

1. Adjust oven rack to middle position and heat oven to 325 degrees. Line rimmed baking sheet with parchment paper and spray with vegetable oil spray. Pulse ½ cup almonds in food processor until coarsely chopped, 8 to 10 pulses; transfer to bowl.

2. Process remaining almonds in now-empty food processor until finely ground, about 45 seconds. Add flour, baking powder, and salt and process to combine, about 15 seconds; transfer to separate bowl.

3. Add whole egg to now-empty food processor. With processor running, slowly add sugar until thoroughly combined, about 15 seconds. Add melted butter, almond extract, and vanilla and process until combined, about 10 seconds; transfer to large bowl.

4. Sprinkle half of flour mixture over egg mixture and, using rubber spatula, fold until just combined. Add remaining flour mixture and chopped almonds and fold until just combined.

5. Using your floured hands, press dough into 8 by 3-inch loaf on prepared baking sheet. Brush loaf with beaten egg white. Bake loaf until golden and just beginning to crack on top, 20 to 25 minutes, rotating sheet halfway through baking.

6. Let loaf cool on sheet for 30 minutes, then transfer loaf to cutting board. Using serrated knife, slice loaf on slight bias into ½-inch-thick slices. Lay slices, cut side down, about ¼ inch apart on wire rack set in rimmed baking sheet. Bake cookies until crisp and light golden brown on both sides, 25 to 30 minutes, flipping slices and rotating sheet halfway through baking. Let biscotti cool completely on rack before serving.

PER COOKIE

Cal 100 • **Total Fat** 5g • **Sat Fat** 1.5g • **Chol** 15mg
Sodium 55mg • **Total Carbs** 11g • **Fiber** 1g • **Total Sugar** 4g
Added Sugar 3g • **Protein** 3g • **Total Carbohydrate Choices** 1

MAKING BISCOTTI

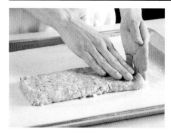

1. Using your floured hands, press dough into 8 by 3-inch loaf on prepared baking sheet.

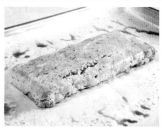

2. Bake loaf until golden and just beginning to crack on top, 20 to 25 minutes.

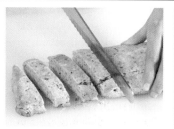

3. Let loaf cool for 30 minutes, then slice on slight bias into ½-inch-thick slices using serrated knife.

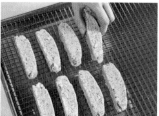

4. Lay slices, cut side down, ¼ inch apart on wire rack set in rimmed baking sheet and bake until crisp and light golden brown, 25 to 30 minutes.

Hazelnut-Orange Biscotti

Substitute lightly toasted and skinned hazelnuts for almonds. Add 1 tablespoon minced fresh rosemary to food processor with flour. Substitute orange-flavored liqueur for almond extract and add 1½ teaspoons grated orange zest to egg mixture.

PER COOKIE

Cal 100 • **Total Fat** 6g • **Sat Fat** 1.5g • **Chol** 15mg
Sodium 55mg • **Total Carbs** 11g • **Fiber** 1g • **Total Sugar** 4g
Added Sugar 3g • **Protein** 2g • **Total Carbohydrate Choices** 1

Pistachio-Spice Biscotti

Substitute shelled pistachios for almonds. Add ½ teaspoon ground cardamom, ¼ teaspoon ground cloves, ¼ teaspoon pepper, ⅛ teaspoon ground cinnamon, and ⅛ teaspoon ground ginger to food processor with flour. Substitute ½ teaspoon water for almond extract and increase vanilla extract to ½ teaspoon.

PER COOKIE

Cal 90 • **Total Fat** 4.5g • **Sat Fat** 1.5g • **Chol** 15mg
Sodium 55mg • **Total Carbs** 11g • **Fiber** 1g • **Total Sugar** 4g
Added Sugar 3g • **Protein** 3g • **Total Carbohydrate Choices** 1

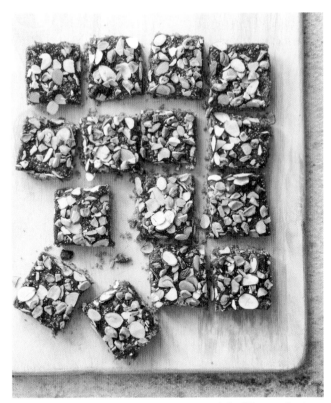

Dried figs are naturally sweet plus they are full of fiber and rich in several vitamins.

Fig Bars
MAKES 16 BARS

WHY THIS RECIPE WORKS Dried figs make a great bar cookie filling: They're naturally supersweet and have great depth of flavor; plus, they're available year-round. Dried figs are relatively low in sugar compared to other dried fruits. We wanted to take advantage of figs' inherent sweetness to create a bar with no added sugar. The filling was simple: We hydrated the figs (soft, sweet Turkish or Calimyrna figs worked best) with a little no-sugar-added apple juice and then pureed the mixture to create a jammy, ultraflavorful fig filling. But we ran into problems with the crust. We wanted a shortbread-like crust and topping that would provide balanced, buttery flavor and nice textural contrast. But with no sugar at all, the crust tasted floury and flat and the texture was far too soft. We first tried incorporating some of the pureed fig mixture into the crust for sweetness, but found it only made the base mushy. The simplest solution turned out to be the best one: We used a bit of the no-sugar-added apple juice to impart a slight sweetness

and give us the shortbread texture we were after. Baking the crust on its own ensured a flaky texture; once it cooled, all we had to do was spread the fig filling over the crust. A simple sprinkling of toasted nuts on top gave us the extra crunch we craved, for a bar that now had only 6 grams of sugar. Do not use dried Black Mission figs in this recipe.

1 cup (5 ounces) all-purpose flour
2 teaspoons ground allspice
½ teaspoon salt
¼ teaspoon baking powder
8 tablespoons unsalted butter, cut into ½-inch pieces and chilled
½ cup plus 3 tablespoons no-sugar-added apple juice
1 cup dried Turkish or Calimyrna figs, stemmed and quartered
¼ cup sliced almonds, toasted
¼ cup shelled pistachios, toasted and chopped

1. Adjust oven rack to middle position and heat oven to 375 degrees. Make foil sling for 8-inch square baking pan by folding 2 long sheets of aluminum foil so each is 8 inches wide. Lay sheets of foil in pan perpendicular to each other, with extra foil hanging over edges of pan. Push foil into corners and up sides of pan, smoothing foil flush to pan. Grease foil.

2. Pulse flour, allspice, salt, and baking powder in food processor until combined, about 3 pulses. Scatter chilled butter over top and pulse until mixture resembles wet sand, about 10 pulses. Add 3 tablespoons apple juice and pulse until dough comes together, about 8 pulses.

3. Transfer mixture to prepared pan and press into even layer with bottom of dry measuring cup. Bake crust until golden brown, 35 to 40 minutes, rotating pan halfway through baking. Let crust cool completely in pan, about 45 minutes.

4. Microwave figs and remaining ½ cup apple juice in covered bowl until slightly softened, about 2 minutes. Puree fig mixture in now-empty food processor until smooth, about 15 seconds. Spread fig mixture evenly over cooled crust, then sprinkle with almonds and pistachios, pressing to adhere. Using foil overhang, lift bars from pan and transfer to cutting board. Cut into 16 squares and serve.

PER BAR

Cal 130 • **Total Fat** 7g • **Sat Fat** 3.5g • **Chol** 15mg
Sodium 80mg • **Total Carbs** 15g • **Fiber** 2g • **Total Sugar** 6g
Added Sugar 0g • **Protein** 2g • **Total Carbohydrate Choices** 1

Carrot Snack Cake
SERVES 12

WHY THIS RECIPE WORKS Simple, sweet, and satisfying, snack cakes will curb just about any cake craving. Instead of a plain vanilla cake, which offers little in the way of nutrition, we wanted a moist, rich carrot snack cake. Carrot cakes typically use oil instead of butter for their fat, another plus. To maximize the nutritional punch of the carrots, we incorporated as many as the batter could handle without making it too difficult to spread or overly vegetal tasting. We tried replacing the standard white flour with whole-wheat and found we preferred whole-wheat flour's earthy, nutty flavor, which complemented the carrots. We included just enough sugar to make our cake pleasantly moist and sweet, but not so much that it overpowered the other flavors. Fragrant, warm spices complemented the carrots' natural sweetness. To streamline the process, we relied on our food processor to both shred the carrots and mix the batter.

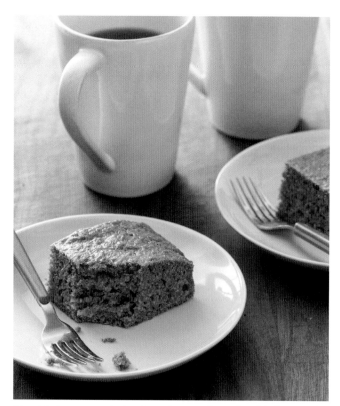

Shredded carrots, whole-wheat flour, and canola oil help to make our carrot snack cake nutritious as well as delicious.

12 ounces carrots, peeled
⅔ cup (4⅔ ounces) sugar
¼ cup canola oil
¼ cup 1 percent low-fat milk
2 large eggs
2 teaspoons vanilla extract
1 teaspoon baking powder
¾ teaspoon ground cinnamon
½ teaspoon baking soda
¼ teaspoon ground nutmeg
¼ teaspoon salt
1⅓ cups (7⅓ ounces) whole-wheat flour

1. Adjust oven rack to middle position and heat oven to 350 degrees. Make foil sling for 8-inch square baking pan by folding 2 long sheets of aluminum foil so each is 8 inches wide. Lay sheets of foil in pan perpendicular to each other, with extra foil hanging over edges of pan. Push foil into corners and up sides of pan, smoothing foil flush to pan. Grease foil. Working in batches, use food processor fitted with shredding disk to shred carrots; transfer carrots to bowl.

2. Fit now-empty processor with chopping blade. Process sugar, oil, milk, eggs, vanilla, baking powder, cinnamon, baking soda, nutmeg, and salt until sugar is mostly dissolved and mixture is emulsified, 10 to 12 seconds, scraping down sides of bowl as needed. Add shredded carrots and pulse until combined, about 3 pulses. Add flour and pulse until just incorporated, about 5 pulses; do not overmix.

3. Scrape batter into prepared pan and smooth top. Bake until cake is light golden and toothpick inserted in center comes out clean, 26 to 30 minutes, rotating pan halfway through baking.

4. Let cake cool in pan on wire rack for 10 minutes. Using foil overhang, remove cake from pan and return to wire rack. Discard foil and let cake cool completely on rack, about 2 hours. Cut cake into 12 pieces and serve.

PER 2-INCH PIECE

Cal 170 • **Total Fat** 6g • **Sat Fat** 0.5g • **Chol** 30mg
Sodium 170mg • **Total Carbs** 27g • **Fiber** 3g • **Total Sugar** 13g
Added Sugar 11g • **Protein** 4g • **Total Carbohydrate Choices** 2

Mini Chocolate Cupcakes with Creamy Chocolate Frosting

MAKES 12 MINI CUPCAKES

WHY THIS RECIPE WORKS An indulgent treat, a good chocolate cupcake should be rich and ultrachocolaty. It also must have a moist and tender yet sturdy crumb. To make this splurge-worthy dessert diabetic-friendly, we reached for our mini muffin tin to bake a more sensibly sized treat. Using less sugar than in our traditional recipe produced a decent cupcake with abundant chocolate flavor. However, with less sugar, the cupcake was still a bit dense: To solve this problem, we turned to higher protein bread flour and increased the amount of baking powder to open up the crumb. This cake was now lighter, but it was also drier and had muted chocolate flavor. We tested cupcakes using butter and oil and found that oil produced a moister cake than butter. We couldn't add more chocolate without sacrificing texture or adding more sugar, so we turned to coffee since its robust flavor enhances chocolate flavor. A few teaspoons of vinegar helped to activate the leavening power of the baking soda, ensuring a perfect texture. The frosting came together in just a couple of minutes with the help of the food processor. The quick cutting motion of the blade emulsified the ingredients into a smooth frosting that didn't break into a greasy mess as we frosted the cupcakes. We were left with party-perfect cupcakes that were mini in size, but not in flavor. If you use natural cocoa powder for this recipe, the cake will be

Chocolate

Chocolate is not off limits as long as it is used judiciously and you make the right choices from among the many types. Semisweet, bittersweet, and milk chocolates usually contain sugar. Depending on the brand, cacao percentage, and other factors, sweetened chocolates can contain variable amounts of sugar, so we suggest using our recommended brands for the best results.

MILK CHOCOLATE Milk chocolate is the sweetest chocolate. Although it must contain at least 10 percent chocolate liquor and 12 percent milk solids, the rest is made up of sweeteners and flavorings (milk chocolate is usually more than 50 percent sugar and contains more saturated fat than other varieties). Our favorite brand is **Dove Silky Smooth Milk Chocolate**.

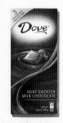

DARK CHOCOLATE Encompassing semisweet and bittersweet chocolates, dark chocolate must contain at least 35 percent chocolate liquor, although most contain more than 55 percent and some go as high as 99 percent. When possible, we use bittersweet chocolate since it generally contains less sugar than semisweet; our favorite brand is **Ghirardelli 60% Cacao Bittersweet Chocolate Premium Baking Bar**. We've also had good luck with **Ghirardelli Semi-Sweet Chocolate Premium Baking Bar**.

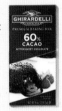

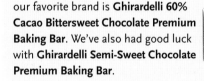

UNSWEETENED CHOCOLATE Unsweetened chocolate contains no sugar and worked well when we wanted a bold chocolate flavor. Our favorite brand is **Hershey's Unsweetened Baking Bar**.

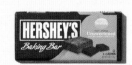

COCOA POWDER Cocoa powder comes in natural and Dutch-processed versions. Dutching raises the powder's pH, which neutralizes its acids and astringent notes and rounds out its flavor; it also darkens the color. Make sure to check the label, as some brands are sweetened. Our favorite Dutch-processed cocoa powder is **Droste Cacao**; the natural cocoa powder we used is **Hershey's Natural Unsweetened Cocoa**.

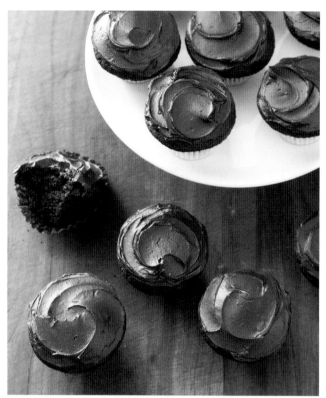

Brewed coffee helps to enhance the flavor of both bittersweet chocolate and cocoa powder in our very chocolaty mini cupcakes.

lighter in appearance and have a milder chocolate flavor. Our favorite brand of bittersweet chocolate is Ghirardelli 60% Cacao Bittersweet Chocolate Premium Baking Bar (see page 361 for more information); other brands may contain different amounts of sugar. You will need a mini muffin tin for this recipe.

CAKE

- 1½ ounces bittersweet chocolate, chopped
- 3 tablespoons Dutch-processed cocoa powder
- ⅓ cup hot brewed coffee
- 6 tablespoons (2 ounces) bread flour
- ¼ cup (3½ ounces) granulated sugar
- ¼ teaspoon salt
- ¼ teaspoon baking soda
- ¼ teaspoon baking powder
- 3 tablespoons canola oil
- 1 large egg
- 1 teaspoon distilled white vinegar
- ½ teaspoon vanilla extract

CHOCOLATE FROSTING

- 2 ounces bittersweet chocolate, chopped
- 6 tablespoons unsalted butter, softened
- ½ cup (2 ounces) confectioners' sugar
- ¼ cup (¾ ounce) Dutch-processed cocoa powder
  Pinch salt
- 1 teaspoon vanilla extract

1. FOR THE CAKE Adjust oven rack to middle position and heat oven to 350 degrees. Line 12 cups of mini muffin tin with paper or foil liners.

2. Place chocolate and cocoa in medium bowl, add hot coffee, and whisk until melted and smooth. Refrigerate mixture until completely cool, about 20 minutes. In separate bowl, whisk flour, granulated sugar, salt, baking soda, and baking powder together.

3. Whisk oil, egg, vinegar, and vanilla into cooled chocolate mixture until smooth. Add flour mixture and whisk until smooth.

4. Portion batter evenly into prepared muffin tin, filling cups to rim. Bake cupcakes until toothpick inserted in center comes out with few crumbs attached, 14 to 16 minutes, rotating muffin tin halfway through baking.

5. Let cupcakes cool in muffin tin on wire rack for 10 minutes. Remove cupcakes from muffin tin and let cool completely on rack, about 1 hour. (Unfrosted cupcakes can be stored at room temperature for up to 2 days.)

6. FOR THE FROSTING Microwave chocolate in bowl at 50 percent power, stirring occasionally, until melted and smooth, 2 to 4 minutes. Let cool slightly. Process butter, confectioners' sugar, cocoa, and salt in food processor until smooth, about 20 seconds, scraping down sides of bowl as needed. Add vanilla and process until just combined, 5 to 10 seconds. Add melted chocolate and pulse until smooth and creamy, about 10 pulses, scraping down sides of bowl as needed. (Frosting can be kept at room temperature for up to 3 hours before using or refrigerated for up to 3 days. If refrigerated, let sit at room temperature for 1 hour before using.)

7. Spread frosting evenly over cupcakes and serve.

PER CUPCAKE (WITH FROSTING)
Cal 210 • **Total Fat** 13g • **Sat Fat** 6g • **Chol** 30mg
Sodium 100mg • **Total Carbs** 22g • **Fiber** 2g • **Total Sugar** 13g
Added Sugar 13g • **Protein** 2g • **Total Carbohydrate Choices** 1.5

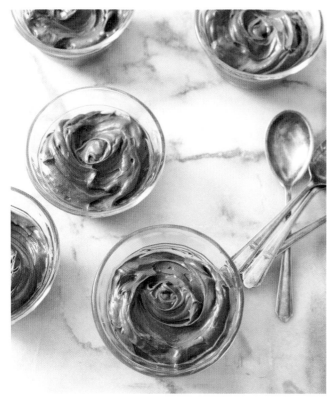

Our rich-tasting—and dairy-free—chocolate pudding uses heart-healthy avocados for its creamy base.

Dark Chocolate–Avocado Pudding
SERVES 8

WHY THIS RECIPE WORKS Making a luscious chocolate pudding by substituting vitamin-rich, heart-healthy avocados for the cream and eggs has become something of a craze. We wanted a pudding that was silky-smooth with blockbuster chocolate flavor that concealed any vegetal notes. And we didn't want the recipe to be too complicated. Rather than start by simply blending everything together, we created a simple hot cocoa syrup in a saucepan (with a touch of espresso powder, vanilla, and salt to enhance the chocolate flavor). Meanwhile, we processed the flesh of two large avocados for a full two minutes until they were absolutely smooth. Next, with the food processor running, we carefully streamed in the cocoa syrup until the mixture was velvety and glossy. We finished by blending in a moderate amount of melted dark chocolate

to give our pudding a wonderfully full chocolate flavor and additional richness. We prefer the flavor of 70 percent dark chocolate in this recipe, though higher cacao percentages will also work.

> 1 cup water
> ¼ cup (1¾ ounces) sugar
> ¼ cup (¾ ounce) unsweetened cocoa powder
> 1 tablespoon vanilla extract
> 1 teaspoon instant espresso powder (optional)
> ¼ teaspoon salt
> 2 large ripe avocados (8 ounces each), halved and pitted
> 3½ ounces 70 percent dark chocolate, chopped

1. Combine water, sugar, cocoa, vanilla, espresso powder (if using), and salt in small saucepan. Bring to simmer over medium heat and cook, stirring occasionally, until sugar and cocoa dissolve, about 2 minutes. Remove saucepan from heat and cover to keep warm.

2. Scoop flesh of avocados into food processor bowl and process until smooth, about 2 minutes, scraping down sides of bowl as needed. With processor running, slowly add warm cocoa mixture in steady stream until completely incorporated and mixture is smooth and glossy, about 2 minutes.

3. Microwave chocolate in bowl at 50 percent power, stirring occasionally, until melted, 2 to 4 minutes. Add to avocado mixture and process until well incorporated, about 1 minute. Transfer pudding to bowl, cover, and refrigerate until chilled and set, at least 2 hours or up to 24 hours. Serve.

PER SERVING
Cal 170 • **Total Fat** 12g • **Sat Fat** 4g • **Chol** 0mg
Sodium 75mg • **Total Carbs** 17g • **Fiber** 5g • **Total Sugar** 10g
Added Sugar 6g • **Protein** 2g • **Total Carbohydrate Choices** 1

MELTING CHOCOLATE IN THE MICROWAVE

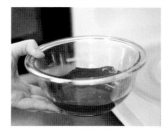

Microwave the chopped chocolate at 50 percent power for the amount of time specified in the recipe. (This will depend on the amount of chocolate.) Stir the chocolate and continue microwaving until melted, stirring occasionally.

Strawberry Mousse
SERVES 8

WHY THIS RECIPE WORKS We set out to create a lighter, healthier mousse with a beautifully fluffy texture and unmistakable strawberry flavor. To enhance the strawberries' natural sweetness, we macerated some of the berries with just a quarter-cup of sugar. This drew out some of the berries' juices; we didn't want to toss the juice (and the flavor) down the drain, but we knew the large amount of liquid would make the mousse too runny. The solution was to reduce some of the juice to a thick syrup, concentrating its flavor. We combined the remaining juice with a small amount of gelatin, which contributed to a more stable texture in the finished mousse. Whipped cream and cream cheese gave the mousse just enough richness and tang while also helping to ensure that the mousse set nicely. Garnishing the finished mousse with fresh diced strawberries was a perfect finishing touch. Be careful not to overprocess the berries in step 1.

2 pounds strawberries, hulled (6½ cups)
¼ cup (1¾ ounces) sugar
 Pinch salt
1¾ teaspoons unflavored gelatin
4 ounces cream cheese, cut into 8 pieces and softened
½ cup heavy cream

1. Dice enough strawberries into ¼-inch pieces to measure 1 cup; refrigerate until serving. Pulse remaining strawberries in food processor in 2 batches until most pieces are ¼ to ½ inch thick, 6 to 10 pulses. Combine processed strawberries, sugar, and salt in bowl. Cover and let strawberries sit, stirring occasionally, for 45 minutes. (Do not clean processor.)

2. Drain processed strawberries in fine-mesh strainer set over bowl (you should have about ⅔ cup juice). Measure out 3 tablespoons juice into small bowl, sprinkle gelatin over top, and let sit until gelatin softens, about 5 minutes. Place remaining juice in small saucepan and cook over medium-high heat until reduced to 3 tablespoons, about 10 minutes. Remove pan from heat, add softened gelatin mixture, and whisk until dissolved. Add cream cheese and whisk until smooth. Transfer mixture to large bowl.

3. While juice is reducing, return drained strawberries to now-empty processor and process until smooth, 15 to 20 seconds. Strain puree through fine-mesh strainer into medium bowl, pressing on solids to remove seeds and pulp (you should have about 1⅔ cups puree). Discard remaining solids. Add strawberry puree to juice-gelatin mixture and whisk until incorporated.

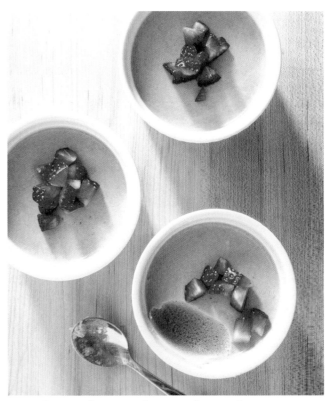

To get the most flavor out of supermarket strawberries, we reduce some of their juice into a concentrated liquid.

4. Using stand mixer fitted with whisk attachment, whip cream on medium-low speed until foamy, about 1 minute. Increase speed to high and whip until stiff peaks form, 1 to 3 minutes. Add whipped cream to strawberry mixture and whisk until no white streaks remain. Portion evenly into 8 dessert dishes and chill for at least 4 hours or up to 2 days. (If chilled longer than 6 hours, let mousse sit at room temperature for 15 minutes before serving.) Garnish with reserved diced strawberries and serve.

PER SERVING
Cal 160 • **Total Fat** 10g • **Sat Fat** 6g • **Chol** 35mg
Sodium 75mg • **Total Carbs** 16g • **Fiber** 2g • **Total Sugar** 12g
Added Sugar 6g • **Protein** 3g • **Total Carbohydrate Choices** 1

No-Fuss Banana Ice Cream

MAKES 1 QUART; SERVES 8

WHY THIS RECIPE WORKS Traditional ice cream relies on sugar for its smooth, creamy texture, so we set out to create a low-sugar ice cream alternative that wouldn't feel like a compromise. While we were at it, we decided to ditch the ice cream machine. Bananas were a perfect choice for our "ice cream" base: Their high pectin content allows them to remain creamy when frozen and their natural sweetness meant that we didn't need to add any sugar. We started by simply freezing whole peeled bananas and then sliced them and processed them into a smooth puree. Letting the bananas come to room temperature for 15 minutes before slicing made them easier to cut through and kept the processing time at only 5 minutes. The end result had good banana flavor, but wasn't quite as creamy as tasters wanted. We decided to try adding a little dairy to help achieve our desired creamy consistency. We tested ice creams made with both milk and heavy cream; the version made with heavy cream produced an unbeatable silky-smooth texture. A teaspoon of lemon juice and a bit of cinnamon gave our ice cream more dimension, while a tablespoon of vanilla rounded out the other flavors. Be sure to use very ripe, heavily speckled (or even black) bananas in this recipe. You can skip the freezing in step 3 and serve the ice cream immediately, but the texture will be softer.

- **6 very ripe bananas**
- **½ cup heavy cream**
- **1 tablespoon vanilla extract**
- **1 teaspoon lemon juice**
- **¼ teaspoon salt**
- **¼ teaspoon ground cinnamon**

1. Peel bananas, place in large zipper-lock bag, and press out excess air. Freeze bananas until solid, at least 8 hours.

2. Let bananas sit at room temperature to soften slightly, about 15 minutes. Slice into ½-inch-thick rounds and place in food processor. Add cream, vanilla, lemon juice, salt, and cinnamon and process until smooth, about 5 minutes, scraping down sides of bowl as needed.

3. Transfer mixture to airtight container and freeze until firm, at least 2 hours or up to 5 days. Serve.

PER ½-CUP SERVING

Cal 160 • **Total Fat** 6g • **Sat Fat** 3.5g • **Chol** 15mg
Sodium 75mg • **Total Carbs** 28g • **Fiber** 3g • **Total Sugar** 18g
Added Sugar 0g • **Protein** 1g • **Total Carbohydrate Choices** 2

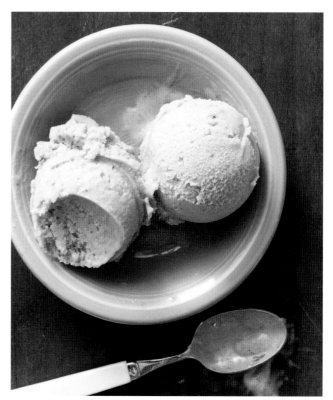

The natural sweetness of ripe bananas makes the perfect ice cream base since it doesn't require any added sugar.

VARIATIONS
No-Fuss Peanut Butter–Banana Ice Cream

Reduce amount of heavy cream to ¼ cup. Add ¼ cup unsweetened natural peanut butter to food processor with bananas in step 2.

PER ½-CUP SERVING

Cal 170 • **Total Fat** 7g • **Sat Fat** 2.5g • **Chol** 10mg
Sodium 110mg • **Total Carbs** 26g • **Fiber** 3g • **Total Sugar** 14g
Added Sugar 1g • **Protein** 3g • **Total Carbohydrate Choices** 2

No-Fuss Chocolate-Banana Ice Cream with Walnuts

Add ½ cup unsweetened cocoa powder to food processor with bananas in step 2. Before removing ice cream from processor, add 1 cup walnuts, toasted and chopped, and pulse to combine, about 5 pulses.

PER ½-CUP SERVING

Cal 260 • **Total Fat** 16g • **Sat Fat** 5g • **Chol** 20mg
Sodium 75mg • **Total Carbs** 29g • **Fiber** 5g • **Total Sugar** 14g
Added Sugar 0g • **Protein** 5g • **Total Carbohydrate Choices** 2

Conversions and Equivalents

Some say cooking is a science and an art. We would say that geography has a hand in it, too. Flours and sugars manufactured in the United Kingdom and elsewhere will feel and taste different from those manufactured in the United States. So we cannot promise that the loaf of bread you bake in Canada or England will taste the same as a loaf baked in the States, but we can offer guidelines for converting weights and measures. We also recommend that you rely on your instincts when making our recipes. Refer to the visual cues provided. If the dough hasn't "come together in a ball" as described, you may need to add more flour—even if the recipe doesn't tell you to. You be the judge.

The recipes in this book were developed using standard U.S. measures following U.S. government guidelines. The charts below offer equivalents for U.S. and metric measures. All conversions are approximate and have been rounded up or down to the nearest whole number.

Example

1 teaspoon	=	4.9292 milliliters, rounded up to 5 milliliters
1 ounce	=	28.3495 grams, rounded down to 28 grams

Volume Conversions

U.S.	METRIC
1 teaspoon	5 milliliters
2 teaspoons	10 milliliters
1 tablespoon	15 milliliters
2 tablespoons	30 milliliters
¼ cup	59 milliliters
⅓ cup	79 milliliters
½ cup	118 milliliters
¾ cup	177 milliliters
1 cup	237 milliliters
1¼ cups	296 milliliters
1½ cups	355 milliliters
2 cups (1 pint)	473 milliliters
2½ cups	591 milliliters
3 cups	710 milliliters
4 cups (1 quart)	0.946 liter
1.06 quarts	1 liter
4 quarts (1 gallon)	3.8 liters

Weight Conversions

OUNCES	GRAMS
½	14
¾	21
1	28
1½	43
2	57
2½	71
3	85
3½	99
4	113
4½	128
5	142
6	170
7	198
8	227
9	255
10	283
12	340
16 (1 pound)	454

Conversions for Common Baking Ingredients

Baking is an exacting science. Because measuring by weight is far more accurate than measuring by volume, and thus more likely to produce reliable results, in our recipes we provide ounce measures in addition to cup measures for many ingredients. Refer to the chart below to convert these measures into grams.

INGREDIENT	OUNCES	GRAMS
Flour		
1 cup all-purpose flour*	5	142
1 cup cake flour	4	113
1 cup whole-wheat flour	5½	156
Sugar		
1 cup granulated (white) sugar	7	198
1 cup packed brown sugar (light or dark)	7	198
1 cup confectioners' sugar	4	113
Cocoa Powder		
1 cup cocoa powder	3	85
Butter†		
4 tablespoons (½ stick or ¼ cup)	2	57
8 tablespoons (1 stick or ½ cup)	4	113
16 tablespoons (2 sticks or 1 cup)	8	227

* U.S. all-purpose flour, the most frequently used flour in this book, does not contain leaveners, as some European flours do. These leavened flours are called self-rising or self-raising. If you are using self-rising flour, take this into consideration before adding leaveners to a recipe.

† In the United States, butter is sold both salted and unsalted. We generally recommend unsalted butter. If you are using salted butter, take this into consideration before adding salt to a recipe.

Oven Temperatures

FAHRENHEIT	CELSIUS	GAS MARK
225	105	¼
250	120	½
275	135	1
300	150	2
325	165	3
350	180	4
375	190	5
400	200	6
425	220	7
450	230	8
475	245	9

Converting Temperatures from an Instant-Read Thermometer

We include doneness temperatures in many of the recipes in this book. We recommend an instant-read thermometer for the job. Refer to the table above to convert Fahrenheit degrees to Celsius. Or, for temperatures not represented in the chart, use this simple formula:

Subtract 32 degrees from the Fahrenheit reading, then divide the result by 1.8 to find the Celsius reading.

Example:
"Roast chicken until thighs register 175 degrees."
To convert:

$175\,°F - 32 = 143\,°$

$143\,° \div 1.8 = 79.44\,°C$, rounded down to $79\,°C$

Index

Note: Page references in *italics* indicate photographs.

D

Dairy products, choosing, 11
Dal (Spiced Red Lentils), 145
Dal with Coconut Milk, 145
Dark Chocolate–Avocado Pudding, 363, *363*
Dark Chocolate Bark with Almonds and
    Cherries, 345
Dark Chocolate Bark with Pepitas and
    Goji Berries, 345, *345*
Deviled Eggs, Herbed, 50, *50*
Diabetes
    diabetes-friendly ingredients, 10–11
    healthy fats and, 6
    limiting refined starch and sugar, 5
    overview of, 3–6
    Plate Method meal planning, 7
    role of carbohydrates in, 4–5
    role of protein in, 5
    sodium guidelines, 6
    statistics on, 2
    Type 1, 3
    Type 2, 3
Dill
    Sauce, Creamy, 243
    Smoked Salmon Rolls, 55, *55*
Dipping Sauces
    Lemon-Tarragon, Coriander Shrimp
        Skewers with, *53*, 53–54
    Yogurt, Curried Chicken Skewers with,
        52, 52–53
Dips
    Artichoke and White Bean, 36–37
    Artichoke-Lemon Hummus, 40
    Beet Tzatziki, 38, *38*
    Classic Hummus, 39, *39*
    Fresh Tomato Salsa, 41–42
    Green Goddess, 36, *36*
    Guacamole, *40*, 40–41
    Roasted Garlic Hummus, 40
    Roasted Red Pepper Hummus, 39
    Spicy Whipped Feta with Roasted Red
        Peppers, 37, *37*
    Toasted Corn and Black Bean Salsa, 42
    Toasted Corn Salsa, 42, *42*
    Tzatziki, 38

Dressings
    Parmesan-Peppercorn, 87
    Tahini-Lemon, 87
    see also Vinaigrettes
Drinks
    Berry Smoothies, 32–33, *33*
    Green Smoothies, 33, *33*
Dukkah and Lemon, Sautéed Spinach with,
    316, 316–17

E

Easy Greek-Style Chickpea Salad, 148
Easy Roast Turkey Breast, *202*, 202–3
Easy Stuffed Pork Loin with Figs and
    Balsamic Vinegar, *226*, 226–27
Edamame
    Noodles with Mustard Greens and
        Shiitake-Ginger Sauce, 170, *170*
    and Shiitakes, Baked Brown Rice with,
        124, *124*
    and Snap Pea Slaw, Seared Scallops with,
        266, *266*
Eggplant
    Broiled, with Basil, 303
    Chinese, about, 303
    globe, about, 303
    Grilled Flank Steak with Summer
        Vegetables, *211*, 211–12
    Indian-Style Vegetable Curry, *281*, 281–82
    Involtini, 270, *270*
    Italian, about, 303
    Marinated, with Capers and Mint, 302, *302*
    One-Pan Roasted Chicken Breasts with
        Ratatouille, *184*, 184–85
    Pasta alla Norma with Olives and Capers,
        156, 156–57
    Squash, and Tomato Tian, 319
    Stuffed, with Bulgur, *273*, 273–74
    Thai, about, 303
    Tomato, and Chickpea Salad, Grilled
        Swordfish with, 258–59
    and Tomatoes, Stewed Chickpeas with,
        284, 284
    Tunisian-Style Grilled Vegetables with
        Couscous and Eggs, *279*, 279–80

Egg(s)
    Breakfast Tacos, 21, *21*
    buying, 15
    and Couscous, Tunisian-Style Grilled
        Vegetables with, *279*, 279–80
    farm-fresh and organic, 15
    Fried, with Garlicky Swiss Chard and
        Bell Pepper, 16
    Fried, with Sweet Potatoes and Turkey
        Sausage, 17, *17*
    Frittata with Asparagus, Mushrooms, and
        Goat Cheese, 20
    Frittata with Spinach, Bell Pepper, and
        Basil, *19*, 19–20
    Herbed Deviled, 50, *50*
    Mushroom and Gruyère Omelets, 19
    omega-3s in, 15
    pack by date, 15
    Poached, Open-Faced Sandwiches, *12*, 20
    Scrambled, with Feta, Shallot, and Basil, 14
    Scrambled, with Goat Cheese, Sun-Dried
        Tomatoes, and Oregano, 14, *14*
    Scrambled, with Herbs, 14
    Scrambled, with Parmesan and Asparagus, 15
    sell-by date, 15
    shell color, 15
    Spinach and Feta Omelets, 18–19
Enchiladas
    Beef, *220*, 220–21
    Chicken, 196, *196*
Endive
    and Cucumber, Bibb Lettuce Salad with, 89
    preparing, for crudités, 43
Escarole
    and Meatball Soup, Italian, *328*, 328
    and White Beans, Sicilian, 150–51

F

Fajitas, Stovetop Chicken, 194–95, *195*
Farro
    about, 11, 129
    Bowl with Tofu, Mushrooms, and Spinach,
        274–75, *275*
    cooking methods, 136
    health benefits, 126

Fried Eggs with Sweet Potatoes and
Turkey Sausage, 17, *17*

Frisée
Parmesan-Crusted Chicken Breasts
with Warm Bitter Greens and Fennel
Salad, 178–79, *179*
and Strawberries, Spinach Salad with, 92

Frittatas
with Asparagus, Mushrooms, and Goat
Cheese, 20
with Spinach, Bell Pepper, and Basil,
19, 19–20

Fruit
Fresh, and Coconut, Chia Pudding with,
28, 28–29
in Plate Method meal, 7
see also specific fruits

Fusilli
with Skillet-Roasted Cauliflower, Garlic,
and Walnuts, 155–56
with Zucchini, Tomatoes, and Pine
Nuts, 155

G

Garden Minestrone, 72, *72*
Garlic
about, 294
and Anchovies, Roasted Broccoli with, 293
buying and storing, 294
-Chicken and Wild Rice Soup, 65, 65–66
Chips, Spinach, Beans, and Tomatoes,
Spaghetti with, *158*, 158–59
Chips and Spinach, Lentils with, *144*, 144–45
cooking, 294
Cumin, and Cilantro, Sautéed Snow
Peas with, 311
Ginger, and Scallion, Sautéed Snow
Peas with, 311
and Herbs, Sautéed Green Beans with, 304–5
-Lemon Potatoes, Greek-Style, 313, *313*
Marinated Artichokes, *51*, 51–52
and Parmesan, Spaghetti Squash with,
319, 319–20
and Parsley, Chickpeas with, *149*, 149
Pork Roast, 225–26

Garlic *(cont.)*
Potatoes, Lemon-Herb Cod Fillets with,
249–50
preparing, 294
Roasted, and Smoked Paprika, Roasted
Mushrooms with, 309
Roasted, Hummus, 40
roasting, 40
Sautéed Swiss Chard with, 317, *317*
Skillet-Roasted Cauliflower, and Walnuts,
Fusilli with, 155–56
and Walnuts, Roasted Beets with, 291
and Warm Spices, Popcorn with, 45
and White Wine, Braised Cauliflower
with, 299–300

Garlicky Braised Kale, 306
**Garlicky Yogurt and Chickpeas, Sautéed
Spinach with**, 278, *278*
Gazpacho Salad, 99, *99*
Ginger
-Carrot Soup, Creamy, 59
Garlic, and Scallion, Sautéed Snow
Peas with, 311
and Lemon Grass, Cod in Coconut
Broth with, *248*, 248–49
and Scallions, Boiled Carrots with, 297
-Shiitake Sauce and Mustard Greens,
Noodles with, 170, *170*
-Tomato Vinaigrette, Warm, Poached
Chicken Breasts with, 174, *174*

Glycemic control, 6
Goat Cheese
and Almonds, Mesclun Salad with, 88, *88*
Asparagus, and Mushrooms, Frittata with, 20
Asparagus, Red Pepper, and Spinach
Salad with, 95
Fennel, Apple, and Chicken Chopped
Salad, *112*, 112–13
Fennel, Cucumber, and Apple Chopped
Salad, 97
and Hazelnuts, Lentil Salad with, 143
and Honey, Warm Figs with, 350–51, *351*
Open-Faced Poached Egg Sandwiches,
12, 20
Strawberries, and Almonds, Warm
Spinach Salad with, 93–94
Sun-Dried Tomatoes, and Oregano,
Scrambled Eggs with, 14, *14*

Goji Berries
and Chocolate, Oatmeal Cookies with,
355, 355–56
health benefits, 32
Muesli, 32
and Pepitas, Dark Chocolate Bark with,
345, *345*

Grains
boiling directions, 136
microwave directions, 136
pilaf-style directions, 136
rinsing, 127
storing, 128
whole, choosing, 11
whole, health benefits, 126
whole, in Plate Method meal, 7
whole, test kitchen favorites, 129
see also specific grains

Granola
Bars, 31
Omega-3, 29–30
Omega-3, with Cherries, 30
Omega-3, with Peanut Butter, 30
Quinoa, *30*, 30–31

Grapefruit
and Avocado, Shrimp Salad with, 116, *116*
-Basil Relish, 242, *243*
Grilled Sea Bass with Citrus and Black
Olive Salad, 256–57
Sesame Salmon with Napa Cabbage Slaw,
239–40

Grapes and Feta, Bulgur Salad with, 130–31
Greek-Style Braised Pork with Leeks, 228, *228*
Greek-Style Garlic-Lemon Potatoes, 313, *313*
Green Bean(s)
Beef and Garden Vegetable Soup, 327, *327*
and Bok Choy, Stir-Fried Beef with, 216–17
cooking methods and cooking times, 292
Garden Minestrone, 72, *72*
Indian-Style Vegetable Curry, *281*, 281–82
and Potatoes, One-Pan Roasted Pork
Tenderloin with, 224–25, *225*
preparing, for crudités, 43
Quick Beef and Vegetable Soup, 64, 64–65
Roasted, with Almonds and Mint, 306
Roasted, with Pecorino and Pine Nuts,
305, 305–6
Salad with Cilantro Sauce, 100–101

J

Jícama

Salmon Tacos with Super Slaw, 244–45, *245*

Slaw, Steak Tacos with, *217*, 217–18

K

Kale

Beef and Vegetable Stew, *76*, 76–77

and Brussels Sprout Salad with Herbs and Peanuts, 102

and Butternut Squash, One-Pan Roasted Chicken Breasts with, 183

Chicken Thighs with Black-Eyed Pea Ragout, 334–35

and Chickpea Soup, 73, *73*

Chips, 44, *44*

Garlicky Braised, 306

Green Smoothies, 33, *33*

massaging, 96

Pesto, Tomatoes, and Chicken, Pasta with, *161*, 161–62

Salad with Sweet Potatoes and Pomegranate Vinaigrette, 95–96, *96*

selecting and storing, 307

Kidney beans

Refried Beans, 151, *151*

Turkey Chili, 331–32

Vegetarian Chili, 83, *83*

L

Lamb

boneless leg of, preparing, 235

Braised, with Tomatoes and Red Wine, 232

Harissa-Rubbed Roast Boneless Leg of, with Warm Cauliflower Salad, 234–35

internal cooking temperatures, 209

Roast Butterflied Leg of, with Coriander, Cumin, and Mustard Seeds, 233–34, *234*

Roast Butterflied Leg of, with Coriander, Fennel, and Black Pepper, 234

Lamb *(cont.)*

Roast Butterflied Leg of, with Coriander, Rosemary, and Red Pepper, 234

Shish Kebabs, Grilled, *232*, 232–33

Lasagna

Spinach, 167–68, *168*

Turkey and Cheese, 168–69, *169*

Latin-Style Chicken and Brown Rice, 190–91

Latin-Style Chicken with Tomatoes and Olives, 332

Leek(s)

Fennel, and Saffron, Hearty Chicken Stew with, 75–76

Greek-Style Braised Pork with, 228, *228*

and Lemon, Baked Scallops with, 266–67

and Mustard, Braised Halibut with, 252, *252*

preparing, 326

and Saffron, Baked Scallops with, 267

and White Wine Pan Sauce, Pan-Seared Chicken Breasts with, 175

Lemon Grass

and Basil, Sautéed Snow Peas with, 311

and Ginger, Cod in Coconut Broth with, *248*, 248–49

Lemon(s)

-Artichoke Hummus, 40

-Basil Dressing, Grilled Zucchini and Red Onion with, *323*, 323

-Caper Sauce, Roasted Root Vegetables with, *315*, 315–16

Chicken Piccata, 176, *176*

-Garlic Potatoes, Greek-Style, 313, *313*

-Herb Cod Fillets with Garlic Potatoes, 249–50

and Herbs, Barley with, 128

Marinated Artichokes, *51*, 51–52

No-Fuss Quinoa with, 340–41, *341*

and Parsley, Sautéed Snow Peas with, *310*, 310–11

-Tahini Dressing, 87

-Tarragon Dipping Sauce, Coriander Shrimp Skewers with, *53*, 53–54

-Tarragon Gremolata, Roasted Asparagus with, 291

and Thyme, Quinoa Pilaf with, 139

Vinaigrette, 86

Lemony Penne with Chicken, Sun-Dried Tomatoes, and Artichokes, 163, *163*

Lemony Steamed Spa Fish, 247

Lentil(s)

brown and green, about, 142

and Chard, Pomegranate Roasted Salmon with, 240

Dal with Coconut Milk, 145

Lentilles du Puy, about, 142

Red, Spiced (Dal), 145

red and yellow, about, 142

Salad, Spiced, with Winter Squash, *143*, 143–44

Salad with Carrots and Cilantro, 143

Salad with Hazelnuts and Goat Cheese, 143

Salad with Olives, Mint, and Feta, 142

Salad with Radishes, Cilantro, and Pepitas, 341

Salad with Spinach, Walnuts, and Parmesan, 143

Soup, Classic, 70–71, *71*

with Spinach and Garlic Chips, *144*, 144–45

Lettuce

Basic Green Salad, 88

Bibb, about, 90

Bibb, Salad with Endive and Cucumber, 89

Chicken Caesar Salad, *109*, 109–10

Classic Wedge Salad, *90*, 90–91

Cobb Salad, *110*, 110–11

Fennel, Apple, and Chicken Chopped Salad, *112*, 112–13

Fennel, Cucumber, and Apple Chopped Salad, 97

iceberg, about, 90

loose-leaf, about, 90

Mediterranean Chopped Salad, 96–97, *97*

Radish, Orange, and Avocado Chopped Salad, 98

romaine, about, 90

Romaine Salad with Chickpeas and Feta, 89

Shrimp Salad with Avocado and Grapefruit, 116, *116*

whole heads, buying, 94

Wraps, Asian Chicken, 193–94, *194*

Lime

Cherry, Coconut, and Chili Trail Mix, 46

-Orange Dressing, Seared Scallops with, 265, *265*

Linguine with Meatless "Meat" Sauce, 160–61

M

Mango and Nut Chocolate Clusters, 344
Maple-Caramel Apples, 349
Marinated Artichokes, *51*, 51–52
Marinated Eggplant with Capers and Mint, 302, *302*
Marsala-Porcini Pan Sauce, 206
Mayonnaise, choosing, 10
Mayonnaise-based sauces
    Chipotle Crema, 276, *276*
    Creamy Chipotle Chile Sauce, 243
    Creamy Dill Sauce, 243
    Horseradish Sauce, 213, *213*
    Parmesan-Peppercorn Dressing, 87
    Tartar Sauce, 243
Meal planning
    breakfast sample menus, 8
    dinner sample menus, 9
    lunch sample menus, 9
    Plate Method, 7
Meat
    internal cooking temperatures, 209
    in Plate Method meal, 7
    resting, before slicing, 210
    shredding, 326
    see also Beef; Lamb; Pork
Meatball and Escarole Soup, Italian, 328, *328*
Meatballs, Spaghetti and, *165*, 165–66
Meatloaf with Mushroom Gravy, *218*, 218–19
Mediterranean Chopped Salad, 96–97, *97*
Mediterranean Tuna Salad, 119
Mediterranean Tuna Salad with Carrots, Radishes, and Cilantro, 119
Melon, Plums, and Cherries with Mint and Vanilla, 346, *346*
Mesclun
    about, 90
    Salad with Goat Cheese and Almonds, 88, *88*
Mexican Pork and Rice, 231, *231*
Mexican-Style Spaghetti Squash Casserole, 272, *272*
Milk, low-fat, choosing, 11
Minestrone, Garden, 72, *72*
Mini Chocolate Cupcakes with Creamy Chocolate Frosting, 361–62, *362*

Mint
    and Almonds, Roasted Green Beans with, 306
    Barley with Lemon and Herbs, 128
    Bulgur Salad with Carrots and Almonds, 130, *130*
    Bulgur Salad with Grapes and Feta, 130–31
    and Capers, Marinated Eggplant with, 302, *302*
    Cucumber, and Yogurt, Farro Salad with, 135
    Easy Greek-Style Chickpea Salad, 148
    Fattoush, 104, *104*
    Olives, and Feta, Lentil Salad with, 142
    -Orange Gremolata, Roasted Asparagus with, 290, *290*
    and Paprika, Boiled Carrots with, 297
    and Pistachios, Sautéed Zucchini Ribbons with, 323
    Saffron, and Yogurt, Chickpeas with, 149–50
    Shallots, and Cucumber, Swordfish en Cocotte with, 258
    Spiced Tabbouleh, 131
    and Sumac, Braised Cauliflower with, 300
    Tabbouleh, 131, *131*
    Thai Grilled-Steak Salad, 115, *115*
    and Vanilla, Melon, Plums, and Cherries with, 346, *346*
    Warm Cabbage Salad with Chicken, 114, *114*
    -Yogurt Cucumber Salad, 103
    Zucchini Ribbon Salad with Shaved Parmesan, 108, *108–9*
Monounsaturated fats, 6
Moroccan Chickpea Soup, 73–74
Moroccan-Style Carrot Salad, *102*, 102–3
Mousse, Strawberry, 364, *364*
Mozzarella
    Caprese Skewers, 49, *49*
    Fresh, and Basil, Cherry Tomato Salad with, 108
    Spinach Lasagna, 167–68, *168*
    Turkey and Cheese Lasagna, 168–69, *169*
Muesli, 32
Muesli, Sunflower Seed, Hazelnut, and Cherry, 32
Muffins, Whole-Wheat Blueberry, *354*, 354–55

Mushroom(s)
    Asparagus, and Goat Cheese, Frittata with, 20
    Baked Brown Rice with Shiitakes and Edamame, 124, *124*
    Beef en Cocotte with, 212
    Braised Swiss Chard with Shiitakes and Peanuts, 339–40
    buying and storing, 47
    Catalan Beef Stew, *329*, 329–30
    cleaning, 47
    Cobb Salad, *110*, 110–11
    Gravy, Meatloaf with, *218*, 218–19
    and Gruyère Omelets, 19
    and Harissa, Seared Tuna with, 261–62
    Hearty Ten Vegetable Stew, *78*, 78–79
    Linguine with Meatless "Meat" Sauce, 160–61
    Noodles with Mustard Greens and Shiitake-Ginger Sauce, 170, *170*
    Porcini-Marsala Pan Sauce, 206
    Portobello, and Shallots, Grilled, with Rosemary-Dijon Vinaigrette, *309*, 309–10
    portobello, preparing for the grill, 310
    preparing, 309
    Rigatoni with Turkey Ragu, 166–67, *167*
    Roasted, with Harissa and Mint, 308
    Roasted, with Parmesan and Pine Nuts, 308, *308*
    Roasted, with Roasted Garlic and Smoked Paprika, 309
    Soup, Creamy, 63
    Stir-Fried Tofu with Shiitakes and Green Beans, *280*, 280–81
    Stuffed, 46–48, *47*
    and Thyme, Warm Farro with, 137, *137*
    Tofu, and Spinach, Farro Bowl with, 274–75, *275*
    and Tomatoes, Braised Chicken Thighs with, *188*, 188–89
    Turkey Shepherd's Pie, *201*, 201–2
    Ultimate Beef Chili, 79–80, *80*
    and Wheat Berry Soup, 69, *69*
    Wild, Pan-Roasted Sea Bass with, 254–55, *255*
Mustard
    -Balsamic Vinaigrette, 86
    and Cognac Pan Sauce, 206
    French Potato Salad with Dijon and Fines Herbes, 104–5, *105*

Warm Spinach Salad with Strawberries,
Goat Cheese, and Almonds, 93–94
Warm Wheat Berries with Zucchini, Red
Bell Pepper, and Oregano, *141,* 141–42
Weeknight Skillet Roast Chicken, *192,* 192–93
Wheat Berry(ies)
about, 11, 129
cooking methods, 136
and Mushroom Soup, 69, *69*
Salad with Roasted Red Pepper, Feta, and
Arugula, 140–41
Warm, with Zucchini, Red Bell Pepper,
and Oregano, *141,* 141–42
White Bean(s)
and Artichoke Dip, 36–37
Asparagus and Arugula Salad with
Cannellini Beans, 94, *94*–95
and Butternut Squash Soup with Sage
Pesto, 74–75, *75*
and Escarole, Sicilian, 150–51
Garden Minestrone, 72, *72*
Italian Meatball and Escarole Soup, 328, *328*
Salad with Bell Peppers, 150
Salad with Oranges and Celery, 150
Spinach, Tomatoes, and Garlic Chips,
Spaghetti with, *158,* 158–59
White Chicken Chili, 80–81, *81*
White Chicken Chili, 80–81, *81*
White wine vinegar, about, 112
Whole-Wheat Blueberry Muffins, *354,* 354–55
Wild Rice
and Garlic-Chicken Soup, *65,* 65–66
health benefits, 126
Pilaf with Scallions and Almonds,
125, 125–26

Y

Yams, about, 287
Yogurt
Beet Tzatziki, 38, *38*
Berry Smoothies, 32–33, *33*
Chipotle Crema, 276, *276*
Coriander Shrimp Skewers with
Lemon-Tarragon Dipping Sauce,
53, 53–54
Cucumber, and Mint, Farro Salad with, 135
-Cucumber Sauce, 286, *286*
-Cumin Dressing, Tomato Salad with,
106, 106–7
Dipping Sauce, Curried Chicken
Skewers with, *52,* 52–53
and Dukkah, Sautéed Spinach with,
316, 316–17
Garlicky, and Chickpeas, Sautéed
Spinach with, *278,* 278
Green Smoothies, 33, *33*
low-fat, choosing, 11
-Mint Cucumber Salad, 103
Orange-Honey, *24,* 25
Parfaits, 28
Saffron, and Mint, Chickpeas with, 149–50
Sauce and Warm Bulgur Salad, Herbed
Chicken with, 333–34, *334*
Turkish Stuffed Apricots with Rose
Water and Pistachios, 348, *348*
Tzatziki, 38

Z

Za'atar
Chickpeas, and Spinach, Bulgur with,
132, *132*
and Parsley, Roasted Winter Squash
Salad with, 106
Zucchini
buying, 320
Grilled, and Red Onion with Lemon-Basil
Dressing, 323, *323*
Grilled Flank Steak with Summer
Vegetables, *211,* 211–12
Grilled Lamb Shish Kebabs, *232,* 232–33
Hearty Ten Vegetable Stew, 78, 78–79
Italian Vegetable Soup, 67, *67*
Moroccan Chickpea Soup, 73–74
One-Pan Roasted Chicken Breasts with
Ratatouille, *184,* 184–85
Red Bell Pepper, and Oregano, Warm
Wheat Berries with, *141,* 141–42
ribbons, creating, 109
Ribbons, Sautéed, 322, *322*
Ribbons, Sautéed, with Mint and
Pistachios, 323
Ribbon Salad with Shaved Parmesan,
108, 108–9
seeding, 74
Squash and Tomato Tian, 318, *318*
storing, 320
Tomato, and Potato Tian, 319
Tomatoes, and Pine Nuts, Fusilli with, 155
and Tomatoes, Chicken Baked in Foil
with, 181
and Tomatoes, Halibut Baked in Foil
with, 253–54
Tunisian-Style Grilled Vegetables with
Couscous and Eggs, *279,* 279–80
Vegetarian Chili, 83, *83*